Alzheimer's Disease and Related Disorders

ETIOLOGY, PATHOGENESIS AND THERAPEUTICS

This publication was
supported by an educational grant from
Janssen Pharmaceutica and Research Foundation

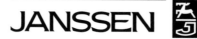

Alzheimer's Disease and Related Disorders

ETIOLOGY, PATHOGENESIS AND THERAPEUTICS

Edited by
KHALID IQBAL
New York State Institute for Basic Research, New York, USA

DICK F. SWAAB
The Netherlands Institute for Brain Research, Amsterdam, The Netherlands

BENGT WINBLAD
Karolinska Institute, Stockholm, Sweden

HENRY M. WISNIEWSKI
New York State Institute for Basic Research, New York, USA

JOHN WILEY & SONS, LTD
Chichester · New York · Weinheim · Brisbane · Singapore · Toronto

Other Wiley Editorial Offices

John Wiley & Sons, Inc., 605 Third Avenue,
New York, NY 10158-0012, USA

WILEY-VCH Verlag GmbH, Pappelallee 3,
D-69469 Weinheim, Germany

Jacaranda Wiley Ltd, 33 Park Road, Milton,
Queensland 4064, Australia

John Wiley & Sons (Asia) Pte Ltd, 2 Clementi Loop #02-01,
Jin Xing Distripark, Singapore 129809

John Wiley & Sons (Canada) Ltd, 22 Worcester Road,
Rexdale, Ontario M9W 1L1, Canada

Library of Congress Cataloging-in-Publication Data

Alzheimer's disease and related disorders / edited by Khalid Iqbal . . .
[et al.].
    p.   cm.
  Includes bibliographical references and indexes.
  ISBN 0-471-98683-6 (cased)
    1. Alzheimer's disease—Congresses. 2. Dementia—Congresses.
I. Iqbal, Khalid.
  [DNLM: 1. Alzheimer Disease. 2. Dementia.   WT 155 A4778 1999]
RC523.A3888   1999
616.8'31—dc21
DNLM/DLC
for Library of Congress   98–44809
                                                                            CIP

British Library Cataloguing in Publication Data

A catalogue record for this book is available from the British Library

ISBN 0-471-98683-6

Typeset in 10/12pt Plantin by Dorwyn Ltd, Rowlands Castle, Hants.
Printed and bound in Great Britain by Bookcraft (Bath) Ltd, Midsomer Norton, Somerset
This book is printed on acid-free paper responsibly manufactured from sustainable forestry, in which at least two trees are planted for each one used for paper production.

Contents

CONTENTS

Contributors

A. Akaike *Department of Pharmacology, Graduate School of Pharmaceutical Sciences, Kyoto University, Kyoto, Japan*

T.A. Ala *Alzheimer's Research Center, Health Partners at Regions Hospital, 640 Jackson Street, St Paul, MN 55101, USA*

I. Alafuzoff *Department of Neuroscience and Neurology, University of Kuopio, PO Box 1627, FIN-70211 Kuopio, Finland*

D. Allsop *SmithKline-Beecham Pharmaceuticals, Harlow, Essex, UK*

B. Almberg *Stockholm Gerontology Research Center, Box 6401, SE–113 82 Stockholm, Sweden*

A. del C. Alonso *Universidad Nacional de Cordoba, Fac. de Ciencias Quimicas Dpto Qca, CC61 AP4 CP5000, Cordoba, Argentina*

G. Amari *Department of Pharmacology and Chemistry, Chiesi Pharmaceuticals S.p.A., Via Palermo 26/A, 43100 Parma, Italy*

P. Amouyel *INSERM CJF95-05, Institut Pasteur de Lille, 1 rue du Professeur Calmette, BP 245, 59019 Lille Cedex, France*

K. Andersen *c/o EURODEM, Department of Epidemiology and Biostatistics, Erasmus University Medical School, PO Box 1738, 3000 DR Rotterdam, The Netherlands*

L. Anderson *Department of Biochemistry and Cell Biology, Institute of Gerontology, Nippon Medical School, 1–396 Kosugi-cho, Nakahara-ku, Kawasaki 211–0061, Japan*

B.H. Anderton *Department of Neuroscience, Institute of Psychiatry, De Crespigny Park, London SE5 8AF, UK*

S. Arakawa *1–4–3 Asahimachi, Abenoku, Osaka 545–8585, Japan*

S. Arlt *Medical Clinic, University Hospital Eppendorf, Martinistrasse 52, 20246 Hamburg, Germany*

R. Asok Kumar *Department of Pathology, New York University Medical Center, 550 First Avenue, New York, NY 10016, USA*

C.S. Atwood *Laboratory for Oxidation Biology, Harvard Medical School, Massachusetts General Hospital, Boston, MA 02114, USA*

H. Backhovens *Laboratory of Neurogenetics, Flanders Interuniversity of Biotechnology, Born Bunge Foundation, University of Antwerp, Department of Biochemistry, Universiteitsplein 1, B-2610 Antwerp, Belgium*

R. Baumeister *Central Institute of Mental Health, Department of Molecular Biology, J5, 68159 Mannheim, Germany*

C. Behl *Max Planck Institute of Psychiatry, Kraepelinstrasse 2–16, 80804 Munich, Germany*

U. Beisiegel *Medical Clinic, University Hospital Eppendorf, Martinistrasse 52, 20246 Hamburg, Germany*

O. Berger *UCLA School of Medicine, Research Institute, 710 Westwood Plaza, Los Angeles, CA 90098-1769, USA*

C. Berr *INSERM U360, Hôpital de la Salpetriere, 75651 Paris, Cedex 13, France*

J. Betts *Department of Neuroscience, Institute of Psychiatry, De Crespigny Park, London, SE5 8AF, UK*

K. Beyer *EuroEspes Biomedical Research Center, Institute for CNS Disorders, 15166 Bergondo, La Coruña, Spain*

K. Beyreuther *Zentrum fur Molekulare Biologie Heidelberg, Universitat Heidelberg, Im Neuenhelmer Feld 282, D-69120 Heidelberg, Germany*

J. Biernat *Max Planck Research Unit for Structural Molecular Biology, Notkestrasse 85, D-22603 Hamburg, Germany*

T.D. Bird *Department of Biochemistry and Cell Biology, Institute of Gerontology, Nippon Medical School, 1–396 Kosugi-cho, Nakahara-ku, Kawasaki 211–0061, Japan*

W. Blackstock *Department of Neuroscience, Biomolecular Structure Unit, Glaxo Wellcome Research and Development, Stevenage SG1 2NY, UK*

D. Blum-Degen *Clinical Neurochemistry, Department of Psychiatry, University of Würtzburg, Füchsleinstrasse 15, 97080 Würtzburg, Germany*

M. Boberg *Department of Public Health and Caring Sciences/Geriatrics, PO Box 609, SE–751 25 Uppsala, Sweden*

M. Bobinski *Institute for Basic Research, Staten Island, New York, NY 10314, USA*

F. Boller *U324 INSERM, Neuropsychologie et Neurobiologie du Vieillissement Cerebral, Centre Paul Broca, Paris, France*

P.T. Bolzoni *Department of Pharmacology and Chemistry, Chiesi Pharmaceuticals S.p.A., Via Palermo 26/A, 43100 Parma, Italy*

D.R. Borchelt *Department of Pathology, 558 Ross Building, 720 Rutland Avenue, Johns Hopkins University School of Medicine, Baltimore, MD 21205, USA*

G.L. Boulianne *Program in Developmental Biology, Hospital for Sick Children, 555 University Avenue, Toronto M5G 1X8, Canada*

A. Bouma *Department of Clinical Psychology, Netherlands Institute for Brain Research, Amsterdam, The Netherlands*

P. Bozner *Department of Pathology, University of South Alabama College of Medicine, 2451 Fillingim Street, Mobile, AL 36617, USA*

E. Braak *Department of Anatomy, J.W. Goethe University, Theodor Stern Kai 7, 60590 Frankfurt am Main, Germany*

H. Braak *Department of Anatomy, J.W. Goethe University, Theodor Stern Kai 7, 60590 Frankfurt am Main, Germany*

D.E. Brenneman *Section on Developmental and Molecular Pharmacology, Laboratory of Developmental Neurobiology, National Institute for Child Health and Human Development, National Institutes of Health, Bethesda, MD 20892, USA*

M.M.B. Breteler *EURODEM Research Group, c/o EURODEM, Department of Epidemiology and Biostatistics, Erasmus University Medical School, PO Box 1738, 3000 DR Rotterdam, The Netherlands*

G. Brewer *Southern Illinois University School of Medicine, Springfield, IL, USA*

J.-P. Brion *Department of Neuroscience, Université Libre de Bruxelles, Faculté de Médicine, B1070 Bruxelles, Belgium*

M. Brockhaus *F. Hoffmann-La Roche Ltd, Pharma Division, Preclinical CNS Research—Gene Technology, Basel, Switzerland*

P. Brown *Laboratory of CNS Studies, NINDS, NIH Bethesda, MD 20892, USA*

M.E. Bruce *Institute for Animal Health, Neuropathogenesis Unit, Ogston Building, West Mains Road, Edinburgh EH9 3JF, UK*

G. Bu *Department of Neurology, Washington University, School of Medicine, 660 S. Euclid Avenue, Box 8111, St. Louis, MO 63110, USA*

C. Buhmann *Medical Clinic, Neurological Clinic and Psychiatric Clinic, University Hospital Hamburg, Hamburg, Germany*

A.I. Bush *Laboratory for Oxidation Biology, Genetics and Aging Unit, Harvard Medical School, Massachusetts General Hospital—East, Building 149, 13th Street, Charlestown, MA 02129, USA*

J. Busser *University Alzheimer Center, Department of Neurology, Case Western Reserve University, 10900 Euclid Avenue, Cleveland, OH 44106, USA*

D. Allan Butterfield *Department of Chemistry, Center of Membrane Sciences, Sanders–Brown Center on Aging, University of Kentucky, Lexington, KY 40506-0055, USA*

R. Cacabelos *EuroEspes Biomedical Research Center, Institute for CNS Disorders, 15166 Bergondo, La Coruña, Spain*

A. Capell *Central Institute of Mental Health, Department of Molecular Biology, J5, 68159, Mannheim, Germany*

S. Capellari *Division of Neuropathology, Case Western Reserve University, Cleveland, OH 44106, USA*

P. Caruso *Departments of Pharmacology and Chemistry, Chiesi Pharmaceuticals S.p.A., Via Palermo 26/A, 43100 Parma, Italy*

E.M. Castaño *IDEHU, University of Buenos Aires, Argentina*

A. Cattaneo *Institute of Neuroimmunology, Slovak Academy of Sciences, Dubravska, Cesta 9, 84246 Bratislava, Slovak Republic*

B. Caughey NIAID, NIH, Rocky Mountain Laboratories, Hamilton, MT 59840, USA

W.S. Caughey NIAID, NIH, Rocky Mountain Laboratories, Hamilton, MT 59840, USA

D. Cécyre McGill Centre for Studies in Aging, 6875 La Salle Boulevard, Verdun, Quebec H4H 1R3, Canada

R.H. Cha Department of Health Sciences Research, Mayo Clinic and Mayo Foundation, 200 First Street SW, Rochester, MN 55905, USA

J. Chabry NIAID, NIH, Rocky Mountain Laboratories, Hamilton, MT 59840, USA

M.-C. Chartier-Harlin INSERM CJF95-05, Institut Pasteur de Lille, 1 rue du Professeur Calmette, BP 245, 59019 Lille Cedex, France

O. Chatzizisi Immunology Department, 3rd Department of Neurology, Aristotle University of Thessaloniki, Despere 3, Thessaloniki 54621, Greece

J. Chen Genetics and Aging Unit, Department of Neurology, Massachusetts General Hospital East, Harvard Medical School, 149 13th Street, Charlestown, MA 02129, USA

P.P. Chen Sepulveda VAMC GRECC11E, UCLA Departments of Medicine and Neurology (SFVP), 16111 Plummer Street, Sepulveda, CA 91343, USA

X.-Q. Chen Department of Pharmaceutics, College of Pharmacy, University of Minnesota, 308 Harvard Street SE, Minneapolis, MN 55101, USA

B. Chesebro NIAID, NIH, Rocky Mountain Laboratories, Hamilton, MT 59840, USA

R. Chiesa Department of Cell Biology and Physiology, Washington University School of Medicine, St. Louis, MO 63110, USA

D.W. Choi Washington University School of Medicine, Box 8111, 660 S. Euclid Avenue, St. Louis, MO 63110, USA

Y.-J. Chyan Department of Pathology, University of South Alabama, College of Medicine, 2451 Fillingim Street, Mobile, AL 36617, USA

M. Civelli Departments of Pharmacology and Chemistry, Chiesi Pharmaceuticals S.p.A., Via Palermo 26/A, 43100 Parma, Italy

G.M. Cole Sepulveda VAMC GRECC 11E, UCLA Departments of Medicine (SFVP) and Neurology, 16111 Plummer Street, Sepulveda, CA 91343, USA

M.-A. Colle Ecole Nationale Veterinaire d'Alfort, Laboratorie de Neuropathologie R. Escourolle, Hôpital de la Salpetriere, 47 Blvd de l'Hôpital, 75651 Paris Cedex 13, France

A. Convit Department of Psychiatry, New York University Medical Center, NY 10016, USA

R.J.M. Copeland EURODEM Research Group, Department of Epidemiology and Biostatistics, Erasmus University Medical School, PO Box 1738, 3000 DR Rotterdam, The Netherlands

D. Cottel INSERM CJF 95-05, Institut Pasteur de Lille, 1 rue du Professeur Calmette, BP 245-59019 Lille Cedex, France

F. Crawford Roskamp Institute, 3515 E. Fletcher Avenue, University of South Florida, Tampa, FL 33613, USA

R.A. Crowther MRC Laboratory of Molecular Biology, Hills Road, Cambridge CB2 2QH, UK

M. Cruts Laboratory of Neurogenetics, Flanders Interuniversity of Biotechnology, Born Bunge Foundation, University of Antwerp, Department of Biochemistry, Universiteitsplein 1, B-2610 Antwerp, Belgium

W. Cui Department of Psychiatry and Fishberg Research Center for Neurobiology, Mount Sinai School of Medicine, New York, USA

J.G. Culvenor Department of Pathology, University of Melbourne, Mental Health Research Institute, Parkville, Victoria 3052, Australia

D. Daher Medical Clinic, University Hospital Eppendorf, Martinistrasse 52, 20246 Hamburg, Germany

D. Damon INSERM U 330, Université de Bordeaux II, 146 rue Leo Saignat, 33076 Bordeaux Cedex, France

J.-F. Dartigues EURODEM Research Group, Department of Epidemiology and Biostatistics, Erasmus University Medical School, PO Box 1738, 3000 DR Rotterdam, The Netherlands

D.R. Davis Department of Neuroscience, Institute of Psychiatry, De Crespigny Park, London SE5 8AF, UK

C.J.A. De Groot Graduate School of Neurosciences Amsterdam, Faculty of Medicine, Department of Pathology, Van der Boechorststraat 7, 1081 BT Amsterdam, The Netherlands

G.I. De Jong Department of Animal Physiology, Graduate School of Behavioral and Cognitive Neurosciences, University of Groningen, Groningen, The Netherlands

C. De Jonghe *Laboratory of Neurogenetics, Flanders Interuniversity of Biotechnology, Born Bunge Foundation, University of Antwerp, Department of Biochemistry, Universiteitsplein 1, B-2610 Antwerp, Belgium*

M.J. de Leon *Department of Psychiatry, New York University Medical Center, NY 10016, USA*

S.K. DebBurman *Dept. Molecular Genetics and Biology, University of Chicago, Howard Hughes Medical Institute N339, MC1028 5841 S. Maryland Avenue, Chicago, IL 60637, USA*

N.M. de Vos *Graduate School Neurosciences Amsterdam, Faculty of Medicine, Department of Psychiatry, Vrije Universiteit, Van der Boechorstsraat 7, 1081 BT Amsterdam, The Netherlands*

R.A.I. de Vos *Laboratory of Pathology, University of Groningen, Groningen, The Netherlands*

A. Delacourte *INSERM U422 Place de Verdun, 59045 Lille Cedex, France*

M. Delcanale *Departments of Pharmacology and Chemistry, Chiesi Pharmaceuticals S.p.A., Via Palermo 26/A, 43100 Parma, Italy*

R. Demaimay *Dept. Molecular Genetics and Biology, University of Chicago, Howare Hughes Medical Institue N339, MC1028 5841 S. Maryland Avenue, Chicago, IL 60637, USA*

B. Dermaut *Laboratory of Neurogenetics, Flanders Interuniversity of Biotechnology, Born Bunge Foundation (BBS), University of Antwerp (UIA), Department of Biochemistry, Universiteitsplein 1, B-2610 Antwerp, Belgium*

S. De Santi *Department of Psychiatry, New York University Medical Center, NY 10016, U SA*

A. Di-Carlo *EURODEM Research Group, Department of Epidemiology and Biostatistics, Erasmus University Medical School, PO Box 1738, 3000 DR Rotterdam, The Netherlands*

E.J.G. Dubelaar *Netherlands Institute for Brain Research, Meibergdreef 33, 1105 AZ Amsterdam, The Netherlands*

U. Dürrwang *Zentrum fur Molekulare Biologie Heidelberg, Universitat Heidelberg, Im Neuenheimer Feld 282, D-69120 Heidelberg, Germany*

C. Duyckaerts *Laboratoire de Neuropathologie R. Escourolle, Hôpital de la Salpêtrière, 47 Blvd de l'Hôpital, 75651 Paris Cedex 13, France*

E. Efremidou *Department of Cognitive Psychology, Aristotle University of Thessaloniki, Greece*

S. Efthimiopoulos *Departments of Psychiatry and Neurobiology, Mount Sinai School of Medicine, One Gustave Levy Place, Box 1229, New York, NY 10029, USA*

P. Eikelenboom *Graduate School of Neurosciences Amsterdam, Faculty of Medicine, Department of Psychiatry, Van der Boechorststraat 7, 1081 BT Amsterdam, The Netherlands*

U. Eloniemi-Sulkava *Department of Public Health and General Practice, University of Kuopio, PO Box 1627, 70211 Kuopio, Finland*

G. Erin *Department of Pathology, University of Melbourne, Parkville, Victoria 3052, Australia*

R.A. Faber *South Texas Veterans Health Care Systems, Department of Psychiatry, University of Texas Health Science Center at San Antonio, 116A, 7400 Merton Minter, San Antonio, TX 78284, USA*

C. Fabrigoule *INSERM U 330, Université de Bordeaux II, 146 rue Leo Saignat, 33076 Bordeaux, France*

A.M. Fagan *Department of Neurology, Washington University School of Medicine, 660 8111, St Louis, MO 63110, USA*

C. Fang *Roskamp Institute, 3515 E. Fletcher Avenue, University of South Florida, Tampa, FL 3313, USA*

E. Farkas *Department Animal Physiology, PO Box 14, 9750 AA Haren, The Netherlands*

J. Fastbom *Department of Geriatric Medicine, Karolinska Institute and Stockholm Gerontology Research Center, Stockholm, Sweden*

L. Fasulo *Institute of Neuroimmunology, Slovak Academy of Sciences, Dubravska Cesta 9, 84246 Bratislava, Slovak Republic*

J.R. Fawcett *Alzheimer's Research Center, Health Partners at Regions Hospital, 640 Jackson Street, St Paul, MN 55101, USA*

A. Ferland *Genetics and Aging Unit, Department of Neurology, Massachusetts General Hospital East, Harvard Medical School, 149 13th Street, Charlestown, MA 02129, USA*

L. Fernández-Novoa *EuroEspes Biomedical Research Center, Institute for CNS Disorders, 15166 Bergondo, La Coruña, Spain*

M. Fiala *Department of Medicine, UCLA School of Medicine, Los Angeles, CA, USA*

A. Fisher *The Israel Institute for Biological Research, Ness Ziona, Israel*

E. Floor *Department of Physiology and Cell Biology, University of Kansas Lawerence, KS, USA*

F. Forette *Service de Gérontologie, Hôpital Broca, CHU Cochin, Université Paris V, 54–56 rue Pascal, 75 013 Paris, France*

B. Frangione *Department of Pathology, New York University Medical Center, 550 1st Avenue, New York, NY 10016, USA*

H. Fraser *Institute for Animal Health, Neuropathogenesis Unit, Ogston Building, West Mains Road, Edinburgh EH9 3JF, UK*

L. Fratiglioni *Department of Geriatric Medicine, Karolinska Institute and Stockholm Gerontology Research Center, Stockholm, Sweden*

S.A. Frautschy *Sepulveda VAMC GRECC 11E, UCLA Departments of Medicine and Neurology (SFVP), 16111 Plummer Street, Sepulveda, CA 91343, USA*

W.H. Frey II *Department of Pharmaceutics, College of Pharmacy, University of Minnesota, 308 Harvard Street, SE Minneapolis, MN 55455, USA*

M. Fridkin *Department of Organic Chemistry, Weizmann Institute of Science, Rehovot, Israel*

B. Frigard *Centre de Geriatrie de Wasquehal, rue Salvador Allende, B.P. 165, 59444 Wasquehal, France*

S.J. Fuller *Department of Pathology, University of Melbourne, Mental Health Research Institute, Parkville, Victoria 3052, Australia*

D. Galasko *Department of Neurosciences, University of California at San Diego, 3350 La Jolla Village Drive, San Diego, CA 9216, USA*

P. Gambetti *Division of Neuropathology, Case Western Reserve University, Cleveland, OH 44106, USA*

X. Gan *Department of Neurology, UCLA School of Medicine, Research Institute, 719 Westward Plaza, Los Angeles, CA 90098-1769, USA*

D.S. Geldmacher *University Alzheimer Center, Department of Neurology, Case Western Reserve University, 10900 Euclid Avenue, Cleveland, OH 44106, USA*

I. Genis *Department of Neurobiochemistry, The Israel Institute for Biological Research, Ness Ziona, Israel*

A. Georgakopoulos *Department of Psychiatry and Fishberg Research Center for Neurobiology, Mount Sinai School of Medicine, New York, USA*

E. Ghebremedhin *Department of Anatomy, J.W. Goethe University, Theodor Stern Kai 7, 60590 Frankfurt am Main, Germany*

B. Ghetti *Division of Neuropathology, Indiana University School of Medicine, Indianapolis, IN 46202, USA*

J. Ghiso *Department of Pathology, New York University Medical Center, 550 1st Avenue, New York, NY 10016, USA*

G. Gibb *Department of Neuroscience, Institute of Psychiatry, De Crespigny Park, London SE5 8AF, UK*

C.J. Gibbs Jr *Laboratory of CNS Studies, NINDS, NIH Bethesda, MD 20892, USA*

I. Gineke *Department of Animal Physiology, PO Box 14, 9750 AA Haren, The Netherlands*

R. Godemann *Max Planck Research Unit for Structural Molecular Biology, Notkestrasse 85, D-22603 Hamburg, Germany*

M. Goedert *MRC Laboratory of Molecular Biology, Hills Road, Cambridge CB2 2QH, UK*

A. Golabek *New York State Institute for Basic Research in Developmental Disabilities, 1050 Forest Hill Road, Staten Island, New York 10314, USA*

L.E. Goldstein *Laboratory for Oxidation Biology, Harvard Medical School, Massachusetts General Hospital, Boston, MA 02114, USA*

C.-X. Gong *Chemical Neuropathology Laboratory, New York State Institute for Basic Research in Developmental Disabilities, 1050 Forest Hill Road, Staten Island, NY 10314-6399, USA*

P. Gorevic *Department of Medicine, Mount Sinai Medical Center, One Gustave Levy Place, New York, NY 10029, USA*

M.E. Götz *Karolinska Institute of Environmental Medicine , Doktorsringen 16C, 17177 Stockholm, Sweden*

J.A. Gondal *Chemical Neuropathology Laboratory, New York State Institute for Basic Research in Developmental Disabilities, 1050 Forest Hill Road, Staten Island, NY 10314-6399, USA*

S. Govoni *Institute of Pharmacology, University of Pavia, Italy*

I. Gozes *Department of Clinical Biochemistry, Sackler School of Medicine, Tel Aviv University, Tel Aviv 69978, Israel*

M. Grafström *Stockholm Gerontology Research Center, Box 6401, SE 113 82 Stockholm, Sweden*

M.C. Graves *Department of Neurology, UCLA School of Medicine, Research Institute, 710 Westwood Plaza, Los Angeles, CA 90098-1769, USA*

C.W. Gray *SmithKline-Beecham Pharmaceuticals, Harlow, Essex, UK*

J. Grünberg *Central Institute of Mental Health, Department of Molecular Biology, J5, 68159 Mannheim, Germany*

I. Grundke-Iqbal *New York State Institute for Basic Research in Developmental Disabilities, Staten Island, NY 10314, USA*

S.Y. Guénette *Genetics and Aging Unit, Department of Neurology, Massachusetts General Hospital East, Harvard Medical School, 149 13th Street, Charlestown, MA 02129, USA*

M. Guerriero Austrom *Department of Psychiatry and Indiana Alzheimer Disease Center, 541 Clinical Drive, CL 590, Indiana University School of Medicine, Indianapolis, IN 46202-5111, USA*

Y. Guo *Program in Developmental Biology, Hospital for Sick Children, 555 University Avenue, Toronto, Ontario M5G 1X8, Canada*

Z. Guo *Department of Geriatric Medicine, Karolinska Institute and Stockholm Gerontology Research Center, Stockholm, Sweden*

C. Haass *Central Institute of Mental Health, Department of Molecular Biology, J5, 68155 Mannheim, Germany*

M. Hallupp *Garvan Institute of Medical Research, Neurobiology Program, 384 Victoria Street, Darlinghurst, NSW 2010, Australia*

D.P. Hanger *Department of Neuroscience, Institute of Psychiatry, De Crespigny Park, London SE5 8AF, UK*

L. Hansson *Department of Public Health and Caring Sciences/Geriatrics, PO Box 609, SE–751 25 Uppsala, Sweden*

N. Haque *Chemical Neuropathology Laboratory, New York State Institute for Basic Research in Developmental Disabilities, 1050 Forest Hill Road, Staten Island, NY 10314-6399, USA*

J. Hardy *Birdsall Building, Mayo Clinic Jacksonville, 4500 San Pablo Road, Jacksonville, FL 32224, USA*

D.A. Harris *Department of Cell Biology and Physiology, Washington University School of Medicine, 660 South Euclid Avenue, St. Louis, MO 63130, USA*

T. Hartmann *Center for Molecular Biology, INF 282 University of Heidelberg, D-69120, Germany*

M.A. Hartshorn *Harvard Medical School, Massachusetts General Hospital, Boston, MA 02114, USA*

M. Hasegawa *MRC Laboratory of Molecular Biology, Hills Road, Cambridge CB2 2QH, UK*

J.-J. Hauw *Laboratorie de Neuropathologie R. Escourelle, Hôpital de la Salpêtrière, 47 Blvd de l'Hôpital, 75651 Paris Cedex 13, France*

N. Helbecque *INSERM CJF 95-05, Institut Pasteur de Lille, 1 rue du Professeur Calmette, F-59019 Lille, France*

C. Helmer *INSERM U 330, Université de Bordeaux II, 146 rue Leo Saignat, 33076 Bordeaux Cedex, France*

L. Hendriks *Neurogenetics Laboratory, Flanders Interuniversity Institute for Biotechnology (VIB), Universiteitsplein 1, B-2610 Antwerp, Belgium*

L.M. Herrmann *NIAID, NIH, Rocky Mountain Laboratories, Hamilton, MT 59840, USA*

K. Herrup *University Alzheimer Center, Department of Neurology, Case Western Reserve University, 10900 Euclid Avenue, Cleveland, OH 44106, USA*

A. Hofman *EURODEM Research Group, Department of Epidemiology and Biostatistics, Erasmus University Medical School, PO Box 1738, 3000 DR Rotterdam, The Netherlands*

E.M. Hol *Graduate School for Neurosciences Amsterdam, Netherlands Institute for Brain Research, Meibergdreef 33, 1105 AZ Amsterdam, The Netherlands*

D.M. Holtzman *Department of Neurology, Washington University School of Medicine, 660 S. Euclid Ave, Box 8111, St. Louis, MO 63110, USA*

T. Honda *Laboratory for Alzheimer's Disease, Brain Science Institute, Riken, 2–1 Hirosawa, Wakoshi, Saitama 351–0198, Japan*

M. Horiuchi *NIAID, NIH, Rocky Mountain Laboratories, Hamilton, MT 59840, USA*

S. Hozumi *Institute of Mental Health, NCNP, Department of Psychophysiology, Kohnadai 1–7–3, 272-0827 Ichikawa-Shi, Japan*

K. Hsiao *Sepulveda VAMC GRECC 11E, UCLA Departments of Medicine and Neurology (SFVP), 16111 Plummer Street, Sepulveda, CA 91343, USA*

X. Huang *Laboratory for Oxidation Biology, Genetics and Aging Unit, Harvard Medical School, Massachusetts General Hospital—East, Building 149, 13th Street, Charlestown, MA 02129, USA*

J. Humphrey   *Roskamp Institute, USF, 3515 E. Fletcher Avenue, Tampa, FL 33613, USA*

R. Igata-Yi   *Department of Neuropsychiatry, Kumamoto University School of Medicine, Honjo 1–1–1, Kumamoto 860–8556, Japan*

S. Illenberger   *Max Planck Research Unit for Structural Molecular Biology, Notkestr. 85, D-22603 Hamburg, Germany*

K. Iqbal   *Chemical Neuropathology Laboratory, New York State Institute for Basic Research in Developmental Disabilities, 1050 Forest Hill Road, Staten Island, NY 10314-6399, USA*

J.W. Ironside   *National CJD Surveillance Unit, Western General Hospital, Edinburgh EH4 2XU, UK*

K. Ishizuka   *Department of Neuropsychiatry, Kumamoto University School of Medicine, Honjo 1–1–1, Kumamoto 860–8556, Japan*

T.A. Ishunina   *Netherlands Institute for Brain Research, Meibergdreef 33, 1105 AZ Amsterdam, The Netherlands*

T. Iwatsubo   *Laboratory for Alzheimer's Disease, Brain Science Institute, Riken, 2–1 Hirosawa, Wako-shi, Saitama 351–0198, Japan*

H. Jacobsen   *Central Institute of Mental Health, Department of Molecular Biology, J5, 68159 Mannheim, Germany*

C. Jagger   *c/o EURODEM, Department of Epidemiology and Biostatistics, Erasmus University Medical School, PO Box 1738, 3000 DR Rotterdam, The Netherlands*

P. Jäkälä   *Department of Neuroscience and Neurology, University and University Hospital of Kuopio, PO Box 1627, FIN-70211 Kuopio, Finland*

R. Jakes   *MRC Laboratory of Molecular Biology, Hills Road, Cambridge CB2 2QH, UK*

W. Jansson   *Stockholm Gerontology Research Center, PO Box 6401, SE–113 82 Stockholm, Sweden*

K. Kamino   *Department of Biochemistry and Cell Biology, Institute of Gerontology, Nippon Medical School, 1–396 Kosugi-cho, Nakahara-ku, Kawasaki 211–8533, Japan*

C. Kampitsis   *Department of Physical Education and Sport Science, Democritus University of Thrace, 40 Mikras Asias Str., 55 132 Kalamaria, Greece*

E. Kardalinou   *Department of Psychiatry, De Crespigny Park, London SE5 8AF, UK*

E.H. Karran   *SmithKline-Beecham Pharmaceuticals, Harlow, Essex, UK*

S. Katsuragi   *Department of Neuropsychiatry, Kumamoto University School of Medicine, Honjo 1–1–1, Kumamoto 860–8556, Japan*

A. Kazis   *3rd Department of Neurology, Aristotle University of Thessaloniki, Despere 3, Thessaloniki 54621, Greece*

S. Khatoon   *Chemical Neuropathology Laboratory, New York State Institute for Basic Research in Developmental Disabilities, 1050 Forest Hill Road, Staten Island, NY 10314-6399, USA*

E. Kida   *New York State Institute for Basic Research in Developmental Disabilities, 1050 Forest Hill Road, Staten Island, New York, NY 10314, USA*

T. Kihara   *Department of Neurology, Graduate School of Medicine, Graduate School of Pharmaceutical Sciences, Kyoto University, Kyoto, Japan*

L. Kilander   *Department of Public Health and Caring Sciences/Geriatrics, PO Box 609, SE–751 25, Sweden*

T.-W. Kim   *Genetics and Aging Unit, Department of Neurology, Massachusetts General Hospital—East, Harvard Medical School, 149 13th Street, Charlestown, MA 02129, USA*

T. Kimura   *Department of Neuropsychiatry, Kumamoto University School of Medicine, Honjo 1–1–1, Kumamoto 860–8556, Japan*

G. Koenig   *Bayer AG, CNS Research, Wuppertal, Germany*

E. Kokmen   *Department of Health Sciences Research, Mayo Clinic and Mayo Foundation, 200 First Street SW, Rochester, MN 55905, USA*

A. Kontush   *Medical Clinic, University Hospital Eppendorf, Martinistrasse 52, 20246 Hamburg, Germany*

D.M. Kovacs   *Genetics and Aging Unit, Department of Neurology, Massachusetts General Hospital—East, Harvard Medical School, 149 13th Street, Charlestown, MA 02129, USA*

A. Kundtz   *Roskamp Institute, 3513 E. Fletcher Avenue, University of South Florida, Tampa, FL 33613, USA*

J.B.J. Kwok   *Garvan Institute of Medical Research, Neurobiology Program, 384 Victoria Street, Darlinghurst, NSW 2010, Australia*

G. Kyriazis   *Immunology Department, 3rd Department of Neurology, Aristotle University of Thessaloniki, Despere 3, Thessaloniki 54621, Greece*

M.P. Laakso *Department of Radiology, University and University Hospital of Kuopio, PO Box 1627, FIN-70211 Kuopio, Finland*

M.J. LaDu *University of Chicago, Department of Cell and Molecular Biology, Northwestern Drug Discovery Program, Chicago, IL, USA*

J.-C. Lambert *INSERM CJF 95-05, Institut Pasteur de Lille, 1 rue Calmette, F-59019 Lille, France*

P.L. Lantos *Institute of Psychiatry, King's College London University, De Crespigny Park, Denmark Hill, London SE5 8AF, UK*

J.I. Lao *EuroEspes Biomedical Research Center, Institute for CNS Disorders, 15166 Bergondo, La Coruña, Spain*

L.J. Launer *EURODEM Research Group, Department of Epidemiology and Biostatistics, Erasmus University Medical School, PO Box 1738, 3000 DR Rotterdam, The Netherlands*

G. Lee *Brigham and Women's Hospital, 77 Avenue Louis Pasteur—HIM 758, Boston MA 02115, USA*

M.K. Lee *Department of Pathology, 558 Ross Building, 720 Rutland Avenue, Johns Hopkins Univeristy School of Medicine, Baltimore, MD 21205, USA*

M. Lehtovirta *Department of Neuroscience and Neurology, University of Kuopio, PO Box 1627, FIN-70211 Kuopio, Finland*

U. Leimer *Central Institute of Mental Health Department of Molecular Biology, J5, 68159 Mannheim, Germany*

C. Lendon *Department of Psychiatry, Neurology and Genetics, Washington University School of Medicine, St Louis, MI 63310, USA*

L. Letenneur *INSERM U 330, Université de Bordeaux II, 146 rue Leo Saignat, 33076 Bordeaux Cedex, France*

E. Levy *Departments of Pharmacology and Pathology, New York University Medical Center, 550 First Avenue, New York, NY 10016, USA*

F. Lezoualc'h *Max Planck Institute of Psychiatry, Kraepelinstrasse 2–16, 80804 Munich, Germany*

Q.-X. Li *Department of Pathology, University of Melbourne Mental Health Research Institute, Parkville, Victoria 3052, Australia*

S.F. Lichtenthaler *Center for Molecular Biology, INF 282, University of Heidelberg, D-69120 Heidelberg, Germany*

S. Lindquist *NIAID, NIH, Rocky Mountain Laboratories, Hamilton, MT 59840, USA*

H. Lithell *Department of Public Health and Caring Sciences/Geriatrics, PO Box 609, SE 751–25 Uppsala, Sweden*

I. Livne Bar *Program in Developmental Biology, Hospital for Sick Children, 555 University Avenue, Toronto, Ontario M5G 1X8, Canada*

A. Lobo *c/o EURODEM, Department of Epidemiology and Biostatistics, Erasmus University Medical School, PO Box 1738, 3000 DR Rotterdam, The Netherlands*

H. Loetscher *Central Institute of Mental Health, Department of Molecular Biology, J5, 68159 Mannheim, Germany*

S. Lovestone *Department of Neuroscience, Institute of Psychiatry, De Crespigny Park, London SE5 8AF, UK*

P.J. Lucassen *Leiden/Amsterdam Center for Drug Research, Leiden, The Netherlands*

P.G.M. Luiten *Department of Animal Physiology, University of Groningen, Groningen, The Netherlands*

N. Machiel de Vos *Eijkman–Winkler Institute, Section of Neuroviroimmunology, Utrecht University, Heidelberglaan 100, 3584 CX Utrecht, The Netherlands*

R. Mancini *Genetics and Aging Unit, Department of Neurology, Massachusetts General Hospital East, Harvard Medical School, 149 13th Street, Charlestown, MA 02129, USA*

E.-M. Mandelkow *Max Planck Research Unit for Structural Molecular Biology, Notkestrasse 85, D-22603 Hamburg, Germany*

D. Mann *Department of Pathological Sciences, Stopford Building, University of Manchester, Oxford Road, Manchester M13 9PT, UK*

U. Mann *Medical Clinic, University Hospital Eppendorf, Martinistrasse 52, 20246 Hamburg, Germany*

J. Martinez-Lage *c/o EURODEM, Department of Epidemiology and Biostatistics, Erasmus University Medical School, PO Box 1738, 3000 DR Rotterdam, The Netherlands*

C.L. Masters *Department of Pathology, University of Melbourne, Mental Health Research Institute, Parkville, Victoria 3052, Australia*

E. McGeer *Kinsmen Laboratory of Neurological Research, University of British Columbia, 2255 Wesbrook Mall, Vancouver, BC V6T 1Z3, Canada*

P.L. McGeer *Kinsmen Laboratory of Neurological Research, University of British Columbia, 2255 Wesbrook Mall, Vancouver, BC V6T 1Z3, Canada*

C. McLendon *Woodlands Medical and Research Center, 3150 Tampa Road, Oldsmar, FL 34677, USA*

D. Meier *Memory Clinic, Geriatric University Clinic, Hebelstrasse 10, 4031 Basel, Switzerland*

M.D. Mesa *EuroEspes Biomedical Research Center, Institute for CNS Disorders, 15166 Bergondo, La Coruña, Spain*

D.M. Michaelson *Department of Neurobiochemistry, George S. Wise Faculty of Life Sciences, Tel Aviv University, Tel Aviv 69978, Israel*

L. Milward *CERA, Department of Immunology, Concord Hospital, Concord, NSW 2139, Australia*

K. Mishima *Institute of Mental Health, NCNP, Department of Psychophysiology, Kohnadai 1–7–3, 272–0827 Ichikawa-shi, Japan*

T. Miyakawa *Department of Neuropsychiatry, Kumamoto University School of Medicine, Honjo 1–1–1, Kumamoto 860–8556, Japan*

H.-J. Möbius *Merz & Co., Frankfurt am Main, Germany*

M. Mohr *Institut de Pathologie, 1 Place de l'Hôpital, BP 22, 67064 Strasbourg Cedex, France*

R.D. Moir *Departments of Psychiatry and Neurology, Harvard Medical School, Massachusetts General Hospital, Boston, MA 02114, USA*

L. Morelli *Department of Pathology, New York University Medical Center, 550 First Avenue, New York, NY 10016, USA*

H. Mori *Tokyo Institute of Psychiatry and Molecular Biology, 2–1–8 Kamikitazawa, Setagay-Ku, 156-0057 Tokyo, Japan*

V. Mouroux *Birdsall Building, Mayo Clinic Jacksonville, 4500 San Pablo Road, Jacksonville, FL 32224, USA*

C. Mouzakidis *Department of Physical Education and Sport Science, Democritus University of Thrace, 40 Mikras Asias Str., 55 132 Kalamaria, Greece*

M. Mullan *Roskamp Institute, University of South Florida, 3515 E. Fletcher Avenue, Tampa, FL 33613, USA*

T. Müller-Thomsen *Medical Clinic, University Hospital Eppendorf, Martinistrasse 52, 20246 Hamburg, Germany*

M. Murayama *Laboratory for Alzheimer's Disease, Brain Science Institute, Riken, 2–1 Hirosawa, Wako-shi, Saitama 351–0198, Japan*

O. Murayama *Laboratory for Alzheimer's Disease, Brain Science Institute, Riken, 2–1 Hirosawa, Wako-shi, Saitama 351–0198, Japan*

J.R. Murrell *c/o M. Goedert, MRC Laboratory of Molecular Biology, Hills Road, Cambridge CB2 2QH, UK*

S. Na *Genetics and Aging Unit, Department of Neurology, Massachusetts General Hospital East, Harvard Medical School, 149 13th Street, Charlestown, MA 02129, USA*

P.J. Negro *South Texas Veterans Health Care Systems, Department of Psychiatry, University of Texas Health Science Center at San Antonio 116A, 7400 Merton Minter, San Antonio, TX 78284, USA*

E. Nemens *Department of Biochemistry and Cell Biology, Institute of Gerontology, Nippon Medical School, 1–396 Kosugi-cho, Nakahara-ku, Kawasaki 211–0061, Japan*

H. Nomiyama *Department of Biochemistry, Kumamoto University School of Medicine, Kumamoto, Japan*

H.S.L.M. Nottet *Eijkman–Winkler Institute, Section of Neuroviroimmunology, Utrecht University, Heidelberglaan 100, 3584 CX Utrecht, The Netherlands*

M. Novák *Institute of Neuroimmunology, Slovak Academy of Sciences, Dubravska str. 9, 842 46 Bratislava, Slovak Republic*

H. Nyman *Department of Public Health and Caring Sciences/Geriatrics, PO Box 609, SE–751 25, Sweden*

S. Ohta *Department of Biochemistry and Cell Biology, Institute of Gerontology, Nippon Medical School, 1–396 Kosugi-cho, Nakahara-ku, Kawasaki 211–0061, Japan*

M. Okawa   *National Institute of Mental Health, NCNP, Akita University School of Medicine, Akita, Japan*

J.-M. Orgogozo   *Department of Neurology, CHU Pellegrin, Neuroepidemiology Research Unit IN-SERM U 330, University of Bordeaux II, 33076 Bordeaux Cedex, France*

M. Ovečka   *Institute of Neuroimmunology, Slovak Academy of Sciences, Dubravska, Cesta 9, k84246 Bratislava, Slovak Republic*

K. Paliga   *Zentrum fur Molekulare Biologie Heidelberg, Universitat Heidelberg, Im Neuenheimer Feld 282, D-69120 Heidelberg, Germany*

J. Papanastasiou   *Department of Neurology, NIMTS, Athens, Greece*

M.A. Pappolla   *University of South Alabama College of Medicine, Mobile, AL, USA*

P. Parchi   *Division of Neuropathology, Institute of Pathology, Case Western Reserve University, 2085 Adelbert Road, Cleveland, OH 44106, USA*

D. Paris   *Roskamp Institute, USF, 3515 E. Fletcher Avenue, Tampa, FL 33613, USA*

T. Parker   *Roskamp Institute, USF, 3515 E. Fletcher Avenue, Tampa, FL 33613, USA*

F. Pasquier   *CHR et U de Lille, Clinique Neurologique, Centre de la Mémoire, Hôpital Salengro, 59037 Lille Cedex, France*

S. Patel   *Department of Neurology, Washington University School of Medicine, 660 S. Euclid Avenue, Box 8111, St Louis, MO 63110, USA*

J. Pearce   *Department of Neuroscience, Institute of Psychiatry, De Crespigny Park, London SE5 8AF, UK*

J. Pérez-Tur   *Birdsall Building, Mayo Clinic Jacksonville, 4500 San Pablo Road, Jacksonville, FL 32224, USA*

P. Piccardo   *Division of Neuropathology, Indiana University School of Medicine, Indianapolis, IN 46202, USA*

C. Pieträ   *Department of Pharmacology, Chiesi Pharmaceuticals S.p.A., Via Palermo 26/A, 43100 Parma, Italy*

T. Pirttilä   *Department of Neuroscience and Neurology, University of Kuopio, PO Box 1627, FIN-70211 Kuopio, Finland*

A. Placzek   *Roskamp Institute, 3515 E. Fletcher Avenue, University of South Florida, Tampa, FL 33613, USA*

J. Poirier   *McGill Centre for Studies in Aging, 6875 La Salle Boulevard, Verdun, Quebec H4H 1R3, Canada*

P. Pompl   *Roskamp Institute, 3515 E. Fletcher Avenue, University of South Florida, Tampa, FL 33613, USA*

N. Poritis   *Latvian Study Group, Riga, Latvia*

U. Preuss   *Max Planck Research Unit for Structural Molecular Biology, Notkestrasse 85, D-22603 Hamburg, Germany*

D.L. Price   *Department of Pathology, 558 Ross Building, 720 Rutland Avenue, Johns Hopkins University School of Medicine, Baltimore, MD 21205, USA*

A. Probst   *Institute of Pathology, Division of Neuropathology, Basel University, Basel, Switzerland*

M. Racchi   *Institute of Pharmacology, Viale Taramelli 14, I-27100 Pavia, Italy*

Y.-E. Rahman   *Department of Pharmaceutics, College of Pharmacy, University of Minnesota, 308 Harvard Street, SE Minneapolis, MO 55455, USA*

G.J. Raymond   *NIAID, NIH, Rocky Mountain Laboratories, Hamilton, MT 59840, USA*

L.D. Raymond   *NIAID, NIH, Rocky Mountain Laboratories, Hamilton, MT 59840, USA*

G. Reed   *Department of Pathology, The University of Melbourne Mental Health Research Institute, Parkville, Victoria 3052, Australia*

F.B.M. Reinhard   *Zentrum fur Molekulare Biologie Heidelberg, Universitat Heidelberg, Im Neuenheimer Feld 282, D-69120 Heidelberg, Germany*

R.J. Reiter   *University of Texas Health Science Center at San Antonio, TX, USA*

C.H. Reynolds   *Department of Neuroscience, Institute of Psychiatry, De Crespigny Park, London SE5 8AF, UK*

F. Richard   *INSERM CJF 95-05, Institut Pasteur de Lille, 1 rue Calmette, F-59019 Lille, France*

M. Riekkinen   *Department of Neuroscience and Neurology, University Hospital of Kuopio, PO Box 1627, FIN-70211, Kuopio, Finland*

P. Riekkinen Jr   *Department of Neuroscience and Neurology, University Hospital of Kuopio, PO Box 1627, FIN-70211, Kuopio, Finland*

P. Riekkinen Sr *A.I. Virtanen Institute, University of Kuopio, PO Box 1627, FIN-70211 Kuopio, Finland*

N.K. Robakis *Department of Psychiatry and Fishberg Research Center for Neurobiology, Mount Sinai School of Medicine, New York, USA*

W.A. Rocca *Department of Health Sciences Research, Mayo Clinic and Mayo Foundation, 200 First Street SW, Rochester, MN 55905, USA*

S. Röhrig *Genzentrum, Feodor-Lynen Strasse 25, 81377 Munich, Germany*

J.M. Rozemuller-Kwakkel *Graduate School Neurosciences Amsterdam, Faculty of Medicine, Department of Psychiatry, Vrije Universiteit, Van der Boechorststraat 7, 1081 BT Amsterdam, The Netherlands*

G.C. Ruben *Department of Biological Sciences, Dartmouth College, Hanover, NH 03766, USA*

D.C. Rubinsztein *Department of Medical Genetics, University of Cambridge, Box 158, Addenbrooke's NHS Trust, Hills Road, Cambridge CB2 2QQ, UK*

G.P. Saborio *Department of Pathology, New York University Medical Center, 550 First Avenue, New York, NY 10016, USA*

M. Sadowski *New York State Institute for Basic Research in Developmental Disabilities, 1050 Forest Hill Road, Staten Island, New York, NY 10314, USA*

N. Sahara *Tokyo Institute of Psychiatry and Molecular Biology, 2-1-8 Kamikitazawa, Setagay-Ku, 156-0057 Tokyo, Japan*

P. Sakka *Department of Neurology, NIMTS, Athens, Greece*

A. Salehi *Netherlands Institute for Brain Research, Meibergdreef 33, 1105 AZ Amsterdam, The Netherlands*

I. Sassin *Department of Anatomy, J.W. Goethe University, Theodor Stern Kai 7, 60590 Frankfurt am Main, Germany*

M. Sastre *Departments of Pharmacology and Pathology, New York University Medical Center, 550 First Avenue, New York, NY 10016, USA*

A.J. Saunders *Laboratory for Oxidation Biology, Harvard Medical School, Massachusetts General Hospital, Boston, MA 02214, USA*

G.D. Schellenberg *c/o K. Kamino, Department of Biochemistry and Cell Biology, Institute of Gerontology, Nippon Medical School, 1-396 Kosugi-cho, Nakahara-ku, Kawasaki 211-8533, Japan*

E.J.A. Scherder *Department of Clinical Psychology, Vrije Universiteit, De Boelelaan 1109, 1081 HV Amsterdam, The Netherlands*

A. Schindzielorz *Central Institute of Mental Health, Department of Molecular Biology, J5, 68159 Mannheim, Germany*

S. Schippling *Medical Clinic, University Hospital Eppendorf, Martinistrasse 52, 20246 Hamburg, Germany*

B. Schmidt *IRCCS, Centro San Giovanni di Dio FBE, Via Pilastroni 4, 25135 Brescia, Italy*

R. Schmidt *EURODEM Research Group, Department of Epidemiology and Biostatistics, Erasmus University Medical School, PO Box 1738, 3000 DR Rotterdam, The Netherlands*

P.R. Schofield *Garvan Institute of Medical Research, Neurobiology Program, 384 Victoria Street, Darlinghurst, NSW 2010, Australia*

C. Schultz *Department of Anatomy, J.W. Goethe University, Theodor Stern Kai 7, 60590 Frankfurt am Main, Germany*

M. Schulzer *Kinsmen Laboratory of Neurological Research, University of British Columbia, 2255 Westbrook Mall, Vancouver, BC V6T 1Z3, Canada*

C. Schwab *Kinsmen Laboratory of Neurological Research, University of British Columbia, 2255 Westbrook Mall, Vancouver, BC, V6T 1Z3, Canada*

R. Scott Turner *Departments of Pharmacology and Pathology, New York University Medical Center, 550 First Avenue, New York, NY 10016, USA*

A. Sengupta *Chemical Neuropathology Laboratory, New York State Institute for Basic Research in Developmental Disabilities, 1050 Forest Hill Road, Staten Island, NY 10314-6399, USA*

H. Shao *Case Western Reserve University, 10900 Euclid Avenue, Cleveland, OH 44106, USA*

X. Shao *Department of Medicine, Mount Sinai Medical Center, One Gustave Levy Place, New York, NY 10029, USA*

B. Sherry *The Picower Institute, Manhasset, New York, USA*

S. Shimohama *Department of Neurology, Graduate School of Medicine, Kyoto University, 54 Shogoin-Kawaharacho, Sakyoku, Kyoto 606, Japan*

J. Shioi   *Department of Psychiatry and Fishberg Research Center for Neurobiology, Mount Sinai School of Medicine, New York, USA*

E. Shohami   *Department of Pharmacology, The Hebrew University of Jerusalem, Jerusalem, Israel*

E.M. Sigurdsson   *Department of Pathology, New York University Medical Center, 550 First Avenue, New York, NY 10016, USA*

S.S. Sisodia   *Department of Pharmacological and Physiological Sciences, 947 E. 58th Street, Abbott 316, University of Chicago, Chicago, IL 60637, USA*

J. Sivenius   *Department of Neurology, University of Kuopio and Neuron Rehabilitation Center, Kuopio, Finland*

I. Skoog   *Department of Psychiatry, Sahlgrenska University Hospital, S–413 45 Göteborg, Sweden*

A.J.C. Slooter   *Department of Epidemiology and Biostatistics, Erasmus Medical School, PO Box 1738, 3000 DR Rotterdam, The Netherlands*

J.A. Sluijs   *Graduate School of Neurosciences Amsterdam, Netherlands Institute for Brain Research, Meibergdreef 33, 1105 AZ Amsterdam, The Netherlands*

A.B. Smit   *Department of Molecular and Cellular Neurobiology, Research Institute Neurosciences, Free University Amsterdam, The Netherlands*

M.J. Smith   *MRC Laboratory of Molecular Biology, Hills Road, Cambridge CB2 2QH, UK*

H.A. Smits   *Eijkman–Winkler Institute, Section of Neuroimmunology, Utrecht University, Heidelberglaan 100, 3584 CX Utrecht, The Netherlands*

H. Soininen   *Department of Neurology, University of Kuopio, PO Box 1627, FIN-70211 Kuopio, Finland*

M.A.F. Sonnemans   *Graduate School for Neurosciences Amsterdam, Netherlands Institute for Brain Research, Meibergdreef 33, 1105 AZ Amsterdam, The Netherlands*

C. Soto   *Department of Pathology, New York University Medical Center, 550 First Avenue, New York, NY 10016, USA*

D.L. Sparks   *Sun Health Research Institute, 10515 West Santa Fe Drive, Sun City, AZ 85351, USA*

R. Spiegel   *Memory Clinic, Geriatric University Clinic, Hebelstrasse 10, 4031 Basel, Switzerland*

M.G. Spillantini   *MRC Brain Repair Centre, University of Cambridge, Forvie Site, Robinson Way, Cambridge CB2 2PY, UK*

K. Stamer   *Max Planck Research Unit for Structural Molecular Biology, Notkestrasse 85, D-22603 Hamburg, Germany*

J.C. Steele   *Guam Memorial Hospital, Agana, Guam; and Kinsmen Laboratory of Neurological Research, University of British Columbia, 2255 Wesbrook Mall, Vancouver, BC V6T 1Z3, Canada*

H. Steiner   *Central Institute of Mental Health, Department of Molecular Biology, 15, 68159 Mannheim, Germany*

E.N.H. Jansen Steur   *Medisch Spectrum Twente, Enschede, The Netherlands*

H.J. Stürenburg   *Medical Clinic, University Hospital Eppendorf, Martinistrasse 52, 20246 Hamburg, Germany*

G. Su   *Roskamp Institute, 3515 E. Fletcher Avenue, University of South Florida, Tampa, FL 33613, USA*

R. Sulkava   *Department of Public Health and General Practice, Department of Medicine, University of Kuopio, Kuopio, Finland*

Y. Sun   *Department of Neurology, Washington University School of Medicine, 660 S. Euclid Avenue, Box 8111, St Louis, MO 63110, USA*

Z. Suo   *Roskamp Institute, University of South Florida, 3515 E. Fletcher Avenue, Tampa, FL 33613, USA*

D.F. Swaab   *Netherlands Institute for Brain Research, Meibergdreef 33, 1105 AZ Amsterdam, The Netherlands*

J. Takamatu   *National Kikuchi Hospital, Kumamoto, Japan*

A. Takashima   *Laboratory for Alzheimer's Disease, Brain Science Institute, Riken, 2–1 Hirosawa, Wako-shi, Saitama 351–0198, Japan*

J. Tan   *Roskamp Institute, 3515 E. Fletcher Avenue, University of South Florida, Tampa, FL 33613, USA*

J.E. Tanner   *Department of Pathology, University of Melbourne, Mental Health Research Institute, Parkville, Victoria 3052, Australia*

R.E. Tanzi   *Department of Neurology, Genetics and Aging Unit, Massachusetts General Hospital East, Harvard Medical School, 149 13th Street, Charlestown, MA 02129, USA*

T. Tapiola Department of Neurology, University of Kuopio, PO Box 1627, FIN-70211 Kuopio, Finland

D. Taub National Institute on Aging, Baltimore, MD, USA

L. Teri Department of Psychosocial and Community Health, Box 357263, University of Washington, Seattle, WA 98195-7263, USA

G. Tesco Genetics and Aging Unit, Massachusetts General Hospital and Harvard Medical School, Charlestown, MA 02129, USA

J. Theodorakis Department of Physical Education and Sport Science, Democritus University of Thrace, 40 Mikras Asias Str., 55 132 Kalamaria, Greece

G. Thinakaran Department of Pathology, 558 Ross Building, 720 Rutland Avenue, Johns Hopkins University School of Medicine, Baltimore, MD 21205, USA

G. Thomas Woodlands Medical and Research Center, 3150 Tampa Road, Oldsmar, FL 34677, USA

T. Thomas Woodlands Medical and Research Center, 3150 Tampa Road, Oldsmar, FL 34677, USA

M. Tolnay Institute of Pathology, Division of Neuropathology, Schoenbeinstrasse 40, CH-4003 Basel, Switzerland

T. Tomita Laboratory for Alzheimer's Disease, Brain Science Institute, RIKEN, 2–1 Hirosawa, Wako-shi, Saitama 351–0198, Japan

T. Town Roskamp Institute, USF, 3515 E. Fletcher Avenue, University of South Florida, Tampa, FL 33613, USA

B. Trinczek Max Planck Research Unit for Structural Molecular Biology, Notkestrasse 85, D-22603 Hamburg, Germany

M. Tsolaki 3rd Department of Neurology, Aristotle University of Thessaloniki, Despere 3, Thessaloniki 54621, Greece

C. Tysoe Department of Medical Genetics, University of Cambridge, Box 158, Addenbrooke's NHS Trust, Hills Road, Cambridge CB2 2QQ, UK

G. Ugolini Institute of Neuroimmunology, Slovak Academy of Sciences, Dubravska, Cesta 9, 84246 Bratislava, Slovak Republic

F.W. Unverzagt Department of Psychiatry, Indiana Alzheimer Disease Center, 541 Clinical Drive, CL 590 Indiana University School of Medicine, Indianapolis, IN 46202-5111, USA

C. Van Broeckhoven Laboratory of Neurogenetics, University of Antwerp (UIA), Universiteitsplein 1, B-2610 Antwerp, Belgium

R.C. van der Schors Department of Molecular and Cellular Neurobiology Research Institute Neurosciences, Free University, Amsterdam, The Netherlands

C.M. van Duijn Department of Epidemiology and Biostatistics, Erasmus Medical School, PO Box 1738, 3000 DR Rotterdam, The Netherlands

L. van Eldik Northwestern University School of Medicine, USA

S. van Gestel Laboratory of Neurogenetics, Flanders Interuniversity of Biotechnology, Born Bunge Foundation, University of Antwerp, Department of Biochemistry, Universiteitsplein 1, B-2610 Antwerp, Belgium

F.W. van Leeuwen Graduate School for Neurosciences Amsterdam, Netherlands Institute for Brain Research, Meibergdreef 33, 1105 AZ Amsterdam, The Netherlands

F.L. van Muiswinkel Graduate School Neurosciences Amsterdam, Faculty of Medicine, Department of Psychiatry, Vrije Universiteit, Van der Boechorststraat 7, 1081 BT Amsterdam, The Netherlands

E.J.W. Van Someren Department of Clinical Psychology, Vrije Universteit, De Boelelaan 1109, 1081 HV Amsterdam; and Netherlands Institute for Brain Research, Meibergdreef 33, 1105 AZ Amsterdam, The Netherlands

I. Vanderhoeven Neurogenetics Laboratory, Flanders Interuniversity Institute for Biotechnology (VIB), Universiteitsplein 1, B-2610 Antwerp, Belgium

H. Vanderstichele Innogenetics Inc., Zwijnaarde, Belgium

E. Vanmechelen Innogenetics Inc., Zwijnaarde, Belgium

J. Verhoef Eijkman–Winkler Institute, Section of Neuroviroimmunology, Utrecht University, Heidelberglaan 100, 3584 CX Utrecht, The Netherlands

R.W.H. Verwer Netherlands Institute for Brain Research, Meibergdreef 33, 1105 AZ Amsterdam, The Netherlands

R.G. Vidal   *Department of Pathology, TH 429 New York University School of Medicine, 550 1st Avenue, New York, NY 10016, USA*

M. Viitanen   *Department of Geriatric Medicine, Karolinska Institute and Stockholm Gerontology Research Center, Stockholm, Sweden*

G. Villetti   *Department of Pharmacology and Chemistry, Chiesi Pharmaceuticals S.p.A., via Palermo 26/A, 43100 Parma, Italy*

M. Visintin   *Institute of Neuroimmunology, Slovak Academy of Sciences, Dubravska, Cesta 9, 84246 Bratislava, Slovak Republic*

V. Vodoz   *Memory Clinic, Geriatric University Clinic, Hebelstrasse 10, 4031 Basel, Switzerland*

H. Wadsworth   *SmithKline-Beecham Pharmaceuticals, Harlow, Essex, UK*

J. Walter   *Central Institute of Mental Health, Department of Molecular Biology, J5, 68159 Mannheim, Germany*

J.-Z. Wang   *Wuhan, People's Republic of China*

R.V. Ward   *SmithKline-Beecham Pharmaceuticals, Harlow, Essex, UK*

M.-T. Webster   *Department of Neuroscience, Institute of Psychiatry, De Crespigny Park, London SE5 8AF, UK*

J. Wegiel   *New York State Institute for Basic Research in Developmental Disabilities, 1050 Forest Hill Road, Staten Island, New York, NY 10314, USA*

A. Weidemann   *Center for Molecular Biology, Heidelberg (ZMBH), INF 282, University of Heidelberg, D-69120 Heidelberg, Germany*

S. Whyte   *CERA, Department of Immunology Concord Hospital, Concord, NSW 2139, Australia*

E. Wijsman   *Department of Biochemistry and Cell Biology, Institute of Gerontology, Nippon Medical School, 1-396 Kosugi-cho, Nakahara-ku, Kawasaki 211-0061, Japan*

R.G. Will   *National CJD Surveillance Unit, Western General Hospital, Edinburgh EH4 2XU, UK*

B. Winblad   *Stockholm Gerontology Research Center, Box 6401, SE–113 82 Stockholm, Sweden*

H.M. Wisniewski   *Chemical Neuropathology Laboratory, New York State Institute for Basic Research in Developmental Disabilities, 1050 Forest Hill Road, Staten Island, NY 10314-6399, USA*

T. Wisniewski   *Department of Pathology, New York University School of Medicine, NY, USA*

N. Wittenburg   *Central Institute of Mental Health, Department of Molecular Biology, J5, 68159 Mannheim, Germany*

P.C. Wong   *Department of Pathology, 558 Ross Building, 720 Rutland Avenue, Johns Hopkins University School of Medicine, Baltimore, MD 21205, USA*

S. Wu   *Department of Neurology, Washington University School of Medicine, 660 S. Euclid Avenue, Box 8111, St Louis, MO 63110, USA*

T. Yamada   *Laboratory for Alzheimer's Disease, Brain Science Institute, Riken, 2–1 Hirosawa, Wako-shi, Saitama 351–0198, Japan*

H. Yamagata   *Department of Biochemistry and Cell Biology, Institute of Gerontology, Nippon Medical School, 1-396 Kosugi-cho, Nakahara-ku, Kawasaki 211-0061, Japan*

F. Yang   *Sepulveda VAMC GRECC 11E, UCLA Departments of Medicine and Neurology (SFVP), 16111 Plummer Street, Sepulveda, CA 91343, USA*

K. Yasojima   *Kinsmen Laboratory of Neurological Research, University of British Columbia, 2255 Wesbrook Mall, Vancouver, BC V6T 1Z3, Canada*

S.P. Yu   *Center for the Study of Nervous System Injury and Department of Neurology, Box 8111, Washington University School of Medicine, St. Louis, MO 63110, USA*

M.G. Zagorski   *Case Western Reserve University, 10900 Euclid Avenue, Cleveland, OH 44106, USA*

P. Zambenedetti   *Department of Biology, University of Padova, Via G. Colombo 3, 35131 Padova, Italy*

R. Zamostiano   *Department of Organic Chemistry, Weizmann Institute of Science, Rehovot, Israel*

P. Zatta   *CNR Center on Metalloproteins, University of Padova, Via G. Colombo 3, 35131 Padova, Italy*

L. Zhang   *Department of Neurology, UCLA School of Medicine, Research Institute, 710 Westward Plaza, Los Angeles, CA 90098-1769, USA*

Q. Zheng-Fischhöfer   *Max Planck Research Unit for Structural Molecular Biology, Notkestrasse 85, D-22603 Hamburg, Germany*

L. Zhu   *Department of Geriatric Medicine, Karolinska Institute and Stockholm Gerontology Research Center, Stockholm, Sweden*

Scientists Honored for Pioneering Research in Europe

EVA BRAAK PhD AND HEIKO BRAAK MD

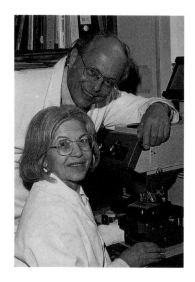

Professor Heiko Braak graduated from the Christian Albrecht University School of Medicine, Kiel, Germany, in 1964. After receiving his postdoctoral clinical training, he started his career in neuroanatomy at the Anatomic Institute in Kiel, where he was Associate Professor until 1979, when he moved to his present position as the Professor and Chairman of Neuroanatomy, J.W. Goethe University of Frankfurt am Main.

Professor Eva Braak received her PhD in Biology from the Georg August University, Göttingen, Germany, in 1967. It was at the Anatomic Institute in Kiel (around 1970) that this great husband-and-wife team of neuroanatomists started studying the cytoarchitecture of the human brain. In 1979 Professor Eva Braak also moved to the J.W. Goethe University of Frankfurt am Main to work in the Department of Neuroanatomy.

In the 1970s Professors Eva and Heiko Braak developed the special histological techniques required to study whole brain sections of humans and introduced the use of immunocytochemistry and advanced silver impregnation methods for these 100 µm sections to study the histopathology of Alzheimer's disease and related disorders. They successfully employed these techniques not only to correlate distinctive pigmentation patterns of several types of nerve cells with the features of these cells in Golgi and immunostained sections but also, in 1989, identified a new, not infrequently occurring tauopathy, argyrophilic grain disease, which is often marked by cognitive impairment. In 1991 they developed a now widely used staging system for the evaluation of Alzheimer histopathology, called the Braak Staging System.

KURT A.C. JELLINGER MD

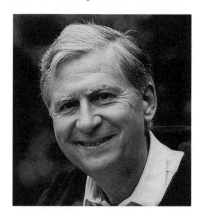

Professor Kurt Jellinger graduated from the University of Vienna School of Medicine in 1956. He held the positions of Assistant Professor from 1966 to 1971, Associate Professor from 1971 to 1973 and Full Professor from 1973 to the present, at the Neurological Institute University of Vienna. In addition he was Director, Department of Neurology, Lainz Hospital, from 1976 to 1997. Since 1977 he has been the Director of the Ludwig Boltzmann Institute of Clinical Neurobiology in Vienna.

Professor Jellinger's pioneering studies include the clinico-pathological correlations of dementing disorders and especially Alzheimer's disease, and the elucidation of the structural bases of dementia in aging, movement disorders, including Parkinson's disease, and different types of non-Alzheimer dementias. He has been one of the major contributors in developing the consensus recommendations for the pathological diagnosis of Alzheimer's disease, dementia with Lewy bodies, frontal lobe dementia, and atypical movement disorders such as progressive supranuclear palsy, multiple system atrophy and cortico-basal degeneration using neuronal networks. More recently, he and his associates have defined senile dementia with tangles, a rare type of dementia in the oldest-old, morphologically featured by neurofibrillary tangles in the absence of amyloid deposits and with very low prevalence of the apolipoprotein E4 allele.

MICHAEL KIDD MB BS

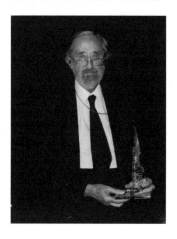

Professor Michael Kidd received his medical degree from University College London Medical School in 1956. After two years of medical practice, Professor Kidd started his research career in anatomy and human morphology as Lecturer at the Institute of Neurology, London, from 1961 to 1968. He was Lecturer in Anatomy from 1968 to 1975 at the University of Bristol and Senior Lecturer in Human Morphology from 1975 to 1995 at the University of Nottingham. Since 1995 Professor Kidd has been an Honorary Research Fellow at St George's Hospital Medical School, London, where he continues his research on Alzheimer's disease.

Professor Kidd's pioneering studies in Alzheimer's disease included the identification of paired helical filaments and the ultrastructure of senile plaques in the early 1960s. In 1969 he also showed the very first images of negative-stained paired helical filaments. The term 'paired helical filaments' was coined by Professor Kidd in 1963. He also reported one of the first accounts of the ultrastructure of spongiform encephalopathy and other cortical diseases.

CARL-GERHARD GOTTFRIES MD PhD

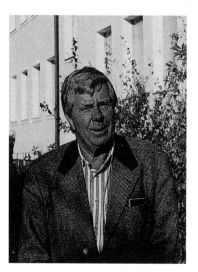

Professor Carl-Gerhard Gottfries received his MD and PhD degrees in 1958 and 1967, respectively, from the University of Lund in Sweden. He held the positions of Associate Professor of Psychiatry at the University of Lund from 1968 to 1971, Professor of Psychiatry and Head Physician at the Psychiatric Clinic, University of Umea, from 1971 to 1977 and Professor and Head Physician at the Department of Psychiatry and Neurochemistry, University of Göteborg, from 1977 to 1994. Since 1994 he has been Professor Emeritus at the University of Göteborg.

Professor Gottfries has spent his entire academic career studying neurotransmitter abnormalities and the clinical course of Alzheimer's disease and related conditions. In 1962, he developed the Gottfries Brane–Steen Rating Scale and Confusional State Evaluation (CSE) for geriatric patients. His pioneering studies include the demonstration, in postmortem human brain investigations, of multiple neurotransmitter deficits in Alzheimer's disease in the 1970s. He was also the first to observe that monoamine oxidase B activity was significantly increased in aged and Alzheimer's disease brains. Subsequent studies showed this monoamine oxidase activity in blood platelets as well, indicating that Alzheimer's disease is not only localized to the CNS. These monoaminergic deficits may explain the emotional disturbances that are part of the symptomatology of Alzheimer's disease. In subsequent studies, Professor Gottfries showed that selective serotonin reuptake inhibitors improved emotional disturbances in Alzheimer's disease patients.

Preface

Improvement in modern medicine, combined with better health education, continues to improve the human life span throughout the world. Alzheimer's disease, the prevalence of which increases sharply with age, thus poses one of the major public health problems, not only to the present society but even more to coming generations. Fortunately, research interest in Alzheimer's disease and related disorders is growing at a marked rate and there are significant new and important research findings which were not available at the time of our previous book on Alzheimer's disease two years ago. The present book describes advances in epidemiology, diagnosis, disease mechanisms, genetic factors and in both therapeutic opportunities and new therapeutic drugs. The articles in this book were selected from over 1300 papers presented at the Sixth International Conference on Alzheimer's Disease and Related Disorders, held in Amsterdam, The Netherlands. We believe this volume will be useful not only to basic scientists but also to clinicians and caregivers interested in Alzheimer's disease and related disorders.

Khalid Iqbal PhD
Dick F. Swaab MD PhD
Bengt Winblad MD PhD
Henry M. Wisniewski MD PhD

Acknowledgements

We would like to thank the chapter contributors for prompt submission of their manuscripts and the following individuals who played a major role in the ground work that materialized in this book. Professors Brian H. Anderton, Eva A.G. Braak, Charles J.C. Duyckaerts, Albert Hofman, Daniel Michaelson, Michal Novák, Jean-Marc Orgogozo, Paavo Riekkinen Sr, Ingmar G. Skoog, Sangram Sisodia, Dick F. Swaab and Christine L. Van Broeckhoven helped select the papers from over 1300 presented at the Sixth International Conference on Alzheimer's Disease and Related Disorders, Amsterdam, The Netherlands. Milet Verberne, Abey Jaarsma and Kim deJong of Congrex Holland BV provided outstanding logistical support. Dr Al Snider provided the most meticulous necessary coordination that facilitated the smooth and timely editorial process.

Financial support for the book was generously provided by Janssen Pharmaceutica and Research Foundation.

Khalid Iqbal PhD
Dick F. Swaab MD PhD
Bengt Winblad MD PhD
Henry M. Wisniewski MD PhD

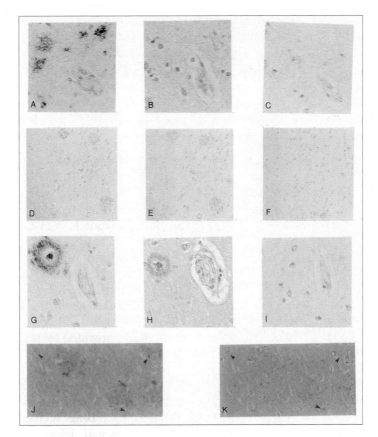

Plate I. Immunohistochemical staining for MCP-1 in SP and reactive microglia. Serial sections containing diffuse, primitive and classic plaques (A–C, D–F and G–I), stained with anti-ß AP antibody (A, D, G), MCP-1 (B, E, H) and non-immune mouse IgG as a negative control (C, F, I). Note MCP-1-positive reactivity in primitive plaques and classic plaques (E, H) but not in diffuse plaques (B) and negative control sections (C, F, I). Double-immunostaining with anti-MCP-1 antibody (blue in J) and then, after decolorization, with anti-ferritin antibody (brown in K) demonstrated that ferritin-positive microglia were also positive for MCP-1 (arrowheads in J, K). A–C × 400, D–F × 80, G–I × 400, J,K × 200

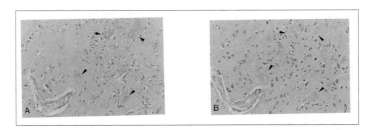

Plate II. Immunohistochemical staining for CCR2 in SP. Serial sections stained with anti-MCP-1 antibody (A) and anti-CCR2 antibody (B). Note CCR2 immunoreaction in senile plaques, which were positive for MCP-1 (arrowheads in A, B). A,B × 165

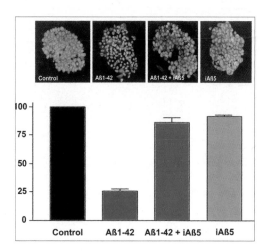

Plate III. Prevention of Aß neurotoxicity by iAß5. IMR-32 human neuroblastoma cells were used and cell viability was evaluated by DNA/RNA cell staining with AO/EtBr, as described [13]. Top panel shows photomicrographs of cell cultures treated with the peptide mixtures for 48 h and then stained with AO/EtBr and visualized by fluorescent microscopy. Cells that stain green are alive and those that stain orange are dead. The graph shows the quantitation of cell viability under different conditions. Each bar represents the mean + SD of three separate experiments. Reproduced with permission from reference [2]

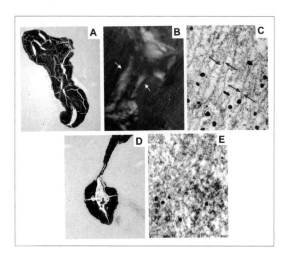

Plate IV. Reduction of cerebral Aß deposition and prevention of amyloid fibril formation *in vivo* by iAß5. Immunohistochemical staining of amygdaloid Aß deposits (× 50) at 8 days postoperatively of rats treated with Aß–42 alone (A) and a mixture of Aß1–42 and iAß5 (D). A Congo red-stained (× 100) adjacent section to that shown in (A) is presented in (B). Note the Congo red-positive birefringence (arrows) under polarized light (B). In the animals injected with Aß1–42 and iAß5, Congo red staining was completely negative (data not shown). Electron microscopic analysis (× 82 000) of the ultrastructure of immunogold-labelled Aß aggregates obtained in the absence (C) and presence (E) of iAß5. Note that the size of the gold particles was increased by the silver intensification Amyloid-like fibrils in (C) are indicated by arrows. Reproduced with permission from reference [2]

I Epidemiology and Risk Factors

1 Time Trends in the Prevalence of Dementia and Alzheimer's Disease in Rochester, Minnesota

EMRE KOKMEN, RUTH H. CHA AND WALTER A. ROCCA

INTRODUCTION

It is important to know whether the prevalence of dementia or Alzheimer's disease (AD) is increasing over time or not. However, studying time trends in prevalence requires repeated prevalence studies in a defined community and is, therefore, extremely time-consuming. There have been only a few studies that have reported time trends in the prevalence of dementia [1–4]. We report here the results of our most recent studies in Rochester, MN.

MATERIALS AND METHODS

We used the records-linkage system of the Rochester Epidemiology Project to identify all subjects whose records contained one or more diagnostic rubrics associated with any form of dementia. We identified 112 such rubrics from the *International Classification of Diseases*, 9th edn (ICD-9). This search covered the 15 years of the study (1975–1989) plus five additional years to allow for delayed diagnoses. Nurse abstractors screened all records of potential cases for evidence of cognitive decline and dementia and, when applicable, a dementia specialist (E.K.) determined the presence of dementia and the year of onset. Our criteria for dementia and AD have been published before and are shown in Table 1. Our criteria for dementia are similar to those in DSM-III [5].

Once a case met the criteria for dementia, we assessed whether the patient was a resident of Rochester, Minnesota, on a given prevalence date. Only subjects with onset of dementia before the prevalence date and alive and resident of the community on that day were counted. Population denominators were derived from census data [5].

Alzheimer's Disease and Related Disorders
Edited by K. Iqbal, D.F. Swaab, B. Winblad and H.M. Wisniewski
© 1999 John Wiley & Sons Ltd

Table 1. Diagnostic criteria for dementia and Alzheimer's disease

---

Diagnostic criteria for dementia
Documented evidence of:
  Previously normal intellectual and social function
  Irreversible decline in intellectual and social function
  Dementia as a predominant symptom
  Definite evidence of memory impairment
Documentation of at least two of the following (patient must be completely
    alert):
  Disorientation
  Decline in personality and/or behavior
  Dyscalculia
  Apraxia and/or agnosia
  Problems with language
  Impairment in judgment and/or abstract thinking
If diagnosis is based on clinical information only (that is, without autopsy
    confirmation), dementia must have been present for 6 months

Clinical diagnosis of Alzheimer's disease
Dementia as previously defined
Insidious onset
Slow progression
Other causes for dementia ruled out

Pathologic diagnosis of Alzheimer's disease
Dementia as previously defined
Presence of abundant neuritic plaques and/or neurofibrillary tangles in one or
    more cortical regions other than the hippocampus

RESULTS

We assessed the prevalence of dementia and AD for the population aged 30 years and above at four points in time, i.e. January 1 of 1975, 1980, 1985 and 1990. On January 1 1975, prevalent cases were 300 with dementia and 220 with AD. On January 1 1980, prevalent cases were 365 with dementia and 285 with AD. On January 1 1985, prevalent cases were 557 with dementia and 457 with AD. On January 1 1990, prevalent cases were 613 with dementia and 496 with AD. Tables 2 and 3 provide age-specific prevalence figures for dementia and AD at four points in time. These prevalence figures are also presented graphically in Figure 1.

DISCUSSION AND CONCLUSIONS

Comparing age-specific prevalence over time, we found no consistent trend for the age classes 65–84 years (65–69; 70–74; 75–79; 80–84 years). However, the age classes 85–89 and 90–94 years showed some increase over time for

Table 2. Time trends in age-specific prevalence of dementia (cases/1000) in Rochester, MN, 1975–1990

Age class (years)	Prevalence date*			
	1975	1980	1985	1990
65–69	10.5	7.7	8.5	14.0
70–74	21.7	22.2	23.1	20.0
75–79	46.0	42.3	53.6	51.2
80–84	102.8	97.0	128.0	119.8
85–89	145.1	184.5	237.9	209.9
90–94	224.2	276.2	300.4	302.9

* Prevalence refers to January 1 of each year.

Table 3. Time trends in age-specific prevalence of Alzheimer's disease (cases/1000) in Rochester, MN, 1975–1990

Age class (years)	Prevalence date*			
	1975	1980	1985	1990
65–69	4.9	3.5	4.2	7.7
70–74	11.9	15.7	14.0	15.4
75–79	36.5	28.8	44.2	37.2
80–84	81.2	70.8	104.3	99.0
85–89	113.4	170.9	210.0	177.3
90–94	181.8	252.4	279.2	271.4

* Prevalence refers to January 1 of each year.

both dementia and AD. The increase was consistent between 1975 and 1985 but did not continue through 1990. We found these increases in prevalence to result primarily from an increased migration of elderly patients with dementia to Rochester, rather than from a trend in incidence or survival. Further analyses of trends in incidence, prevalence, survival and migration are under way using our extensive database.

There are very few studies of time trends in the prevalence of dementia in other communities. The Lundby Study, which ended in 1972, did not indicate specific time trends in prevalence. A study done in Hisayama, Japan, showed a decrease in the prevalence of dementia between 1985 and 1992 for men but not for women. That study included dementia from all causes; the authors attributed their results to a relative decrease in the rates of vascular dementia.

ACKNOWLEDGEMENTS

This study was partially supported by NIA grant AG06786.

6

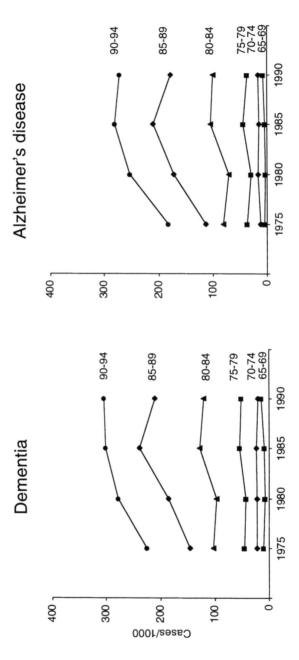

Figure 1. Time trends in age-specific prevalence of dementia and Alzheimer's disease in Rochester, Minnesota, 1975–1990

REFERENCES

1. Hagnell O. Repeated incidence and prevalence studies of mental disorders in a total population during 25 years. The Lundby Study, Sweden. Acta Psychiat Scand 1989; 79 (Suppl 348): 61–78.
2. Kiyohara Y, Yoshitake T, Kato I et al. Changing patterns in the prevalence of dementia in a Japanese community: the Hisayama study. Gerontology 1994; 40 (Suppl 2): 29–35.
3. Beard CM, Kokmen E, Offord K, Kurland LT. Is the prevalence of dementia changing? Neurology 1991; 41: 1911–14.
4. Beard CM, Kokmen E, O'Brien PC, Kurland LT. The prevalence of dementia is changing over time in Rochester, Minnesota. Neurology 1995; 45: 75–9.
5. Kokmen E, Beard CM, O'Brien PC, Kurland LT. Epidemiology of dementia in Rochester, Minnesota. Mayo Clin Proc 1996; 71: 275–82.

Address for correspondence:
Emre Kokmen,
Department of Neurology,
Mayo Clinic and Mayo Foundation,
200 First Street SW,
Rochester, MN 55905, USA

2 Regional Differences in the Incidence of Dementia in Europe: EURODEM Collaborative Analyses

L.J. LAUNER, L. FRATIGLIONI, K. ANDERSEN,
M.M.B. BRETELER, R.J.M. COPELAND,
J.-F. DARTIGUES, A. LOBO, J. MARTINEZ-LAGE,
H. SOININEN AND A. HOFMAN FOR EURODEM
INCIDENCE RESEARCH GROUP

INTRODUCTION

There are two reasons for examining regional differences in the incidence of disease. Such data are important for planners, who must provide for health services in different regions, as will be the case for the future European Union planners. Second, comparisons might provide clues to the etiology of the disease. We studied regional differences in dementia by comparing and pooling population-based studies conducted in Europe. In 1988 a network (EURODEM) of researchers in Europe was formed, with the aim of harmonizing the designs of their newly initiated studies on the incidence of dementia [1]. One important goal of this collaboration was to identify regional differences in the incidence of dementia. The eight studies pooled in these analyses are a part of this collaboration. There is a wide north–south distribution. The studies include the Kuopio Study, Finland [2], Kungsholmen Project, Sweden [3], the Odense Study, Denmark [4], the Rotterdam Study, The Netherlands [5], the MRC-Alpha Study, UK [6], the PAQUID Study, France [7], the Pamplona Study, Spain [8] and the Zaragoza Study, Spain [9].

Alzheimer's Disease and Related Disorders
Edited by K. Iqbal, D.F. Swaab, B. Winblad and H.M. Wisniewski
© 1999 John Wiley & Sons Ltd

METHODS

STUDY DESIGN

The design of all studies consisted of a baseline and one follow-up, with the exception of the PAQUID Study, which had two follow-up examinations. At baseline, the dementia-free cohort was defined by identifying prevalent cases of dementia. At follow-up, newly developed dementia cases (incident cases) were identified. The interval between baseline and follow-up ranged from 2.1 to 4.5 years. All the studies are based on either random or total samples of individuals in a defined geographic residence. More detailed descriptions of the studies can be found in the listed references.

CASE ASCERTAINMENT

Studies used a two-phase study design to ascertain the demented cases. A screening phase was followed by a clinical phase where all subjects who screened positive were clinically examined. Different screening tests were used, although all included the Mini-Mental State Exam [10]. In all studies, the minimal diagnostic work-up consisted of a clinical examination performed by physicians and a neuropsychological assessment. Data from informant interviews, medical records, brain imaging and blood tests were not available in all studies.

DIAGNOSTIC CRITERIA

Dementia diagnosis was made according to DSM-IIIR [11] criteria, or equivalent criteria such as CAMDEX [12] and AGECAT [13]. The use of diagnostic criteria for Alzheimer's disease and vascular dementia were more varied among the studies. Guidelines for Alzheimer's disease included DSM-IIIR [11] and NINCDS–ADRDA [14]. Guidelines for vascular dementia included: DSM-IIIR [11], ICD-10 [15] and the Hachinski score [16].

STATISTICAL ANALYSIS

All studies provided aggregated cell frequency data (number of incident cases and person-years of follow-up) by sex and five-year age group (65 years to 90 and over years). Age- and sex-specific incidence rates for each study were calculated as the number of new cases divided by the person-years at risk. Person-years for non-demented subjects were calculated as the time between the screening test of the baseline and the follow-up examination or death. For the demented subjects, half of this time was assumed, if precise information on dementia onset was not available. A subject who developed a questionable dementia was considered to be still at risk for developing a clinically definite dementia.

To examine differences by region, we created two sets of pooled estimates: the northern estimates are based on data from the Kuopio Study, Finland; Kungsholmen Project, Sweden; Odense Study, Denmark; the Rotterdam Study, The Netherlands; and the MRC-Alpha Study, UK. By pooling the data we increase the sample size and thereby the precision of the estimates. This overcomes some of the problems in interpretation of results from a single study that might have a limited sample size in a particular age or sex group.

RESULTS

Alzheimer's disease comprised the majority of dementia cases (60–70%) in all studies. Vascular dementia (VaD) accounted for about 15–20% of all dementia cases, with similar findings in all studies.

The pooled dementia rates are shown by region for the total sample (Figure 1). When data were analyzed by sex, similar regional patterns were found (data not shown). Pooled data on Alzheimer's disease (Figure 2) as well as VaD (Figure 3) also suggest the rates in the northern studies are higher than in the southern studies.

DISCUSSION

SUMMARY

Data from eight population-based studies of incident dementia were pooled by region. Five studies were included in the northern region and three in the

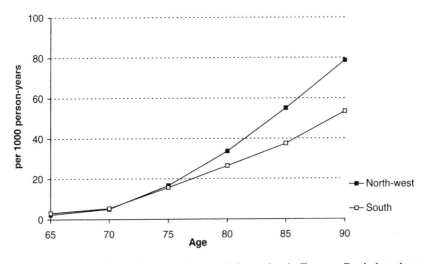

Figure 1. Age-specific incidence of dementia by region in Europe. Pooled analyses

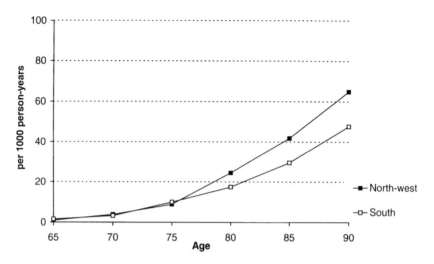

Figure 2. Age-specific incidence of Alzheimer's disease by region in Europe. Pooled analyses

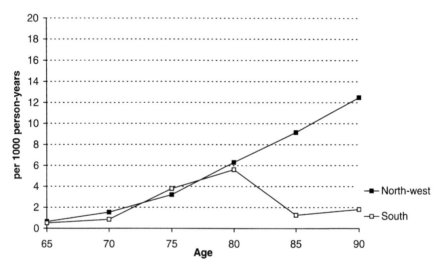

Figure 3. Age-specific incidence rates of vascular dementia by region in Europe. Pooled analyses

southern region. After age 80 years, we find a higher rate of dementia in the northern compared to southern regions. These differences were also evident in the pooled data on Alzheimer's disease and on vascular dementia.

LIMITATIONS

The regional differences have to be interpreted with caution. A comparison of the rates across the individual studies does not reveal large differences. This may be due to the small sample size of individual studies, particularly at the older ages. The northern rate estimates are more stable than the southern because they are based on more person-years of follow-up. Since studies sent data in aggregated form, we could not estimate precise confidence intervals and formally test for statistical differences in the rates. The regional differences are apparent only in the later age strata. Although the pooling increases the precision of these estimates, the sample size is still relatively small compared to those in the younger age strata. With the exception of the Rotterdam Study, there was no ascertainment of case status in persons lost to follow-up between the baseline and follow-up. The extent of bias created by this loss is partly related to the duration of the incidence interval. However, since the average percentage loss to follow-up did not differ by region, this is not likely to have severely biased the comparison. Finally, the regional differences by sub-type of dementia should be interpreted with caution, as there were differences in the criteria and in the protocols used for assessing sub-types.

CONCLUSIONS

These data raise the possibility that there are regional differences in the incidence of dementia. Studies comparing the prevalence of intermediate markers of dementia may help us to understand better the pathology underlying these differences. Neuroimaging with MRI, a tool becoming increasingly accessible to research centers, can provide information on such intermediary markers. For instance, MRI can provide images of vascular disease (infarcts, lacunae infarcts, white matter lesions) and cortical atrophy. Geographic differences or similarities in these brain changes would provide important clues about the risk factors associated with, and the pathology underlying, regional differences (or similarities) in the rates of dementia. The study of anatomical changes can help focus investigations on specific and multiple changes that might eventually lead to a dementia syndrome. It goes beyond the dichotomization of the dementia syndrome into Alzheimer's disease and vascular dementia, and may give us more insight into complex changes leading to the dementia identified in population-based studies. A multi-centre study is currently in progress to examine geographic differences in brain changes measured on MRI. This collaboration, CASCADE, is based on 12 cohorts located in northern, southern, eastern and western Europe [17].

REFERENCES

1. Launer LJ, Brayne C, Dartigues J-F, Hofman A (eds). European Studies on the incidence of dementing diseases. EURODEM Incidence. Neuroepidemiology 1992; 11 (suppl 1): 1–122.
2. Koivisto K. Population based dementia screening program in the city of Kuopio, eastern Finland. Thesis. Series of reports, Dept. Neurology, University of Kuopio, No 33, 1995.
3. Fratiglioni L, Viitanen M, Backman L, Sandman PO, Winblad B. Occurrence of dementia in advanced age: the study design of the Kungsholmen Project. Neuroepidemiology 1992; 11(1): 29–36.
4. Andersen K, Lolk A, Nielsen H, Andersen J, Olsen C, Kragh Sorensen P. Prevalence of very mild to severe dementia in Denmark. Acta Neurol Scand 1997; 96: 872–7.
5. Breteler MM, van den Ouweland FA, Grobbee DE, Hofman A. A community based study of dementia: the Rotterdam Elderly Study. Neuroepidemiology 1992; 11(1): 23–8.
6. Saunders PA, Copeland JRM, Dewey ME, Larkin BA, Scott A. ALPHA: The Liverpool MRC study of the incidence of dementia and cognitive decline. Neuroepidemiology 1992; 11: (S44–7).
7. Gagnon M, Letenneur L, Dartigues J-F, Commenges D, Orgogozo J-M, Barberger Gateau P et al. Validity of the Mini-Mental State examination as a screening instrument for cognitive impairment and dementia in French elderly community residents. Neuroepidemiology 1990; 9(3): 143–50.
8. Manubens JM, Martinez-Lage JM, Lacruz F et al. Prevalence of Alzheimer's disease and other dementing disorders in Pamplona, Spain. Neuroepidemiology 1995; 14: 155–64.
9. Lobo A, Saz P, Marcos G, Dia JL, de la Camara C. The prevalence of dementia and depression in the elderly community in a southern European population. The Zaragoza Study. Arch Gen Psychiat 1995; 52: 497–506.
10. Folstein MF, Folstein SE, McHugh PR. 'Mini-Mental State': a practical method for grading the cognitive state of patients for the clinician. J Psych Res 1975; 12: 189–98.
11. American Psychiatric Association. Diagnostic and Statistical Manual of Mental Disorders, 3rd edn. Washington, DC: American Psychiatric Association, 1987.
12. Roth M, Tym E, Mountjoy CQ, Huppert FA, Hendrie H, Verma S, Goddard R. CAMDEX: A standardized instrument for the diagnosis of mental disorders in the elderly with special reference to the early detection of dementia. Br J Psychiat 196; 149: 698–709.
13. Copeland JRM, Kelleler MJ, Kellett JM et al. A semi-structured clinical interview for the assessment of diagnosis and mental state in the elderly: the Geriatric Mental State Schedule. Psychol Med 1976; 6: 439–49.
14. McKahnn G, Drachman D, Folstein M, Katzman R, Price D, Stadlan EM. Clinical diagnosis of Alzheimer's disease: report of the NINCDS–ADRDA Work Group under the auspices of Department of Health and Human Services Task Force on Alzheimer's Disease. Neurology 984; 34: 939–44.
15. World Health Organization. International Classification of Diseases, 10th edn. Geneva: WHO, 1992.

16. Hachinski VC, Iliff LD, Zilhka E, Du Boulay, McAllister VL, Marshell J et al. Cerebral blood flow in dementia. Arch Neurol 1975; 32: 632–7.
17. Launer LJ, Hofman A. Cardiovascular risk factors for dementia: CASCADE (EU DGXII Biomed2 contract no: BMH4-CT-96-1508).

Address for correspondence:
    L.J. Launer,
    c/o EURODEM,
    Department of Epidemiology and Biostatistics,
    Erasmus University Medical School,
    PO Box 1738,
    3000 DR Rotterdam, The Netherlands

3   Cerebrovascular Risk Factors Are Determinants of Low Cognitive Function: A 20-Year Follow-up of 999 Elderly Men

LENA KILANDER, HÅKAN NYMAN, LENNART HANSSON, MERIKE BOBERG AND HANS LITHELL

INTRODUCTION

The interest in cognitive decline of vascular origin is steadily increasing, due to the possibilities of preventive treatment. Hypertension is a main risk factor for cerebrovascular disease, and there is a strong, linear relation between diastolic blood pressure (DBP) and stroke, even down to low levels [1]. Diabetes and atrial fibrillation are other main determinants of stroke [2, 3]. We investigated the relations between cerebrovascular risk factors and performance in cognitive tests in a population of elderly men who had been followed with respect to vascular risk factors since the age of 50 years.

POPULATION AND METHODS

The study population consisted of 999 men, aged 69–74 years. They were recruited from a cohort study, focusing on cardiovascular risk factors, that was started in the beginning of the 1970s. The original cohort was defined as all 50 year-old men, i.e. born in 1920–1924, who lived in Uppsala at that time-point. The participation rate was 82% (n = 2322). Primary preventive treatment was offered to subjects at high risk for vascular disease. A total of 1221 men (65.2% of all 1874 survivors) took part in the follow-up 20 years later, i.e. at age approximately 70. These participants were also invited to a testing of cognitive functions, in which 999 men agreed to take part. The methods have been described previously [4]. Cognitive functions were assessed by the Mini-Mental State Examination (MMSE) [5] and the Trail Making Tests A and B [6]. After a logarithmic transformation of the test

Alzheimer's Disease and Related Disorders
Edited by K. Iqbal, D.F. Swaab, B. Winblad and H.M. Wisniewski
© 1999 John Wiley & Sons Ltd

results, a z-transformation was applied, and a composite cognitive score was calculated for each subject as the sum of the z-scores, divided by the number of tests performed. Thus, ± 0.0 is equal to the mean result in the population; $+1.0$ is a result one SD over the mean score. The first consecutive 502 men were examined with a more extensive testing, covering performance also in tests on vocabulary [7], verbal learning and delayed recall [8], verbal (Digit Span Test) [7] and non-verbal attention (Block Span Test) [9], verbal fluency (FAS) [9] and visuoconstructional ability (Rey–Osterrieth's Figure) [6].

Office blood pressure (BP) was measured at the baseline examination at age 50. At follow-up at age 70, both office BP and 24 h ambulatory BP were registered. Recordings were made every 20 or 30 minutes during day-time, and every 30 or 60 minutes during the night. The difference between mean day-time and nocturnal systolic BP (SBP) was calculated, and non-dipping was defined as a BP difference between day and night of zero or less. An oral glucose tolerance test (OGTT) classified subjects as having normal or impaired glucose tolerance or diabetes. Peripheral insulin sensitivity was estimated with the hyperinsulinemic euglycemic clamp technique. Body mass index and serum lipids and lipoproteins were measured. Resting standard electrocardiograms (ECGs) were obtained, and coded with regard to presence or absence of atrial fibrillation. Echocardiography was performed in a subgroup (n = 375), and ejection fraction was used as a measurement of systolic function. Any use of BP lowering agents, irrespective of indication, was classified as antihypertensive treatment. Previous stroke cases were identified by the National Inpatient Register and by direct questioning. All statistical analyses were adjusted for age, educational level (low, i.e. elementary school only; medium; or high, i.e. university studies) and previous occupational level, stratified as low, medium or high.

RESULTS

Measurements of socioeconomic status and baseline DBP did not differ between the participants in the cognitive study (n = 999) and the surviving non-participants from the baseline examination (n = 875). A large majority of the men had high scores in the MMSE—77% scored ≥ 28 points. Thirty-four per cent were treated with antihypertensive agents. There was no association between hypertension, or atrial fibrillation, and low education. Seventy men had a hospital diagnosis of previous stroke. Their mean cognitive score was markedly lower (-0.43 ± 1.14) than the mean score in stroke-free participants ($+0.02 \pm 0.78$, p = 0.0001). In the following analyses, men with stroke according to the Inpatient Register are excluded from the analyses; also excluding men with a self-reported stroke did not affect the results.

LONGITUDINAL MEASUREMENTS

Office DBP at age 50 years was inversely related to cognitive test results 20 years later (Figure 1). The mean cognitive z-score in men with low DBP (≤ 70 mmHg) at age 50 was $+0.17 \pm 0.71$, while those with baseline DBP ≥ 105 mmHg had markedly lower results (-0.33 ± 0.82), corresponding to a difference of 0.5 SD between groups. As shown, the rate of treatment in hypertensive subjects was high. Only three men with baseline DBP ≥ 105 mmHg were not treated at follow-up; their mean cognitive score was -1.24.

A further analysis of relationships between baseline BP and performance in different cognitive areas was made in a subgroup (the first consecutive 502 men). Subjects with low DBP (≤ 70 mmHg, n = 63) at age 50 had, 20 years later, better performance in tests on mental speed and flexibility (Trail Making Tests); verbal attention (Digit Span Test); verbal fluency (FAS) and in the MMSE, than men with baseline DBP ≥ 75 mmHg (Table 1). The relationships were significant, independently of age, education and previous occupation, stroke and diabetes. There was no relationship between baseline BP levels and later performance in tasks on vocabulary, non-verbal attention, verbal learning and recall, or visuoconstructional ability.

CROSS-SECTIONAL MEASUREMENTS

There was an inverse relationship between 24 h ambulatory BP and cognitive score; nocturnal DBP showed the strongest linear relation ($r = -0.15$, $p < 0.0001$).

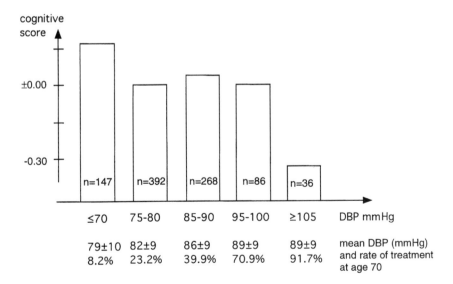

Figure 1. Diastolic blood pressure at age 50 in relation to cognitive function at age 70 years. Test for trend (Spearman): p = 0.0040, adjusted for age, education and occupation

Table 1. Performance in different cognitive areas at age 70 in relation to diastolic blood pressure at age 50 years

Cognitive test	DBP at 50 years		p
	≤ 70 mmHg (n = 63)	≥ 75 mmHg (n = 439)	
MMSE*	29 (27–30)	29 (26–30)	0.048
Vocabulary	47 ± 11	45 ± 11	0.100
Digit span	13 ± 4	12 ± 3	0.013
Block span	13.3 ± 3.0	13.6 ± 3.1	0.466
Verbal learning†	142 ± 71	159 ± 79	0.188
Verbal retention	5.9 ± 2.1	5.6 ± 2.3	0.393
Trail Making A†	39 ± 13	44 ± 17	0.038
Trail Making B†	107 ± 45	122 ± 52	0.009
Figure copying	33.3 ± 3.7	32.3 ± 3.7	0.097
Figure retention	16.2 ± 5.6	16.7 ± 6.2	0.729
Verbal fluency	29.9 ± 10.7	26.2 ± 10.3	0.002

Mean values ± SD, analysis of covariance or *median values (10–90%), partial Spearman rank correlation test. p values are adjusted for age, education, occupation and previous stroke. † High scores indicate low performance.

Figure 2 shows cognitive score by tertiles of mean 24 h DBP, with separate analyses for untreated men (n = 594) and treated men (n = 289). The inverse relation between BP and cognitive score was similar in both categories, but significant for untreated men only. The mean cognitive results did not differ between men with and without antihypertensive treatment.

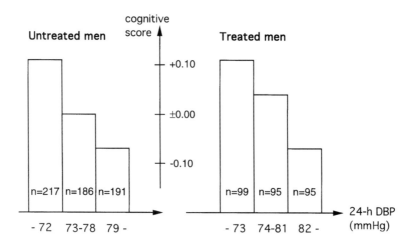

Figure 2. Cognitive score by tertiles of 24 h diastolic blood pressure at age 70. Test for trend (Spearman), adjusted for age, education, occupation and insulin sensitivity index: p = 0.014 in untreated men, p = 0.272 in treated men

Non-dippers, i.e. men with absence of normal nocturnal systolic BP fall (n = 59), had lower test results independently of 24 h DBP. The rate of non-dipping was 5.4% in those with MMSE ≥ 28 p, and 10.8% in those with MMSE ≤ 27 p (p < 0.05). There were no indications of a J-shaped relation between BP, treated or untreated, and cognitive function. Neither was extreme blood pressure dipping during the night associated with low cognitive results.

Cognitive performance in atrial fibrillation is shown in Table 2. Mean cognitive z-score was –0.44 ± 0.96 in the 38 men with atrial fibrillation and +0.04 ± 0.77 in the others, i.e. a difference of 0.5 SD, p = 0.0001. Results in the MMSE and in the Trail Making Tests were equally affected. The relationship between atrial fibrillation and low cognitive score remained after adjusting for 24 h DBP and heart rate, diabetes and ejection fraction. Men with atrial fibrillation who were treated with digoxin (n = 28) performed markedly better than those without treatment (n = 10), while test results were equal between men treated with low-dose aspirin or warfarin and untreated men; and between men with and without antihypertensive treatment.

Men with diabetes according to the OGTT (n = 130) had significantly lower cognitive z-scores than non-diabetic men (n = 779), although the difference between groups was small (–0.16 ± 0.90 vs. +0.06 ± 0.75, p = 0.002). In a multivariate model, high 24 h DBP, atrial fibrillation and diabetes were all independently related to low results. There was no significant relationship between hyperlipidemia or obesity and low cognitive scores, independently of BP and diabetes.

Table 2. Cognitive performance in atrial fibrillation

	Atrial fibrillation	
	Yes	No
	n = 38	n = 845
Composite cognitive score	–0.44 ± 0.96***	+0.04 ± 0.77
Range 10–90%	–1.79–+0.48	–0.95–+0.98
MMSE	28 (24–30) p	29 (27–30) p
Trail Making A	49 (36–99) s	42 (28–69) s
Trail Making B	134 (83–240) s	108 (66–192) s

Mean ± SD (composite score) or median values (range 10–90%) (MMSE and TMT).
*** p = 0.0004 adjusted for age, education and occupation. In a model including age, education, occupation, 24 h DBP, 24 h heart rate, diabetes and ejection fraction (n = 325), the p value for atrial fibrillation was 0.009.

DISCUSSION

In these community-living elderly men, high diastolic blood pressure at age 50 years predicted low cognitive function 20 years later. Cross-sectional measurements showed that high 24 h DBP, atrial fibrillation, a non-dipping nocturnal BP pattern and diabetes all were independently linked to low results in cognitive tests (MMSE and the Trail Making Tests). This was a healthy cohort, where subjects with a clinically manifest stroke had been excluded, and they were representative for the original cohort with regard to education and baseline BP. A majority of the participants had high scores in the MMSE, and it is likely that the rate of preventive treatment is higher than in a general population. Hence, the relationships are likely not to be overestimated.

We chose to use the mean cognitive test results as a continuous outcome variable, since there is no clear-cut borderline between "healthy" and "low cognitive function". Since cognitive functions were measured on one occasion only, low results are not necessarily equal to cognitive decline, and no clear conclusions regarding causality may be drawn. However, an association between DBP in middle age and cognitive performance in late life suggests a causal relationship. Pathophysiological mechanisms may be multifactorial, including silent ischemia, dysfunction of the blood–brain barrier, hemodynamic dysfunction or apoptosis [10]. Specifically, low DBP in midlife predicted higher performance tests on mental speed and flexibility, verbal fluency and attention. In magnetic resonance imaging (MRI) studies, these areas of cognitive function have been related to subcortical white matter lesions [11–13]. Atrial fibrillation may be a cause of silent embolic cerebrovascular lesions, and myocardial dysfunction may also cause periodical disability in maintaining cerebral blood flow, with subsequent ischemic lesions. Interestingly, digoxin treatment in atrial fibrillation was associated with better performance.

Several recent studies have added support to a link between vascular risk factors and cognitive impairment [14–17]. Hypertension may be a determinant not only of vascular dementia, but also of Alzheimer's disease [18, 19]. Conversely, low blood pressure might protect from subclinical cerebrovascular lesions causing cognitive impairment. There is convincing evidence of the importance of adequate antihypertensive treatment in the primary prevention of cerebrovascular disease, even at older ages [20, 21]. The hypothesis that optimal antihypertensive treatment may be beneficial not only in stroke prevention but also in preventing cognitive impairment and dementia remains to be proved in randomized clinical trials.

ACKNOWLEDGEMENTS

This research was supported by grants from the Swedish Medical Research Council (Grant No. 5446), the Thuréus Foundation, the Loo and Hans Osterman Foundation, the Stohne Foundation, the Stroke Foundation, the Dementia Foundation and the Swedish Hypertension Society.

REFERENCES

1. MacMahon S, Peto R, Cutler J, Collins R, Sorlie P, Neaton J et al. Blood pressure, stroke and coronary heart disease, part 1. Lancet 1990; 335: 765–74.
2. Fuller J, Shipley M, Rose G, Jarrett RJ, Keen H. Mortality from coronary heart disease and stroke in relation to degree of glycaemia: the Whitehall study. Br Med J 1983; 287: 867–70.
3. Wolf PA, Dawber TR, Thomas HE, Kannel WB. Epidemiologic assessment of chronic atrial fibrillation and risk of stroke: the Framingham Study. Neurology 1978; 28: 973–7.
4. Kilander L, Nyman H, Hansson L, Boberg M, Lithell H. Hypertension and associated metabolic disturbances are related to cognitive impairment. A 20-year follow-up of 999 men. Hypertension 1998; 31: 780–86.
5. Folstein MF, Folstein SE, McHugh PR. 'Mini-Mental State': a practical method for grading the cognitive state of patients for the clinician. J. Psychiatr Res 1975; 12: 189–98.
6. Lezak M. Neuropsychological Assessment, 3rd edn. New York: Oxford University Press, 1995.
7. Wechsler D. Wechsler Adult Intelligence Scale—Revised. San Antonio, CA: The Psychological Corporation, 1981.
8. Claeson L-E, Dahl E. The Claeson–Dahl learning test for clinical use. Stockholm: Psykologiförlaget, 1971 (in Swedish).
9. Kaplan E, Fein D, Morris R, Delis DC. WAIS-R NI. Manual. San Antonio, CA: The Psychological Corporation, 1991.
10. Hamet P, Richard L, Than-Vinh D, Teiger E, Orlov S, Gaboury L et al. Apoptosis in target organs of hypertension. Hypertension 1995; 26: 642–8.
11. Breteler MM, van Amerongen NM, van Swieten JC, Claus JJ, Grobbee DE, van Gijn J et al. Cognitive correlates of ventricular enlargement and cerebral white matter lesions on magnetic resonance imaging. The Rotterdam Study. Stroke 1994; 25: 1109–15.
12. Schmidt R, Fazekas F, Offenbacher H, Dusek T, Zach E, Reinhart B et al. Neuropsychologic correlates of MRI white matter hyperintensities: a study of 150 normal volunteers. Neurology 1993; 43: 2490–94.
13. Elias MF, Wolf PA, D'Agostino RB, Cobb J, White LR. Untreated blood pressure level is inversely related to cognitive functioning: the Framingham Study. Am J Epidemiol 1993; 138: 353–64.
14. Launer L, Masaki K, Petrovitch H, Foley D, Havlik R. The association between mid-life blood pressure levels and late-life cognitive function. The Honolulu–Asia aging study. JAMA 1995; 274: 1846–51.
15. Kalmijn S, Feskens EJM, Launer LJ, Stijnen T, Kromhout D. Glucose intolerance, hyperinsulinaemia and cognitive function in a general population of elderly men. Diabetologia 1995; 38: 1096–102.
16. Ott A, Breteler M, de Bruyne M, van Harskamp F, Grobbee D, Hofman A. Atrial fibrillation and dementia in a population-based study: the Rotterdam Study. Stroke 1997; 28: 316–21.
17. Skoog I, Lernfelt B, Landahl S, Palmertz B, Andreasson L-A, Nilsson L et al. 15–year longitudinal study of blood pressure and dementia. Lancet 1996; 347: 1141–5.
18. Sparks DL, Scheff SW, Liu H, Landers TM, Coyne CM, Hunsaker JC III. Increased incidence of neurofibrillary tangles in non-demented individuals with hypertension. Neurol Sci 1995; 131: 162–9.

19. Dahlöf B, Lindholm LH, Hansson L, Schersten B, Ekbom T, Wester P-O. Morbidity and mortality in the Swedish trial in old patients with hypertension (STOP-Hypertension). Lancet 1991; 338: 1281–5.
20. Hansson L, Zanchetti A, Carruthers SG, Dahlöf B, Elmfeldt D, Julius S et al. Effects of intensive blood pressure lowering and low-dose aspirin in patients with hypertension: principal results of the Hypertension Optimal Treatment (HOT) randomised trial. Lancet 1998; 351: 1755–62.

Address for correspondence:
Lena Kilander,
Department of Public Health and Caring Sciences/Geriatrics,
PO Box 609,
SE-751 25 Uppsala, Sweden

4 Marital Status and Risk of Alzheimer's Disease: A French Population-based Cohort Study

CATHERINE HELMER, DIDIER DAMON,
LUC LETENNEUR AND JEAN-FRANÇOIS DARTIGUES

INTRODUCTION

Marital status has been shown to be associated with longevity and risk of chronic psychiatric disorders. Singles have been found to have a lower life-expectancy than marrieds [1, 2] and to have a higher risk of developing schizo-phrenia, particularly in men [3]. Despite these findings, marital status was not considered as a possible risk factor for Alzheimer's disease (AD) or dementia until Bickel and Cooper's paper on a population-based cohort from Mannheim [4]. These authors have found that the risk of dementia was significantly increased in single or divorced subjects as compared to married subjects, with a relative risk (RR) of 2.9 after adjustment for age. However, adjustments for other social characteristics like gender, education or occupation were not presented.

More recently, in the Hisayama Study, Yoshitake et al. [5] did not confirm this relationship between marital status and risk of AD or vascular dementia after 7 years of follow-up of 828 elderly Japanese. However, the proportion of 'singles' was completely different in the Mannheim sample (10.2%) as com-pared to the Japanese sample (38%), particularly considering the high percen-tage of 'singles' among elderly Japanese women (more than 55%). In view of these contradictory results, it seems necessary to analyse this relationship again.

The aim of this chapter is to study the relationship between marital status and risk of AD in the PAQUID cohort, a French population-based prospec-tive study conducted in the Bordeaux area [6], taking into account possible confounding factors. We also wish to test the hypothesis that this relationship could be explained by differences in cognitive stimulation related to social network or leisure activities, according to marital status.

Alzheimer's Disease and Related Disorders
Edited by K. Iqbal, D.F. Swaab, B. Winblad and H.M. Wisniewski
© 1999 John Wiley & Sons Ltd

METHODS

The PAQUID cohort was constituted with a representative sample of 5554 subjects living at home in the south-west of France. This cohort is an epidemiological study on normal and pathological ageing after 65 years, particularly focused on non-genetic risk factors in dementia. Subjects were seen at home by a psychologist. The baseline variables registered included socio-demographic factors, social support and network, living conditions and habits, subjective and objective health measures, a functional assessment, depressive symptomatology, and personal medical history. A more complete description of the PAQUID Study has been published previously [6]. Marital status was classified into four categories: married or cohabitant; single; widowed; and divorced or separated. Evolution of marital status has been considered in the analyses: married or cohabitant subjects who became widowed during the follow-up were included in the group of married subjects until their widow(er)hood, and in the group of widowed thereafter.

Intellectual functioning was examined through a series of psychometric tests. After the psychometric evaluation, the psychologists systematically completed a standardized questionnaire designed to obtain the criteria for DSM-IIIR dementia [7]. In a second stage, subjects who met these DSM-IIIR criteria for dementia were seen by a senior neurologist who completed the NINCDS–ADRDA criteria and the Hachinski score for vascular dementia to establish the aetiology—probably or possible Alzheimer's disease or other type of dementia. An informant was consulted by the neurologist when available.

FOLLOW-UP

Subjects were re-evaluated following the same procedure as for the baseline screening 1, 3 and 5 years after the initial visit in Gironde and 3 and 5 years after the initial visit in Dordogne. Marital status was assessed at each follow-up visit.

STATISTICAL ANALYSIS

Age-specific incidence was estimated using the person-years method. The relative risks of AD were estimated using a Cox proportional hazards model with delayed entry, in which the time-scale is the age of the subjects. Marital status was considered as a time-dependent co-variate. Because the age-specific incidence of dementia has been previously found to differ according to gender [8], the analyses were stratified for gender; this allowed us to obtain global relative risks taking into account the effect of gender.

RESULTS

Of the 5554 subjects contacted, a total of 3777 (68.0%) agreed to participate in the study. Non-responders did not differ from responders in age, gender or educational level [9]. Among the 3675 initially non-demented subjects of the cohort, 2133 (58%) were women and 1822 (49.6%) were older than 74. The baseline marital status was distributed as follows: 2106 married or cohabitant (57.3%); 1287 widowed (35.0%); 179 singles (4.9%); and 103 divorced or separated (2.8%).

Of the 3675 subjects, 794 (21.6%) did not participate at any follow-up visit because they died (n = 365, 9.9%) or were either lost to follow-up or refused the follow-up screenings (n = 429, 11.7%). At least one complete follow-up evaluation was performed on 2881 subjects (78.4%). There were no significant differences in follow-up status according to baseline marital status, even if the refusal rate seemed slightly lower in singles (8.9%) and greater in divorced (16.5%) than in married (12.2%) or widowed (10.9%) subjects (χ^2 = 11.8, p = 0.07).

During the 5 years of follow-up, 190 subjects developed an incident dementia, of whom 140 were classified as incident cases of AD and 50 as other types of dementia. Among the 190 incident cases of dementia, 73 were married, 94 were widowed, 19 were singles and 4 were divorced at the time of diagnosis. Among the 140 incident cases of AD, 44 were married, 74 were widowed, 18 were singles and 4 were divorced.

Taking the married subjects as the reference group, the risk of dementia was significantly greater in singles (RR = 1.91, p = 0.018), while it did not change for widowed or divorced subjects (Table 1). Similar trends were observed for the risk of AD, with the RR greatest for singles (RR = 2.68, p < 0.001). On the other hand, the RR of non-AD dementia for singles was lower than one and not significantly different from married subjects. In this last analysis, divorced subjects were excluded due to the absence of incident cases of non-AD dementia in this group.

Table 1. Relative risk of dementia and Alzheimer's disease (AD) according to marital status, stratified for gender. Cox model with delayed entry taking age as the time scale. PAQUID 1989–1996, n = 3675

	RR	95% CI	p value
Risk of dementia			
Married	1	—	—
Widowed	0.95	0.66–1.38	0.803
Singles	**1.91**	**1.12–3.25**	**0.018**
Divorced	0.90	0.33–2.50	0.843
Risk of AD			
Married	1	—	—
Widowed	1.10	0.70–1.72	0.679
Singles	**2.68**	**1.49–4.81**	**<0.001**
Divorced	1.48	0.52–4.20	0.457
Risk of non-AD dementia			
Married	1	—	—
Widowed	0.75	0.38–1.47	0.399
Singles	0.35	0.05–2.64	0.311

The age-specific incidence of AD according to the marital status gave similar results (Figure 1). The incidence increased with age in singles, more than it did in other categories of marital status.

After adjustment for possible confounding factors such as gender, educational level, principal occupation during life and wine consumption, the relationship between marital status and risk of AD remained unchanged. The risk of AD was close to one in widowed subjects (RR = 0.96, 95% CI = 0.61–1.52), significantly increased among singles (RR = 3.08, 95% CI = 1.70–5.58) and non-significant for divorced subjects (RR = 1.78, 95% CI = 0.63–5.06); thus, bias of confusion from the risk factors of AD seemed unlikely. Educational level and wine consumption were also independently significantly related to the risk of AD.

Most of the variables considered as potential mediators in the relationship between marital status and AD were significantly correlated with marital status. Singles were more frequently living alone (χ^2 test, p < 0.001), had a lower number of people in their social network (p < 0.001), were less satisfied with their network (p = 0.01), had fewer leisure activities (p < 0.001) and reported more depressive symptoms than married subjects (p < 0.013). After adjustment for all these factors, in addition to educational level and wine consumption, the RR for AD among singles decreased only from 2.68 to 2.31 and remained significant (95% CI = 1.14–4.68, p = 0.02). The relationship did not seem to be explained by depressive symptomatology and leisure activities, which were independently significantly related to the risk of AD.

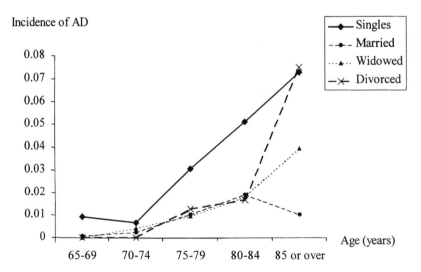

Figure 1. The age-specific incidence of Alzheimer's disease according to marital status. PAQUID 1988–1996, n = 3675

DISCUSSION

Our results, based on the follow-up of 2881 initially non-demented subjects with prospective screening of incident cases of dementia, confirm that singles have a significantly higher risk of dementia or AD than marrieds: a two-fold increase for the risk of dementia and almost three-fold increase for the risk of AD. These relative risks are of the same magnitude as those found in the Mannheim cohort [4]. Moreover, this higher risk seems specific to AD, since the RR of non-AD dementia was lower than one. These results remained unchanged after adjustment for several confounding factors. This relationship seems not to be explained by differences in leisure activities and depressive symptomatology according to marital status.

Several methodological issues may have influenced these results. During the follow-up of the cohort, the refusal rate in singles was slightly lower than in married subjects (8.9% [95% CI = 4.7–13.1] vs. 12.2% [95% CI = 10.8–13.6]). However, this difference was small and not significant, with a large confidence interval for singles. Selective survival could also occur according to marital status. However, the 5-year cumulative death rates were the same in marrieds (9%) and singles (8.9%).

In the statistical analyses we have not taken into account all the known risk factors of dementia or AD. Apolipoprotein genotype was only ascertained on 626 subjects of the cohort. In this subsample, the marital status of apoE4 carriers was similar to the non-apoE4 carriers. Thus the risk of a confounding bias should be weak. Current consumption of non-steroid anti-inflammatory drugs (NSAIDs) or oestrogen replacement therapy were collected at baseline. In our cohort, NSAID consumption was not related to the risk of AD [10]; concerning oestrogen, the proportion of elderly people taking these drugs was very low in France in 1988.

Another methodological problem could be that the clinical diagnosis of AD was different according to marital status. Since the spouse is certainly the best informant, an accurate diagnosis could be more difficult among singles in comparison to marrieds. In fact, our data show that elderly people living alone (in general without an informant) have the same risk of AD as people not living alone (with an informant). Moreover, analysis of the MMSE scores at the time of diagnosis show that the proportion of incident cases of AD with a MMSE score greater than 18 was higher in married subjects (69.4%) than in singles (35.3%). In fact, if a bias exists in the diagnostic procedure, it probably underestimates the risk of AD in singles.

Several explanations could be given for our findings. There could be either a deleterious effect for single subjects, or a protective effect for married subjects. Single subjects could have premorbid personality and premorbid behaviours that could explain both their marital status and the risk of dementia. This explanation was considered as the most credible for schizophrenia [3]. But on the other hand, singles could have less cognitive stimulation due to a less active social network and fewer leisure activities; nevertheless, our results did not confirm this hypothesis. However, the variables used to measure the social network of the subjects may not have been sufficiently precise to correctly adjust for this potential mediator. Singles could also be more likely to be exposed to risk factors of AD not taken into account in our analysis, such as malnutrition or undernutrition. It is also possible, on the other hand, that marriage or cohabitation could be protective for subjects. Previous studies have demonstrated that support and counselling for spouse-caregivers and families could prevent or delay nursing home placement [11]. It is also possible to consider an earlier effect of the spouse before the beginning of the disease. Among marrieds, the spouse may help the subject to carry out his/her activities. The spouse could also stimulate the subject and enable him/her to preserve his/her cognitive capacities, thus protecting against dementia or delaying the clinical stage of dementia. This hypothesis, if confirmed, could incite development of a social network to decrease incidence of dementia.

In conclusion, marital status seems to influence the risk of AD in old age. These findings need to be confirmed by further studies, and should be taken into consideration in the evaluation of risk of AD.

ACKNOWLEDGEMENTS

This study was supported by grants from Fondation de France, Novartis Pharma, Axa Insurance Group, Caisse Nationale d'Assurance Maladie, Caisse Primaire d'Assurance Maladie de Dordogne, Conseil Général de la Dordogne, Conseil Général de la Gironde, Conseil Régional d'Aquitaine, Danone, Ministère de la Recherche et de la Technologie, Mutualité Sociale Agricole de Gironde et Dordogne, Mutuelle Générale de l'Education Nationale, Société Pechiney, 2010 Media, Caisse de Retraite Interentreprise, Capimmec, Institut du Cerveau, Direction Régionale des Affaires Sanitaires et Sociales d'Aquitaine.

REFERENCES

1. House JS, Robbins C, Metzner HL. The association of social relationships and activities with mortality: prospective evidence from the Tecumseh community Health Study. Am J Epidemiol 1982; 116: 123–40.
2. Campbell TL. Family's impact on health: a critical review. Family Systems Med 1986; 4: 135–328.
3. Jablensky A, Cole S. Is the earlier age at onset of schizophrenia in males a confounded finding? Results from a cross-cultural investigation. Br J Psychiatry 1997; 170: 234–40.
4. Bickel H, Cooper B. Incidence and relative risk of dementia in an urban elderly population: findings of a prospective field study. Psychol Med 1994; 24: 179–92.

5. Yoshitake T, Kiyohara Y, Kato I et al. Incidence and risk factors of vascular dementia and Alzheimer's disease in a defined Japanese elderly population: the Hisayama study. Neurology 1995; 45: 1161–8.
6. Fabrigoule C, Letenneur L, Dartigues J-F, Zarrouk M, Commenges D, Barberger-Gateau P. Social and leisure activities and risk of dementia: a prospective longitudinal study. J Am Geriatr Soc 1995; 43: 485–90.
7. American Psychiatric Society. Diagnostic and Statistical Manual of Mental Disorders, 3rd edn (Revised) (DSM-IIIR). Washington, DC: American Psychiatric Association, 1987.
8. Commenges D, Letenneur L, Joly P, Alioum A, Dartigues J-F. Modelling age-specific risk: application to dementia. Stat Med 1998; 17: 1973–88.
9. Dartigues J-F, Gagnon M, Michel P et al. Le programme de recherche PAQUID sur l'épidémiologie de la démence. Méthodologie et résultats initiaux. Rev Neurol 1991; 147: 225–30 (in French).
10. Fourrier A, Letenneur L, Bégaud B, Dartigues, J-F. Nonsteroidal antiinflammatory drug use and cognitive function in the elderly: inconclusive results from a population-based cohort study (letter). J Clin Epidemiol 1996; 49: 1201.
11. Mittelman MS, Steven HF, Shulman E, Steinberg G, Levin B. A family intervention to delay nursing home placement of patients with Alzheimer's disease. JAMA 1996; 276: 1725–31.

Address for correspondence:
J.-F. Dartigues,
INSERM U 330,
Université de Bordeaux II,
33076 Bordeaux Cedex, France.
Fax: (33) 5 56 99 13 60

5 The Influence of Diuretics on the Occurrence and Progression of Dementia in a Community Population Aged 75 Years and Over

MATTI VIITANEN, ZHENCHAO GUO,
LAURA FRATIGLIONI, LI ZHU, JOHAN FASTBOM AND
BENGT WINBLAD

INTRODUCTION

Hypertension has been assigned an important role in the pathogenesis of dementia [1–6]. We examined whether antihypertensive medication affects the occurrence of dementia and cognitive decline in persons with dementia in a community-based cohort aged 75 years and over.

METHODS

Data for this study was derived from the baseline and first follow-up from a longitudinal study of aging and dementia known as the Kungsholmen Project [7]. The study population comprised all inhabitants of the Kungsholmen district of Stockholm who were aged 75 years and older on 1 October 1987. Of the 2369 eligible subjects, 1810 (74.6%) were administered the Mini-Mental State Examination (MMSE) [8]. Two hundred and twenty-five prevalent dementia cases were detected by means of a two-phase design, which included a screening phase and a clinical examination phase [9]. The follow-up evaluation included 1301 non-demented subjects. Of these, 987 were clinically examined at the follow-up. The mean follow-up interval of the cohort was 36.7 months, with a maximum of 63.1 months.

Among the 225 prevalent dementia cases, 115 died before the follow-up examination. Among the 110 who participated in the follow-up evaluation,

Alzheimer's Disease and Related Disorders
Edited by K. Iqbal, D.F. Swaab, B. Winblad and H.M. Wisniewski
© 1999 John Wiley & Sons Ltd

28 with a baseline MMSE score under 6 points were excluded from further analyses. We also excluded three persons who did not use diuretics but who took other antihypertensive drugs. After these exclusions we were left with 79 individuals, including 46 cases with AD, 18 with vascular dementia (VaD), and 15 with other dementias. Dementia was defined according to the Diagnostic and Statistical Manual of Mental Disorders, 3rd edn (Revised) diagnostic criteria [10]. Details of the clinical examination and diagnostic procedure have already been reported [9, 11].

Information on drug use during 2 weeks preceding the baseline interview was collected [12]. Use of both prescription and non-prescription drugs was registered. Drug containers and drug prescription forms were inspected in order to verify this information. Drugs were classified according to the Anatomical Therapeutic Chemical (ATC) classification system [13]. Antihypertensive drugs included all medicines potentially used for lowering blood pressure (ATC codes C02, C03, C07–09).

We used Cox proportional hazards regression analysis to calculate the relative risk (RR) of developing dementia in relation to the use of antihypertensive medication. Rate of decline in the score on the MMSE among dementia patients was calculated using the following formula: (baseline score – follow-up score) ÷ (baseline score) ÷ (years of follow-up).

RESULTS

PREVALENCE OF DEMENTIA

Among the 225 prevalent dementia cases, 121 individuals had AD, 52 had VaD and 52 were diagnosed as having other forms of dementia. Compared with those not taking antihypertensive medication, subjects taking diuretics had a higher score on the MMSE (p = 0.006) and a lower prevalence of dementia (p < 0.004). Logistic regression analysis showed that subjects taking diuretics had an odds ratio of 0.4 (95% confidence interval [CI], 0.3–0.6) for any form of dementia, 0.4 (0.3–0.7) for AD, and 0.3 (0.1–0.6) for VaD, after adjustment for age, sex, education, systolic blood pressure, heart disease and stroke. Subjects taking other antihypertensive drugs but not diuretics also had a lower prevalence of dementia.

INCIDENCE OF DEMENTIA

Among the 1301 non-demented persons at the baseline who were included in the follow-up evaluation, 987 (76%) were subjected to a comprehensive clinical examination which revealed that 199 fulfilled the criteria of dementia according to DSM-IIIR (155 AD, 32 VaD, and 12 other forms of dementia). Among the 314 subjects who died during the follow-up interval, 25 were given a diagnosis of dementia (9 AD, 9 VaD, and 7 other forms of dementia) based on information from medical records and death certificates. At the baseline, 484 (37.2%) individuals used diuretics. Subjects taking diuretics were older (82.6 ± 5.1 years vs. 81.7 ± 4.9 years), more often female (81.4% vs. 70.9%), and they had a higher prevalence of heart disease (26.9% vs. 8.1%) and stroke (9.5% vs. 4.9%) than those not taking antihypertensive medication.

Subjects taking diuretics had a lower incidence of any form of dementia (p = 0.02) and AD (p = 0.005) (Table 1). Among the 484 persons taking diuretics, 139 also took other antihypertensive drugs at the same time. Persons with diuretic monotherapy (n = 345) had an adjusted RR of 0.6 (0.4–0.9) for any form of dementia, 0.6 (0.4–0.8) for AD, and 0.7 (0.3–1.6) for VaD.

Table 1. Use of antihypertensive medication and the relative risk (95% confidence interval)* of dementia at the first follow-up of the Kungsholmen Project

Use of antihypertensive medication at baseline	All forms of dementia	Alzheimer's disease	Vascular dementia
Use of diuretics (n = 484)†	0.7 (0.5–0.95)	0.6 (0.4–0.9)	1.1 (0.6–2.2)
Use of other antihypertensives (n = 100)‡	0.9 (0.5–1.5)	0.7 (0.3–1.3)	1.2 (0.4–3.5)
No use of antihypertensives (n = 717)	1.0	1.0	1.0

* Adjusted for age, sex, education, systolic pressure, heart disease, and stroke.
† 71.3% on diuretic monotherapy; 15.1% also on calcium channel antagonists, and 11.0% also on β-blockers.
‡ 50% on calcium channel antagonists and 45% on β-blockers.

COGNITIVE DECLINE

There was no difference in MMSE score between those using diuretics and those not using antihypertensive medication (26.5 ± 2.9 vs. 26.6 ± 2.7). Subjects not taking diuretics declined 17% from the baseline MMSE score every year. This was twice more than the decline of those taking diuretics (Table 2). By using a multiple stepwise linear regression analysis, it was found that use of diuretics was inversely related to the rate of cognitive decline (regression coefficient = −0.07, p = 0.04).

DISCUSSION

Use of diuretics was related to a lower prevalence of dementia, reduced incidence of dementia and AD, and slower cognitive decline among patients with dementia. The results were derived from a population-based epidemiological

Table 2. Decline in the score on the Mini-Mental State Examination of the 79 baseline patients with dementia according to use of diuretics

	n	Baseline score	Follow-up score	Rate of decline*
Use of diuretics†	23	17.1 ± 5.5	13.4 ± 6.2	0.08 ± 0.13
No use of antihypertensives	56	16.8 ± 5.1	9.5 ± 6.8	0.17 ± 0.13

* Defined as: (baseline score – follow-up score) ÷ (baseline score) ÷ (years of follow-up).
† 18 persons with diuretic monotherapy; three also with calcium channel antagonists and two also with β-blockers.

study of 1810 persons aged 75 years and over in which a number of factors, including potential protectors for AD reported in the literature, were considered.

The antihypertensive effect of diuretics, especially in the elderly, has been proven [14]. It is therefore conceivable that diuretics may reduce the risk of dementia or slow the progress of dementia by reducing the number of cerebrovascular events. We demonstrated that use of diuretics was related to a 30% reduced risk of dementia in the general population. The result is similar to that of a meta-analysis which reported a 34% reduced risk of major cerebrovascular events with low-dose diuretic therapy in hypertensive patients [15]. Hypertension-related silent vascular lesions in the brain, such as white matter changes, have been found to be common in demented persons (both AD and VaD) [16], although they can also occur in normal aging. In addition, a recent study showed an increased incidence of senile plaques and neurofibrillary tangles in individuals with hypertension [17].

Increasing evidence suggests that cerebrovascular dysfunction and damage may also be involved in the pathogenesis of AD [18]. A recent study found that amyloid β-protein, the major component of amyloid plaques in the AD brain [19], enhanced vasoconstriction and resistance to relaxation of endothial cells in intact rat aorta [20]. *In vitro*, this toxicity of amyloid β-protein can be partially prevented by verapamil (a commonly used calcium channel antagonist) [21], probably due to verapamil's anti-oxidative activities. Diuretics, especially thiazides, also have direct vasorelaxant effects on vessel walls [22–24], which may contribute to their antihypertensive properties, and may have potential implications in reducing amyloid β-protein toxicity.

Several limitations of this study should be addressed. Information on the duration of antihypertensive medication was not available. The classification of drug use was made only at baseline. Unlike a clinical trial, our study is not designed specifically to assess the effects of antihypertensive medication. The group using antihypertensive medication in our cohort differs inherently from the group not using antihypertensive medication in a number of factors, such as heart disease, stroke and hypertension that may be related to the risk of dementia. Generally, these limitations may decrease the power to detect a given association or lead to an underestimation of the association. These limitations may particularly affect the results regarding the use of other antihypertensive medication, as this group was relatively small.

In cross-sectional studies, patients with dementia often have a lower blood pressure level than those without dementia [25, 26]. Therefore, current use of antihypertensive medication should be lower in those with clinically manifest dementia. This may explain the much lower relative risks of dementia associated with use of antihypertensive medication estimated from prevalent data, compared to those from incident data. In addition, subjects with cognitive impairment may underestimate their use of medications, although we tried to get information from proxy informants on drug use of the subjects with suspected cognitive dysfunction. However, there was no difference in the use of cardiac glycosides between demented (18.2%) and non-demented individuals (19.2%). This may suggest that recall bias is minimal in this study.

Although we cannot definitely rule out the possibility that our findings are the results of joint effects of antihypertensive medication and lifestyle modifications for hypertension control, we believe it is unlikely that a fat-modified diet can fully explain the slower progression of dementia associated with use of diuretics found in this study.

In summary, this study suggests that use of diuretics protects against dementia and AD. The main mechanism is probably that diuretics significantly reduce the number of cerebrovascular events or lesions which are believed to be important in the pathogenesis of both AD and VaD.

REFERENCES

1. Forette F, Boller F. Hypertension and the risk of dementia in the elderly. Am J Med 1991; 90 (suppl 3A): 14–19S.
2. Hachinski V. Preventable senility: a call for action against the vascular dementias. Lancet 1992; 340: 645–8.
3. Roman GC. Senile dementia of the Binswanger type. A vascular form of dementia in the elderly. JAMA 1987; 258: 1782–8.
4. Guo Z, Viitanen, M, Fratiglioni L, Winblad B. Blood pressure and dementia in the elderly: epidemiologic perspectives. Biomed Pharmacother 1997; 51: 68–73.
5. Yoshitake T, Kiyohara Y, Kato I et al. Incidence and risk factors of vascular dementia and Alzheimer's disease in a defined elderly Japanese population: the Hisayama Study. Neurology 1995; 45: 1161–8.
6. Skoog I, Lernfelt B, Landahl S et al. 15-year longitudinal study of blood pressure and dementia. Lancet 1996; 347: 1141–5.
7. Fratiglioni L, Viitanen M, Bäckman L, Sandman PO, Winblad B. Occurrence of dementia in advanced age: the study design of the Kungsholmen Project. Neuroepidemiology 1992; 11 (suppl 1): 29–36.
8. Folstein MF, Folstein SE, McHugh PR. 'Mini-Mental State.' A practical method for grading the cognitive state of patients for the clinician. J Psychiatr Res 1975; 12: 189–98.

9. Fratiglioni L, Grut M, Forsell Y et al. Prevalence of Alzheimer's disease and other dementias in an elderly urban population: relationship with age, sex, and education. Neurology 1991; 41: 1886–92.
10. American Psychiatric Association. Diagnostic and Statistical Manual of Mental Disorders, 3rd edn (Revised) (DSM-IIIR). Washington, DC: American Psychiatric Association, 1987.
11. Fratiglioni L, Viitanen M, von Strauss E et al. Very old women at highest risk of dementia and Alzheimer's disease: incidence data from the Kungsholmen Project, Stockholm. Neurology 1997; 48: 132–8.
12. Wills P, Fastbom J, Claesson CB et al. Use of cardiovascular drugs in an older Swedish population. J Am Geriatr Soc 1996; 44: 54–60.
13. Nordic Council on Medicines. Guidelines for ATC Classification. (NLN Publication No. 16). Uppsala: Nordic Council on Medicines, 1985.
14. Kaplan NM, Gifford RW Jr. Choice of initial therapy for hypertension. JAMA 1996; 275: 1577–80.
15. Psaty BM, Smith NL, Siscovick DS et al. Health outcomes associated with antihypertensive therapies used as first-line agents. A systematic review and meta-analysis. JAMA 1997; 277: 739–45.
16. Pantoni L, Garcia JH. The significance of cerebral white matter abnormalities 100 years after Binswanger's report: a review. Stroke 1995; 26: 1293–1301.
17. Sparks DL, Scheff SW, Liu H et al. Increased incidence of neurofibrillary tangles in non-demented individuals with hypertension. J Neurol Sci 1995; 131: 162–9.
18. Kalaria R. Cerebral vessels in aging and Alzheimer's disease. Pharmacol Ther 1996; 72: 193–214.
19. Selkoe DJ. Amyloid beta-protein and the genetics of Alzheimer's disease. J Biol Chem 1996; 271: 18295–8.
20. Thomas T, Thomas G, McLendon C, Sutton T, Mullan M. β-Amyloid-mediated vasoactivity and vascular endothelial damage. Nature 1996; 380: 168–71.
21. Suo Z, Fang C, Crawford F, Mullan M. Superoxide free radical and intracellular calcium mediate $A\beta_{1-41}$-induced endothelial toxicity. Brain Res 1997; 762: 144–52.
22. Kool ML, Lustermans FA, Breed JG et al. The influence of perindopril and the diuretic combination amilorid + hydrochlorothiazide on the vessel wall properties of large arteries in hypertensive patients. J Hypertens 1995; 13: 839–48.
23. Kähönen M, Mäkynen H, Arvola P, Wuorela H, Pörsti I. Arterial function after trichlormethiazide therapy in spontaneously hypertensive rats. J Pharmacol Exp Ther 1995; 272: 1223–30.
24. Abrahams Z, Tan LLY, Pang MYM et al. Demonstration of an *in vitro* direct vascular relaxant effect of diuretics in the presence of plasma. J Hypertens 1996; 14: 381–8.
25. Guo Z, Viitanen M, Fratiglioni L, Winblad B. Low blood pressure and dementia in elderly people: the Kungsholmen project. Br Med J 1996; 312: 805–8.
26. Hogan DB, Ebly EM, Rockwood K. Weight, blood pressure, osmolarity, and glucose levels across various stages of Alzheimer's disease and vascular dementia. Dement Geriatr Cogn Disord 1997; 8: 147–51.

Address for correspondence:
Matti Viitanen,
Division of Geriatric Medicine, B84,
Huddinge Hospital,
S-141 86 Huddinge,
Sweden

6 Prognosis with Dementia: Results from a European Collaborative Analysis of Population-based Studies

C. JAGGER, K. ANDERSEN, M.M.B. BRETELER,
J.R.M. COPELAND, J.-F. DARTIGUES, A. DI CARLO,
L. FRATIGLIONI, A. LOBO, R. SCHMIDT, H. SOININEN,
A. HOFMAN AND L.J. LAUNER FOR THE EURODEM
RESEARCH GROUP

INTRODUCTION

Few studies have provided information on the prognosis of individuals who become demented. However, information on prognostic indicators such as survival time and time to institutionalization is needed for resource planning and indeed for counseling of patients and their carers.

In this chapter we present the results of a collaborative analyses of time to death, and time to institutionalization in population-based samples of dementia cases. Data are from nine studies conducted in Europe, that are a part of a collaborative research network of institutions studying risk factors for, and prognosis of, dementia (EURODEM) [1]. The studies included in these analyses are: the Kungsholmen Project, Sweden [2]; the Melton Mowbray Study, UK [3]; the MRC-Alpha Study, Liverpool, UK [4]; the Rotterdam Study, The Netherlands [5]; the Zaragoza Study, Spain [6]; the Kuopio Study, Finland [7]; the Odense Study, Denmark [8]; the ILSA Study, Italy [9]; and the PAQUID Study, France [10].

METHODS

The studies are based either on random or total samples of individuals in a defined geographic residence. The baseline populations included those living in institutions, except for the PAQUID Study in France, which only included

Alzheimer's Disease and Related Disorders
Edited by K. Iqbal, D.F. Swaab, B. Winblad and H.M. Wisniewski
© 1999 John Wiley & Sons Ltd

community dwellers at baseline. The Kuopio Study in Finland excluded those in long-stay hospital beds. Details of the studies can be found in the respective referenced material [1–10].

All studies used a two-phase design with an initial screen of the total study population followed by a clinical examination to detect dementia. Selection criteria for the clinical examination was based upon the Mini-Mental State Examination (MMSE) [11] in all studies, either explicitly by using MMSE cutpoints, by combining MMSE test scores with other tests, or because the MMSE is part of the CAMCOG scale of the CAMDEX [12]. Studies used DSM-IIIR [13] or equivalent [14] criteria for the classification of cases of dementia. A person was considered institutionalized if he/she was living in a facility that provided full medical and care services. Vital status was collected from municipal or medical services. Data were provided by the centers as aggregated cell frequencies for time to institutionalization and death. The cells were defined by sex, five-year age groups (55–90 years and over), case status, and time (years) since baseline.

SURVIVAL WITH DEMENTIA

A number of studies have reported estimates of survival time with dementia. However, most of these studies are based on prevalent cases in institutions or clinic settings. In addition, samples are often too small to provide age- and sex-specific survival curves. A systematic review [15] of the literature on survival with dementia reported 2-year survival rates ranging from 37% to 86% in community-based studies. The variety of diagnostic criteria employed may account for some of the variation.

In the European collaborative data, we found that prevalent cases had a lower survival rate than non-cases. This trend was consistent over time in all age groups. Women with dementia had a consistently higher survival than men with dementia, a pattern that mirrored the male–female differences in the non-demented subjects. For instance, among men 85 years of age or older at baseline, 52% of the cases and 76% of the non-cases were still alive after 2 years' follow-up. Among women, 60% of the cases and 81% of the non-cases were still alive. After five years, 16% of male cases and 44% of male non-cases had survived; in females 27% of the cases and 52% of the non-cases were still alive.

INSTITUTIONALIZATION

As for survival, studies on institutionalization concentrate on demonstrating associations between increased severity and shorter times to institutionalization (see e.g. [16]). Patients from the Consortium to Establish a Registry for

Alzheimer's Disease (CERAD) form the largest sample of patients in whom time to institutionalization has been estimated. In that group of patients, the median time to first institutionalization was 3.1 years from entry into the study; unmarried men had the shortest time [17].

Comparisons of the proportion of cases and non-cases that were institutionalized at baseline provided interesting insights. Women had a higher probability of being in institutional care than men. This sex difference was independent of case status (either prevalent or incident) or age (Table 1). For both men and women, the odds of being in institutional care at baseline was significantly higher for both prevalent and incident cases than non-cases. After adjustment for age and sex, prevalent cases were more likely to have been resident in institutional care at baseline than non-cases. This difference between cases and controls decreased as age increased, reflecting the increasing rate of institutionalization at older ages for reasons other than dementia. We also found that incident cases of dementia were three times more likely than non-cases to live in an institution at baseline. This could reflect an increased incidence of dementia in institutional care. The pattern may also be a result of subjects with milder levels of dementia who did not achieve case status at baseline.

We were not able to examine whether the dementia preceded entry into care or vice versa, because date of admission to nursing home was not available for these analyses. Therefore, entry rates into institutional care were estimated as the rate of admission to institutional care at 2 and 3 years from baseline assessment for prevalent cases, and 4 years from assessment for incident cases (Table 2). Compared to non-cases, prevalent cases of dementia had twice the entry rates to institutional care. There were no differences in transitions to care by sex at any time period, although transition rates did increase

Table 1. Fitted odds (95% CI) of being in institutional care at baseline for prevalent cases compared to non-cases by sex and age group

| Age group in years | Odds (95% CI) of being in institutional care at baseline* | | |
	Total	Men	Women
55	303.82 (64.12–1439.60)	772.14 (60.19–9906.06)	76.74 (36.24–162.50)
60	114.72 (42.73–307.99)	177.68 (35.81–881.59)	53.34 (28.60–99.46)
65	50.00 (28.39–88.07)	53.41 (21.608–132.08)	37.08 (22.53–61.02)
70	25.16 (18.44–34.34)	20.97 (12.71–34.62)	25.77 (17.67–37.59)
75	14.62 (11.64–18.36)	10.76 (7.29–15.87)	17.91 (13.71–23.40)
80	9.80 (8.00–12.02)	7.21 (5.07–10.26)	12.45 (10.34–15.00)
	6.98 (5.73–8.48)	6.62 (4.49–9.77)	6.96 (5.59–8.66)

* Reference is non-cases.
Contributing studies: the Kungsholmen Project [2]; the Melton Mowbray Study [3]; the MRC-Alpha Study, Liverpool [4]; the Rotterdam Study [5]; the Zaragoza Study [6]; the Kuopio Study [7]; the Odense Study [8]; the ILSA Study.

Table 2. Fitted* rates of entry (per 1000 person-years) of prevalent and incident cases of dementia into institutional care

	Rate of entry into institutional care per 1000 person-years					
	In 2 years from baseline assessment		In 3 years from baseline assessment		In 4 years from baseline assessment	
Age group in years	Non-cases	Prevalent cases	Non-cases	Prevalent cases	Non-cases	Prevalent cases
65–69	1.10	2.59	0.71	6.52	2.90	9.23
70–74	6.60	15.50	1.46	13.34	1.34	4.25
75–79	9.97	23.41	7.15	65.26	6.13	19.46
80–84	19.63	46.08	12.37	112.97	11.57	36.76
85+	42.15	98.95	17.02	155.42	30.05	95.46

* Fitted values from log linear modeling of transition rates with age group, sex and case status as co-variates.
Contributing studies: the Kungsholmen Project [2]; the MRC-Alpha Study [4]; the Rotterdam Study [5]; the Kuopio Study [7]; the Odense Study [8]. Only prevalent cases: the Melton Mowbray Study [3]; the Zaragoza Study [6].

significantly with increasing age. Subjects who became demented also had higher rates of entry into care over the 4 years from assessment.

CONCLUSION

To date, individual studies have generally been too small or had insufficient length of follow-up to give age- and sex-specific survival or institutionalization rates. Systematic comparisons [14] have suffered from inconsistency in diagnostic criteria across studies. This problem was reduced in this collaborative reanalysis by using equivalent DSM-IIIR criteria for case definition. However, some caution needs to be exercised when interpreting these results. The analyses based on prevalent cases include a mixture of new and long-existing cases. This may lead to an over-representation of long-existing cases and thus to an over-estimate of survival times and time to institutionalization. Studies based on incident cases are needed to reduce this source of bias. Second, there is a difference among countries in survival and transitions into institutional care, due to factors other than dementia. These factors range from national health care policies to the presence of other illness and the availability of caretakers for the demented. More detailed analyses with information on factors related to institutionalization are needed to understand better what co-factors are related to survival and institutionalization in the demented. Given these limitations, this European collaborative reanalysis of studies of prognosis with dementia provides important information for service planning.

REFERENCES

1. Launer LJ, Brayne C, Dartigues J-F, Hofman A (eds). European studies on the incidence of dementing diseases. EURODEM Incidence. Neuroepidemiol 1992; 1 (suppl 1): 1–122.
2. Fratiglioni L, Viitanen M, Backman L, Sandman PO, Winblad B. Occurrence of dementia in advanced age: the study design of the Kungsholmen Project. Neuroepidemiol 1992; 11(1): 29–36.
3. Clarke M, Jagger C, Anderson J et al. The prevalence of dementia in a total population—the comparison of two screening instruments. Age Ageing 1991; 20: 396–403.
4. Saunders PA, Copeland JRM, Dewey ME, Larkin BA, Scott A. ALPHA: the Liverpool MRC study of the incidence of dementia and cognitive decline. Neuroepidemiology 1992; 11: S44–7.
5. Breteler MM, van den Ouweland FA, Grobbee DE, Hofman A. A community-based study of dementia: the Rotterdam Elderly Study. Neuroepidemiol 1992; 11(1): 23–8.
6. Lobo A, Saz P, Marcos G, Morales F. Incidence of dementia and other psychiatric conditions in the elderly: Zaragoza Study. Neuroepidemiol 1992; 11(1): 52–6.
7. Koivisto K. Population based dementia screening program in the city of Kuopio, eastern Finland. Thesis. Series of reports, Department of Neurology, University of Kuopio, No. 33, 1995.
8. Andersen K, Lolk A, Nielsen H, Andersen J, Olsen C, Kragh Sorensen P. Prevalence of very mild to severe dementia in Denmark. Acta Neurol Scand 1997; 96: 872–7.
9. Maggi S, Zucchetto M, Grigoletto F, Baldereshi M et al. The Italian Longitudinal Study on Aging (ILSA): design and methods. Aging Clin Exp Res 1994; 6: 464–73.
10. Gagnon M, Letenneur L, Dartigues J-F et al. Validity of the Mini-Mental State Examination as a screening instrument for cognitive impairment and dementia in French elderly community residents. Neuroepidemiol 1990; 9(3): 143–50.
11. Folstein MF, Folstein SE, McHugh PR. 'Mini-Mental State': a practical method for grading the cognitive state of patients for the clinician. J Psych Res 1975; 12: 189–98.
12. Roth M, Tym E, Mountjoy CQ et al. CAMDEX: a standardized instrument for the diagnosis of mental disorders in the elderly with special reference to the early detection of dementia. Br J Psych 1986; 149: 698–709.
13. American Psychiatric Association. Diagnostic and Statistical Manual of Mental Disorders, 3rd edn (DSM-III) Washington, DC: American Psychiatric Association, 1987.
14. Copeland JRM, Kelleler MJ, Kellett JM et al. A semi-structured clinical interview for the assessment of diagnosis and mental state in the elderly: the Geriatric Mental State Schedule. Psychol Med 1976; 6: 439–49.
15. van Dijk PTM, Dippel DWJ, Habbema JDF. Survival of patients with dementia. JAGS 1991; 39: 603–10.
16. Brodaty H, McGilchrist C, Harris L, Peters KE. Time until institutionalization and death in patients with dementia. Arch Neurol 1993; 50: 643–50.

17. Heyman A, Peterson B, Fillenbaum G, Pieper C. Predictors of time to institutionalization of patients with Alzheimer's disease: the CERAD experience, Part XVII. Neurol 1997; 48: 1304–9.

Address for correspondence:
    C. Jagger,
    c/o EURODEM,
    Department of Epidemiology and Biostatistics,
    Erasmus University Medical School,
    PO Box 1738,
    3000 DR Rotterdam,
    The Netherlands

II Genetic Factors

7 The Risk of Developing Alzheimer's Disease Associated with the *APOE* Promoter Polymorphisms

JEAN-CHARLES LAMBERT, CLAUDINE BERR,
FLORENCE PASQUIER, ANDRÉ DELACOURTE,
BERNARD FRIGARD, DOMINIQUE COTTEL,
JORDI PÉREZ-TUR, VINCENT MOUROUX,
MICHEL MOHR, DANIELLE CÉCYRE,
DOUGLAS GALASKO, CORINNE LENDON,
JUDES POIRIER, JOHN HARDY, DAVID MANN,
PHILIPPE AMOUYEL AND
MARIE-CHRISTINE CHARTIER-HARLIN

INTRODUCTION

Several epidemiological studies have shown that the apolipoprotein E (*APOE*) gene could be involved in 45–60% of Alzheimer's disease (AD) cases [1]. However, not all individuals carrying either one or two copies of the ε4 allele systematically develop the disease. Other factors, such as family history, cholesterol level, oestrogen and smoking habits, could also modify the risk associated with *APOE* [2, 3]. Complete genetic analysis of the *APOE* locus has suggested the presence of other mutations in this region which may enhance this risk [4]. We hypothesized that genetic variability at this locus could modulate the control of *APOE* expression. We first estimated the relative expression of the ε2 and ε4 alleles relative to the ε3 allele in *APOE* heterozygous brain samples. We reported an allelic distortion of the *APOE* expression in AD compared to control brain tissues reinforcing the hypothesis of the existence of such mutations. Then we analysed the impact of three of the five *APOE* promoter polymorphisms recently described [5–7] in a large AD case-control study.

Alzheimer's Disease and Related Disorders
Edited by K. Iqbal, D.F. Swaab, B. Winblad and H.M. Wisniewski
© 1999 John Wiley & Sons Ltd

RESULTS

APOE ALLELIC EXPRESSION

As can be seen in Figure 1, we confirmed the allelic distortion of the ε2/ε3/ε4 alleles in 43 AD compared to 43 control brain samples, as previously reported in a smaller population [8]. The expression level of the ε3 allele was distinctly higher than the expression of the ε4 allele in AD patients as well as in controls. We observed a relative increased expression of the ε4 allele between ε3/ε4 AD and control brains (35 ± 3% vs. 23 ± 2%, respectively; p < 10⁻⁴) and a relative decrease of expression of the ε2 allele between ε2/ε3 AD and controls (33 ± 5% vs. 48 ± 4, respectively; p = 0.002), as could be expected from the protective effect reported for ε2 [4].

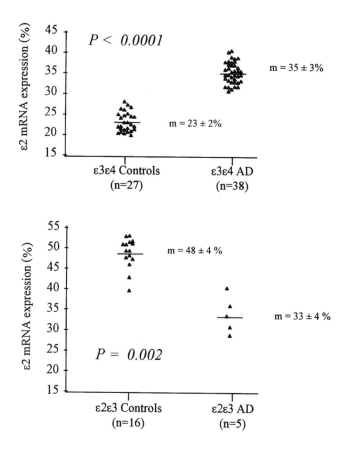

Figure 1. Relative expression (%) of the ε4 and ε2 alleles vs. the ε3 allele in ε3ε4 and ε2ε3 AD control and AD brain tissues, respectively. Calculations have been performed as described in reference [8]

APOE PROMOTER POLYMORPHISMS

The allelic frequencies and genotypes distributions of the Th1/E47cs, −491 AT, −427 CT and *APOE* polymorphisms are presented in Table 1. The analyses were carried out on 573 sporadic AD cases (age = 73.8 ± 8.1 years; age of onset = 70.4 ± 7.9 years) and 509 controls (age = 74.3 ± 9.9 years). No difference of age and sex distribution appeared between these two groups. The genotypes distributions were in Hardy–Weinberg equilibrium in the control population. As expected, the ε4 allele was a strong risk factor for AD and the percentage of subjects carrying at least one ε4 allele was significantly higher in the AD group (36%) than in the control group (11%, p < 0.0001). The odds ratio (OR) for carriers of the ε4 allele was 5.40 (95% confidence interval (CI), 4.11–7.09). Conversely, subjects carrying an ε2 allele were more frequent in the control (7%) than in the AD group (3%) and therefore exhibited a protective effect (OR = 0.47, 95% CI 0.31–0.70). The frequency of the Th1/E47cs T allele was increased in cases compared to controls and the OR for carriers of at least one T allele was 2.13 (95% CI 1.61–2.82, p < 0.0001). Conversely, the frequency of the −491 T allele was decreased in patients compared to controls and the OR to develop AD for individuals with at least a −491 T allele was 0.67 (95% CI 0.52–0.88, p = 0.004). No significant difference in allelic or genotypic distribution between cases and controls was found for the −427 CT polymorphisms. Since the effect of the Th1/E47cs and the −491 AT could only be due to linkage disequilibrium with the *APOE* ε4 allele, we estimated the effect of each allele by using a logistic regression model adjusted for the presence or absence of at least one *APOE* 4 allele. After adjustment, the effect of the Th1/E47cs T allele remained significant (OR = 1.56, 95% CI 5.15–2.11, p = 0.004), while the effect of the −491 T allele did not (OR = 0.82, 95% CI 0.62–1.10, p = 0.19). This data led us to assume that the effect of the Th1/E47cs T allele was statistically independent of that of the ε4 allele.

Table 1. Allele and genotype distributions of the *APOE*, −491 AT, −427 CT and Th1/E47cs polymorphisms

	Allele			Genotype					
APOE	ε2	ε3	ε4	ε2ε2*	ε2ε3	ε2ε4	ε3ε3	ε3ε4	ε4ε4
Controls	75(0.07)	832(0.82)	111(0.11)	4(0.01)	57(0.11)	10(0.02)	344(0.68)	88(0.17)	6(0.01)
AD	40(0.03)	699(0.61)	407(0.36)	—	16(0.03)	24(0.04)	223(0.39)	237(0.41)	73(0.13)
Th1/E47cs	G	T		GG[a]	GT	TT			
Controls	562(0.55)	456(0.45)		162(0.32)	238(0.47)	109(0.21)			
AD	515(0.45)	631(0.55)		103(0.18)	308(0.54)	162(0.28)			
−427 TC[b]	T	C		TT	TC	CC			
Controls	874(0.91)	88(0.09)		396(0.82)	82(0.17)	3(0.01)			
AD	1000(0.92)	86(0.08)		458(0.84)	84(0.16)	1(0.00)			
−491 AT	A	T		AA[c]	AT	TT			
Controls	833(0.82)	185(0.18)		343(0.67)	147(0.29)	19(0.04)			
AD	993(0.87)	153(0.13)		432(0.75)	129(0.23)	12(0.02)			

[a] p < 10⁻⁴. [b] NS. [c] p = 0.005.

DISCUSSION

The allelic distortion of the *APOE* expression suggested that ε3/ε4 individuals expressing high levels of ε4 could have a greater risk of developing AD than those expressing this allele at a lower level. Conversely, individuals expressing a higher level of the ε2 allele may have less risk of developing AD than those expressing this allele at a lower level. Such modulation of the expression could be mediated by sequence variability in the *APOE* promoter. Interestingly, on the five polymorphisms identified in the promoter, the two most frequent presented an association with AD in populations of different origins [5, 6]. Even if we cannot exclude that these two polymorphisms were in linkage disequilibrium with other unknown polymorphisms, their involvement is re-inforced by *in vitro* data: (a) both sequences containing these polymorphisms presented nuclear protein binding; and (b) both modulate the *in vitro* gene reporter expression in hepatoma cells [6, 7].

The differential expression of *APOE* alleles between AD cases and controls could lead to a new approach in our understanding of the role of *APOE* in AD pathogenesis. Several hypotheses have been suggested: the E4 isoform may: (a) be less resistant to oxidative stress conversely to the E2 isoform [9]; (b) not inhibit the aggregation of Tau protein in paired helical filaments, while the E2 and E3 isoforms may [10]; (c) not block the microglia activation by β-APP [11]; (d) promote amyloid deposition. Indeed, the ε4 allele has been described as being linked to increased deposition of amyloid β-peptide in AD and in individuals suffering head injury [12, 13]. Moreover, *APOE* expression has been shown to correlate with Aβ deposition in transgenic mice [14]. In this context, the over-expression of the ε4 allele may be particularly relevant to AD etiology.

Obviously, it is unlikely that the ε4 allele is the only genetic determinant necessary for Aβ deposition. Other components are interesting candidates to interact with the ε4 allele and to contribute to disease risk. In particular, proteins found in senile plaques may act independently or in concert with apoE4. For instance, at least two *APOE* receptors present in senile plaques have been associated with AD in case-control studies [15, 16]. Furthermore, the ε4 allele is associated with higher cholesterol levels that may be important for the generation of β-amyloid formation [17]. All these data indicate the potential impact of *APOE* metabolism on AD development.

In conclusion, together with the qualitative effects of the *APOE* ε2/ε3/ε4 polymorphisms on the occurrence of AD, the quantitative variations of expression of these alleles, possibly due to functional *APOE* promoter mutations, may be a key determinant of AD occurrence. Various combinations of different mutations may confer a large *APOE* expression heterogeneity [18], which may partly explain the heterogeneity of the impact of the ε4 allele in different ethnic groups, for instance [1, 19].

REFERENCES

1. The *APOE* and Alzheimer disease meta-analysis consortium. Effects of age, gender and ethnicity on the association between apolipoprotein E genotype and Alzheimer disease. JAMA 1997; 278: 1349–56.
2. Van Duijn CM, Havekes LM, Van Broeckhoven C, De Knijff P, Hofman A. Apolipoprotein E genotype and association between smoking and early-onset Alzheimer's disease. Br Med J 1995; 310: 627–31.
3. Jarvik GP, Wijsman EM, Kukull WA, Schellenberg GD, Yu C, Larson EB. Interactions of apolipoprotein E genotype, total cholesterol level, age and sex in prediction of Alzheimer's disease: a case-control study. Neurology 1995; 45: 1092–6.
4. Chartier-Harlin M-C, Parfitt M, Legrain S, Pérez-Tur J, Brousseau T, Evans A, Berr C, Vidal O, Roques P, Gourlet V, Fruchart J-C, Delacourte A, Rossor M, Amouyel P. Apolipoprotein E ε4 allele as a major risk factor for sporadic early- and late-onset forms of Alzheimer's disease: analysis of the 19q13.2 chromosomal region. Hum Mol Genet 1994; 3: 569–74.
5. Lambert J-C, Pasquier F, Cottel D, Frigard B, Amouyel P, Chartier-Harlin M-C. A new polymorphism in the *APOE* promoter associated with risk of developing Alzheimer's Disease. Hum Mol Genet 1998; 7: 533–40.
6. Bullido MJ, Artiga MJ, Recuero M, Sastre I, Garcia MA, Aldudo J, Lendon C, Han SW, Morris JC, Frank A, Vazquez J, Goate A, Valdivieso F. A polymorphism in the regulatory region of *APOE* associated with risk for Alzheimer's dementia. Nat Genet 1998; 18: 69–71.
7. Artiga MJ, Bullido MJ, Sastre I, Recuero M, Garcia MA, Aldudo J, Vazquez J, Valdivieso F. Allelic polymorphisms in the transcriptional regulatory region of apolipoprotein E gene. FEBS Lett 1998; 421: 105–8.
8. Lambert J-C, Pérez-Tur J, Dupire M-J, Galasko D, Mann D, Amouyel P, Hardy J, Delacourte A, Chartier-Harlin M-C. Distortion of allelic expression of apolipoprotein E in Alzheimer's disease. Hum Mol Genet 1997; 12: 2151–4.
9. Miyata M, Smith JD. Apolipoprotein E allele-specific antioxidant activity and effects on cytotoxicity by oxidative insults and β-amyloid peptides. Nat Genet 1996; 14: 55–60.
10. Strittmatter WJ, Weisgraber KH, Goedert M, Saunders AM, Huang D, Corder EH, Dong L-M, Jakes R, Alberts MJ, Gilbert JR, Han SH, Hulette C, Einstein G, Schmechel DE, Pericak-Vance MA, Roses AD. Hypothesis: microtubule instability and paired helical filament formation in Alzheimer disease are related to apolipoprotein E genotype. Exp Neurol 1994; 125: 163–71.
11. Barger SW, Harmon AD. Microglial activation by Alzheimer amyloid precursor protein and modulation by apolipoprotein E. Nature 1997; 388: 878–81.
12. Berr C, Hauw J-J, Delaere P, Duyckaerts C, Amouyel P. Apolipoprotein E allele epsilon 4 is linked to increased deposition of the amyloid beta-peptide (A-β) in cases with or without Alzheimer's disease. Neurosci Lett 1994; 178: 221–4.
13. Nicoll JA, Roberts GW, Graham DI. Apolipoprotein E ε4 allele is associated with deposition of amyloid β-protein following head injury. Nat Med 1995; 1: 135–7.
14. Bales KR, Verina T, Dodel RC, Du Y, Altstiel L, Bender M, St George-Hyslop P, Johnstone EM, Little SP, Cummins DJ, Piccardo P, Ghetti B, Paul SM. Lack of apolipoprotein E dramatically reduces amyloid β-peptide deposition. Nat Genet 1997; 17: 263–4.
15. Kang DE, Saitoh T, Chen X, Xia Y, Masliah E, Hansen LA, Thomas RG, Thal LJ, Katzman R. Genetic association of the low-density lipoprotein receptor-related protein gene (LRP), an apolipoprotein E receptor, with late-onset Alzheimer's disease. Neurology 1997; 49: 56–61.

16. Lambert J-C, Wavrant De-Wrièze F, Amouyel P, Chartier-Harlin M-C. Association at LRP locus with sporadic late-onset Alzheimer's disease. Lancet 1998; 351: 1787–8.
17. Simons M, Keller P, De Strooper B, Beyreuther K, Dotti CG, Simons K. Cholesterol depletion inhibits the generation of β-amyloid in hippocampal neurons. Proc Natl Acad Sci USA 1998; 95: 6460–64.
18. Lambert J-C, Berr C, Pasquier F, Delacourte A, Frigard B, Cottel D, Pérez-Tur J, Mouroux M, Mohr M, Cécyre D, Galasko D, Lendon C, Poirier J, Hardy J, Mann D, Amouyel A, Chartier-Harlin M-C. Pronounced impact of Th1/E47cs mutation compared to −491 AT mutation on neural *APOE* gene expression and risk of developing Alzheimer's disease. Hum Mol Genet 1998; in press.
19. Tang MX, Stern Y, Marder K, Bell K, Gurland B, Lantigua R, Andrews H, Feng L, Tucko B, Mayeux R. The *APOE*-ε4 allele and the risk of Alzheimer disease among African-Americans, whites and Hispanics. JAMA 1998; 279: 751–5.

Address for correspondence:
    J.-C. Lambert
    INSERM CJF95-05, Institut Pasteur de Lille,
    1 rue du Professeur Calmette,
    59019 Lille Cédex, France
    Tel: +33 3 20 87 77 10; fax: +33 3 20 87 78 94;
    e-mail: jean-charles.lambert@pasteur-lille.fr

8 Apolipoprotein E, Vascular Factors and Alzheimer's Disease

P. AMOUYEL, F. RICHARD, J.-C. LAMBERT,
M.-C. CHARTIER-HARLIN AND N. HELBECQUE

INTRODUCTION

Several studies have suggested that vascular factors and Alzheimer's disease (AD) may be associated more frequently than expected. Stroke-affected patients seem more prone to develop AD and the brains of patients with dementia often have pathological features of both AD and cerebrovascular disease [1]. Cerebrovascular disease may also influence the development and the degree of severity of AD clinical symptoms [2]. Atherosclerotic risk was recently associated with AD [3], suggesting that vascular risk factors may be potential determinants of AD. Reinforcing this hypothesis, necropsy studies showed that the brains of non-demented patients who died as a result of severe coronary artery disease presented more senile plaques than the brains of subjects without heart disease [4]. Moreover, subjects who developed dementia after age 79 years had higher blood pressure levels, 10–15 years before, than those who did not [5]. Thus, AD and vascular factors could be associated in a causative way or at least share common environmental and genetic determinants. Among the genetic susceptibility risk factors of AD implicated in vascular risk, the polymorphism of the apolipoprotein E gene (*APOE*) may be one of these shared determinants.

APOLIPOPROTEIN E POLYMORPHISM AND VASCULAR RISK

Apolipoprotein E (APOE) is a polymorphic protein playing a major role in lipid and lipoprotein metabolism. Three frequent alleles, ε2, ε3 and ε4, coding for three protein isoforms (E2, E3 and E4, respectively) are associated with low-density lipoprotein cholesterol (LDL-C) plasma concentration variations, involved in vascular risk assessment. With the ε3ε3 genotype as a reference, ε4 allele bearers have higher LDL-C plasma levels; conversely, ε2 allele bearers

Alzheimer's Disease and Related Disorders
Edited by K. Iqbal, D.F. Swaab, B. Winblad and H.M. Wisniewski
© 1999 John Wiley & Sons Ltd

have lower LDL-C plasma levels [6]. Similarly, the risk of myocardial infarction associated with *APOE* genotypes when compared with ε3ε3 bearers is increased in ε4 allele bearers and decreased in ε2 allele bearers, despite higher triglyceride levels (Figure 1). However, at the population level, *APOE* polymorphism seems to explain a modest proportion (12%) of myocardial infarction cases.

Odds Ratio

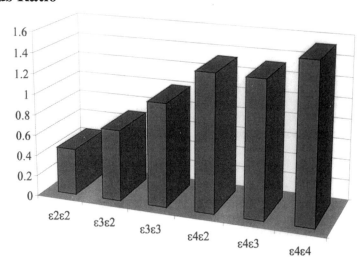

Figure 1. Risk of myocardial infarction according to *APOE* polymorphism (data from [6])

APOLIPOPROTEIN E POLYMORPHISM AND ALZHEIMER'S DISEASE RISK

In the brain of AD and Creutzfeldt–Jakob disease-affected patients, APOE immunoreactivity was detected in cerebral amyloid deposits and kuru plaque amyloid [7]. At the epidemiological level, for individuals bearing the *APOE* ε4 allele, the risk of developing AD is at least four-fold [8]. This observation was confirmed in numerous studies all over the world and extended to other neurodegenerative processes [9]. Thus, the *APOE* polymorphism, a vascular risk factor, has also to be considered as a major AD risk factor. The similarity of the impact of the *APOE* polymorphism in AD with vascular risk can be enlarged to the impact of the *APOE* ε2 allele also. Indeed, individuals bearing the *APOE* ε2 allele have a lower probability of developing AD than ε2 non-bearers [10]. However, at the biochemical and cellular levels, mechanisms by which AD and myocardial infarction occur vary. For vascular disease, the influence of the *APOE* polymorphism seems to be related to its impact on lipid trafficking [6]. In the nervous system, APOE seems to be a cornerstone protein in the maintenance of the brain. *APOE* polymorphism is associated with variations of transport and clearance of hydrophobic compounds such as lipids or amyloid substances or with variation in neurite outgrowth [11]. Given the absence of neural cell replication, membrane and cell repair processes are unavoidable ways to limit the extent of neuronal cell injuries due to vascular damage, progression of unconventional agents, neurotoxic product consequences or any insult involved in the occurrence of AD. Moreover, APOE isoforms are reported to have potential intrinsic antioxidant properties [12] that may influence the occurrence of AD. Finally, the level of expression of the *APOE* alleles [13] under the control of *APOE* promoter mutations [14] is also an additional determinant of AD.

THE RENIN–ANGIOTENSIN SYSTEM COMPONENTS AS POTENTIAL LINKS BETWEEN AD AND VASCULAR RISK

Other potent regulators of the cardiovascular system as the renin–angiotensin system (RAS) may be implicated in nervous system functioning. RAS components are located in the brain [15]. Among the numerous RAS components, the angiotensin I-converting enzyme (ACE) is a key element that promotes the formation of angiotensin II, a potent vasoconstrictor, and the degradation of bradykinin, a vasodilator (Figure 2). Cellular and circulating levels of ACE are partly genetically determined through a deletion (D)/insertion (I)

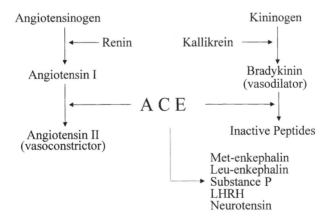

Figure 2. Main biochemical pathways involving the angiotensin I-converting enzyme (ACE)

polymorphism of the ACE gene (*ACE*). Subjects bearing the *ACE* D allele have higher concentration and activity levels of the enzyme than I allele bearers. Moreover, subjects bearing the D allele are at high risk of myocardial infarction and postangioplasty restenosis after coronary stenting [16].

Experimental and clinical evidence suggests that ACE may be implicated in neurodegenerative processes. In humans, the use of ACE inhibitors in the hypertensive elderly was associated with improved cognitive function, while other hypotensive drugs had no such effect, and in a sample of subjects over 60 years, the *ACE* D allele was associated with severe cognitive impairment [17]. All these observations suggest that RAS components, as vascular determinants, may constitute attractive sources of candidate genes for AD susceptibility.

CONCLUSION

Other known proteins or vascular factors may be associated with AD susceptibility. For instance, environmental factors such as alcohol consumption [18] or
hormone replacement therapies in post-menopausal women [19] seem to reduce both vascular and AD risk. Moreover, to further dissect the potential
relationships between vascular factors and AD, the APOE-associated components, involved in lipid and lipoprotein metabolism, may constitute other clues.
For instance, APOE is suspected to act as a ligand implicated in the delivery of
lipids mediated by receptors expressed in the brain; polymorphism of the LDL-
receptor related protein (LRP) gene has been associated with AD risk [20].

The impact of APOE polymorphism on AD and vascular disease is one of the
most consistent evidence for the hypothesis of a link between vascular and neurodegenerative processes. However, whether this association is due to a concomitant increased frequency of both pathologies with age, becoming less probable as
data accumulates, or reflects a causative association, remains open to question. In
any case, both hypotheses have a major impact on the understanding and the
potential ways of treatment and prevention of AD: first, new areas of research in
AD are offered; second, the numerous ways of treatment and prevention that
have existed for several years in vascular risk control may benefit the prevention
strategies of AD and neurodegenerative processes. However, most of these observations have been obtained from retrospective studies, and results from ongoing
prospective studies will help to address these various issues.

REFERENCES

1. Pasquier F, Leys D. Why are stroke patients prone to develop dementia? J Neurol 1997; 244: 135–42.
2. Snowdon DA, Greiner LH, Mortimer JA, Riley KP, Greiner PA, Markesbery WR. Brain infarction and the clinical expression of Alzheimer disease. The Nun Study. JAMA 1997; 277: 813–17.

3. Hofman A, Ott A, Breteler MM, Bots ML, Slooter AJ, van Harskamp F, van Duijn CN, Van Broeckhoven C, Grobbee DE. Atherosclerosis, apolipoprotein E, and prevalence of dementia and Alzheimer's disease in the Rotterdam Study. Lancet 1997; 349: 151–4.

4. Sparks DL, Hunsaker JC, Scheff SW, Kryscio RJ, Henson JL, Markesbery WR. Cortical senile plaques in coronary artery disease, aging and Alzheimer's disease. Neurobiol Aging 1990; 11: 601–7.

5. Skoog I, Lernfelt B, Landahl S, Palmertz B, Andreasson LA, Nilsson L, Persson G, Oden A, Svanborg A. 15-year longitudinal study of blood pressure and dementia. Lancet 1996; 347: 1141–5.

6. Luc G, Bard JM, Arveiler D, Evans A, Cambou JP, Bingham A, Amouyel P, Schaffer P, Ruidavets JB, Cambien F. Impact of apolipoprotein E polymorphism on lipoproteins and risk of myocardial infarction. The ECTIM Study. Arterioscler Thromb 1994; 14: 1412–19.

7. Namba Y, Tomonaga M, Kawasaki H, Otomo E, Ikeda K. Apolipoprotein E immunoreactivity in cerebral amyloid deposits and neurofibrillary tangles in Alzheimer's disease and kuru plaque amyloid in Creutzfeldt–Jakob disease. Brain Res 1991; 541: 163–6.

8. Strittmatter WJ, Saunders AM, Schmechel D, Pericak-Vance M, Enghild J, Salvesen GS, Roses AD. Apoliproprotein E: high-avidity binding to β-amyloid and increased frequency of type 4 allele in late-onset familial Alzheimer disease. Proc Natl Acad Sci USA 1993; 90: 1977–81.

9. Farrer LA, Cupples LA, Haines JL, Hyman B, Kukull WA, Mayeux R, Myers RH, Pericak-Vance MA, Risch N, van Duijn CM. Effects of age, sex, and ethnicity on the association between apolipoprotein E genotype and Alzheimer disease. A meta-analysis. APOE and Alzheimer Disease Meta Analysis Consortium. JAMA 1997; 278: 1349–56.

10. Chartier-Harlin M-C, Parfitt M, Legrain S, Pérez-Tur J, Brousseau T, Evans A, Berr C, Vidal O, Roques P, Gourlet V, Fruchart J-C, Delacourte A, Rossor M, Amouyel P. Apolipoprotein E, ε4 allele as a major risk factor for sporadic early and late-onset forms of Alzheimer's disease: analysis of the 19q13.2 chromosomal region. Hum Mol Genet 1994; 3: 569–74.

11. Weisgraber KH, Mahley RW. Human apolipoprotein E: the Alzheimer's disease connection. FASEB J 1996; 10: 1485–94.

12. Miyata M, Smith JD. Apolipoprotein E allele-specific antioxidant activity and effects on cytotoxicity by oxidative insults and β-amyloid peptides. Nat Genet 1996; 14: 55–61.

13. Lambert J-C, Pérez-Tur J, Dupire M-J, Galasko D, Mann D, Amouyel P, Hardy J, Delacourte A, Chartier-Harlin M-C. Distortion of allelic expression of apolipoprotein E in Alzheimer's diesease. Hum Mol Genet 1997; 6: 2151–4.

14. Lambert J-C, Pasquier F, Cottel D, Frigard B, Amouyel P, Chartier-Harlin M-C. A new polymorphism in the APOE promoter associated with risk of developing Alzheimer's disease. Hum Mol Genet 1998; 7: 533–40.

15. Wright JW, Harding JW. Brain angiotensin receptor for subtypes in the control of physiological and behavioral responses. Neurosci Biobehav Rev 1994; 18: 21–53.

16. Amant C, Bauters C, Bodart JC, Lablanche JM, Grollier G, Danchin N, Hamon M, Richard F, Helbecque N, McFadden EP, Amouyel P, Bertrand ME. D allele of the angiotensin I-converting enzyme is a major risk factor for restenosis after coronary stenting. Circulation 1997; 96: 56–60.

17. Amouyel P, Richard F, Cottel D, Amant C, Codron V, Helbecque N. The deletion allele of the angiotensin I-converting enzyme gene as a genetic susceptibility factor for cognitive impairment. Neurosci Lett 1996; 217: 203–5.

18. Orgogozo J-M, Dartigues J-F, Lafont S, Letenneur L, Commenges D, Salamon R, Renaud S, Breteler MB. Wine consumption and dementia in the elderly: a prospective community study in the Bordeaux area. Rev Neurol (Paris) 1997; 153: 185–92.

19. Tang MX, Jacobs D, Stern Y, Marder K, Schofield P, Gurland B, Andrews H, Mayeux R. Effect of oestrogen during menopause on risk and age at onset of Alzheimer's disease. Lancet 1996; 348: 429–32.

20. Lambert J-C, Wavrant-De Vriese F, Amouyel P, Chartier-Harlin M-C. Association at LRP gene locus with sporadic late-onset Alzheimer's disease. Lancet 1998; 351: 1787–8.

Address for correspondence:
    P. Amouyel,
    INSERM/U 508,
    Institut Pasteur de Lille,
    1 rue Calmette,
    F-59019 Lille, France
    Tel: +33 3 20 87 77 10; fax: +33 3 20 87 78 94;
    e-mail: philippe.amouyel@pasteur-lille.fr

9 Molecular Misreading and Accumulation of +1 Proteins in Alzheimer's and Down's Syndrome Patients

E.M. HOL, J.A. SLUIJS, M.A.F. SONNEMANS, A.B. SMIT, R.C. VAN DER SCHORS AND F.W. VAN LEEUWEN

INTRODUCTION

During the last decade, genetic linkage studies revealed a set of genes that are associated with Alzheimer's disease (AD). Genomic mutations in the genes for β-amyloid precursor protein (β-APP) and the presenilins are rare, but are the major cause of the autosomal dominant (early onset) forms of AD [1]. Furthermore, the presence of two ε4 alleles of the apolipoprotein E (ApoE) gene is associated with the disease [2]. Despite the gain in knowledge on the functional implications of the genetic mutations and the ApoE polymorphism, the primary cause of AD remains unknown [3]. Our recent discovery of the occurrence of dinucleotide deletions in β-APP and ubiquitin-B (UBB) transcripts in non-familial AD cases, which are the most numerous, adds a new vista to the list of genetic and risk factors that are implicated to play a role in the development of AD neuropathology [4–6].

MOLECULAR MISREADING

Molecular misreading can be defined as an inaccurate conversion of the genomic information into correct mRNA [6]. Co- or post-transcriptional errors are introduced in or adjacent to GAGAG motifs present in the mRNA (Figure 1).

Frameshift mutations in vasopressin (VP) transcripts in hypothalamic nuclei of the homozygous Brattleboro rat were a first example of molecular misreading in post-mitotic neurons [7]. In these rats a germ-line mutation in the VP gene (a single base deletion) causes hypothalamic diabetes insipidus, due to the production of a mutant VP-precursor. In a small, but with age

Alzheimer's Disease and Related Disorders
Edited by K. Iqbal, D.F. Swaab, B. Winblad and H.M. Wisniewski
© 1999 John Wiley & Sons Ltd

60

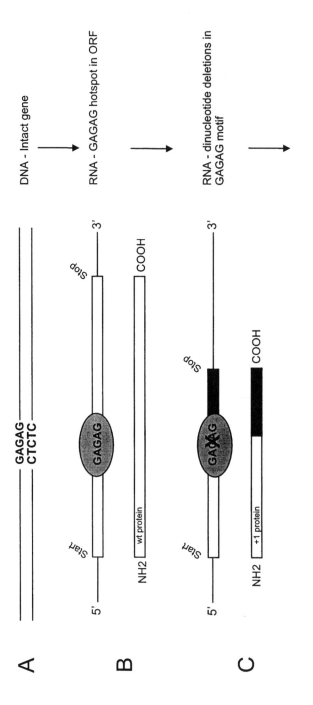

Figure 1. Molecular misreading. A frameshift mutation in mRNA results in the translation of +1 proteins. The diagram presents an intact genomic sequence (A) that is transcribed into an mRNA molecule with a GAGAG motif in the open reading frame (ORF). Normally this sequence is translated into the corresponding wild-type (wt) protein (B). This GAGAG motif, however, is very susceptible for dinucleotide deletions in neurons affected during Alzheimer's disease (C). We provide evidence that a GA deletion indeed occurs in exon 9 or 10 of the β-APP transcripts and that a GU deletion occurs in exon 2 of the UBB transcripts, either co- or post-transcription [4]. The result of these deletions is that the mRNA is translated into a protein, with a wt N-terminus (open bar) and a nonsense C-terminus (solid bar). It is hypothesized that these +1 proteins slowly accumulate in neurons and affect their normal function, leading to neuronal degeneration

increasing, number of neurons that produce the mutant VP-precursor, the VP reading frame appeared to be restored [8]. Further studies revealed that in these cells a proportion of the VP transcripts encountered an additional dinucleotide deletion, which resulted in restoration of the wild-type reading frame downstream from the germ-line deletion [7]. In addition, evidence was provided that a similar process of transcript mutation also occurred in wild-type rats, resulting in the synthesis of frameshifted VP (VP^{+1}) [7]. Subsequent studies demonstrated that molecular misreading was not restricted to rats, as VP^{+1} immunoreactivity could be readily detected in human hypothalami [9]. At that time it was assumed that somatic mutations were the cause for the frameshift mutations in VP [10]. However, no evidence for a somatic mutation could be found (Evans, Burbach, Spence, van Leeuwen, unpublished observations) [6].

ACCUMULATION OF β-APP^{+1} AND UBB^{+1} IN THE NEUROPATHOLOGICAL HALLMARKS OF AD

The observation that the number of neurons producing frameshifted VP increased with aging in rats [7, 8] was an important lead to start the study of the occurrence of molecular misreading in AD. The prevalence of sporadic and familial AD is increasing with age, which prompted us to hypothesize that GAGAG motifs in transcripts of AD-related genes might also be a target for the dinucleotide deletions [6].

β-AMYLOID PRECURSOR PROTEIN

Much AD research has been focused on β-APP, as it is one of the genes that is mutated in a small subset of AD patients [1] and as an error in the enzymatic processing of β-APP causes the accumulation of βA4 peptide in amyloid plaques [11]. In addition, this gene is highly susceptible for molecular misreading. Based upon statistical calculations, the open reading frame of β-APP, which consists of 2234 bases, should comprise 2.2 GAGAG motifs, as one GAGAG motif can be expected in 4^5 bases (i.e. 1:1024). However, in the coding sequence of β-APP, seven GAGAG motifs are present. Three are clustered in exon 9 and 10 and a dinucleotide deletion in either the second or the third GAGAG motif leads to translation into a +1 protein with an identical C-terminus. An antibody was raised against this C-terminus of the β-APP^{+1} protein [4, 5]. The antibody stained: (a) the dystrophic neurites surrounding the neuritic plaques, but not the core of the plaques; (b) the neurofibrillary tangles; and (c) the neuropil threads in cortical and hippocampal sections of early and late onset AD, Down's syndrome (DS) patients and elderly non-demented controls with initial neuropathology (see http://www.knaw.nl/nih/) [4–6].

IDENTIFICATION AND FUNCTIONAL IMPLICATIONS OF β-APP^{+1}

The frameshift mutations in β-APP mRNA were confirmed by a molecular biological approach. Transcripts were found with a GA-deletion in the GAGAG motif of either exon 9 or 10 [4]. These mutations give rise to a premature termination of the β-APP translation. The resulting truncated β-APP^{+1} protein can be detected by Western blotting. The protein band, of the expected 38 kDa size, was clearly stained with an N-terminal β-APP wt antibody and with the β-APP^{+1} antibody [4].

At present, it is only possible to speculate what consequences the accumulation of β-APP^{+1} in neurons will have, as the function of β-APP itself is unknown. However, the truncated β-APP^{+1} has lost the potentially neurotrophic RERMS sequence [12]. Moreover, β-APP^{+1} might interfere with the normal enzymatic processing of β-APP and thus contribute to the neuropathogenesis of AD.

UBIQUITIN-B

UBB is a highly conserved protein that plays an essential role in a number of processes, including protein breakdown by proteasomes [13]. UBB is a component of neurofibrillary tangles and is conjugated to tau protein in paired helical filaments in AD patients [14, 15]. Like β-APP, UBB is also susceptible for dinucleotide deletions in GAGAG motifs. UBB consists of three repeats of 76 residues; a dinucleotide deletion in the GAGAG motifs in the first two repeats will lead to the translation of an aberrant UBB of 93 residues instead of 76. Antibodies were raised against the C-terminus of the putative UBB^{+1} protein [4]. Once again, we obtained strong indications that molecular misreading of the UBB gene occurred in the brains of AD patients. UBB^{+1} immunoreactivity was detected in the frontal and temporal cortex and hippocampus of AD and DS patients and elderly controls (see http://www.knaw.nl/nih/). The antibody again stained the neuropathological hallmarks of AD: neuritic plaques, tangles and neuropil threads [4].

IDENTIFICATION AND FUNCTIONAL IMPLICATIONS OF UBB^{+1}

Cortex homogenate of two severely affected patients, an 81 year-old female AD patient and a 58-year-old female DS patient, were pooled and biochemically analyzed by reverse-phase HPLC followed by an UBB^{+1} radioimmunoassay (Figure 2). The peak fraction (fraction 29) of the crude homogenate co-eluted with recombinant UBB^{+1} (rec-UBB^{+1}) protein. Thus, the human UBB^{+1} protein present in the AD brain has similar properties to the rec-UBB^{+1} protein.

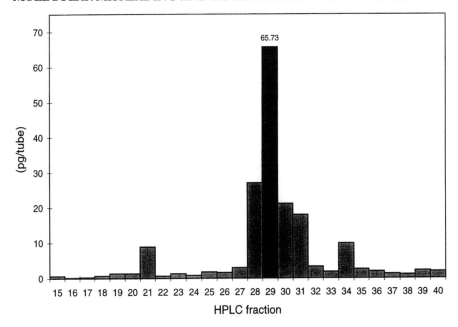

Figure 2. Reverse-phase HPLC fractionation of a pooled cortex homogenate of two severely affected AD patients. The fractions were analyzed using an UBB^{+1} radioimmunoassay. The elution position of the fraction with highest UBB^{+1} immunoreactivity (fraction 29) was identical to the elution position of the reference protein, i.e. recombinant-UBB^{+1} protein

In UBB transcripts of AD and DS patients, GU-deletions occur that result in the translation of UBB^{+1} protein [6]. UBB^{+1} lacks the C-terminal glycin that is essential for multi-ubiquitylation of the proteins. Efficient proteasomal protein breakdown is highly dependent on multi-ubiquitylation [13]. Therefore, accumulation of UBB^{+1} most certainly will interfere with an efficient protein breakdown [6]. Indeed, in tangles of AD brains a lack of multi-ubiquitylation of hyperphosphorylated tau has been demonstrated [16].

DISCUSSION

There are a few important future issues concerning the +1 proteins: (1) are +1 proteins a cause or consequence of AD neuropathology?; (2) what is the mechanism that causes the dinucleotide deletion?; (3) why are the aberrant mRNA molecules not efficiently degraded?; and (4) what causes the accumulation of +1 proteins?

1. An important question is whether molecular misreading and the subsequent production and accumulation of β-APP^{+1} and UBB^{+1} can cause

AD neuropathology or whether it is a mere consequence of AD. This is presently addressed in transgenic mice that over-express β-APP^{+1} and/or UBB^{+1}.

2. Intact genomic information is misinterpreted, especially when high expression levels of a gene are observed. Dinucleotide deletions occur in a subpopulation of the mRNA. The mutation might be the result of slippage or stuttering of the RNA polymerase during transcription (Figure 3D) or the result of a post-transcriptional RNA-editing event (Figure 3E).

3. This mutant mRNA is not degraded (Figure 3F) and is translated in +1 proteins (Figure 3G). Frameshift mutations, such as the dinucleotide deletions in GAGAG motifs, result in premature termination codons (PTCs) in the mRNA. In yeast [17] and mammals [18], a vast amount of data exists on the presence of an RNA surveillance system that detects these PTCs in a coding sequence and subsequently degrades the mutant mRNA [19]. An inefficient degradation of the +1 transcripts in AD and DS patients and elderly controls indicates a failure in the RNA surveillance system (Figure 3F).

4. Finally, the +1 proteins are inefficiently degraded and accumulate in the neurons (Figure 3H and I). The production of UBB^{+1} and β-APP^{+1} might be an early event in the development of AD neuropathology, as the proteins are already present in elderly controls with initial neuropathology [4] and β-APP^{+1} is produced in young DS patients without any neuropathology [20]. Increasing amounts of UBB^{+1} may slowly interfere with the ubiquitylation of aberrant proteins by wild-type UBB. Thus, an initial mutation in UBB mRNA might be followed by an inefficient protein breakdown via the proteasomal pathway and a subsequent gradual accumulation of other aberrant proteins.

In conclusion, aberrant RNA molecules do not seem to be efficiently degraded in AD patients, thus UBB^{+1} is produced and as a consequence many aberrant proteins gradually accumulate in the affected neurons. A similar role for transcript variability in neurodegeneration has been described in non-familiar amyotrophic lateral sclerosis patients [21, 22]. In these patients a part of exon 3 of the EAAT2 transporter has been skipped, which results in a dominant negative phenotype [21]. Similar mutations, present in β-APP and UBB transcripts in AD, may also be present in other transcripts expressed in neurons, but also proliferating cell types [23], and thus may underlie other (neuro)pathologies as well. A combination with a failure in detecting the aberrant transcripts will lead to the accumulation of aberrant proteins, which may gradually affect neuronal integrity and contribute to the pathological changes in AD and other age-related pathologies.

MOLECULAR MISREADING

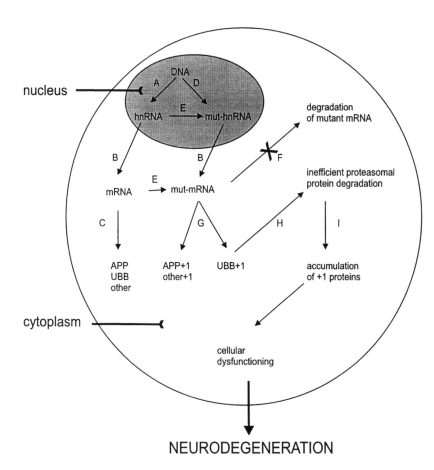

Figure 3. Working hypothesis. This model explains how frameshift mutations in RNA and the subsequent +1 proteins could accumulate in the neurons of AD patients. In the cell nucleus the genomic information is intact and is transcribed into heteronuclear RNA (hnRNA) (A). This hnRNA is spliced and transported to the cytoplasm (B), where it is translated into wild-type β-APP, UBB and other proteins (B). In the event that the coding sequence contains GAGAG motifs, the sequence is susceptible for dinucleotide deletions (D, E). Molecular misreading can be caused by stuttering or slippage of the RNA polymerase during transcription (D) or by editing of the mRNA or hnRNA after transcription (E). In AD patients the mRNA decay pathway may be impaired (F) and therefore the +1 mRNA is translated into +1 protein (G). In particular, UBB^{+1} may have a prominent role as it will probably directly interfere with the ubiquitin/proteasome system and lead to an inefficient protein breakdown through the proteasomal pathway (H). Together, these changes lead to a gradual accumulation of aberrant proteins in neurons, cellular dysfunction and ultimately neurodegeneration (I)

REFERENCES

1. Van Broeckhoven CL. Molecular genetics of Alzheimer disease: identification of genes and gene mutations. Eur Neurol 1995; 35: 8–19.
2. Corder EH, Saunders AM, Strittmatter WJ, Schmechel DE, Gaskell PC, Small GW et al. Gene dose of apolipoprotein E type 4 allele and the risk of Alzheimer's disease in late onset families. Science 1993; 261: 921–3.
3. Itzhaki RF. Possible factors in the etiology of Alzheimer's disease. Mol Neurobiol 1994; 9: 1–13.
4. Van Leeuwen FW, De Kleijn DPV, Van den Hurk HH, Neubauer A, Sonnemans MAF, Sluijs JA, Köycü S, Ramdjielal RDJ, Salehi A, Martens GJM et al. Frameshift mutants of β-amyloid precursor protein and ubiquitin-B in Alzheimer's and Down's patients. Science 1998; 279: 242–7.
5. Hol EM, Neubauer A, De Kleijn DPV, Sluijs JA, Ramdjielal RDJ, Sonnemans MAF, Van Leeuwen FW. Dinucleotide deletions in neuronal transcripts: a novel type of mutation in non-familial Alzheimer's disease and Down's syndrome patients. Prog Brain Res 1998; 117: 379–95.
6. Van Leeuwen FW, Burbach JPH, Hol EM. Mutations in RNA: a first example of molecular misreading in Alzheimer's disease. Trends Neurosci 1998; 21: 331–5.
7. Evans DAP, Van der Kleij AAM, Sonnemans MAF, Burbach JPH, Van Leeuwen FW. Frameshift mutations at two hotspots in vasopressin transcripts in postmitotic neurons. Proc Natl Acad Sci USA 1994; 91: 6059–63.
8. Van Leeuwen FW, Van der Beek EM, Seger M, Burbach JPH, Ivell R. Age-related development of a heterozygous phenotype in solitary neurons of the homozygous Brattleboro rat. Proc Natl Acad Sci USA 1989; 86: 6417–20.
9. Evans DAP, Burbach JPH, Swaab DF, Van Leeuwen FW. Mutant vassopressin precursors in the human hypothalamus: evidence for neuronal somatic mutations in man. Neuroscience 1996; 71: 1025–30.
10. Evans DAP, Burbach JPH, Van Leeuwen FW. Somatic mutations in the brain: relationship to aging? Mutation Res 1995; 338: 173–82.
11. Selkoe DJ. Alzheimer's disease: genotypes, phenotypes, and treatments. Science 1997; 275: 630–31.
12. Jin L-W, Ninomiya H, Roch J-M, Schubert D, Masliah E, Otero DAC, Saitoh T. Peptides containing the RERMS sequence of amyloid β/A4 protein precursor bind cell surface and promote neurite extension. J Neurosci 1994; 14: 5461–70.
13. Varshavsky A. The ubiquitin system. Trends Biochem Sci 1997; 22(10): 383–7.
14. Mori H, Kondo J, Ihara Y. Ubiquitin is a component of paired helical filaments in Alzheimer's disease. Science 1987; 235: 1641–4.
15. Mayer RJ, Tipler C, Arnold J, Lásló L, Al-Khedhairy A, Lowe J, Landon M. Endosome-lysosomes, ubiquitin and neurodegeneration. Adv Exp Med Biol 1996; 389: 261–9.
16. Morishima-Kawashima M, Hasegawa M, Takio K, Suzuki M, Titani K, Ihara Y. Ubiquitin is conjugated with amino-terminally processed tau in paired helical filaments. Neuron 1993; 10: 1151–60.
17. Ruiz-Echevarría MJ, González CI, Peltz SW. Identifying the right stop: determining how the surveillance complex recognizes and degrades an aberrant mRNA. EMBO J 1998; 17(2): 575–89.
18. Nagy E, Maquat LE. A rule for termination-codon position within intron-containing genes: when nonsense affects RNA abundance. Trends Biochem Sci 1998; 23: 198–99.
19. Ruiz-Echevarría MJ, Czaplinski K, Peltz SW. Making sense of nonsense in yeast. Trends Biochem Sci 1996; 21: 433–8.

20. Van Leeuwen FW, Mann DM, Sonnemans MF, Hol EM. Frameshift mutations in amyloid precursor protein precede neuropathology in young Down's syndrome patients. Soc Neurosci Abstracts 1998; 24.
21. Lin C-L, Bristol LA, Jin L, Dykes-Hoberg M, Crawford T, Clawson L, Rothstein JD. Aberrant RNA processing in a neurodegenerative disease: the cause for absent EAAT2, a glutamate transporter, in amyotrophic lateral sclerosis. Neuron 1998; 20: 589–602.
22. Bai G, Lipton SA. Aberrant RNA splicing in sporadic amyotrophic lateral sclerosis. Neuron 1998; 20: 363–6.
23. Van Leeuwen FW, Hermanussen RWH, Sonnemans MAF, Evans DAP, Chooi K-F, Burbach JPH, Murphy D. Molecular misreading in proliferating cells (submitted, 1998).

Address for correspondence:
Elly M. Hol,
Netherlands Institute for Brain Research,
Meibergdreef 33,
1105 AZ Amsterdam, The Netherlands
Tel: +31 20 5665515; fax: +31 20 6961006; e-mail: e.hol@nih.knaw.nl

.

10 Novel Familial Early-onset Alzheimer's Disease Mutation (Leu723Pro) in Amyloid Precursor Protein (APP) Gene Increases Production of 42(43) Amino Acid Isoform of Amyloid-β Peptide

JOHN B.J. KWOK, QIAO-XIN LI, MARIANNE HALLUPP, LIZ MILWARD, SCOTT WHYTE AND PETER R. SCHOFIELD

INTRODUCTION

Analyses of the heritable forms of early-onset AD (EOAD) have identified key genetic mutations in the APP gene (Figure 1). All the mutations appear to cluster within or adjacent to the sequence which encodes β-AP (reviewed in [1]). Each mutation has a subtly different biochemical effect, either altering the nature of the β-AP sequence or the metabolism of APP, which increases production of the insoluble β-AP$_{42}$ isoform. For example, the Swedish double mutation (codons 670/671 from Lys/Met to Asn/Leu in the 770 amino acid isoform) results in overall increased secretion of the normal 40 amino acid residue peptide (β-AP$_{40}$) and a longer and more insoluble 42 amino acid residue isoform of β-AP (β-AP$_{42}$), most probably by enhancing β-secretase activity [2, 3]. The London mutation at codon 717 (Val to Ile), which is situated outside the β-AP sequence, alters γ-secretase activity to favour the specific secretion of the β-AP$_{42}$ isoform [3]. In an Australian pedigree with hereditary presumptive AD, we screened exons 16 and 17 of the APP gene to determine the presense of pathogenic missense mutations. In the present study, we present a novel mutation (Leu723Pro) in the APP gene and its effects on APP metabolism in transfected Chinese hamster ovarian (CHO) cell lines, using either constitutive or inducible promoter systems.

Alzheimer's Disease and Related Disorders
Edited by K. Iqbal, D.F. Swaab, B. Winblad and H.M. Wisniewski
© 1999 John Wiley & Sons Ltd

70

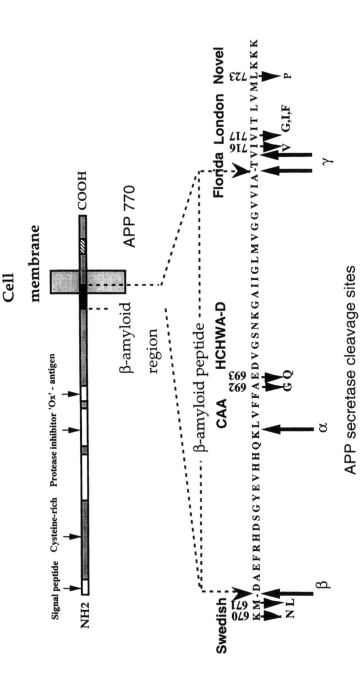

Figure 1. Schematic diagram of APP. The protein is a multi-domain cell-surface molecule. The β-amyloid peptide region (black box) contains part of the transmembrane domain and part of the extracellular domain of APP. The putative G$_o$ binding motif of APP involved in the transduction of apoptotic signal is shown (hatched box). Mutations that cause AD are indicated at the bottom of the figure by thin vertical arrows. Secretase cleavage sites are indicated by thick vertical arrows

IDENTIFICATION OF A NOVEL FAMILIAL MUTATION IN CODON 723 (Leu TO Pro) OF THE APP GENE

The Australian pedigree consisted of three generations where presenile dementia was inherited in a clearly autosomal dominant manner, with the disease being transmitted through both maternal and paternal lines. The male proband has shown clinical manifestations of AD, as determined by the NINCDS–ADRDA criteria for probable AD [4]. Intronic were used to amplify, by polymerase chain reaction (PCR), portions of the APP gene [5] from genomic DNAs isolated from seven individuals of the putative EOAD family, consisting of the proband and six of his unaffected relatives (Figure 2A). As shown in the nucleotide sequence analysis of the proband PCR product (Figure 2B), there is a band in both the T and C lane at a position corresponding to codon 723 (as numbered for the 770 amino acid residue isoform) which is not found in the unaffected controls (Figure 2B). This indicates that the proband contains a heterozygote missense mutation which converted a T to a C nucleotide at a codon in one of his APP gene alleles, corresponding to a substitution of leucine for a proline residue. The Leu723Pro mutation was only found in the proband and not in any of the unaffected members analysed, or in 50 other chromosomes analysed.

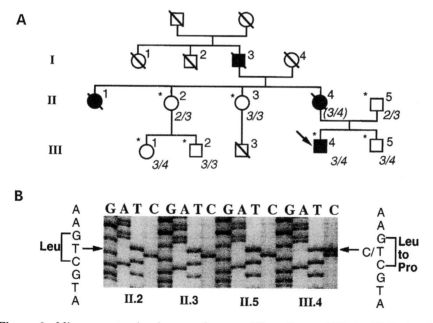

Figure 2. Missense mutation in an early-onset AD pedigree, AUS-2. (A) Proband (arrow) is part of a three-generation pedigree. (B) Sequence analysis of exon 17 of the APP gene revealed that proband (III.4) is heterozygotic for a missense mutation in codon 723 which substitutes a leucine for a proline residue

MEASUREMENT OF AMYLOID-β PEPTIDE (β-AP) LEVELS IN CHO CLONES EXPRESSING APP cDNAS

CONSTITUTIVE EXPRESSION OF APP USING CMV PROMOTER

CHO.K1 cells were transfected with expression vectors which contain either the wild-type or mutant forms (Leu723Pro, Swedish, and London mutations) of the APP cDNAs under the control of the constitutive cytomegalovirus (CMV) promoter (pCMV–APPs). Over-expressions of APP cDNAs in stably transfected clones were determined by Northern analysis (data not shown). Three clones transfected with each construct were chosen and metabolically labelled and immunoprecipitated [6] with mouse monoclonal antibodies, which are specific for either the 40 amino acid (G2-10) or 42–43 amino acid β-AP isoform (G2-11) [7]. As shown in Figure 3A, the 4 kDa band corresponds to β-AP. Elevation of β-AP_{42} levels are expressed as a ratio of β-AP_{42}:β-AP_{40} to take into account variations in the amount of protein loaded onto each lane. As shown in Figure 3B, there was an average 1.89 ± 0.82-fold (p < 0.14, using Student's t-test) increase in production of β-AP_{42} in the three Leu723Pro expressing clones compared with the clones expressing the wild-type cDNA. As a comparison with the Leu723Pro mutation, the Swedish and London mutations were also examined using the same system. As shown in Figure 3C, clones over-expressing the Swedish and London mutations also resulted in a similar increase (1.88 ± 0.91 and 1.89 ± 0.60, respectively) in production of β-AP_{42}. These results are comparable to other studies [3, 8].

INDUCIBLE EXPRESSION OF APP USING THE TET-OFF SYSTEM

CHO.AA8 cells which stably express the tetracycline-responsive transcriptional activator were transfected with pBI-G vectors (Clonetech) carrying either the normal or mutant (Leu723Pro) version of APP cDNAs (pBI-G/APP) under the control of a tetracycline response element and the immediate early promoter of CMV. This allows clones which carry integrated copies of the constructs to be induced by the removal of tetracycline from the growth medium. Two clones from each construct that demonstrated inducible expression of APP, as determined by Western blotting using the amino-terminal APP specific antibody 22C11, were selected (data not shown). Levels of β-AP_{42} from each clone were determined using the immunoprecipitation procedure, as described above.

Each clone was induced by exposure to low concentrations of tetracyclin (0.2 µg/ml) for 24 h, followed by 3 h of metabolic labelling in the absence of tetracyclin. This was necessary to avoid excessive cell mortality in one of the APP (Leu723Pro) clones. The conditioned medium from each clone was collected and examined for the secretion of β-AP_{42}. As shown in Figure 3,

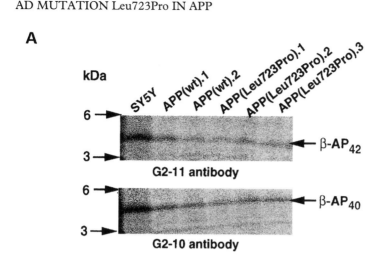

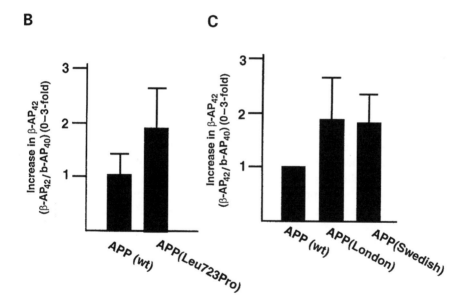

Figure 3. Elevated production of β-AP$_{42}$ in CHO clones which constitutively over-express APP Leu723Pro mutation. (A) Conditioned media were immunoprecipitated with monoclonal antibodies G2-10 or G2-11. Samples were electrophoresed on a 10–15% Tris–Tricine gel and blotted onto PVDF membrane before exposure for auto-radiography. Presence of a 4 kDa band indicates presence of β-AP. (B) Quantification of β-AP levels. 2, 3 = two-fold, three-fold increase. Clones over-expressing APP Leu723Pro mutation gave, on average, a two-fold increase in β-AP$_{42}$ levels compared with the wild-type (wt) APP clones. (C) Similar levels were achieved for the clones expressing the APP London or Swedish mutations

expression of either the wild-type or Leu723Pro-mutant version of APP cDNA resulted in the same level of production of β-AP_{42} (a value of approximately 4.0 for the ratio between β-AP_{42} and β-AP_{40} in all four clones examined). The apparent lack of β-AP_{42} elevation in the inducible clones expressing Leu723Pro APP needs to be investigated by looking at other APP mutations.

CYTOTOXICITY OF THE Leu723Pro MUTATION

Both the London mutations of the APP gene and several mutations in the presenilin genes have been shown to induce apoptosis when expressed in transiently transfected cells [9, 10]. Apoptoses induced by the mutant genes were reversed by the addition of pertussis toxin (PTX), an inhibitor of heteromeric G proteins. We examined whether the APP Leu723Pro mutation was capable of inducing apoptosis in the same manner as the APP London mutation. CHO.K1 cells were transiently transfected with each of the pCMV–APP constructs. After 24 h, the cells were harvested and examined for the presence of a key feature of apoptosis, the cleavage of genomic DNA into nucleosomal-length fragments. Genomic DNAs from each transfection were harvested and end-labelled with [^{32}P]dCTP [11]. After electrophoresis on a 2% agarose gel, the DNAs were blotted onto a filter and exposed for autoradiography. As shown in Figure 4A, the distinctive DNA 'ladder' is present in CHO.K1 cells treated with 1 mM staurosporine, a potent inducer of apoptosis. The same laddering pattern is found in comparable levels in all the mutant APP cDNAs, suggesting that the Leu723Pro mutation, like the London mutation, may induce apoptosis as part of its cytotoxic mechanism. The level of apoptotic cells was quantified using a sandwich ELISA assay (Cell Death Detection ELISA^{PLUS}, Boehringer-Mannheim) which detects histone-associated DNA fragments found in apoptotic bodies released from dying cells. As shown in Figure 4B, transient expression of the Leu723Pro APP cDNA resulted in a marked increase in apoptotic cells compared with cells transfected with the parental vector or the 'No DNA' control. Moreover, the level of apoptosis was reduced to basal levels with the addition of PTX.

We also examined the inducible APP clones for the presence of apoptosis at set time points after the removal of tetracycline. As shown in Figure 5A, 24 h after induction of the clone TO.APPL723P-1, the level of apoptosis was increased eight-fold compared with the other clonal lines, as determined by the ELISA assay. However, this level of apoptosis was not seen in the other Leu723Pro mutant line, TO.APPL723P-3. This may indicate clonal variation in sensitivity to the cytotoxic effects of the Leu723Pro APP mutation. To verify that the cells were dying through the apoptotic pathway, genomic DNAs were purified and electrophoresed as described above. As shown in Figure 5B, the TO.APPL723P-1 clone clearly has apoptotic cells, as indicated by the distinctive DNA ladder pattern.

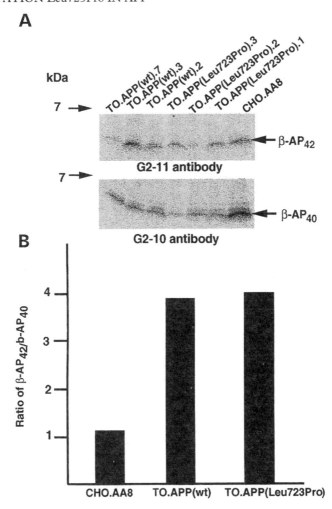

Figure 4. (A) Secretion of β-AP$_{42}$ in inducible clones expressing APP Leu723Pro mutation. Conditioned media from three clones expressing either the wild-type or Leu723Pro mutation were immunoprecipitated with either G2-10 or G2-11. Samples were electrophoresed on a 16% Tris–Tricine gel. (B) Quantification of β-AP levels averaged from the three clones. There does not appear to be a difference between wild-type and mutant inducible APP clones

DISCUSSION

The amyloid cascade hypothesis postulates that the deposition of β-AP is the central causative event in AD and that other features of AD, the neuro-fibrillary tangles, neuronal cell death and dementia, follow as a direct result of this deposition [12]. Studies on the biochemical effect of the familial

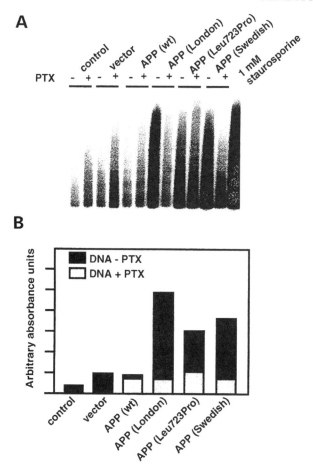

Figure 5. Transient transfection of pCMV-APP mutant constructs into CHO cells induced high levels of apoptotic cells. (A) Cells were seeded onto 24-well plates at a density of 5×10^4 cells/well and transfected with 2 µg of each construct the next day using calcium phosphate precipitation. Genomic DNAs were harvested 48 h after transfection by lysis *in situ* with 7 M guanidine HCl and purified using Wizard Miniprep resin (Promega). 1 µg of genomic DNA from each transfection was endlabelled with [^{32}P]dCTP, electrophoresed on 2% gel and exposed for autoradiography. Apoptosis is indicated by the DNA ladder generated by cleavage of genomic DNA into nucleosome length multimers. (B) Level of apoptosis induced by each construct was quantified using an ELISA assay. Cells were transfected in the same manner as above and contents from each well were harvested and analysed for apoptotic bodies according to the manufacturer's instructions

mutations in the AD genes strongly support the amyloid cascade hypothesis, since a consistent effect of these mutations is the elevated production of β-AP$_{42}$, the more amyloidogenic isoform, since it is highly insoluble and the peptide appears to be the major component of the diffuse plaques seen in both presymptomatic and AD patients [13]. In this study, biochemical analysis of the APP Leu723Pro mutation also supports the amyloid cascade, since clonal lines which constitutively express the mutant APP also result in elevated production of β-AP$_{42}$.

What is also of interest is the implication for the size or sequence specificity of the cleavage site of the γ-secretase in the APP molecule, since the Leu723Pro mutation is located much further downstream of the other known APP mutations (Figure 6). Further functional study is needed to determine

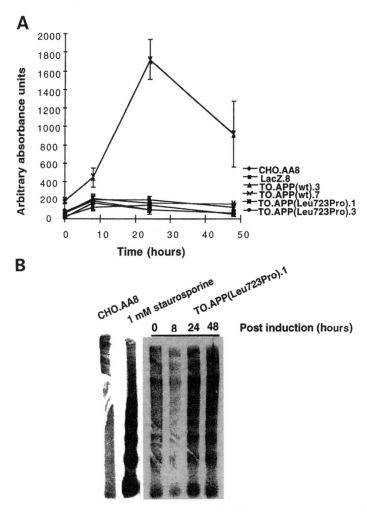

Figure 6. High levels of apoptosis in an inducible clone expressing the APP Leu723Pro mutation. (A) Each clone was seeded in 24-well plates at a density of 5 × 10⁴ cells/well. Tetracycline was removed from the growth medium 24 h later and the level of apoptosis for each time point was quantified by ELISA. (B) Distinctive DNA ladder after gel electrophoresis of genomic DNA isolated from the inducible TO.APP Leu723Pro.1 clone is indicative of apoptosis

the exact nature of the change to the secondary structure of the mutant APP molecule, since the substitution of a proline for the leucine residue at the transmembrane junction is predicted to result in a 'kink' in the protein at the point of substitution, thus altering slightly the position of the APP trans-membrane domain within the cell surface.

Although the β-AP$_{42}$ peptide and the amyloid cascade hypothesis appears to be the underlying biochemical pathway in AD aetiology, yet it is still poss-ible that another neurodegenerative mechanism, apoptosis, may also play a role. Our analysis of the Leu723Pro mutation also indicates that it is capable of inducing apoptosis in CHO cells. To determine the relevance of apoptosis in AD, transgenic mice models which carry various AD mutations can be examined for increased levels of apoptotic neurones. Other APP mutations, such as the Swedish mutation, should also be examined for their ability to induce apoptosis. The challenge is to determine whether the two phenomena of amyloid deposition and apoptosis are indeed independent or, perhaps, are different steps in the same pathway.

ACKNOWLEDGEMENTS

Work in the author's laboratory has been supported by NHMRC through a Block Grant, the Network of Brain Research into Mental Disorders and an Australian Post-Doctoral Fellowship in Dementia. Additional support has been provided by the Vincent Fairfax Family Foundation, the Rebecca L. Cooper Medical Research Foundation, and the Alzheimer's Association (Australia).

REFERENCES

1. Hardy J. Amyloid, the presenilins and Alzheimer's disease. Trends Neurosci 1984; 20: 154–9.
2. Cai X-D, Golde TE, Younkin SG. Release of excess amyloid β-protein from mutant amyloid β-protein precursor. Science 1993; 25: 514–16.
3. Suzuki N et al. An increased percentage of long amyloid β-protein secreted by familial amyloid β-protein precursor (βAPP717) mutant. Science 1994; 264: 1336–40.
4. McKhann G, Drachman D, Folstein M et al. Clinical diagnosis of Alzheimer's disease: report of the NINCDS–ADRDA Work group under the auspices of De-partment of Health and Human Services Task Force on Alzheimer's Disease. Neurology 1984; 34: 939–44.
5. Brooks WS et al. A mutation in codon 717 of the amyloid precursor protein gene in an Australian family with Alzheimer's disease. Neurosci Lett 1995; 199: 183–6.
6. Fuller S et al. Intracellular production of βA4 amyloid of Alzheimer's disease. Biochemistry 1995; 34: 8091–8.

7. Ido N et al. Analaysis of heterogeneous βA4 peptides in human cerebrospinal fluid and blood by a newly developed sensitive Western blot assay. J Biol Chem 1996; 271: 22908–14.

8. Eckman CB et al. A new pathogenic mutation in the APP gene (I716V) increases the relative proportion of Aβ42(43). Hum Mol Genet 1997; 6: 2087–9.

9. Yamatsuji T et al. Expression of V642 APP mutant causes cellular apoptosis as Alzheimer trait-linked phenotype. EMBO J 1996; 15: 498–509.

10. Wolozin B et al. Participation of presenilin 2 in apoptosis. Science 1996; 274: 1710–13.

11. Rosl F. A simple and rapid method for detection of apoptosis in human cells. Nucleic Acids Res 1992; 20: 5243.

12. Hardy JA, Higgins GA. Alzheimer's disease: the amyloid cascade hypothesis. Science 1992; 256: 184–5.

13. Jarrett JT et al. The carboxy-terminus of the β-amyloid protein is critical for the seeding of amyloid formation: implications for the pathogenesis of Alzheimer's disease. Biochemistry 1993; 32: 4693–7.

Address for correspondence:
Peter R. Schofield,
Garvan Institute of Medical Research, Neurobiology Program,
384 Victoria Street, Darlinghurst,
NSW, Australia 2010

11 A Presenilin-1 Truncating Mutation Causing Alzheimer's Disease

C. DE JONGHE, C. TYSOE, M. CRUTS,
I. VANDERHOEVEN, H. VANDERSTICHELE,
E. VANMECHELEN, C. VAN BROECKHOVEN,
D.C. RUBINSZTEIN AND L. HENDRIKS

INTRODUCTION

Mutations in the presenilin-1 (PS-1) gene have been identified that are causative for Alzheimer's disease (AD) [1]. Except for one in-frame deletion of exon 9 ($\Delta9$), all PS-1 mutations are missense mutations. PS-1 mutations are thought to be pathogenic by a gain-of-function mechanism, since it was shown that they alter amyloid precursor protein (APP) processing in such a way that more of the longer 42 amino acids form of Aβ (Aβ_{42}) is secreted [2]. We recently described, in two autopsy-confirmed early-onset AD cases, the first PS-1 truncating mutation, resulting from a base-pair deletion in the consensus sequence of the splice-donor site of intron 4 [3]. The mutation has further been observed independently in three other cases; in one it clearly segregates in a family in an autosomal dominant manner [4] (Hardy et al., unpublished results).

This mutation gave rise to abnormally spliced transcripts lacking the entire exon 4 ($\Delta4$) or part of exon 4 ($\Delta4_{cryptic}$), due to exon skipping or cryptic splicing within exon 4, respectively (Figure 1). In both deletion transcripts the reading frame is shifted, resulting in a premature stop codon. Both $\Delta4$ and $\Delta4_{cryptic}$ transcripts are detected in AD patients, although at a much lower abundance than wild-type PS-1 mRNA. Based on the truncation site and the location of the premature stop codon, we predicted the formation of a C-truncated PS-1 protein, corresponding to a peptide of approximately 7 kDa (Figure 1). We hypothesized that this truncating mutation most likely led to AD pathology through haplo-insufficiency of full-length PS-1. This

Alzheimer's Disease and Related Disorders
Edited by K. Iqbal, D.F. Swaab, B. Winblad and H.M. Wisniewski
© 1999 John Wiley & Sons Ltd

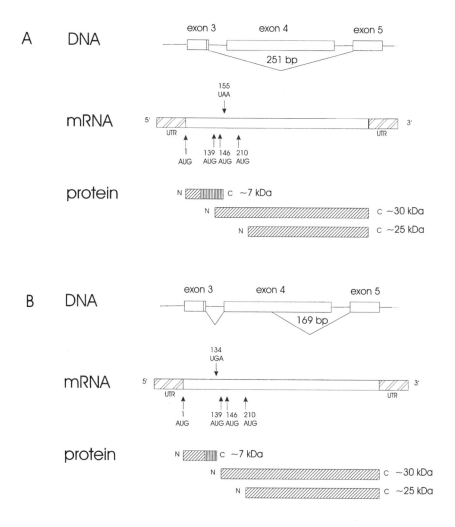

Figure 1. Schematic representation of the truncated proteins generated by PS-1 Δ4 (A) and PS-1 Δ4$_{cryptic}$ (B). Premature stop codons and alternative initiation codons are indicated. Truncated proteins are represented as hatched boxes. Frameshifted regions are vertically hatched

contrasts with the PS-1 missense mutations, which are thought to confer a gain-of-function.

In this study we examined the cell biology of this PS-1 truncating mutation *in vitro* by Western blotting of transient and stable cDNA transfectants and *in vivo* by Western blotting and immunoprecipitation of brain tissue.

IN VITRO EXPRESSION OF PS-1 Δ4 AND Δ4$_{cryptic}$ cDNA CONSTRUCTS

Δ4 and Δ4$_{cryptic}$ cDNA constructs were generated by site-directed mutagenesis of the wild-type (WT) PS-1 cDNA cloned downstream of the cytomegalovirus promotor in pCDNA3. The Δ4 and Δ4$_{cryptic}$ constructs were identical to the mutant PS-1 cDNAs, present in the brains of the two AD patients with the truncating mutation.

WT, Δ4 and Δ4$_{cryptic}$ PS-1 cDNAs were used to transiently transfect CHO.K1 cells and to generate monoclonal stable HEK-293 cell lines. Cell lysates from transfected cells were analysed by Western blotting using SB129, an antiserum directed against the N-terminus (amino acids 3–18) of PS-1, and αPS1loop antiserum, directed against the large sixth hydrophilic loop of PS-1 [5]. SB129 only recognized a band of 46 kDa in WT PS-1 transfectants, corresponding to the full-length PS-1. In the stable cell lines, the ~28 kDA N-terminal PS-1 fragment (NTF), resulting from endoproteolytic processing of the endogenous PS-1, was also observed. The predicted ~7 kDa C-truncated PS-1 peptide (PS-1$_{Ctrunc}$) was not detected. Immunoprecipitation on the medium of Δ4 and Δ4$_{cryptic}$ transfectants excluded that the PS-1$_{Ctrunc}$ peptide was secreted. Upon inhibiting non-lysosomal degradation in stably transfected cells by treating them with 50 μM ALLN, the ~7 kDa PS-1$_{Ctrunc}$ was observed in cells expressing Δ4$_{cryptic}$ but not in those expressing Δ4. These data indicate that PS-1$_{Ctrunc}$ is formed but is rapidly degraded under normal cell culture conditions.

Immunoblotting with αPS-1 loop showed two aberrant bands of ~30 kDa and ~25 kDa in lysates of Δ4 and Δ4$_{cryptic}$ transfectants, next to the ~18 kDa C-terminal PS-1 fragment (CTF) in the stable cell lines. Both bands were also present in the cell lysates of WT PS-1, although at significantly lower expression levels compared to the full-length 46 kDa PS-1 band.

Since the aberrant ~30 kDa and ~25 kDa PS-1 bands are negative for the SB129 N-terminal antiserum, we hypothesized that they correspond to N-truncated PS-1 proteins (PS-1$_{Ntrunc}$), resulting from alternative translation initiation. To test this hypothesis, we used site-directed mutagenesis of the Δ4 and Δ4$_{cryptic}$ cDNA constructs to replace the putative alternative initiation codons (ATG) codons by Ala (GCG) codons. After transient transfection of these mutant constructs in CHO cells, cell lysates were analysed by Western blotting with αPS1loop. Our mutagenesis data are consistent with the two aberrant proteins of ~30 kDa and ~25 kDA being N-truncated proteins resulting from alternative initiation of translation at, respectively, Met139 and Met210 in the deletion mutants.

IN VIVO ANALYSIS OF PS-1 EXPRESSION

Frozen brain tissue of the two patients with the truncating mutation was homogenized and analysed by Western blotting and immunoprecipitation with SB129 and αPS1loop antisera. No full-length PS-1 was detected; only the ~28 kDa NTF and ~18 kDa CTF fragments derived from conventional endoproteolytic processing of PS-1 were observed. The PS-1$_{Ctrunc}$ and PS-1$_{Ntrunc}$ were not observed.

EFFECT OF Δ4 AND Δ4$_{cryptic}$ ON SECRETED Aβ_{42} LEVELS

Aβ_{42} concentrations were measured in conditioned media of stable Δ4 and Δ4$_{cryptic}$ transfectants, using an adapted version of the INNOTEST β-amyloid$_{1-42}$ ELISA test [6]. No significant increase in secreted Aβ_{42} concentrations was observed. However, three different PS-1 mutations, I143T, G384A and Δ9, giving rise to AD with similar onset ages and disease progression as the PS-1 truncating mutation, were analysed for Aβ_{42} secretion, using the same ELISA, and showed significant increases in secreted Aβ_{42} (~5.5-fold for G384A, $p = 0.0009$; ~2-fold for I143T, $p = 0.0115$; and for Δ9, $p = 0.0117$). We also measured Aβ_{40} concentrations in the same media of transfectants using an Aβ_{40} ELISA assay. No significant differences were observed for any of the PS-1 mutant transfectants compared to WT PS-1 transfectants.

DISCUSSION

To investigate how the intron 4 truncating mutation leads to AD, we generated Δ4 and Δ4$_{cryptic}$ cDNA transcripts and transfected them into mammalian cells. We showed that the predicted PS-1 C-truncated peptide of ~7 kDa (PS-1$_{Ctrunc}$) is formed, although only in the Δ4$_{cryptic}$ transfectants, but is rapidly degraded since it was only detectable after inhibiting the non-lysosomal degradation pathway of the cell. This rapid degradation is not unexpected because PS-1$_{Ctrunc}$ is a short peptide containing several hydrophilic or charged residues and is not inserted in the membrane. PS-1$_{Ctrunc}$ is therefore not likely to be functionally active. In addition to PS-1$_{Ctrunc}$ N-truncated PS-1 peptides of ~30 and ~25 kDa (PS-1$_{Ntrunc}$), resulting from alternative translation initiation at Met139 and to a lesser extent at Met210, are formed from both truncating cDNA constructs. For Δ4$_{cryptic}$, Met139 is located downstream of the premature stop codon at codon 134 (Figure 1), allowing the ribosomes to reinitiate translation at Met139 (or Met210) with the formation of both PS-1$_{Ctrunc}$ and PS-1$_{Ntrunc}$. For Δ4, however, Met139 is located upstream of the premature stop codon 155 (Figure 1), implying that PS-1$_{Ctrunc}$ and PS-1$_{Ntrunc}$ cannot be translated from the same transcript in this case. Only PS-1$_{Ntrunc}$ but no PS-1$_{Ctrunc}$ were detected in cells expressing Δ4 cDNA, suggesting that translation initiation immediately took place at Met139, skipping Met1 completely.

Missense PS-1 mutations are believed to be pathogenic by a gain-of-function in which $A\beta_{42}$ secretion is selectively increased. We measured $A\beta_{42}$ concentrations in media from $\Delta4$ and $\Delta4_{cryptic}$ stable transfectants and observed no significant increase in $A\beta_{42}$ secretion when compared to WT PS-1. Since all PS-1 mutations tested so far have shown an increase in $A\beta_{42}$ secretion [2], the lack of increased $A\beta_{42}$ secretion in $\Delta4$ and $\Delta4_{cryptic}$ transfectants may suggest that the intron 4 truncating mutation is unrelated to AD pathology. Another explanation is that secreted $A\beta_{42}$ levels are an epiphenomenon. We and others [7] have shown that secreted $A\beta_{42}$ levels do not correlate with onset age in AD patients. Our data on $A\beta_{42}$ secretion in the truncating mutation, as well as the missense mutants, do not imply that altered APP metabolism is not involved in AD pathophysiology in PS-1 mutation patients. All these patients show extensive accumulation in the brain of particularly $A\beta_{42}$ in senile plaques [8, 9] (Singleton et al., unpublished results). It is possible that PS-1 mutations lead to intracellular accumulation of $A\beta_{42}$ and/or $A\beta_{40}$. Intracellular $A\beta_{40}$ or $A\beta_{42}$ concentrations have not been reported for PS-1 mutations. However, decreased intracellular $A\beta_{42}$ could be measured in primary hippocampal neurones of PS-1 null mice [6]. In these cells, loss of PS-1 activity is believed to prohibit APP processing into $A\beta_{42}$.

Since PS-1_{Ntrunc} proteins are made, at least in the cell systems we used, the intron 4 truncating mutation is not a nonsense mutation *sensu stricto*. In brains of patients with this mutation, the truncating transcripts are present at much lower levels than the WT PS-1 transcript of the normal allele [3]. Therefore, it can be expected that the PS-1_{Ctrunc} and PS-1_{Ntrunc} are formed at minor concentrations. The PS-1_{Ctrunc} are most likely rapidly degraded through the non-lysosomal pathway, as suggested by our *in vitro* experiments. The PS-1_{Ntrunc}, on the other hand, have respectively six and four intact TM domains, suggesting that they may be integrated into the membrane. However, in brain homogenates of two patients with the intron 4 truncating mutation [3], we could not detect the PS-1_{Ntrunc} proteins. In brain, PS-1 is endoproteolytically cleaved, leaving no or almost no full-length PS-1 [5, 10]. Possibly the proteolytic products of PS-1_{Ntrunc} are rapidly degraded, leaving only the NTF and CTF corresponding to the normal PS-1 allele. In this case, AD pathophysiology in the intron 4 truncating mutation would result from haplo-insufficiency of PS-1, as we have previously hypothesized [3]. Haplo-insufficiency of PS-1 was also suggested by the functional assays in *Caenorhabditis elegans* indicating that PS-1 mutant proteins (missense and $\Delta9$) have a reduced capacity to rescue the sel-12 mutant phenotype [11, 12].

Our *in vivo* and *in vitro* data on the intron 4 truncating mutation provide evidence that in humans, reduced activity of PS-1 may lead to AD in the absence of increased secreted $A\beta_{42}$. Whether the reduced activity of PS-1 relates to an altered APP metabolism remains to be determined.

ACKNOWLEDGEMENTS

This work was supported by the Fund for Scientific Research—Flanders (Belgium) (FWO-F), the Flemish Biotechnology Program COT-04, the Inter-University Attraction Poles (IUAP P4/17), the International Alzheimer's Research Foundation (IARF), the EC BIOTECH Program (BIO2-CT96-0743), the Focused Giving Program of Johnson & Johnson, and Addenbrooke's NHS Trust. Part of the work was performed at the Mayo Clinic, Jacksonville, USA, and was sponsored by a travel and accommodation award to C.D.J. from the FWO-F. C.D.J. is a research assistant of the FWO-F. D.C.R. is a Glaxo Wellcome Research Fellow. We thank S.S. Sisodia and G. Thinakaran for providing us with the αPS1loop and F. Checler for the FCA3340 antiserum.

REFERENCES

1. Cruts M, Van Broeckhoven C. Presenilin mutations in Alzheimer's disease. Hum Mut 1998; 11: 183–90.
2. Kim T-W, Tanzi R. Presenilins and Alzheimer's disease. Curr Opin Neurobiol 1997; 7: 683–8.
3. Tysoe C et al. A presenilin-1 truncating mutation is present in two cases with autopsy-confirmed early-onset Alzheimer's disease. Am J Hum Genet 1998; 62: 70–76.
4. Mullan M et al. A locus for familial early-onset Alzheimer's disease on the long arm of chromosome 14, proximal to the α1-antichymotrypsin gene. Nature Genet 1992; 2: 340–42.
5. Thinakaran G et al. Endoproteolysis of presenilin 1 and accumulation of processed derivatives *in vivo*. Neuron 1996; 17: 181–90.
6. De Strooper B et al. Deficiency of presenilin-1 inhibits the normal cleavage of amyloid precursor protein. Nature 1998; 391: 387–90.
7. Mehta N et al. Increased $A\beta_{42(43)}$ from cell lines expressing presenilin-1 mutations. Ann Neurol 1998; 43: 256–8.
8. Mann DM et al. Amyloid β-protein (Aβ) deposition in chromosome 14-linked Alzheimer's disease: predominance of $A\beta_{42(43)}$. Ann Neurol 1996; 40: 149–56.
9. Lemere CA et al. The E280A presenilin 1 Alzheimer mutation produces increased $A\beta_{42}$ deposition and severe cerebellar pathology. Nat Med 1996; 2: 1146–50.
10. Hendriks L et al. Processing of presenilin 1 in brains of patients with Alzheimer's disease and controls. Neuroreport 1997; 8: 1717–21.
11. Levitan D et al. Assessment of normal and mutant human presenilin function in *Caenorhabditis elegans*. Proc Natl Acad Sci USA 1996; 93: 14940–44.
12. Baumeister R et al. Human presenilin-1, but not familial Alzheimer's disease (FAD) mutants, facilitate *Caenorhabditis elegans* Notch signally independently of proteolytic processing. Genes Funct 1997; 1: 149–59.

Address for correspondence:
Professor C. Van Broeckhoven,
Neurogenetics Laboratory, University of Antwerp (UIA),
Department of Biochemistry, Universiteitsplein 1,
B-2610 Antwerpen, Belgium
Tel: +32 3 8202601; fax +32 3 8202541;
e-mail: CV.broek@uia.ua.ac.be

12 Glu318Gly in Presenilin-1 Is a Neutral Mutation in Relation to Dementia: The Rotterdam Study

BART DERMAUT, MARC CRUTS, ARJEN J.C. SLOOTER,
SOFIE VAN GESTEL, CHRIS DE JONGHE,
HUBERT BACKHOVENS, HUGO VANDERSTICHELE,
EUGEEN VANMECHELEN, MONIQUE M.B. BRETELER,
ALBERT HOFMAN, LYDIA HENDRIKS,
CORNELIA M. VAN DUIJN AND
CHRISTINE VAN BROECKHOVEN

INTRODUCTION

Presenilin-1 (PSEN = gene; psen = protein) missense mutations are generally considered fully penetrant disease-causing mutations [1]. Mostly they are found in patients with a positive family history of early-onset Alzheimer's disease (AD) compatible with autosomal dominant inheritance. Patients within PSEN1 families and unrelated individuals carrying the same mutation usually display very similar onset ages [2]. The PSEN1 gene consists of 10 coding (exons 3–12) and three non-coding exons (exons 1A, 1B and 2) transcribed into a major messenger of 2.7 kb [3] that codes for a 467 amino acid protein. The psen are predominantly localized in the membranes of the rough endoplasmic reticulum and are predicted to have 6–8 transmembrane (TM) domains and 1 large hydrophilic loop (HL) between TM-VI and TM-VII. HL-VI as well as the N- and C-termini of Psen1 are located cytoplasmically [4]. Notably, 60% of all mutations involve TM-II and HL-VI. The other mutations are spread over the rest of Psen1, with the exception of those regions that are not conserved in Psen2: the N-terminal domain (exon 3), the middle part of HL-VI (exon 10) and the C-terminal region (exon 12).

The mechanisms by which variations in the PSEN genes lead to AD remains largely unknown. However, an increasing amount of *in vivo* and *in vitro* evidence suggests that missense mutations in PSEN1 and PSEN2 express their pathogenic effect by (in)directly processing the amyloid precursor protein (app) in such a way that increased levels of the fibrillogenic 42 amino

Alzheimer's Disease and Related Disorders
Edited by K. Iqbal, D.F. Swaab, B. Winblad and H.M. Wisniewski
© 1999 John Wiley & Sons Ltd

acid form of the amyloid β-peptide (A$β_{42}$) are produced [5]. A$β_{42}$ is believed to be pathogenic, since it is more prone to aggregation and therefore leads to accelerated accumulation in AD brain lesions, the senile plaques.

An A to G transition at codon 318 in exon 9 of PSEN1 resulting in the non-conserved Glu to Gly substitution has been reported by us [6] and others [7, 8] in familial AD, with onset ages varying between 46 and 68 years. However, owing to lack of sufficient family members, no proven co-segregation of PSEN1 Glu318Gly with AD has been demonstrated. Also, in contrast to the majority of the other psen1 amino acid substitutions, Glu318Gly is located in a region of psen1 (the middle part of HL-VI) that is not conserved between human psen1 or psen2, or in the psen-homologues *Drosophila* psen1 and *C. elegans* sel-12 [2]. Together, (a) the wide range of onset ages of AD; (b) the lack of well-demonstrated co-segregation of the mutation with AD; and (c) its location in a non-conserved region of the protein, led us to hypothesize that PSEN1 Glu318Gly is incompletely penetrant and that its expression might be modified by other genetic and/or environmental factors. Alternatively, it could represent a rare polymorphism potentially associated with an increased risk of developing AD or other types of dementia.

The present study aimed at assigning a more conclusive role to the PSEN1 Glu318Gly mutation in relation to AD and other types of dementia. In order to evaluate the frequency of Glu318Gly and its contribution to the dementia phenotype, we screened incident and prevalent demented cases and age- and sex-matched controls derived from the Rotterdam Study, a population-based study of elderly people [9]. The potential role of this mutation in app processing was assessed by measuring the secretion of A$β_{42}$ in media of cell lines stably transfected with the Glu318Gly cDNA.

RESULTS

MUTATION SCREENING

All 10 275 residents of a Rotterdam suburb who were 55 years and older were eligible; 7983 (78%) agreed to take part in the study and cognitive functioning was assessed in 7528 (73%) [9]. Screen-positive persons were further evaluated using an interview with a close relative, neuropsychological tests, neurological examination and, if possible, neuro-imaging. A panel of physicians, a neurologist and a neuropsychologist diagnosed dementia based on the DSM-IIIR definition [10]. AD was diagnosed and subtyped according to the NINCDS–ADRDA criteria [11]. Both possible and probable AD cases were grouped in this category. Vascular dementia was diagnosed according to NINCDS–AIREN criteria [12]. For the other dementias the DSM-IIIR definition was used; 474 prevalent demented cases were diagnosed [13] and during mean follow-up of 2.1 (range 1.5–3.4) years, another 146 incident cases of dementia were detected [14]. For 345 prevalent cases, 134 incident cases and 256 controls, blood samples for DNA extraction were available. Controls were randomly selected from participants in the Rotterdam Study and group-matched on age (per 5 years) and sex. To facilitate rapid screening for the mutation, we developed a mismatch PCR assay that allows detection of the mutation by *BstNI* digestion of the mismatch PCR product.

The mutation was observed in two incident (1.5%), 11 prevalent (3.4%) demented cases and nine (4.1%) non-demented aged subjects (Table 1). Out of 13 demented Glu318Gly carriers, 10 were diagnosed with AD (four possible AD and six probable AD), one with Parkinson's disease dementia, one with vascular dementia and one with dementia associated with multiple sclerosis. However, the mutation frequencies were not statistically different between incident/prevalent demented cases and controls (p = 0.22 and p = 0.65, respectively), or between incident and prevalent cases (p = 0.37). Mean age at onset was similar in demented Glu318Gly carriers (83.4 ± 4.7 years) vs. demented non-carriers (81.0 ± 7.7 years) (p = 0.22). As reflected in the Mini-Mental State Examination scores, cognitive functioning of aged non-demented subjects was similar in Glu318Gly-carriers (26.4 ± 2.9) vs. non-carriers (27.0 ± 2.0) (p = 0.71).

Table 1. Identification of the Glu318Gly substitution in subjects from the Rotterdam Study

	Subjects investigated (n)	Subjects with the Glu318Gly mutation [n (%)]
Incident demented patients	131	2 (1.5%)[a]
Prevalent demented patients	326	11 (3.4%)[b]
Controls	219	9 (4.1%)

[a] Fisher exact test: p = 0.22 compared to controls.
[b] χ^2 = 0.25; p = 0.65 compared to controls.

$A\beta_{42}$ SECRETION

$A\beta_{42}$ levels were measured in conditioned media of human embryonic kidney cells (HEK-293) stably expressing Glu318Gly PSEN1 and cell lines transfected with wild-type (WT) PSEN1 were used as reference. No significant differences in $A\beta_{42}$ levels were observed (p = 0.12).

DISCUSSION

To evaluate the contribution of Glu318Gly in AD and other types of dementia, we screened a set of incident as well as prevalent demented cases vs. sex-

and age-matched controls derived from a population-based study, the Rotterdam Study. We found the mutation in cases as well as controls with a frequency for the mutant allele of 1.6%. The Glu318Gly mutation was less frequent in the dementia patients than in the control subjects, although the difference was not statistically significant. We detected no influence of the mutation on onset age of dementia or cognitive functioning of aged non-demented control subjects. Also, the similar mutation frequencies in incident and prevalent cases suggests that there is no influence of Glu318Gly on the duration of disease. Interestingly, allele sharing analysis in Glu318Gly carriers with polymorphic markers within and near PSEN1 revealed common alleles shared by all mutation carriers from The Netherlands, Belgium, Germany and Colombia (data not shown). The latter suggests that the Glu318Gly mutation is an ancient mutation originating from one common founder. Our *in vitro* data, showing no increase in secreted $A\beta_{42}$ levels in conditioned media of stable transfected cells, are consistent with our findings at the population level. Together, these findings strongly suggest that the Glu318Gly mutation is not causally related to AD or dementia in general.

Nevertheless, a few possibilities have remained unexplored in the present study. First, as we detected the mutation only in the heterozygous state, we cannot exclude that Glu318Gly is associated with dementia in an autosomal recessive way. However, there is no evidence supporting autosomal recessive inheritance in familial AD [15]. The allele frequency as observed in the studied population predicts a very low *a priori* probability (1/5000) of detecting a homozygous carrier, which makes it very hard to exclude the possibility of Glu318Gly being a recessive mutation. Another as-yet unexcluded possibility is that all PSEN1 Glu318Gly mutation carriers share a (disease) phenotype that is different from dementia and has remained undetected in the present study. This seems unlikely, since no non-dementia phenotypes have been associated with genetic variations in PSEN1. However, with respect to these considerations, we believe that it is premature to call Glu318Gly a neutral polymorphism but rather, in relation to the studied phenotype 'dementia', a neutral mutation.

In conclusion, we report that Glu318Gly is the first missense mutation in PSEN1 that is not causally related to AD or other types of dementia. Therefore, the occurrence of AD in Glu318Gly cases has another genetic and/or environmental aetiology. Since PSEN1 Glu318Gly is currently considered a causative mutation in AD and frequently found all over the world, our results have major implications in genetic counselling.

ACKNOWLEDGEMENTS

We are grateful to Marleen Van den Broeck and Sally Serneels for their skilled technical assistance in the mutation screening and genotyping. We thank

Alewijn Ott, Frans van Harskamp, Inge de Koning, Maarten de Rijk and Sandra Kalmijn for their contribution in the dementia diagnosis. This work was funded in part by a special research project of the University of Antwerp (UA), the Fund for Scientific Research in Flanders (FWO) and the International Alzheimer's Disease Research Fund (IARF), Belgium; and by the NESTOR stimulation programme for scientific research in The Netherlands (Ministry of Health and Ministry of Education), The Netherlands Organization for Scientific Research (NOW), The Netherlands Prevention Fund, and the municipality of Rotterdam, The Netherlands.

REFERENCES

1. Van Broeckhoven C. Presenilins and Alzheimer disease. Nature Genet 1995; 11: 230–32.
2. Cruts M, Van Broeckhoven C. Presenilin mutations in Alzheimer's disease. Hum Mutat 1998; 11: 183–90.
3. Rogaev EI et al. Analysis of the 5' sequence, genomic structure, and alternative splicing of the presenilin-1 gene (PSEN1) associated with early onset Alzheimer disease. Genomics 1997; 40: 415–24.
4. Li X, Greenwald I. Membrane topology of the *C. elegans* SEL-12 presenilin. Neuron 1996; 17: 1015–21.
5. Hardy J. Amyloid, the presenilins and Alzheimer's disease. Trends Neurosci 1997; 20: 154–9.
6. Cruts M et al. Estimation of the genetic contribution of presenilin-1 and -2 mutations in a population based study of presenile Alzheimer disease. Hum Mol Genet 1998; 7: 43–51.
7. Forsell C et al. A novel pathogenic mutation (Leu262Phe) found in the presenilin 1 gene in early-onset Alzheimer's disease. Neurosci Lett 1997; 234: 3–6.
8. Sandbrink R et al. Missense mutations of the PS-1/S182 gene in German early-onset Alzheimer's disease patients. Ann Neurol 1996; 40: 265–6.
9. Hofman A et al. Determinants of disease and disability in the elderly: the Rotterdam Elderly Study. Eur J Epidemiol 1991; 7: 403–22.
10. American Psychiatric Association. Diagnostic and Statistical Manual of Mental Disorders, 3rd edn, Revised. Washington, DC, American Psychiatric Association.
11. McKhann G et al. Clinical diagnosis of Alzheimer's disease: report of the NINCDS–ADRDA Work Group under the auspices of Department of Health and Human Services Task Force on Alzheimer's Disease. Neurology 1984; 34: 939–44.
12. Roman GC et al. Vascular dementia: diagnostic criteria for research studies. Report of the NINDS–AIREN International Workshop. Neurology 1993; 43: 250–60.
13. Ott A et al. Prevalence of Alzheimer's disease and vascular dementia: association with education. The Rotterdam Study. Br Med J 1995; 310: 970–73.
14. Ott A et al. The incidence and risk of dementia. The Rotterdam Study. Am J Epidemiol 1998; 147: 574–80.

15. Rao Vs et al. Multiple etiologies for Alzheimer disease are revealed by segregation analysis. Am J Hum Genet 1994; 55: 991–1000.

Address for correspondence:
    Professor Christine Van Broeckhoven,
    Laboratory of Neurogenetics, University of Antwerp (UIA),
    Department of Biochemistry, Universiteitsplein 1,
    B-2610 Antwerpen, Belgium
    Tel: +32 3 8202601; fax: +32 3 8202541;
    e-mail: cv.broeck@uia.ua.ac.be

13 Association of Genetic Risk Factors in Alzheimer's Disease and a Novel Mutation in the Predicted TM2 Domain of the Presenilin-2 Gene in Late-onset AD

RAMÓN CACABELOS, KATRIN BEYER, JOSÉ I. LAO, MARÍA D. MESA AND LUCÍA FERNÁNDEZ-NOVOA

INTRODUCTION

The most important factors for Alzheimer's disease (AD) include advanced age, family history of dementia, and the inheritance of AD-related genotypes. In population studies, a family history of dementia appears in 40–65% of cases; however, this frequency varies according to the most prevalent genotypes present in AD families. At the present time there are at least seven different genetic profiles (or defects) associated with AD, including genetic loci on chromosomes 1 (presenilin-2 gene (PS2), 1q31–42), 12 (A2M, LRP1 genes), 14 (presenilin-1 gene (PS1), 14q24.3, and c-FOS gene, 14q24.3–31), 19 (apolipoprotein (APOE) gene, 10q12–23.3), 21 [amyloid precursor protein (APP) gene, 21q11.1–21.1] and mutations in the mitochondrial DNA (Table 1) [1–2]. Specific mutations in the APP, PS1 and PS2 genes can lead to autosomal dominant forms of early-onset AD (EOAD). The intronic polymorphism of the PS1 locus shows the following frequencies: (a) PS1-1/1, 47% in EOAD, 26.5% in late-onset AD (LOAD) and 11.1% in controls; (b) PS1-1/2, 38.2% in EOAD, 53% in LOAD and 55.6% in controls; and (c) PS1-2/2, 14.7% in EOAD, 18.1% in LOAD and 33.3% in controls [2, 3]. Homozygosity for the allele of the PS1 gene seems to confer an increased risk for AD. More than 30 mutations have been described in the PS1 locus [4] (Table 1). Mutations at the PS2 locus account for a small number of autosomal dominant EOAD cases [2, 5] and some mutations in the TM domains are

Alzheimer's Disease and Related Disorders
Edited by K. Iqbal, D.F. Swaab, B. Winblad and H.M. Wisniewski
© 1999 John Wiley & Sons Ltd

also associated with LOAD [2, 5, 6]. PS1 and PS2 share extensive amino acid sequence homology and contain between seven and nine transmembrane (TM) domains where most mutations occur. Several missense mutations in the amyloid precursor protein gene (APP) on chromosome 21 have been found in about 3% of familial EOAD, in which about 50% of the relatives appear affected across several generations. This familial pattern is consistent with an autosomal dominant inheritance. In the Spanish population the presence of APP mutations is approximately 1/1000. The most extensively studied susceptibility gene for AD is APOE [6–13]. The frequencies of the major APOE genotypes in dementia are the following: (a) APOE-2/3, 4.3% in AD, 7.6% in vascular dementia (VD) and 5.1% in controls; (b) APOE-2/4, 0.5% in AD, 0.8% in VD and 1.7% in controls; (c) APOE-3/3, 46.5% in AD, 38.1% in VD and 69.5% in controls; (d) APOE-3/4, 36.2% in AD, 43.2% in VD and 22.6% in controls; and (e) APOE-4/4, 12.4% in AD, 10.2% in VD and 1.1% in controls [1, 2, 14]. The risk of AD increases from 20% to 90%, and the mean age at onset decreases from 84 to 68 years, as the number of APOE-4 alleles increases in families with LOAD [1, 7, 14]. The frequency of the APOE-4 allele is also 2.3 times higher among EOAD cases (35%) than in controls (15%), and is 1.6 times higher in those EOAD cases with a family history of dementia (41%) than in those with a negative family history (25%) [8]. APOE-4 may also be a risk factor for VD.

In the present study we have investigated the frequency of the association of different genetic risk factors (APOE, PS1, PS2, c-FOS, APP) in Spanish AD cases and the potential influence of the coexistence of defective genetic loci on the phenotypic expression of AD (age at onset). Furthermore, we report here the identification of a novel mutation in the PS2 locus in a LOAD case. At present, 33 missense mutations have been detected in the PS1 gene of 61 AD kindreds, and a point mutation upstream of a splice acceptor site which results in an in-frame deletion of exon 9 in several AD pedigrees linked to chromosome 14 [15]. However, in the PS-2 gene only two missense mutations have been identified in eight pedigrees [5, 16]. The N141I mutation within the transmembrane 2 (TM2) domain, consisting of an A to T substitution, was detected in seven Volga-German pedigrees with a disease onset between 44 and 75 years of age [5]. The M239V mutation within the TM5 domain was described in an Italian pedigree (age at onset: 50 years), consisting in an A to G substitution [16]. In our case, we have detected a new mutation (V148I) in the TM2 domain of the PS2 locus in a patient with LOAD.

MATERIAL AND METHODS

The frequency of different AD genotypes was studied in 82 patients with the clinical diagnosis of AD according to DSM-IV and NINCDS–ADRDA

Table 1. Alzheimer's disease-associated genetic risk factors

Chromosome	Locus	Mutation	Gene	Frequency (%)
1	1q31–42/TM2	N141I	PS2	<5
	TM5	M239V	PS2	
	TM2/E5	V148I	PS2	
12	D12S373	?	?	?
	D12S1057			
	D12S1042			
	D12S390			
	12p	–	A2M	10–20?
	12q	–	LRP1	10?
14	14q24.3/TM1	V82L	PS1	60–80
	IL-1	Y115H	PS1	
	TM2	M139T		
	TM2	M139V		
	TM2	M139I		
	TM2	I143T		
	TM2	M146L		
	TM2	M146V		
	TM3	H163R		
	TM3	H163Y		
	TM5	A231T		
	TM6	A246E		
	TM6	A260V		
	TM6	C263R		
	TM6	P264L		
	EL-3	P267S		
	EL-3	E280A		
	EL-3	E280G		
	EL-3	A285V		
	EL-3	L286V		
	EL-3	G384A		
	EL-3	L392V		
	EL-3	C410Y		
14	14q24.3–31	c-Fos(–/+)(+/+)	c-Fos	10–40
19	19q12–23.3		APOE-4/4	5–20
			APOE-3/4	35–50
			APOE-3/3	30–45
			APOE-2/4	1–3
			APOE-2/3	2–5
			APOE-2/2	1–5
21	21q11.1–21.1	APP717 V/I	APP	2–3
		APP717 V/P		
		APP717 V/G		
		APP670–671		
Mitochondrial	MtDNA	Maternal	CO I	5–10?
		Heteroplasmy	CO II	

criteria, in whom the genetic screening of the APOE, PS1, PS2, cFOS, and APP genes was simultaneously assessed as described elsewhere [1, 2, 14, 17] (Tables 2 and 3). We have also analyzed the TM2 and TM5 domains of the PS2 gene in AD patients (n = 128, age: 66 ± 12.3 years; range: 44–81 years) who were clinically diagnosed according to *Diagnostic and Statistical Manual of Mental Disorders*, 4th edn (DMS-IV) and National Institute of Neurological and Communicative Disorders and Stroke and the Alzheimer's Disease and Related Disorders Association (NINCDS–ADRDA) criteria, and in a group of age-matched healthy controls (n = 95, age: 65 ± 11.2 years; range: 40–82 years). DNA was purified from peripheral blood lymphocytes by a method without phenol–chloroform extraction. We have designed a new method to detect all possible mutations on the TM2 and TM5 domains of the PS2 gene. A multiplex polymerase chain reaction (PCR) of these regions was carried out using primers previously described [5, 16]. PCR products were visualized by agarose gel electrophoresis to discard possible large deletions affecting all or parts of these regions. In a genetic screening for point mutations, we developed a single-strand conformation polymorphism (SSCP) analysis of multiplex PCR products. Mutations detected by this screening procedure were characterized by DNA sequencing using the ALFexpress DNA sequencer (Pharmacia Biotech).

Table 2. Frequency of genetic risk factors in Alzheimer's disease

APOE	Frequency (n) %	PS1 (1/1) (n) %	PS1 (1/2) (n) %	PS1 (2/2) (n) %	PS2 (–) (n) %	PS2 (+) (n) %	cFOS (–/–) (n) %	cFOS (+/–) (n) %	cFOS (+/+) (n) %
2/2	(0) 0	(0) 0	(0) 0	(0) 0	(0) 0	(0) 0	(0) 0	(0) 0	(0) 0
2/3	(1) 1.2	(1) 3.6	(0) 0	(0) 0	(0) 0	(0) 0	(1) 1.6	(0) 0	(0) 0
2/4	(3) 3.7	(1) 3.6	(0) 0	(2) 12.5	(2) 4.4	(1) 2.8	(2) 3.1	(1) 6.3	(0) 0
3/3	(33) 40.2	(11) 39.3	(18) 47.4	(4) 25.0	(14) 31.1	(19) 52.8	(28) 43.8	(5) 31.3	(0) 0
3/4	(35) 42.7	(11) 39.3	(16) 42.1	(8) 50.0	(21) 46.7	(14) 38.9	(26) 40.6	(7) 43.8	(2) 100
4/4	(10) 12.2	(4) 14.3	(4) 10.5	(2) 12.5	(8) 17.8	(2) 5.6	(7) 10.9	(3) 18.8	(0) 0
Total	(82) 100	(28) 34.14	(38) 46.84	(16) 19.51	(45) 54.87	(36) 43.90	(64) 78.04	(16) 19.51	(2) 2.44

Table 3. Frequency of associated genetic risk factors in Alzheimer's disease

Genetic risk factors	Frequency (n)%	Onset years(range)
APOE-3/4	(12) 14.6	68 ± 9 (53–77)
APOE-4/4	(3) 3.6	69 ± 2 (67–71)
APOE-3/4 + PS1(1/1)	(4) 4.9	67 ± 4 (63–73)
APOE-4/4 + PS1(1/1)	(2) 2.4	54 ± 6 (50–59)
APOE-3/4 + PS2(+)	(5) 6.1	68 ± 4 (64–73)
APOE-4/4 + PS2(+)	(1) 1.2	56 (56)
APOE-3/4 + cFOS(+)	(4) 4.9	62 ± 6 (53–68)
APOE-4/4 + cFOS(+)	(2) 2.4	63 ± 5 (60–67)
APOE-3/4 + PS1(1/1) + PS2(+)	(5) 6.1	63 ± 10 (49–73)
APOE-4/4 + PS1(1/1) + PS2(+)	(1) 1.2	72 (72)
APOE-3/4 + PS1(1/1) + PS2(+) + cFOS(+)	(1) 1.2	50 (50)
APOE-4/4 + PS1(1/1) + PS2(+) + cFOS(+)	(0) 0	—

RESULTS

ASSOCIATION OF GENETIC RISK FACTORS

The distribution of frequencies for the APOE genotype in AD patients was the following: 0% APOE-2/2; 1.2% APOE-2/3; 3.7% APOE-2/4; 40.2% APOE-3/3; 42.7% APOE-3/4; and 12.2% APOE-4/4 (Table 2). The frequencies for the intronic polymorphism in the PS1 locus were: 34.14% PS1-1/1; 46.84% PS1-1/2; and 19.51% PS1-2/2 (Table 2). The PS2+ frequency was 43.9%, while the PS2– frequency was 54.87% (Table 2). No cases with APP mutations were found among these 82 patients. The c-FOS locus showed 78.04% of the AD cases with c-FOS–/–, 19.51% with c-FOS+/–, and 2.44% with c-FOS+/+ (Table 2). The most frequent associations of genetic risk factors were APOE-3/4 and PS1-1/1 (4.9%), APOE-3/4 and PS2+ (6.1%), APOE-3/4 and c-FOS+ (4.9%), and APOE-3/4 plus PS1-1/1 plus PS2+ (6.1%), with no apparent statistical significance. However, in those cases with the association of APOE-4/4 and PS1-1/1 as well as those with APOE-4/4 plus PS2+, the age at onset seemed to be anticipated by approximately 10 years as compared with the age at onset of cases with single genetic profiles (Table 3). Although the number of cases is very small to reach conclusions, it appears very plausible that the association of APOE-4/4 with PS1-1/1 or PS2+ genotypes constitutes the highest risk genetic factor for AD.

A NOVEL MISSENSE MUTATION IN THE PS2 LOCUS IN LATE-ONSET ALZHEIMER'S DISEASE

We detected an abnormal SSCP pattern affecting only one patient of our sample who had been clinically diagnosed as a LOAD case (Figure 1). A missense mutation consisting of a G to A substitution on exon 5 of the PS2 gene (Figure 2) was found by DNA sequencing; this results in a Val to Ile substitution at codon 148 within the predicted TM2 domain of the presenilin 2 protein. None of the other subjects of the present study carried the mutation. At the time of the clinical diagnosis, at 76 years of age, the patient was in a stage of moderately severe cognitive impairment according to the Global Deterioration Scale (GDS-3). The age at disease onset was 71 years.

There were no first-degree relatives known with dementia in this family pedigree. However, this case cannot be considered a sporadic case, since there were at least two other members of the family who had exhibited symptoms of possible dementia.

In addition to PS2 screening, we carried out a similar genetic screening of this patient at the level of APP and PS1 genes, excluding further mutations. Since the patient had an APOE-3/3 genotype, we excluded the influence of the allele ε4 or the possible epistatic effect of the APOE-2/3 genotype with the PS2 mutation, which might delay the onset of the disease [18]. Therefore, it

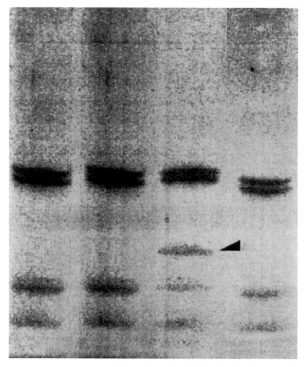

Figure 1. Single-strand conformation polymorphism (SSCP) of the TM2 domain of the PS2 gene. PCR products. Arrowhead = abnormal SSCP pattern

seemed that the V148I mutation by itself might have a pathogenic effect in the origin and clinical course of the AD exhibited by the carrier patient that we describe here.

DISCUSSION

This is the first time that a full screening of genetic risk factors has been investigated in AD patients to study the frequency of potential epistatic effects resulting from the association of genetic risk factors in different segments of the genome. In our study we found that more than 50% of AD patients are carriers of an APOE-4 genotype. Approximately 35% of our patients show a PS1-1/1 genotype and 40% are carriers of a PS2+ genotype. The c-FOS+/+ genotype is very rare in AD (< 3%). With this full genetic screening, we can demonstrate that practically 100% of the AD cases are carriers of some genetic risk factor detectable with molecular markers. In addition, the associations of APOE-4/4 plus PS1-1/1 genotypes and APOE-4/4 plus PS2+ show an anticipation in the age at onset of about 10 years, as compared with APOE-4/4

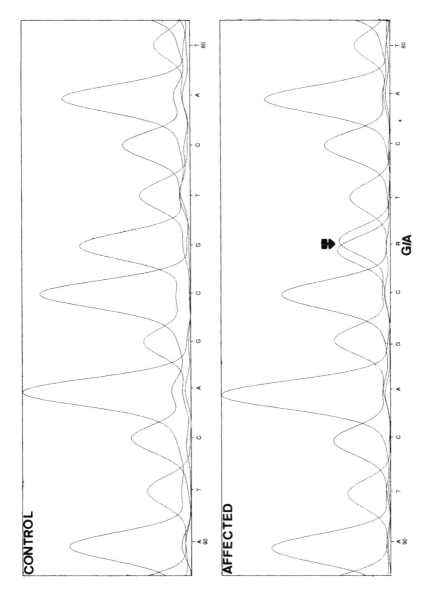

Figure 2. DNA sequence detected in the affected AD patient in comparison with a control sample. G/A = guanine to adenine substitution

alone or PS1-1/1 and PS2+ alone. The youngest case (49 years) was found in a patient with the APOE-3/4 plus PS1-1/1 plus PS2+. According to these preliminary results, it appears that the association of the APOE-4 allele with potential defects in the PS1 or PS2 loci constitute a major susceptibility factor for neurodegeneration and early phenotypic expression of AD. The present report is in agreement with the N141I mutation previously described by others within the predicted TM2 domain of the PS2 gene, since both mutations have been described in LOAD kindreds [5], whereas the mutation within the predicted TM5 domain was found in an EOAD pedigree [18]. Carriers of mutations within the TM2 domain of the PS1 locus have a mean age at onset of 40 years, while the other mutations described in the PS1 gene occur in families with a mean age at onset of 47 years [15]. In our case, the novel mutation (V148I) described here was present in a LOAD patient with no apparent family history of dementia in first-degree relatives, although some members of the family are showing clinical symptoms of mild mental deterioration compatible with a possible dementia. These data suggest that different mutations in specific regions of the TM domains of the PS2 gene might have differential implications in the etiopathogenesis of AD as potential inducers of the neurodegeneration and/or the phenotypic expression of AD at a given age. In addition, the association of homozygocity for APOE-4 plus mutations or specific intronic polymorphisms in the presenilin genes might account for the anticipation of the disease onset following an exponential pattern. Finally, this novel mutation is the third mutation reported in the PS2 gene world-wide and the first presenilin mutation detected in a Spanish AD patient.

ACKNOWLEDGEMENTS

This study was supported by the EuroEspes Foundation.

ABSTRACT

The major risk factors for suffering AD include age, a family history of AD, and the inheritance of a series of potential genetic defects and/or a specific AD-related genotype. In population studies, a family history of AD appears in 40–65% of the cases, but this frequency varies depending upon the AD-genotype present in a particular family. The frequencies of the most common AD-related genotypes in AD patients are the following: APOE-3/3, 40.2%; APOE-3/4, 42.7%; APOE-4/4, 12.2%; PS-1/1, 34.14%; PS1-1/2, 46.34%; PS1-2/2, 19.51%; PS2–, 54.87%; PS2+, 43.9%; c-FOS–/–, 78.04%; c-FOS+/–, 19.51%; and c-FOS+/+, 2.44%. The association of APOE-4/4 and PS1-1/1, as well as the association of APOE-4/4 and PS2+, tend to induce an anticipation of the disease onset of approximately 10 years. However, mutations in the PS1 and PS2 loci are present in both early- and late-onset AD cases. Mutations in the PS2 gene are less frequent than mutations in the PS1 gene. Most mutations (> 30) described in the PS1 gene were found in early-onset AD patients, and two missense mutations have been described in the PS2 locus in some AD pedigrees. We have analyzed the TM2 and TM5 domains of the PS2 gene in Spanish AD patients and in a group of age-matched healthy controls and found one patient with late-onset AD with a novel missense mutation consisting of a guanine-to-adenine substitution on exon 5 of the PS2 gene, which results in a Val to Ile substitution at codon 148 within the predicted TM2 domain of the PS2 protein. This is the third muta-tion described in the PS2 gene and the first presenilin mutation detected in a Spanish AD patient. Both the N141I mutation and the V148I mutation de-scribed here are located within the predicted TM2 domain and both were found in late-onset AD kindreds, whereas the mutation within the predicted TM5 domain was found in an early-onset AD pedigree. Carriers of mutations within the TM2 domain of the PS1 gene have a mean age at onset of 40 years, while the other mutations in the PS1 locus occur in families with a mean age at onset of 47 years. These results seem to indicate that both specific mutations in the PS1 and PS2 loci and the association of genetic defects in the PS genes with the APOE-4/4 genotype are risk factors of maximum vulnerability for neurodegeneration and the early phenotypic expression of AD clinical symptoms.

REFERENCES

1. Cacabelos R. Diagnosis of Alzheimer's disease: defining genetic profiles (genotype vs. phenotype). Acta Neurol Scand 1996; suppl 165: 72–84.
2. Beyer K, Lao JI, Cacabelos R. Molecular genetics and genotyping in Alzheimer's disease. Ann Psychiat 1996; 6: 173–87.
3. Wragg M, Hutton M, Talbot C and the Alzheimer's Disease Collaborative Group. Genetic association between intronic polymorphism in presenilin-1 gene and late-onset Alzheimer's disease. Lancet 1996; 347: 509–12.
4. Murgolo NJ, Brown JE, Bayne ML, Strader CD. Presenilin mutations in Al-zheimer's disease: molecular models suggest a potential functional locus. Trends Pharmacol Sci 1996; 17: 389–93.
5. Levy-Lahad E, Wijsman EM, Nemens E et al. A familial Alzheimer's disease locus on chromosome 1. Science 1995; 269: 970–73.
6. Cacabelos R. Dementia. In: Jobe TH, Gaviria M, Kovilparambil A (eds) Clinical Neuropsychiatry. Malden: Blackwell Scientific, 1997; 73–122.
7. Corder EH, Saunders AM, Strittmatter WJ et al. Gene dose of apolipoprotein E type 4 allele and the risk of Alzheimer's disease in late onset families. Science 1993; 261: 921–3.
8. Van Duijn CM, de Knijff P, Cruts M, Wehnert A, Havekos LM, Hofman A, Van Broeckhoven C. Apolipoprotein E4 allele in a population-based study of early-onset Alzheimer's disease. Nature Genet 1994; 7: 74–8.

9. Roses AD, Strittmatter WJ, Pericak-Vance A, Corder EH, Saunders AM, Schmechel DE. Clinical application of apolipoprotein E genotyping to Alzheimer's disease. Lancet 1994; 343: 1564–5.

10. Saunders AM, Hulette C, Welsh-Bohmer KA et al. Specificity, sensitivity, and predictive value of apolipoprotein E genotyping for sporadic Alzheimer's disease. Lancet 1996; 348: 90–93.

11. Cacabelos R, Rodríguez B, Carrera C, Beyer K, Lao JI, Sellers MA. Behavioral changes associated with different apolipoprotein E genotypes in dementia. Alzheimer Dis Assoc Dis 1997; 11 (suppl 4): S27–34.

12. Roses AD, Saunders AM. Apolipoprotein E genotyping as a diagnostic adjunct for Alzheimer's disease. Int Psychogeriat 1997; 9 (suppl 1): 277–88.

13. Mayeux R, Saunders AN, Shea S et al. Utility of the apolipoprotein E genotype in the diagnosis of Alzheimer's disease. New Engl J Med 1998; 338: 506–11.

14. Beyer K, Lao JI, Alvarez XA, Cacabelos R. Different implications of APOE-4 in Alzheimer disease and vascular dementia in the Spanish population. Alzheimer Res 1996; 2: 215–20.

15. Tanzi RE, Kovacs DM, Kim T-W. The gene defects responsible for familial Alzheimer's disease. Neurobiol Dis 1996; 3: 159–68.

16. Rogaev EI, Sherington R, Rogaeva EA et al. Familial Alzheimer's disease in kindreds with missense mutation in a gene on chromosome 1 related to Alzheimer's disease type 3 gene. Nature 1995; 376: 775–8.

17. Beyer K, Lao JL, Alvarez XA, Cacabelos R. A general method for DNA polymorphism identification in genetic assessment and molecular diagnosis. Meth Find Exp Clin Pharmacol 1997; 19: 87–91.

18. Roses AD. A model for susceptibility polymorphisms for complex diseases. Neurogenetics 1997; 1: 3–11.

Address for correspondence:
    Professor Dr. Ramón Cacabelos,
    EuroEspes Biomedical Research Center,
    Institute for CNS Disorders,
    Sta. Marta de Babío s/n,
    15166-Bergondo, La Coruña, Spain
    Tel: 34 981 780505; fax: 34 981 780511

III Diagnosis, Clinical and Histopathological

14 Structural Neuroimaging: Early Diagnosis and Staging of Alzheimer's Disease

M.J. DE LEON, A. CONVIT, S. DE SANTI AND
M. BOBINSKI

INTRODUCTION

By the year 2030 it is estimated that between 17% and 20% or about 50 million of the US population will be over age 65 [1]. Dementia affects 1–6% of the population over the age of 65 and 10–20% over the age of 80 [2], with its annual incidence approximately doubling for every 5 years of age between the ages of 75 and 89 years [3]. Other data currently show that for every demented patient there are approximately eight non-demented individuals with cognitive deterioration adversely affecting their quality of life [4]. Therefore, with respect to the above estimates, a staggering number of elderly with mild to severe cognitive impairments, perhaps 10–20 million, can be expected in the next 35 years, representing a great human and economic toll.

Recent neuropathology studies identify the neurons of the hippocampal formation as most vulnerable to the age-related deposition of neurofibrillary tangles (NFT), a diagnostic feature of AD [5]. Moreover, for many non-demented elderly patients, especially those with mild cognitive impairments (MCI), NFT deposition in the hippocampal formation is a relatively focal insult [6]. With the progression of the clinical disease (based on cross-sectional observation), there is a correlated progression of the neuropathology with increasing involvement of the neocortex. These observations have led to the proposition that AD-related neuropathology follows over time a relatively fixed pattern that enables one to identify stages of involvement [5]. *In vivo* structural neuroimaging studies have begun to demonstrate similar brain region–time relationships. Neuroimaging studies, although lacking in pathologic specificity, have provided longitudinal observations on the size of the hippocampal formation and neocortical areas. These observations, when combined with post-mortem correlations, have proved to be very informative.

Alzheimer's Disease and Related Disorders
Edited by K. Iqbal, D.F. Swaab, B. Winblad and H.M. Wisniewski
© 1999 John Wiley & Sons Ltd

The purpose of this review is to: (a) briefly describe the normal anatomy of the hippocampal formation as relevant to neuroimaging; (b) to present structural imaging data collected *in vivo* that supports the hypothesis that hippocampal formation atrophy is a relatively specific change that occurs early in the natural history of AD and actually precedes neocortical involvement.

HIPPOCAMPAL FORMATION NEUROANATOMY

The hippocampal formation is one of the major parts of the allocortex (a phylogenetically older cortex that is part of the rhinencephalon). It comprises the hippocampus proper (hippocampus), dentate gyrus, subicular complex, and the entorhinal cortex [7, 8].

In the human brain the hippocampus is particularly well developed, occupying in the temporal lobe the floor of the temporal (inferior) horn of the lateral ventricle. The hippocampus is known for its seahorse-like appearance and much of its gross anatomy can be viewed with MRI (see Figure 1). The length of the hippocampus is about 4–5 cm, with a maximal width of about 2 cm and a maximal height of about 1.5 cm [9].

The boundaries of the hippocampus vary along its rostro-caudal length. The individual fields of the hippocampus can be pictured as a stacked bundle of tissue strips running rostro-caudally in the temporal lobe. The distinctive C-shape of the hippocampus is presented when the bundled strips fold over each other mediolaterally, as seen in the mid-portion or body of the hippocampus. At caudal levels (hippocampal tail), the hippocampus bends dorsally and ascends toward the splenium. The more rostral levels of the hippocampal structure are complex in shape, mostly due to a varied number of rostro-caudal flexures. As part of the allocortex, the hippocampus proper (cornu Ammonis) has three major layers: (a) the stratum oriens; (b) the stratum pyramidale; and (c) a layer which blends the strata radiatum, lacunosum and moleculare. Aspects of these layers and the dentate gyrus can be appreciated using MRI (Figure 2).

Cerebrospinal fluid (CSF) marks the boundary of the hippocampus over a large surface area. This includes the temporal horn of the lateral ventricle and a complex of CSF containing fissures and cisterns. Figure 3 depicts in three orthogonal planes the orientation of the transverse fissure relative to the hippocampus, parahippocampal gyrus, thalamic structures and ventricular CSF. These CSF landmarks are of particular interest for *in vivo* imaging, as they provide high contrast boundaries between the hippocampus and surrounding structures such as the thalamus. In addition, increases in these CSF spaces reflect regional tissue atrophy and they are therefore of interest in clinical evaluation. In the coronal view (Figure 3, top panel) the lateral boundaries of the transverse fissure or Bichat (also known as the lateral transverse fissure, LTF) is the medial aspect of the dentate gyrus (DG) and the fimbria (Fi). The

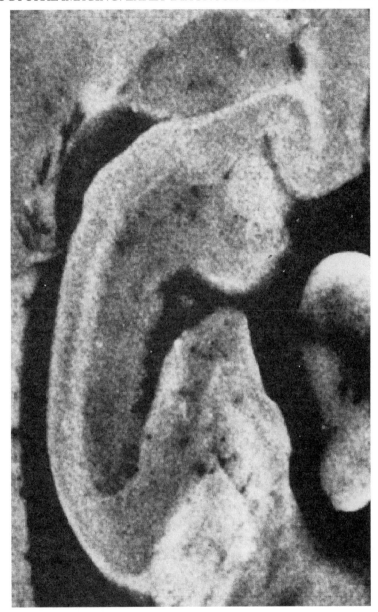

Figure 1. Post-mortem axial plane section depicting the long axis of the hippocampus

coronal view best permits separation of the choroidal (CF) and hippocampal fissure (HF) extensions of the LTF. In the horizontal or axial view, the LTF begins at the posterior border of the pes hippocampus or uncus (Un) (Figure 3, middle panel). Medially the LTF communicates with the ambient cistern

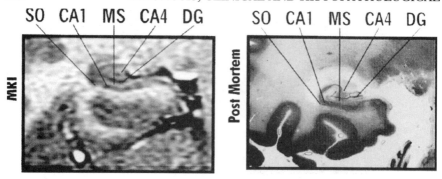

Figure 2. High resolution coronal MRI image with corresponding post-mortem slice depicting the alveus and the stratum oriens (SO); the stratum pyramidale of the CA1; a multi-strata area (MS) that includes the stratum radiatum, stratum lacunosum and stratum moleculare of the cornu Ammonis; the dentate gyrus (DG); and the stratum pyramidale of CA4

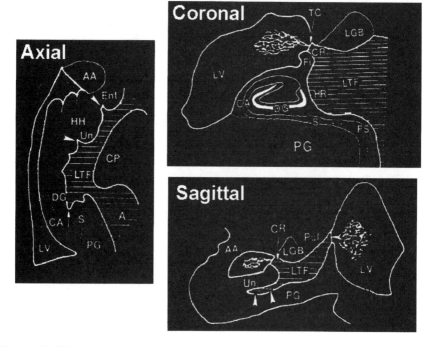

Figure 3. Schematic representations of axial, coronal and sagittal views of the right hippocampal region. AA, amygdala; HH, head of hippocampus; Ent, entorhinal cortex; Fi, fimbria; UN, uncus; DG, dentate gyrus; LTF, lateral transverse fissure of Bichat; CR, choroid fissure recess; HR, hippocampal fissure recess; A, ambient cistern; LV, lateral ventricle; PG, parahippocampal gyrus; CP, cerebral peduncle; S, subiculum; PS, parasubiculum; TC, tela choroidea; LGB, lateral geniculate body; Pul, pulvinar

(A) which borders the cerebral peduncles (CP). Both the coronal and sagittal planes (Figure 3, right panels) of section permit identification of the structures bounding the ventral surface of the transverse fissure, namely the subiculum (S) of the parahippocampal gyrus (PG), as well as the identification of those thalamic structures bounding the dorsal margin, the lateral geniculate body (LGB) and the pulvinar (Pul).

ENTORHINAL CORTEX

The entorhinal cortex and the transentorhinal cortex form a major part of the anterior parahippocampal gyrus. Phylogenetically, they are relatively old structures. Based on histology and connectivity, the entorhinal cortex is transitional between the hippocampus and the neocortex, and is made up of six layers [7, 10]. The term 'entorhinal cortex' was introduced by Brodmann [11] as a synonym for his 'area 28'.

The entorhinal cortex is adjacent to the more lateral perirhinal cortex (areas 35 and 36 of Brodmann). There is no clear-cut border between area 35 and the entorhinal cortex, and these two fields appear to have an obliquely orientated boundary, where the deep layers of the entorhinal cortex extend somewhat more laterally than the superficial layers. This distinctly angled border between area 35 and the entorhinal cortex has been emphasized by Braak [12], who has labeled the region of overlap the 'transentorhinal cortex'. With serial coronal MRI sections, one may reliably identify gyral landmarks that are approximate boundaries for the entorhinal cortex region [70]. These landmarks include, on the medial surface, the semilunar gyrus and the gyrus semiannularis. The lateral boundary, at anterior levels, is approximated by the rhinal sulcus and posteriorly by the collateral sulcus.

HIPPOCAMPAL FORMATION CONNECTIONS

The entorhinal cortex, the gateway to the hippocampus, receives massive synaptic input from neocortical association areas and less pronounced input from primary sensory areas [13, 14]. The entorhinal cortex provides the major source of afferent information to the hippocampus via the perforant path [15]. The predominant component of the perforant path has been regarded as the projection from the stellate layer II neurons of the entorhinal cortex, which synapse in the molecular layer on the dendrites of the granular cells of the dentate gyrus. In the classical model of the 'trisynaptic circuit', this is the first link, followed by the mossy fiber connections to CA3 pyramidal cells and completed by the Schaffer collateral input to CA1. Hippocampal output is also directed back to the entorhinal cortex and neocortex directly from the CA1 and the subiculum. Thus, the entorhinal cortex occupies the key position with respect to gating the communications between the hippocampus and the rest of the brain.

NEUROPATHOLOGY

HIPPOCAMPAL FORMATION PATHOLOGY IN AD

Neuronal pathology in the hippocampal formation appears to be a major component of the memory impairment seen in AD [16, 17]. Looming in the background of these neuronal changes in symptomatic patients are observations that normal elderly patients often show age-related depositions of NFT, lesions that have a predilection for entorhinal cortex and hippocampal neurons [6, 18–20]. Unfortunately, very little is known regarding an association between age-related memory loss and mild age-related neuronal pathology. Recent studies show that, with increasing disease severity, the anatomical distribution of pathological changes progresses from the more localized entorhinal cortex and the hippocampal involvement to the neocortex [5]. Postmortem histopathological studies show that the hippocampal formation, especially the entorhinal and transentorhinal cortex, is one of the earliest and most affected structures in AD [5, 16]. Morphological studies of the hippocampal formation reveal neurofibrillary changes and granulovacuolar degeneration of the neurons, synaptic and neuronal loss, and amyloid β deposition in plaques and vascular walls [5, 21]. Neurofibrillary degeneration and the loss of projection neurons responsible for the majority of afferent and efferent connections of the hippocampal formation cause both the disruption of intrahippocampal connections and functional isolation of the hippocampal formation from other parts of the memory system [16]. Neurofibrillary degeneration has been put forth as a cause of neuronal loss and atrophy of the hippocampal formation [16, 17, 22, 23]. Over the estimated duration of clinically manifest AD, our calculations projected a decrease of 60% in the volume of the hippocampus and of 51% in the volume of the entorhinal cortex [24]. The impact of amyloid deposits on hippocampal formation atrophy is not known.

HIPPOCAMPAL FORMATION NEURONAL LOSS IN AD

Neuronal loss in the hippocampal formation in AD has been described by many investigators. The entorhinal cortex, CA1, and subiculum were found consistently to be severely affected, and the granular layer of the dentate gyrus has generally been found to be spared [22, 25, 26]. The number of hippocampal subdivisions that are found to evidence neuronal loss depends to a great extent on the duration and clinical stage of AD in the patients investigated [17]. In the relatively less affected patient group, significant neuronal loss was found only in the CA1 sector and in the subiculum. In the group of patients with more severe AD, significant neuronal loss was observed in CA1, CA2, CA3, CA4 and the subiculum.

Despite the complex connectivity in the hippocampal formation, neurofibrillary pathology and neuronal loss develop in a structure-specific fashion.

Braak and Braak described a staging scheme of neurofibrillary changes in the brain based on the temporal and topographical distribution of these lesions [5]. According to these authors, neurofibrillary changes develop first in the transentorhinal cortex, then in the entorhinal cortex (transentorhinal stages). Further progression involves CA1, the subiculum and CA4, then sectors CA2 and CA3 of the cornu Ammonis and the parvopyramidal layer of the pre-subiculum (the limbic stage). Changes in the dentate gyrus and the isocortical association areas appear in the last stage of this classification (the isocortical stage). At present, there is little neuropathological information regarding the earliest neocortical areas involved.

Structure-specific neuronal loss in AD was also reported by West et al. who, using unbiased stereological techniques, estimated the total numbers of neurons in several hippocampal formation subdivisions [25]. Among normals they found neuronal losses in two subdivisions, the hilus (CA4) and the subiculum. In the AD group they observed the additional loss of neurons in CA1. Therefore, the regional pattern of neuronal loss in AD is qualitatively and quantitatively different from that observed in normal aging.

Moreover, it has been suggested that the degeneration of much of the neuronal architecture of the entorhinal cortex destroys a large functional part of hippocampal input and output and that this destruction results in the memory and cognitive deficits associated with AD [16]. In a detailed stereological study, Gomez-Isla et al. [26] found that subjects with very mild cognitive impairment (Clinical Dementia Rating, CDR = 0.5) had 32% fewer neurons in the entorhinal cortex than controls. In the entorhinal cortex layer II, neuronal loss reached 60%. In the more severe dementia cases (CDR = 3) the total number of neurons in layer II was decreased by 90%. This study showed that a significant neuronal loss in layer II of the entorhinal cortex distinguished even very mild AD from non-demented aging [26]. Over all the AD cases, the entorhinal cortex volume was reduced by 40%. In summary, these neuropathological findings encourage the comprehensive *in vivo* examination of the hippocampal formation and its relationships to cognitive functioning in aging and AD.

NEUROIMAGING STUDIES OF THE HIPPOCAMPAL REGION

With the nearly simultaneous observations in the late 1980s by several laboratories that the hippocampal region could be reliably studied with structural neuroimaging [27–31] (an advance partly facilitated with the availability of MRI), numerous research efforts were directed away from more general markers of brain atrophy (ventricular size and cortical sulcal prominence) to anatomically better defined regional assessments. In today's neuroimaging literature, a consensus of reports demonstrate the involvement of the hippocampus in AD. All studies report increased hippocampal atrophy in AD relative to aged controls. These results are reflected in: measures of parenchymal volume loss [27, 30, 32–39]; linear 2-D estimates of size [40, 41]; measures of medial temporal lobe gray matter volume [42]; the qualitative rating of the amount of CSF accumulating in the hippocampal fissures [28, 31, 43, 44]; the size of the suprasellar cistern [45]; and the increased distance between the right and left uncus (see [46] for review). However, before hippocampal atrophy can be considered as a diagnostic marker for early (preclinical) AD, several lines of investigation need to be developed further. Specifically, we need to improve our understandings of the prevalence and severity of hippocampal atrophy over the clinical stages of AD, the diagnostic specificity of hippocampal atrophy for AD, and the relationship between hippocampal atrophy and known risk factors for AD, such as age, gender and genetic factors. Moreover, very little is known of the longitudinal course of AD from the standpoint of structural neuroimaging evidence of global atrophy in general and hippocampal atrophy in particular. Only a small number of studies have investigated change over two time points [47–54] and with only a few exceptions [55–57] there are virtually no data examined over three or more time points. Nevertheless, a considerable body of information has accumulated that strongly encourages the continuation and further development of these efforts.

In the studies below, we will review several of our clinical structural neuroimaging studies of the hippocampal formation. These cross-sectional and longitudinal studies show that hippocampal formation imaging is of potential use in the early diagnosis of AD, in the clinical evaluation of age-related memory changes and in the prediction of future brain damage, dementia and a diagnosis of AD. Moreover, the most recent neuroimaging data are supportive of the Braak et al. [58] model that proposes the staging of the brain involvement of AD. With this model, the earliest stages of AD are marked by selective involvement of the entorhinal cortex, followed by a hippocampal stage and finally by stages involving the progressive involvement of the neocortex.

STUDIES OF THE HIPPOCAMPUS

CROSS-SECTIONAL HIPPOCAMPAL STUDIES OF NORMAL AGING AND AD

Over a decade ago, prior to the availability of MRI, the first imaging studies of the hippocampal region were conducted using X-ray computed tomography (CT). Limited by the range of gantry rotation, axial plane rather than coronal plane images were acquired. In order to maximize the amount of the hippocampus visible on any single axial slice, we developed a CT plane of acquisition to parallel the long axis of the hippocampus, resulting in a so-called 'negative angulation view' [28]. With the negative angulation view, one can observe the transverse fissure and the associated choroidal–hippocampal fissures as a continuous CSF space that enlarges with volume losses in the hippocampus and subiculum. When using a 4 mm slice thickness, it is possible to evaluate these atrophic hippocampal changes on 1–3 slices. Moreover, as these procedures are easy to carry out, it is possible to examine large numbers of subjects.

In the first study of the hippocampal region in aging and AD we examined 175 subjects. In this and all the studies below, the patients received an extensive research protocol of medical, neurologic, psychiatric and neuropsychologic examinations, which enabled us to exclude from the study individuals with evidence for conditions that could affect brain functioning or structure, and to include individuals with changes presumably only related to age or AD. We used CT images derived from the negative angulation protocol, and used a subjective four-point assessment scale to rate the extent of CSF accumulation in the fissures surrounding the hippocampus [31]. The hippocampal atrophy (HA) scale points included: 0 = no atrophy, 1 = questionable, 2 = mild, 3 = moderate to severe. The cut-off rating of definite atrophy (≥ 2) in either hemisphere was used to define definite HA (see Figure 4). This qualitative measure has since been validated using MRI against the actual hippocampal volume [34], and is now considered to reflect the extent of HA. The results of this study demonstrated that HA was typically found in AD independent of severity level and age and, in a small sample of MCI patients, HA was predictive of future AD.

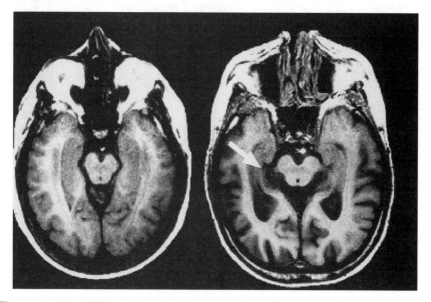

Figure 4. Axial MRI depicting the hippocampal area from a normal control (left) and an age-matched AD patient (right). White arrow points to the CSF accumulation in the area of the hippocampus in the AD patient's brain

More recently, in a CT and MRI study using the negative angle protocol, we studied 405 patients [44]. Four clinical groups were defined using NINCDS–ADRDA criteria and the Global Deterioration Scores (GDS) [59]. The groups identified included: normal elderly (GDS 1 and 2), n = 130; mild AD (GDS 4), n = 73; and moderate to severe AD (GDS 5 and 6), n = 130. The fourth group, the minimal impairment group (MCI), n = 72, was defined as having GDS = 3 and Mini-Mental State Examination (MMSE) scores > 23 [60].

A validation study showed that HA was equivalently determined with CT as with MRI (T1-weighted 4 mm thick axial images). The clinical data showed that HA was significantly more prevalent in all the patient groups as compared with control; 78% of the MCI (GDS = 3), 84% of the mild AD (GDS = 4) and 96% in the moderate to severe AD (GDS ≥ 5) groups showed HA. 29% of the controls (GDS 1–2) showed HA (see Figure 5).

The same study showed that normal controls showed a striking age dependence for HA while the cognitively impaired groups showed prevalence rates independent of age (see Figure 6). In a related study comparing normals with and without HA, we observed, after controlling for age and years of education,

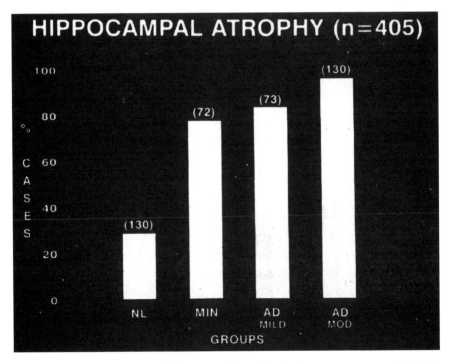

Figure 5. The prevalence of hippocampal atrophy in four groups: normal elderly, minimally impaired elderly, and two AD groups with different severity levels of cognitive impairment

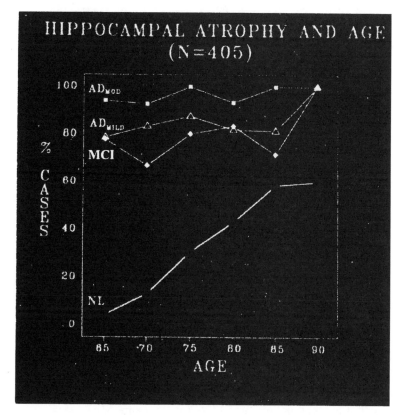

Figure 6. The prevalence of hippocampal atrophy for normals (NL), individuals with mild cognitive impairment (MCI), and two levels of AD as a function of age

that HA was associated with significant reductions in performance on tests of delayed verbal memory (p < 0.01) but not to the tests of immediate memory [61]. This result was consistent with the pattern of memory dysfunction reported in subjects with circumscribed hippocampal lesions.

LONGITUDINAL STUDIES PREDICTING THE DEVELOPMENT OF DEMENTIA

The results of our cross-sectional studies of HA showed that hippocampal changes occur with a high frequency in MCI patients, known to be at increased risk for AD [62]. We therefore reasoned that HA may be predictive of cognitive deterioration and the diagnosis of AD. In order to assess the prognostic value of HA, a 4-year follow-up CT study was carried out in a normal elderly group (n = 54, aged 70 ± 8 SD) and a MCI group (n = 32, aged 71 ± 9 SD) [43]. Over the interval, 23 (72%) of the MCI group and two (4%) of the normal elderly deteriorated to receive the diagnosis of AD (GDS ≥ 4). For the MCI group, baseline hippocampal atrophy was present in 91% of the declining group and in 11% of the non-declining group. The results also showed that the prediction of decline was not related to age or gender. Both cortical sulcal prominence and ventricular enlargement at baseline were related to the observation of decline. However, as compared with the overall prediction accuracies of 91% for HA, these global measures of brain atrophy yielded overall prediction accuracy scores of 70% and 69%, respectively. In summary, the relatively high accuracy of HA for the prediction of decline, and the high rate of preservation in the group not showing HA, suggests the unique potential of HA in the clinical examination of early AD.

The results of these studies pointed to the need for longitudinal study of the temporal relation between hippocampal atrophy, neocortical atrophy and the development of intellectual dysfunction. As only 4% of our normal elderly sample deteriorated to dementia, while 15% had baseline hippocampal atrophy, this study also suggested that in order to evaluate carefully the predictive risk of hippocampal atrophy, we must also: (a) extend the period of observation beyond the four years; (b) use more sensitive and anatomically specific indices of neocortical and hippocampal integrity; and (c) utilize assessments of neuropsychological performance that are more fine-grained.

THE ANATOMIC SPECIFICITY OF HIPPOCAMPAL VOLUME LOSS IN PATIENTS AT RISK FOR AD

A recent validation study, comparing histologically derived hippocampal volume with hippocampal volume determined from MRI imaging of post-mortem materials, showed that the methods produced virtually equivalent results (n = 16, r = 0.97, p < 0.001; see Figure 7) [63]. Both the MRI-based hippocampal volume and the histology-based volume correlated significantly with the numbers of neurons. Moreover, another study reported that normal elderly individuals with NFT lesions in the hippocampus showed hippocampal volume reductions when compared with normal age-matched elderly without NFT [64]. Overall, these findings suggest that the inverse relationships between NFT deposition and both neuronal number and hippocampal volume extends from confirmed clinical AD cases to cognitively normal elderly that do not reach criteria for a brain AD diagnosis.

Using MRI volume data we investigated the hypothesis that hippocampal parenchymal volume reductions, rather than regional neocortical reductions, best characterize MCI patients. We conducted the volumetric MRI and neuropsychological study of 27 normal elderly, 22 elderly MCI patients and 27 AD patients [35]. As in the above normal aging study [65], we used 4 mm thick T1-weighted coronal MRI images. Here, we measured five major regions, encompassing the entire temporal lobe, starting anteriorly from the level of the posterior pes hippocampus and ending posteriorly at the level of

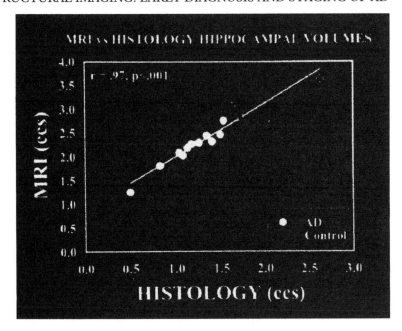

Figure 7. Scattergram depicting the relationship between the hippocampal volume as determined from histologic section and from post-mortem MRI

the posterior pulvinar. The regions included the hippocampus, para-hippocampal gyrus, fusiform gyrus, the superior temporal gyrus, and the combined middle and inferior temporal gyri. All groups were matched for age, gender and education. As compared with the normal elderly group, the MCI patients showed a 14% volume loss that was anatomically specific to the hippocampus (see Figure 8). The AD group, on the other hand, showed significant differences relative to the normal group for all temporal lobe volumes. The reduction in the hippocampus was 22% and in the neocortical regions the reductions ranged from 9% to 14%. These data also

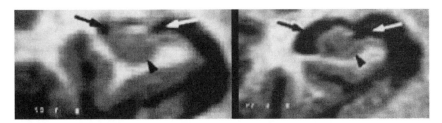

Figure 8. Coronal MRI of the hippocampus showing a representative normal (left) and a representative MCI (right) patient. Arrowhead points to the hippocampus, the white arrow to the transverse fissure and the black arrow to the temporal horn of the lateral ventricle

demonstrated, in the MCI group, an anatomically unique relationship between hippocampus volume and delayed recall performance. In addition, because the entire temporal lobe was studied, these data additionally support the hypothesis that the hippocampal–delayed recall relationship is anatomically specific.

The results also clearly showed that lateral temporal lobe volume losses were necessary to correctly classify cases with dementia. Using logistic regression to classify the MCI and AD patients, lateral temporal lobe volume measurements significantly added information, over and above measurements from the hippocampus and the parahippocampal gyrus (medial temporal lobe). The medial temporal lobe volume correctly classified 67% of MCI and AD patients and inclusion of the lateral regions raised this value to 80%. In the classification of normal and AD patients, the medial temporal lobe correctly classified 87% and, with addition of lateral temporal lobe measurements, the classification significantly improved to 91% correct. In the classification of the normal and the minimal groups, the lateral temporal lobe did not increase classification accuracy.

HIPPOCAMPAL VOLUME PREDICTION STUDIES

MRI volume studies also enable direct examination of the anatomic specificity of the prediction of reduced memory performance in normals and in the clinical decline to dementia in non-demented elderly. In a recent longitudinal study we observed that in elderly normal subjects (MMSE > 27, n = 54) the baseline volume of the hippocampus, but not the superior temporal gyrus, was related to delayed paragraph recall performance [65]. After a follow-up interval of 4 years we observed, in this same normal elderly cohort, that the smaller baseline hippocampal volumes were predictive of disproportionately greater reductions in delayed recall performance [66]. Although the strength of this relationship was significant (r = 0.54, p < 0.01), the results were not sufficiently compelling to provide clinically relevant predictions for the transition between normal and MCI.

On the other hand, the volume data contributes to the prediction of future AD from MCI. Based on a very recent study, we now have preliminary evidence to indicate that baseline fusiform and middle inferior temporal lobe gyri volume reductions predict, over 3 years, decline in MCI to AD with a very high degree of accuracy [67]. The baseline lateral temporal lobe volumes predicted who was going to decline to AD much more accurately than the medial temporal lobe volumes alone and significantly added to it, reaching an overall diagnostic accuracy greater than 90%. These data indicate that the fusiform and middle-inferior temporal lobe gyri may be among the first temporal lobe neocortical sites affected in AD; atrophy in this area among non-demented individuals may herald the presence of future AD. Below we highlight some of our recent findings on the entorhinal cortex that appear to hold additional promise for the prognosis of decline among the normal elderly.

ENTORHINAL CORTEX STUDIES

ANATOMIC VALIDATION OF THE MRI ENTORHINAL CORTEX MEASUREMENTS

Using MRI, several attempts have been made to measure the volume of the entorhinal cortex in AD [68, 69]. As the boundaries of the entorhinal and perirhinal cortices are poorly visible on MRI, the variability associated with the volume study probably accounts for the absence of reports of entorhinal cortex changes early in the course of AD. Recently, we described a method to estimate the surface area of the entorhinal cortex on MRI [70]. In order to validate our method, we used serial 3 mm sections stained with cresyl violet to define actual histological measures of entorhinal cortex volume and entorhinal cortex surface area, as well as to estimate the cortical length using gyral landmarks visible on both the histologic sections and on MRI. Sixteen AD patients and four normal controls were studied. The true entorhinal cortex histologic surface area was measured between the most medial boundary (pyriform cortex, or amygdala, or presubiculum, or parasubiculum) and the most lateral points (referred to as perirhinal or transentorhinal cortex). Using the gyral landmarks, the measurements were made across all slices from 3 mm posterior to the fronto-temporal junction to the rostral pole of the lateral geniculate body. Across slices, the medial boundary of the entorhinal cortex was defined as the depth of the gyrus semiannularis on anterior sections and the medial parahippocampal gyrus on posterior sections. The lateral boundary was the depth of the rhinal sulcus in anterior sections and the depth of the collateral sulcus in the posterior sections (see Figure 9). As the lateral boundaries of the entorhinal cortex landmark lengths go beyond the entorhinal

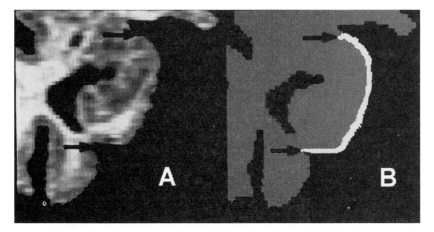

Figure 9. MRI-based entorhinal cortex boundaries depicting, at an anterior level, the medial and the lateral boundaries. (A) shows the MRI and (B) is a schematic drawing based on the MRI

cortex histological lengths, our studies show that this segment consists entirely of perirhinal cortex. The results showed a strong relationship between the volume of the entorhinal cortex and both the histological surface area ($r = 0.95$, $p < 0.001$) and the landmark length ($r = 0.87$, $p < 0.001$). Relative to normals, the entorhinal measurements were significantly reduced in AD ($p < 0.01$): volume 61%, histological surface area 41%, landmark surface area 45%.

ENTORHINAL CORTEX ATROPHY—DIAGNOSTIC ACCURACY IN MILD AD AND THE RELATIONSHIP TO HIPPOCAMPAL ATROPHY

In the clinical *in vivo* study, MRI scans were obtained on eight normal controls [Global Deterioration Scale (GDS) 1–2; Mini-Mental State Exam (MMSE) (28.8 ± 1.0), range 28–30; age 78.1 ± 5.4 years, 4/8 male] and eight patients with very mild to mild AD that were age- and gender-matched to the controls (GDS 4, MMSE (27.1 ± 2.2), range 24–30; age 80.4 ± 4.8 years, 4/8 male). All AD patients were randomly selected from consecutive referrals to a clinic specializing in age-related cognitive impairments, on the basis of age, gender, GDS and MMSE without any knowledge of MRI assessments of atrophy. Patients with other conditions known to cause cognitive impairment were excluded. Controls were volunteers interested in aging or spouses of the patients.

To parallel the neuropathology EC protocol, MRI images were acquired perpendicular to a plane instersecting the inferior frontal lobe and the inferior occipital lobe. Images were reformatted to a 2 mm slice thickness. Landmark EC length measurements were made from all the slices that spanned from 4 mm posterior to the frontotemporal junction to the anterior margin of the lateral geniculate body. The landmark length of the EC was measured along its boundary with the subarachnoid CSF. Subsequently, the landmark EC surface area was computed. For reference, the volumes of the body of the hippocampus and the superior temporal gyrus were measured using previously published procedures [36]. Intracranial volumes, spanning the coronal sections that encompass the regions of interest, were determined by outlining the dural and tentorial margins and used to correct for individual differences in head size.

For each brain measure, to correct for individual differences in head size, the ratio of the regional size divided by the head size was calculated. The EC landmark surface area ratio showed a 27% difference between AD and control groups, ($p < 0.001$). The hippocampal volume ratios were significantly different by 12% between AD and control groups, ($p < 0.05$). No differences were observed between AD and control groups for the superior temporal gyrus volume ratios. In a series of univariate logistic regression models, the EC ratio correctly classified 100% of the control and 75% of the AD group (p < 0.05) The superior temporal gyrus ratio classified 62.5% of the controls and 62.5% of the AD groups (p > 0.05). In addition, in two regression models, each with three steps (variables), the EC and the hippocampal ratios were contrasted to identify their individual contributions to predicting group membership. In both models the superior temporal gyrus ratio was entered as the first step and resulted in a 62.5% overall classification accuracy. The order of entry of the EC and hippocampal ratios in the subsequent steps alternated across the models. For model 1, the hippocampal ratio entered in the second step classified overall 75% correct (χ^2 increase = 6.1, p < 0.01) and the EC ratio in the third step increased the statistical significance of the model and raised the overall classification accuracy to 100% correct (p < 0.001). In model 2, with the EC ratio entered on the second step, the overall classification accuracy reached 100% correct (p < 0.001) and the addition of the hippocampus was not required.

This study indicates that a simple *in vivo* MRI measurement of the surface area of the EC has anatomic validity and is of potentially unique utility in the early diagnosis of AD.

CONCLUSIONS

In vivo examination of the hippocampal region appears to be of descriptive value over the clinical course of AD. The data indicate that atrophic entorhinal and hippocampal changes appear early in the natural history of AD and are progressive. Atrophy of the hippocampus proper is relatively uncommon in the normal elderly. However, when such atrophic changes are present, they are associated with memory deficits. The data suggest that in mildly impaired individuals, hippocampal atrophy appears to be related to the AD process, as it predicts with high sensitivity and specificity the decline to AD levels of cognitive performance [31, 43]. While the frequency of *in vivo*-detected entorhinal cortex atrophy is currently unknown, entorhinal atrophy in both the normal elderly and in MCI patients is associated with progressive memory deterioration and the progressive atrophy of the hippocampus. These observations are in part supported by post-mortem studies that show increased numbers of NFT and reduced numbers of neurons in the entorhinal cortex and hippocampus in both MCI patients [19] and the normal elderly [26].

In summary, it is universally observed at post-mortem examination that hippocampal atrophy occurs in AD. We now extend these observations by showing *in vivo* a remarkably high frequency of hippocampal atrophy among individuals with probable and mild AD and MCI. The imaging data also shows the consistent and necessary involvement of the lateral temporal lobe, particularly the fusiform gyrus, in the statistical classification of AD patients relative to MCI patients. Perhaps most importantly, the recent neuropathology and neuroimaging evidence points to an even earlier lesion that can be detected in the entorhinal cortex. Entorhinal cortex lesions may actually antedate the lesions of the hippocampus proper. Overall, these findings suggest a soon-to-be-reached clinical capability for identifying and measurement of the brain changes in non-demented patients that place them at increased risk for memory decline, further brain damage and AD. It is anticipated that future therapeutic studies will probably use brain-imaging measures, which are relatively free of education and cultural bias, both for study selection purposes and as treatment outcome measures.

ACKNOWLEDGEMENTS

This work was made possible with grants from the National Institute on Aging, Numbers P30 AG08051, RO1 AG12101, AG13616, AG03051 and PO1 AG04220; and the New York State Office of Mental Retardation and Developmental Disabilities.

REFERENCES

1. Schoenberg BS. Epidemiology of Alzheimer's disease and other dementing disorders. J Chron Dis 1986; 39: 1095–104.
2. Clark RF, Goate AM. Molecular genetics of Alzheimer's disease. Arch Neurol 1993; 50: 1164–72.
3. Paykel ES, Brayne C, Huppert FA, Gill C, Barkley C, Gehlhaar E, Beardsall L, Girling DM, Pollitt P, O'Connor D. Incidence of dementia in a population older than 75 years in the United Kingdom. Arch Gen Psychiat 1994; 51: 325–32.
4. Larrabee GJ, Crook TH. Estimated prevalence of age-associated memory impairment derived from standardized tests of memory function. Int Psychogeriat 1994; 6: 95–104.
5. Braak H, Braak E. Neuropathological staging of Alzheimer-related changes. Acta Neuropathol 1991; 82: 239–59.
6. Giannakopoulos P, Hof PR, Mottier S, Michel JP, Bouras C. Neuropathological changes in the cerebral cortex of 1258 cases from a geriatric hospital: retrospective clinicopathological evaluation of a 10-year autopsy population. Acta Neuropathol 1994; 87: 456–68.
7. Amaral DG, Insausti R. Hippocampal formation. In: Paxinos G (ed.) The Human Nervous System. San Diego: Academic Press, 1990; 711–55.
8. Rosene DL, Van Hoesen GW. The hippocampal formation of the primate brain: a review of some comparative aspects of cytoarchitecture and connections. In: Jones EG, Peters A (eds) Cerebral Cortex. New York: Plenum, 1987; 345–456.
9. Duvernoy HM. The Human Hippocampus: An Atlas of Applied Anatomy. Munich: J.F. Bergmann Verlag, 1988; 1–166.
10. Insausti R, Tunon T, Sobreviela T, Insausti AM, Gonzalo LM. The human entorhinal cortex: a cytoarchitectonic analysis. J Comp Neurol 1995; 355: 171–98.
11. Brodmann K. Vergleichende lokalisationslehr der grosshirnrinde in ihren prinzipien dargestellt auf grund des zellenbaues. Leipzig: Barth, 1909.

12. Braak H. Architectonics of the Human Telencephalic Cortex. Berlin: Springer-Verlag, 1980: 1–147.
13. Suzuki WA, Amaral DG. Perirhinal and parahippocampal cortices of the macaque monkey: cortical afferents. J Comp Neurol 1994; 350: 497–533.
14. Van Hoesen GW. The parahippocamal gyrus: new observations regarding its cortical connections in the monkey. Trends Neurosci 1982; 345–50.
15. Witter MP, Amaral DG. Entorhinal cortex of the monkey: V. Projections to the dentate gyrus, hippocampus, and subicular complex. J Comp Neurol 1991; 307: 437–59.
16. Hyman BT, Van Hoesen GW, Damasio AR, Barnes CL. Alzheimer's disease: cell-specific pathology isolates the hippocampal formation. Science 1984; 225: 1168–70.
17. Bobinski M, Wegiel J, Tarnawski M, Reisberg B, de Leon MJ, Miller DC, Wisniewski HM. Relationships between regional neuronal loss and neurofibrillary changes in the hippocampal formation and duration and severity of Alzheimer disease. J Neuropath Exp Neurol 1997; 56: 414–20.
18. Langui D, Probst A, Ulrich J. Alzheimer's changes in non-demented and demented patients: a statistical approach to their relationships. Acta Neuropathol 1995; 89: 57–62.
19. Price JL, Davis PB, Morris JC, White DL. The distribution of tangles, plaques and related immunohistochemical markers in healthy aging and Alzheimer's disease. Neurobiol Aging 1991; 12: 295–312.
20. Arriagada PV, Marzloff K, Hyman BT. Distribution of Alzheimer-type pathologic changes in nondemented elderly individuals matches the pattern in Alzheimer's disease. Neurology 1992; 42: 1681–8.
21. Ball MJ, Hachinski V, Fox A, Kirshen AJ, Fisman M, Blume W, Kral VA, Fox H. A new definition of Alzheimer's disease: a hippocampal dementia. Lancet 1985; i: 14–16.
22. Davies DC, Horwood N, Isaacs SL, Mann DMA. The effect of age and Alzheimer's disease on pyramidal neuron density in the individual fields of the hippocampal formation. Acta Neuropathol 1992; 83: 510–17.
23. Bobinski MJ, Wegiel J, Wisniewski HM, Tarnawski B, Bobinski M, Reisberg B, de Leon MJ, Miller DC. Neurofibrillary pathology—correlation with hippocampal formation atrophy in Alzheimer disease. Neurobiol Aging 1996; 17: 909–19.
24. Bobinski M, Wegiel J, Wisniewski HM, Tarnawski M, Reisberg B, Mlodzik B, de Leon MJ, Miller DC. Atrophy of hippocampal formation subdivisions correlates with stage and duration of Alzheimer disease. Dementia 1995; 6: 205–10.
25. West MJ, Coleman PD, Flood DG, Troncoso JC. Differences in the pattern of hippocampal neuronal loss in normal ageing and Alzheimer's disease. Lancet 1994; 344: 769–72.
26. Gomez-Isla T, Price JL, McKeel DW Jr, Morris JC, Growdon JH, Hyman BT. Profound loss of layer II entorhinal cortex neurons occurs in very mild Alzheimer's disease. J Neurosci 1996; 16: 4491–500.
27. Seab JP, Jagust WS, Wong SFS, Roos MS, Reed BR, Budinger TF. Quantitative NMR measurements of hippocampal atrophy in Alzheimer's disease. Magnet Resonance Med 1988; 8: 200–208.
28. de Leon MJ, McRae T, Tsai JR, George AE, Marcus DL, Freedman M, Wolf AP, McEwen B. Abnormal cortisol response in Alzheimer's disease linked to hippocampal atrophy. Lancet 1988; 2: 391–2.
29. Press GA, Amaral DG, Squire LR. Hippocampal abnormalities in amnesic patients revealed by high-resolution magnetic resonance imaging. Nature 1989; 341: 54–7.

30. Kesslak JP, Nalcioglu O, Cotman CW. Quantification of magnetic resonance scans for hippocampal and parahippocampal atrophy in Alzheimer's disease. Neurology 1991; 41: 51–4.

31. de Leon MJ, George AE, Stylopoulos LA, Smith G, Miller DC. Early marker for Alzheimer's disease: the atrophic hippocampus. Lancet 1989; 2: 672–3.

32. Jack CR, Petersen RC, O'Brien PC, Tangalos EG. MR-based hippocampal volumetry in the diagnosis of Alzheimer's disease. Neurology 1992; 42: 183–8.

33. Jernigan TL, Salmon DP, Butters N, Hesselink JR. Cerebral structure on MRI, Part II: specific changes in Alzheimer's and Huntingdon's diseases. Biol Psychiat 1991; 29: 68–81.

34. Convit A, de Leon MJ, Golomb J, George AE, Tarshish CY, Bobinski M, Tsui W, De Santi S, Wegiel J, Wisniewski HM. Hippocampal atrophy in early Alzheimer's disease: anatomic specificity and validation. Psychiat Qu 1993; 64: 371–87.

35. Convit A, de Leon MJ, Tarshish C, De Santi S, Kluger A, Rusinek H, George A. Hippocampal volume losses in minimally impaired elderly. Lancet 1995; 335: 266.

36. Convit A, de Leon MJ, Tarshish C, De Santi S, Tsui W, Rusinek H, George AE. Specific hippocampal volume reductions in individuals at risk for Alzheimer's disease. Neurobiol Aging 1997; 18: 131–8.

37. Deweer B, Lehericy S, Pillon B, Baulac M, Chiras J, Marsault C, Agid Y, Dubois B. Memory disorders in probable Alzheimer's disease: the role of hippocampal atrophy as shown with MRI. J Neurol Neurosurg Psychiatry 1995; 58: 590–97.

38. Ikeda M, Tanabe H, Nakagawa Y, Kazui H, Oi H, Yamazaki H, Harada K, Nishimura T. MRI-based quantitative assessment of the hippocampal region in very mild to moderate Alzheimer's disease. Neuroradiology 1994; 36: 7–10.

39. Lehericy S, Baulac M, Chiras J, Pierot L, Martin N, Pillon B, Deweer B, Dubois B, Marsault C. Amygdalohippocampal MR volume measurements in the early stages of Alzheimer disease. Am J Neuroradiol 1994; 15: 929–37.

40. Jobst KA, Smith AD, Szatmari M, Esiri MM, Jaskowski A, Hindley N, McDonald B, Molyneux AJ. Rapidly progressing atrophy of medial temporal lobe in Alzheimer's disease. Lancet 1994; 343: 829–30.

41. Scheltens P, Leys D, Barkhof F, Huglo D, Weinstein HC, Vermersch P, Kuiper M, Steinling M, Wolters EC, Valk J. Atrophy of medial temporal lobes on MRI in 'probable' Alzheimer's disease and normal aging: diagnostic value and neuropsychological correlates. J Neurol Neurosurg Psychiat 1992; 55: 967–72.

42. Stout JC, Jernigan TL, Archibald SL, Salmon DP. Association of dementia severity with cortical gray matter and abnormal white matter volumes in dementia of Alzheimer type. Arch Neurol 1996; 53: 742–9.

43. de Leon MJ, Golomb J, George AE, Convit A, Tarshish CY, McRae T, De Santi S, Smith G, Ferris SH, Noz M, Rusinek H. The radiologic prediction of Alzheimer's disease: the atrophic hippocampal formation. Am J Neuroradiol 1993; 14: 897–906.

44. de Leon MJ, George AE, Golomb J, Tarshish C, Convit A, Kluger A, De Santi S, McRae T, Ferris SH, Reisberg B, Ince C, Rusinek H, Bobinski M, Quinn B, Miller DC, Wisniewski HM. Frequency of hippocampus atrophy in normal elderly and Alzheimer's disease patients. Neurobiol Aging 1997; 18: 1–11.

45. Aylward EH, Rasmusson DX, Brandt J, Raimundo L, Folstein M, Pearlson GD. CT measurement of suprasellar cistern predicts rate of cognitive decline in Alzheimer's disease. J Int Neuropsychol Soc 1996; 2: 89–95.

46. de Leon MJ, George AE, Convit A, De Santi S, Golomb J, Tarshish C, Rusinek H, Ferris SH, Bobinski M, Arena L. MR measurement of the medial temporal lobe changes in Alzheimer disease: the case for the interuncal distance. Am J Neuroradiol 1994; 15: 1286–90.

47. Reinikainen KJ, Koivisto K, Mykkanen L, Hanninen T, Laakso M et al. Age-associated memory impairment in aged population: an epidemiologic study. Neurology 1990; 40: 177.
48. Wippold IFJ, Mokhtar HG, Morris JC, Duchek JM, Grant EA. Senile dementia and healthy aging: a longitudinal CT study. Radiology 1991; 179: 215–19.
49. de Leon MJ, George AE, Reisberg B, Ferris SH, Kluger A, Stylopoulos LA, Miller JD, La Regina ME, Chen C, Cohen J. Alzheimer's disease: longitudinal CT studies of ventricular change. Am J Neuroradiol 1989; 10: 371–6.
50. Bird JM, Levy R, Jacoby RJ. Computed tomography in the elderly changes over time in a normal population. Br J Psychiat 1986; 148: 80–85.
51. Shear PK, Sullivan EV, Mathalon DH, Lim KO, Davis LF, Yesavage JA, Tinklenberg JR, Pfefferbaum A. Longitudinal volumetric computed tomographic analysis of regional brain changes in normal aging and Alzheimer's disease. Arch Neurol 1995; 52: 392–402.
52. Luxenberg JS, Haxby JV, Creasey H, Sundaram M, Rapoport SI. Rate of ventricular enlargement in dementia of the Alzheimer type correlates with rate of neuropsychological deterioration. Neurology 1987; 37: 1135–40.
53. Fox NC, Freeborough PA, Rossor MN. Visualisation and quantification of rates of atrophy in Alzheimer's disease. Lancet 1996; 348: 94–7.
54. Wahlund L-O, Almkvist O, Basun H, Julin P. MRI in successful aging, a 5-year follow-up study from the eighth to ninth decade of life. Magnet Reson Imaging 1996; 14: 601–8.
55. Smith DA, Jobst KA. Use of structural imaging to study the progression of Alzheimer's Disease. Br Med Bull 1996; 52: 575–86.
56. Fox NC, Warrington EK, Freeborough PA, Hartikainen P, Kennedy AM, Stevens JM, Rossor MN. Presymptomatic hippocampal atrophy in Alzheimer's disease: a longitudinal MRI study. Brain 1996; 119: 2001–7.
57. Kaye JA, Swihart T, Howieson D, Dame A, Moore MM, Karnos T, Camicioli R, Ball M, Oken B, Sexton G. Volume loss of the hippocampus and temporal lobe in healthy elderly persons destined to develop dementia. Am Acad Neurol 1997; 48: 1287–304.
58. Braak H, Braak E, Bohl J. Staging of Alzheimer-related cortical destruction. Eur Neurol 1993; 33: 403–8.
59. Reisberg B, Ferris SH, de Leon MJ, Crook T. The global deterioration scale for assessment of primary degenerative dementia. Am J Psychiat 1982; 139: 1136–9.
60. Folstein MF, Folstein SE, McHugh PR. Mini-mental state: a practical method for grading the cognitive state of patients for the clinician. J Psychiat Res 1975; 12: 189–98.
61. Golomb J, de Leon MJ, Kluger A, George AE, Tarshish C, Ferris SH. Hippocampal atrophy in normal aging: an association with recent memory impairment. Arch Neurol 1993; 50: 967–73.
62. Flicker C, Ferris SH, Reisberg B. Mild cognitive impairment in the elderly: predictors of dementia. Neurology 1991; 41: 1006–9.
63. de Leon MJ. Neuroimaging and the early diagnosis of Alzheimer Disease. 6th International Conference on Alzheimer's Disease and Related Disorders, 1998. Amsterdam: Rai.
64. de la Monte SM. Quantitation of cerebral atrophy in preclinical and end-stage Alzheimer's disease. Ann Neurol 1989; 25: 450–59.
65. Golomb J, Kluger A, de Leon MJ, Ferris SH, Convit A, Mittelman MS, Cohen J, Rusinek H, De Santi S, George A. Hippocampal formation size in normal human aging: a correlate of delayed secondary memory performance. Learning and Memory 1994; 1: 45–54.

66. Golomb J, Kluger A, de Leon MJ, Ferris SH, Mittelman MS, Cohen J, George AE. Hippocampal formation size predicts declining memory performance in normal aging. Neurology 1996; 47: 810–13.
67. Convit A, de Asis J, de Leon MJ, Tarshish C, De Santi S, Daisley K, Rusinek H. The fusiform gyrus as the first neocortical site in Alzheimer's Disease. 6th International Conference on Alzheimer's Disease and Related Disorders, 1998. Amsterdam: Rai.
68. Pearlson GD, Harris GJ, Powers RE, Barta PE, Camargo EE, Chase GA, Noga JT, Tune LE. Quantitative changes in mesial temporal volume, regional cerebral blood flow, and cognition in Alzheimer's disease. Arch Gen Psychiat 1992; 49: 402–8.
69. Juottonen K, Laakso MP, Insausti R, Lehtovirta M, Pitkanen A, Partanen K, Soininen H. Volumes of the entorhinal and perirhinal cortices in Alzheimer's disease. Neurobiol Aging 1998; 19: 15–22.
70. Bobinski M, de Leon MJ, Convit A, De Santi S, Wegiel J, Tarshish CY et al. MRI of entorhinal cortex in mild Alzheimer disease. Lancet 1999; 38–40.

Address for correspondence:
    Dr Mony J. de Leon,
    New York University Medical Center,
    Department of Psychiatry, Neuroimaging Laboratory,
    New York, NY 10016, USA.
    Tel: 212 263 5805; fax: 212 263 6991

15 Early Diagnosis of Alzheimer's Disease with Simple Neuropsychological Tests

J.-M. ORGOGOZO, C. FABRIGOULE AND
J.-F. DARTIGUES

INTRODUCTON

Early diagnosis of dementia, the first step to the diagnosis of Alzheimer's disease (AD), still relies entirely on the documentation of mild impairments of cognitive functions. By definition, dementia can be diagnosed only when these impairments reach a sufficient degree to induce disability in the more complex activities of daily life and/or handicap in social roles [1]. Therefore, one faces a conceptual dilemma when speaking of 'preclinical dementia' and most authors now use instead the term 'mild cognitive impairment' [2]. This concept refers to a set of objective deficits in different cognitive domains, not severe enough to qualify for a diagnosis of dementia but associated with a high probability of conversion to a full dementia syndrome in the near future. Impairment of memory, particularly verbal episodic memory, is a key feature of the early AD syndrome [3] but neither at an earlier stage nor to a higher degree than other cognitive impairments [4].

Detection of subjects at high risk of developing dementia in the short term is a major issue of research, in the hope of slowing the progression to an overt stage of dementia. Among the predictors of dementia and AD, minor/mild cognitive impairments represent a 'preclinical' stage of the disease. Unfortunately, their detection is difficult because they are easily confounded by those occurring in normal aging or by a low IQ, a poor education, or even depression. Specific norms have been provided in various geographical populations for the Wechsler Adult Intelligence Scale (WAIS-R) [5], e.g. by Ivnick et al. in Rochester [6] and for the Mini-Mental State Examination (MMSE) [7], e.g. by Commenges et al. in Gironde [8]. However, the specificity of the MMSE as a diagnostic test for dementia is low at the early stages of AD [9, 10], even if, at the conventional threshold of 24/30, its sensitivity is high.

Alzheimer's Disease and Related Disorders
Edited by K. Iqbal, D.F. Swaab, B. Winblad and H.M. Wisniewski
© 1999 John Wiley & Sons Ltd

Among the many memory tests available, those which assess both new learning and retrieval of stored information may be more contributive to the early diagnosis of AD than more focused tests [11]. Other neuropsychological tests [12] have a reasonably good predictive value, but they do not contribute independently to the diagnosis of dementia as they are constructs which explore, in fact, similar dimensions of cognitive impairment. So the ideal screening test or the optimal battery of tests to detect early AD remains to be determined.

SURVEY OF THE LITERATURE

Memory function is particularly affected in early AD [3] and is often the first subjective complaint and the first objectively detected change [13]. But other minor/mild cognitive impairments can also be 'premonitory' signs or 'predictors' of dementia. The short-term predictive value of such impairments was assessed in several studies [14–20] by measuring the correlation between the baseline scores of a number of neuropsychological tests with the occurrence of overt dementia, particularly AD, within 1–5 years.

The neuropsychological tests used in these studies were two comprehensive cognitive tests: the Information–Memory–Concentration test [21] or the MMSE [7]; several types of episodic memory tests: the Fuld Object Memory Evaluation (FOSE) [22], the Buschke Selective Reminding Test (BSRT) [23], the Rey Auditory Recall Test [22], the CERAD Word List [24], the Benton Visual Retention Test (BVRT) [25, 26], the California Verbal Learning Test [27] and the WAIS Memory Tests [28, 29]; two verbal category fluency tests [30]; and several subtests from the WAIS [5].

As the majority of these tests were successful in predicting the short-term occurrence of dementia, it is likely that the low performances measured in different cognitive domains represent sub-clinical impairments due to an ongoing dementia process. In that sense they may contribute to the early diagnosis of dementia or AD, rather than really 'predict' the later occurrence of the disease. A practical clinical question is, then, which tests are better suited, i.e. more predictive of subclinical dementia and easier to use?

Potential candidates are the BSRT [31], the BVRT and the Isaac's Set Test (IST) [30] of verbal fluency. Other simple tests are the Zazzo's Cancellation Tests (ZCT) [32], the Wechsler Digit Symbol Substitution Test (DSST), the Wechsler Similarities Test (WST) and the Wechsler Paired Associates Test (WPAT) [5]. In the selection of a battery of instruments it should be kept in mind that they do not always contribute independently to the diagnosis of early AD: many of them explore several dimensions of cognitive impairment, particularly attention and control of information [5, 33], in addition to specific modalities like memory. In the paper by Masur et al. [19] the combination of the BSRT, the FOME, the DSST and the IST identified, among normal elderly volunteers, one subgroup with an 85% probability of converting to dementia within 4 years (sensitivity) and another with a 95% probability of remaining free of dementia (sensitivity). The overall positive and negative predictive values were 68% and 88%, respectively, which is already quite good but leaves way for more efficient screening methods.

RESULTS FROM THE PAQUID STUDY

PAQUID [34, 35] is a prospective study of a representative random sample of more than 4000 elderly people aged 65 years and over, living at home in Gironde and Dordogne, two administrative areas around Bordeaux (France). It was initiated in 1998 and follow-ups were carried out at 1 year (Gironde), 3 years, 5 years and 8 years (both Gironde and Dordogne). The 10-year follow-up is ongoing.

At baseline sociodemographic data, age and gender were recorded, as well as education, with four levels from no schooling to university level. Cognition was examined through a battery of psychometric tests: MMSE, BVRT, WPAT, IST, ZCT, WST and DSST. When the subjects were not willing to perform the tests, were too tired or were unable to understand the instructions, only the MMSE, BVRT and IST, the three simplest tests, were administered.

After this testing, at baseline and at follow-up, the psychologists completed a standardized questionnaire which allowed to obtain the A (memory impairment), B (impairment of at least one other cognitive function) and C (interference with social or professional life) DSM-IIIR [36] criteria for dementia. Then subjects who met these criteria were seen by a senior neurologist, who checked the DSM-IIIR criteria and filled in the NINCDS–ADRDA criteria [37] and the Hachinski score [38], to make the diagnosis of dementia and specify the aetiology.

In a first paper [39] the three easiest tests, MMSE, BVRT and IST, were systematically performed by the vast majority of the subjects studied in Gironde at the beginning of the study (n = 2792). So they were tested for their value as *screening tools* for the diagnosis of *prevalent dementia*. Albeit empirical, this selection was based on the applicability of these tests in the elderly population, making it of practical value.

A MMSE additive score was derived by summing the items. The BVRT was applied with the multiple-choice form. The IST was used with four semantic categories (colours, animals, fruits and cities) in a limited time and the test was stopped if the subject generated more than 10 words, so the total scores ranged from 0 to 40, from 15 s intervals data.

With the MMSE, at the traditional cut-off point of 23–24, the sensitivity was 1.0 and the specificity 0.77. When the results of the BVRT and of the IST were added into the calculation, the sensitivity remained at 1.0 but the specificity rose to 0.90. Adjusting for age and educational level in the model did not change these results. The addition of two simple tests therefore notably increased the reliability of screening for prevalent dementia when compared to the MMSE alone. However, the conditions of the study meant that the process leading to the diagnosis of dementia was not independent from the results of the neuropsychological testing.

A second paper [40] examined the *predictive value* of the WAIS Similarities Test (WST) [5], which involves abstract thinking (a cognitive process not usually considered a predictor of dementia), obtained at 1 year of follow-up of the cohort, for the subsequent *occurrence of dementia* at 3 years of follow-up, i.e. 2 years later. This procedure aimed at minimizing the bias associated with the first exposure to the test situation. The study was restricted to the 1290 non-demented subjects from Gironde seen at 1 year after baseline. To keep its administration short, the test was limited to the first five items, the subjects being asked to identify relevant similarities or superordinate categories for five pairs of items (e.g. orange and banana). The case finding and the aetiological diagnosis of incident cases of dementia was as described above.

The WST scores were significantly related to age ($p < 0.001$), educational level ($p < 0.001$) and sex ($p < 0.05$). Among the non-demented subjects seen at 1 year, 44 developed an incident dementia at the 3-year follow-up. A logistic regression analysis showed a significant relationship between WST scores at 1 year and the risk of dementia 2 years later (OR per one point = 0.75, 95% CI = 0.69–0.83, $p < 10^{-8}$). This relationship remained significant after adjustment on age, sex, and education (OR = 0.78, 95% CI = 0.71–0.87, $p < 10^{-5}$).

The five first-item score of the WST was a strong predictor of 2-year subsequent dementia. This was explained neither by its relation to age and educational level nor by its relation to global cognitive level, as tested by the MMSE, or to semantic memory, as tested by the IST categorical fluency test. This result demonstrates that abstractional abilities can be impaired early in the preclinical phase of dementia, at least as early as semantic memory abilities or global cognitive abilities.

The third study [41] explored the *predictive value* of the MMSE and its combinations with the BVRT and the IST at baseline for the *occurrence of dementia and AD* after 1 year and 3 years of follow-up. The population studied was the same as in the first paper [39], except that the prevalent cases of dementia at baseline were excluded. The administration and scoring of the psychometric tests and the case finding procedure were also the same, except that the results of the baseline neuropsychological testing did not play a role in the diagnosis of dementia at follow-up. Of the 2726 subjects not demented at baseline, 2043 had at least one follow-up, at 1 year or 3 years. At 1 year there were 21 incident cases of dementia (13 AD) and at 3 years 63 new cases (46 AD). Thus, 84 subjects (4.1%) developed dementia and 59 (2.9%) developed possible or probable AD during the time of observation.

The baseline MMSE values were categorized as low when < 24 and normal otherwise; low values of the BVRT and IST were defined as < 9 and < 23 respectively, i.e. the values of the lower quartile of the distribution for these variables in the study sample. The correlation between the combination of normal and low values for the three tests and the occurrence of AD at 1 and 3 years is shown in Table 1. While the probability of AD increases dramatically with the number of tests being rated low, the MMSE is the least discriminant: when it is low in isolation, the probability of AD is only slightly increased as compared to all tests normal (Table 1, last line vs. first line).

Based on the number of low values among the three tests (0 to 3), the sensitivity and specificity were respectively at 90.8% and 52.2% for a cut-off of 1; at 81.2% and 80.4% for a cut-off of 2; and at 52.2% and 91.3% for a cut-off of 3. The predictive value of the IST by itself is interesting because it is an extremely easy test, which can be administered by general practitioners (GPs) or other health professionals without any particular equipment. So its high negative predictive value when normal (Table 1) can be used to reassure anxious patients presenting with subjective cognitive complaints. Conversely, when two or more tests including the IST are abnormal, a more complete work-up in search of an early dementia is justified.

The fourth paper [42] addressed more specifically this issue of early dementia screening by GPs. The objective was to identify very simple tests which can discriminate, in the population, individuals with either a high or a very low risk of dementia. Such tests could then be administered to patients who present with subjective cognitive complaints or are anxious because of a family history of dementia, in order to decide whether or not to pursue further investigations.

Two previously validated tests [40, 41] were selected for being easy and quick to perform and hence adapted to busy GPs' clinical practice: one verbal fluency test (the IST) and the first five items of the WST. Both tests can be usually performed in less than 5 min. The subjects were selected at 1 year and

Table 1. Combination of tests to detect/predict early AD in the PAQUID Study

MMSE/BVRT/IST (N, normal; L, low*)	Prediction of AD (%)	
	1 year	3 years
N/N/N	0.1	0.5
N/N/L	0.2	1.5
N/L/N	0.4	2.5
N/L/L	1.3	8.2
L/L/L	3.2	19.2
L/N/N	0.2	1.1

* Low: MMSE < 24; BVRT < 9; IST < 23 (lower quartile in the sample).
Adapted from reference [45].

followed up at 3 years, as in the previous paper on the WST alone [40]. The association between low vs. normal IST and WST scores at 1 year on the one hand and the risk of incident dementia 2 years later was assessed through odds ratios (OR) and their confidence intervals (95% CI), while the conditional probability of incident dementia was determined by logistic regression. Low values of the tests were defined as those in the lower quartile of the distribution in the study sample.

During follow-up, 44 out of 1297 subjects became demented (3.2%). Low scores at IST and WST were significantly and independently correlated with a higher risk of dementia at 2 years. The OR for low IST was 1.29 (95% CI = 1.18–1.38; $p < 0.001$) and the OR for low WST was 1.15 (95% CI = 1.03–1.29; $p < 0.01$). The probability of incident dementia, computed for the four possible combinations of test results, is shown in Table 2. When at least one score was low, 40 out of the 44 conversions to dementia were predicted, i.e. the sensitivity was 90%. When the two scores were normal the specificity was 92%. This model yielded a positive predictive value of 18.5% when both scores were low (i.e. the observed conversion rate at 2 years shown in Table 2) and a negative predictive value of 99.5% when both scores were normal. These excellent receiver/operator characteristics make the combined use of the IST and the WST, in the conditions described, a powerful tool for primary screening of subjects at risk of developing dementia.

Table 2. Two simple tests to detect preclinical dementia in the PAQUID Study

IST/WST (N, normal; L, low*)	Probability of AD (%) at 2 years
N/N	0.5
N/L	1.65
L/N	7.73
L/L	18.50

IST, Isaacs Set Test; WST, Wechsler Similarities Test.
* Low; IST < 25; WST < 6 (lower quartile in the sample).
Adapted from reference [46].

CONCLUSION

In the elderly, self-reported subjective complaints with memory and other cognitive abilities are correlated more often with psychological problems than with organic causes like AD [43]. However, in the population, non-depressed subjects with subjective memory complaints are more likely to have objective memory impairments [44, 45], and these complaints are indeed predictors of subsequent development of dementia [46], particularly so when confirmed by objective testing [13].

This overview shows that many different neuropsychological tests, not primarily exploring memory, are also able to predict a short-term conversion to dementia. Due to its simplicity and ease of use, the IST seems particularly useful, at least when combined with other tests. The selection of a particular combination of tests should be based on the objective of the assessment (e.g. diagnosis vs. epidemiology or pharmacological research) and on practical considerations, but also on theoretical neuropsychological grounds [4].

REFERENCES

1. Zaudig M. A new systematic method of measurement and diagnosis of 'mild cognitive impairment' and dementia according to ICD-10 and DSM-IIIR criteria. Int Psychogeriatr 1992; 4 (suppl 2): 203–19.
2. Flicker C, Ferris SH, Reisberg B. Mild cognitive impairment in the elderly: predictors of demetia. Neurology 1991; 41: 1006–9.
3. Petersen RC, Smith G, Ivnik RJ, Kokmen E, Tangalos EG. Memory function in very early Alzheimer's disease. Neurology 1994; 44: 867–72.
4. Fabrigoule C, Rouch I, Taberly A, Letenneur L, Commenges D, Mazaux JM, Orgogozo J-M, Dartigues J-F. Cognitive process in preclinical phase of dementia. Brain, 1998; 121: 135–41.
5. Wechsler D. WAIS-R Manual. New York: Psychological Corporation, 1981.
6. Ivnik RJ, Malec JF, Smith GE, Tangalos EG, Petersen RC, Kokmen E, Kurland LT. Mayo's Older Americans Normative Studies: WAIS-R norms for ages 56 to 97. Clin Neuropsychol 1992; 6 (suppl): 1–30.
7. Folstein M, Folstein S, McHugh P. 'Mini-Mental State': a practical method for grading the cognitive state of patients for the clinician. J Psychiat Res 1975; 12: 189–98.
8. Commenges D, Gagnon M, Letenneur L, Dartigues J-F, Barberger-Gateau P, Salamon R. Statistical description of the Mini-Mental State Examination (MMS) for French elderly community residents. J Nerv Ment Dis 1992; 180: 28–32.
9. Gagnon M, Letenneur L, Dartigues J-F, Commenges D, Orgogozo J-M, Barberger-Gateau P, Alperovitch A, Décamps A, Salamon R. The validity of the Mini-Mental State Examination (MMS) as a screening instrument for cognitive impairment and dementia in French elderly community residents. Neuroepidemiology 1990; 9: 143–50.
10. Galasko D, Klaubert MR, Hofstetter CR, Salmon DP, Lasker B, Thal LJ. The Mini-Mental State Examination in the early diagnosis of Alzheimer's disease. Arch Neurol 1990; 47: 49–52.
11. Buschke H, Sliwinski MJ, Kuslansky G, Lipton RB. Diagnosis of early dementia by the Double Memory Test: encoding specificity improves diagnostic sensitivity and specificity. Neurology 1997; 48: 989–97.
12. Stuss D, Meiran N, Guzman A, Lafleche G, Willmer J. Do long tests yield a more accurate diagnosis of dementia than short tests? Arch Neurol 1996; 53: 1033–9.
13. Bowen J, Teri L, Kukull W, McCormick W, McCurry S, Larson E. Progression to dementia in patients with isolated memory loss. Lancet 1997; 349: 763–5.
14. Fuld P, Masur D, Blau A, Crystal H, Aronson M. Object-memory evaluation for prospective detection of dementia in normal functioning elderly: predictive and normative data. J Clin Exp Neuropsychol 1990; 12, 520–28.

15. Masur D, Fuld P, Blau A, Crystal H, Aronson M. Predicting development of dementia in the elderly with the Selective Reminding Test. J Clin Exp Neuropsychol 1990; 529–38.
16. Masur DM, Sliwinski M, Lipton RB, Blau AD, Crystal HA. Neuropsychological prediction of dementia and the absence of dementia in healthy elderly persons. Neurology 1994; 44: 1427–32.
17. Bondi MW, Mosch AU, Galasko D, Butters N, Salmon DP, Delis DC. Preclinical cognitive markers of dementia of Alzheimer type. Neuropsychology 1994; 8: 374–84.
18. Jacobs DM, Sano M, Dooneief G, Marder K, Bell KL, Stern Y. Neuropsychological detection and characterization of preclinical Alzheimer's disease. Neurology 1995; 45: 957–62.
19. Tierney MC, Szalai JP, Snow WG, Fisher RH, Nores A, Nadon G, Dunn E, St George-Hyslop PH. Prediction of probable Alzheimer's disease in memory-impaired patients: a prospective longitudinal study. Neurology 1996; 46: 661–5.
20. Howieson DB, Dame A, Camicioli R, Sexton G, Payami H, Kaye JA. Cognitive markers preceding Alzheimer's dementia in the healthy oldest old. J Am Geriat Soc 1997; 45(5): 584–9.
21. Blessed G, Tomlinson B, Roth M. The association between quantitative measures of dementia and of senile changes in the cerebral grey matter of elderly subjects. Br J Psychiat 1968; 114: 797–811.
22. Fuld PA. The Fuld Object Memory Test. Chicago: The Stoelting Instrument Company, 1981.
23. Buschke H. Selective reminding for analysis of memory and learning. J Verbal Learn Verbal Behav 1973; 12: 543–50.
24. Morris JC, Heyman A, Mohs RC, Hughes JP, VanBelle G, Fillenbaum G, Mellits ED, Clark C. The Consortium to Establish a Registry for Alzheimer's Disease (CERAD). Part I. Clinical and neuropsychological assessment of Alzheimer's disease. Neurology 1989; 39: 1159–65.
25. Benton AL. Manuel pour l'application du test de rétention visuelle. Applications cliniques et expérimentales, 2nd edn (in French). Paris: Centre de Psychologie Appliquée, 1965.
26. Benton AL. The Revised Visual Retention Test, 4th edn. New York: Psychological Corporation, 1974.
27. Delis DC, Kramer JH, Kaplan E, Ober BA. The California Verbal Learning Test. New York: Psychological Corporation, 1987.
28. Wechsler DA, Stone CP. Wechsler Memory Scale. New York: Psychological Corporation, 1973.
29. Wechsler DA. Wechsler Memory Scale—Revised. San Antonio: Psychological Corporation, 1987.
30. Isaacs B, Kennie A. The Set Test as an aid to the detection of dementia in old people. J Psychiat 1973; 123: 467–70.
31. Masur D, Fuld O, Blau A, Thal L, Levin H, Aronson M. Distinguishing normal and demented elderly with the selective reminding test. J Clin Exp Neuropsychol 1989: 615–30.
32. Zazzo R. Test des deux barrages. Actualités pédagogiques et psychologiques, Vol. 7. Neuchâtel: Delachaux et Niestlé, 1974.
33. Parasuraman R, Haxby JV. Attention and brain function in Alzheimer's disease: a review. Neuropsychology 1993; 7: 242–72.
34. Dartigues J-F, Gagnon M, Barberger-Gateau P, Letenneur L, Commenges D. The PAQUID epidemiological program on brain aging. Neuroepidemiology 1992; 11 (suppl 1): 14–18.

35. Dartigues J-F, Gagnon M, Michel P, Letenneur L, Commenges D, Barberger-Gateau P, Auriacombe S, Rigal B, Bedry R, Alperovitch A, Orgogozo J-M, Henry P, Loiseau P, Salamon R. Le programme de recherche PAQUID sur l'épidémiologie de la démence: méthodologie et résultats initiaux. Rev Neurol 1991; 147: 225–30.
36. DSM-IIIR: Diagnostic and Statistical Manual of Mental Disorders: 3rd edn, Revised. Washington, DC: American Psychiatric Association, 1987.
37. McKhann G, Drachman D, Folstein M, Katzmann R, Price D, Stadian EM. Clinical diagnosis of Alzheimer's disease: report of the NINCDS–ADRDA Work Group under the auspices of Department of Health and Human Services Task Force on Alzheimer's disease. Neurology 1984; 34: 939–44.
38. Hachinski V, Iliff L, Duboulay G et al. Cerebral blood flow in dementia. Arch Neurol 1975; 32: 632–7.
39. Commenges D, Gagnon M, Letenneur L, Dartigues J-F, Barberger-Gateau P, Salamon R. Improving screening for dementia in the elderly using Mini-Mental State Examination subscores, Benton's Visual Retention Test and Isaacs Set Test. Epidemiology 1992; 3: 185–8.
40. Fabrigoule C, Lafont S, Letenneur L, Dartigues J-F. WAIS similarities subtest performances as predictors of dementia in elderly community residents. Brain and Cognition, 1996; 30: 323–6.
41. Dartigues J-F, Commenges D, Letenneur L, Barberger-Gateau P, Gilleron V, Fabrigoule C, Mazaux JM, Orgogozo J-M, Salamon R. Cognitive predictors of dementia in elderly community residents. Neuroepidemiology 1997; 16: 29–39.
42. Rouch-Leroyer I, Fabrigoule C, Letenneur L, Commenges D, Orgogozo J-M, Dartigues J-F. A practical psychometric approach to detect preclinical stage of dementia. J Am Geriat Soc, 1998; 46: 394–5.
43. Smith GE, Petersen RC, Ivnik RJ, Malec JF, Tangalos EG. Subjective memory complaints, psychological distress, and longitudinal changes in objective memory performance. Psychol Aging 1996; 11: 272–9.
44. Gagnon M, Dartigues J-F, Mazaux JM, Dequae L, Letenneur L, Giroire JM, Barberger-Gateau P. Self-reported memory complaints and memory performance in elderly French community residents: results of the PAQUID Research Program. Neuroepidemiology 1994; 13: 145–54.
45. Jonker C, Launer L, Hoouijer C, Lindeboom J. Memory complaints and impairments in older individuals. J Am Geriat Soc 1996; 44: 44–9.
46. Schmand B, Jonker C, Hooijer C, Lindeboom J. Subjective memory complaints may announce dementia. Neurology 1996; 46: 121–5.

Address for correspondence:
J.-M. Orgogozo,
Department of Neurology, CHU Pellegrin,
Neuroepidemiology Research Unit INSERM U 330,
University of Bordeaux II, 33076 Bordeaux cedex, France

16 A Sketch of Alzheimer's Disease Histopathology

CHARLES DUYCKAERTS, M.-A. COLLE AND
J.-J. HAUW

INTRODUCTION

We shall successively consider the morphology of the lesions observed in the brains of Alzheimer's disease patients, the composition of those lesions as revealed by immunohistochemistry, their topography, their relationship with the clinical symptoms and finally their hypothetical course.

MORPHOLOGY OF THE LESIONS

FIBRILLARY ALTERATIONS

The neuronal cytoskeleton, as revealed by silver stains, appears extensively altered in Alzheimer's disease. The changes include neurofibrillary tangles, neuropil threads and the crown of senile plaque. A neurofibrillary tangle is an abnormal meshwork of filamentous material stained in black by the deposit of metallic silver and located in the cell body of the neuron. At the ultrastructural level [1], the neurofibrillary tangle appears to be made of bundles of pairs of filaments (paired helical filaments or 'PHF') or, as more recently suggested, of a twisted ribbon [2, 3]. Neuropil threads [4] are short and tortuous neurites [5] loaded with tau-positive [6] PHF. Most of them are probably dendrites but up to 10% have been identified as myelinated axons by electron microscopy [7, 8]. The crown of the senile plaque is made of neuronal processes, some of them dilated. Ultrastructurally, they contain presynaptic vesicles, a characteristic of axon terminals [9].

DEPOSITS

The extracellular deposit that makes up the core of the senile plaque is inconspicuous after standard staining by haematoxylin–eosin, but Congo red

Alzheimer's Disease and Related Disorders
Edited by K. Iqbal, D.F. Swaab, B. Winblad and H.M. Wisniewski
© 1999 John Wiley & Sons Ltd

and thioflavin stain it. These staining properties define the 'amyloid' substances, i.e. proteins or peptides with a high content of β-pleated sheets responsible for their uncommon insolubility [10].

Large vessels (mainly arteries) in the subarachnoid spaces may also contain amyloid deposits (congophilic angiopathy) as small vessels in the parenchyma to which plaques seem sometimes to be attached, as if the amyloid was coming from the vessel to the parenchyma—a process attributed by Scholz [11], who described it, to a disturbance of the blood–brain barrier. There has been some discussion concerning the frequency of amyloid angiopathy in AD: it is undoubtedly very frequent but probably not always present. The factors that influence the balance between the parenchymal and the vascular deposition of amyloid are not known.

IMMUNOCYTOCHEMICAL ASPECTS

FIBRILLARY PATHOLOGY

Abnormally Phosphorylated Tau

Antibodies directed against tau protein, involved in the stabilization of neurotubules, strongly label the neurofibrillary tangles and the crowns of plaques [12] as well as the neuropil threads [6]. Several lines of evidence suggest that tau is indeed the main constituent of the PHF seen in those three lesions [13, 14]. Tau in the NFT is abnormally phosphorylated [15]—a fact that may be attributed to an exaggerated kinase or to a decreased phosphatase activity. However, it has been shown that normal samples contain a high proportion of phosphorylated tau that rapidly decreases after death (in post-mortem material) or after surgery (in biopsies). Part of the hyperphosphorylation may thus be due to the inaccessibility of tau protein to phosphatase [16].

Abnormally phosphorylated tau may be found in the cell body and its processes, the axon and dendrites [17]. The secondary detachment of dendrites filled by abnormally phosphorylated tau has been observed in the CA1 sector [18]. However, continuity between the cell body and the axons innervating the senile plaque has never been fully demonstrated. On the contrary, the continuity between neuropil threads and both tangle-free and tangle-bearing neurons has been documented [19]. The proportion of volume occupied by the neurofibrillary alterations in an AD brain is high, sometimes higher than the proportion of volume occupied by the Aβ peptide—up to 37% [20].

Ubiquitin

Some neurofibrillary tangles and some of the neurites of the senile plaque are ubiquitinated [21]. Ubiquitination occurs secondarily [22]. In the series of cases that we have studied, at the most 33% of the NFT in the CA1 sector of the hippocampus were ubiquitinated and 53% in Brodmann's area 22 (unpublished data). The neuropil threads are probably less ubiquitinated, but quantitative data are lacking.

Epitopes of Extracellular NFT

Some tangle-bearing neurons finally die. The NFT are then free in the neuropil. Those extracellular tangles (eNFT) contain epitopes of the amyloid P component and some complement factors (C4d) that may trigger an inflammatory response [23]. The frequency of the eNFT varies according to the region. They are common in Ammon's horn, rare in the isocortex and absent in the hypothalamus.

Neurofilaments

Immunoreactivity to middle and high molecular weight neurofilament subunits has also been found in the neurofibrillary tangles [24, 25]. Moreover, a monoclonal antibody (SMI32) directed against non-phosphorylated epitopes of the same subunits has been shown to label a population of pyramidal neurons, located in layers III and V, that are vulnerable to Alzheimer's disease [26].

THE SENILE PLAQUES

The Crown of the Senile Plaque

The neurites that are present in the crowns of the senile plaques are stained by antibodies directed against middle molecular weight neurofilament subunits (abundant in axons) and do not contain epitopes of MAP2 (microtubule associated protein abundant in dendrites) [27], data that favour their axonal origin. Some neurites of the senile plaques are labelled by antibodies directed against the precursor protein of the Aβ peptide (amyloid precursor protein: APP) and some are ubiquitinated. Ubiquitin-positive tau-negative neurites have been called 'dystrophic-type neurites' [28]. They are probably present at an early stage of plaque formation [29].

Neurites containing tau-epitopes or 'PHF-type neurites' [28] are present in the crown of the senile plaque only when neurofibrillary tangles are located nearby [30]. The density of senile plaques containing tau-positive neurites is correlated with the density of the neurofibrillary tangles. Some neurites of the crown are enriched in butyryl cholinesterase activity [31] and in various neuromediators [32]. The protein GAP43, present in the axonal growth cone, is also found in the axons of the senile plaque crown, where it is colocalized with APP [33]. This expression shows that the senile plaque is also the site of the regenerative processes and cannot be considered as an inactive scar.

The Core of the Senile Plaque and the Diffuse Deposits

The peptide that precipitates in the core of the senile plaque—the Aβ peptide—is made of 42 or 40 amino acids [34]. The core of the senile plaque is strongly labelled by the Aβ antibodies and appears as a massive and dense spheroid mass ('focal deposit'), usually exhibiting amyloid properties and appearing as fibrils— hence the term 'fibrillized Aβ' [35]. They contain a high proportion of $A\beta_{40}$ [36]. Other alterations labelled by the Aβ antibody have also been called plaque, al- though they are—at least in our opinion—of a different nature. They are more weakly stained and are also much larger than the core. They have indistinct contours and are not surrounded by degenerating neurites. They do not have the tinctorial affinity of amyloid and were called preamyloid [37] or non-fibrillized [35]. Those 'diffuse deposits of Aβ' [38] should be clearly distinguished from neuritic plaques, since they do not have the same clinical consequences. They are, indeed, sometimes present in old patients who were not considered to be de- mented [39] and have been called 'benign plaques' [35] or thought to character- ize 'pathological aging' [40]. Diffuse deposits have been considered an early stage of plaque formation; however, this is certainly not always the case. There are indeed regions—such as the striatum and the cerebellum—where diffuse deposits are abundant and senile (neuritic) plaques are absent. The proportion of total volume occupied by the Aβ deposits (so-called 'amyloid load') [20] may reach 25% in Alzheimer's disease [41], the focal deposits (core plaques) accounting for half this value. There have been hints that some senile plaques may not contain Aβ peptides but instead another yet unidentified peptide [42].

ApoE is present in the senile plaques, especially in the core and in the microglial cells [43–45]. Its deposition appears to be a secondary event [44], as it has been shown in transgenic mice [46]. It could play the role of chap- erone in amyloidogenesis [47].

Activated microglia [48], early components of the complement cascade [49, 50], alpha-antichymotrypsin and various types of interleukin have been identi- fied in the senile plaques, indicating an ongoing inflammation. The activated microglia seem to be better correlated with the neurofibrillary alterations than with the density of Aβ peptide[51]. Microglia could play an important role in the production of the amyloid fibrils [52].

Various components of the extracellular matrix have been shown to ac- cumulate in the senile plaque such as ICAM1 [53], thrombospondin [54], heparan sulphate proteoglycan [55].

PROTEINS THAT ARE MUTATED IN FAMILIAL ALZHEIMER'S DISEASE

A few hundred families have been identified around the world in which AD is transmitted on an autosomal dominant mode. Three mutated proteins are pres- ently known: the amyloid protein precursor (APP), presenilin 1 and 2, their genes being respectively located on chromosomes 21, 14 and 1. Immunohistochemistry with antibodies against APP has shown that its distribution is not severely affected by AD: APP is present in neurones, in both controls and patients. It is not found in the plaque core but might accumulate in some neurites of the crown [56, 57]. That observation has led to different interpretations: the accumulated APP has been considered the source of the deposited Aβ peptide; alternatively, it could be evidence of altered axonal transport, with no direct relationship with the Aβ accumulation. Presenilin 1 is seen in neurons, in both AD and controls [44]. An epitope of presenilin, located at the carboxyterminal of the protein, associated with the Aβ peptide, is found in the core of the senile plaque [58].

QUANTITATIVE ASPECTS: THE LOSSES

NEURONES

Neuronal loss is difficult to quantify. It is masked by atrophy that restores the neuronal density to normal, by shrinking the volume in which the neurones are distributed [59, 60]. It is selective and involves only specific areas, and within them, specific layers. Small neurones having a lower probability of being included in a microscopical section than large ones, the atrophy of the cell body artificially decreases the neuronal density on sections [60]—a stereological bias that is presently prevented by using special techniques of counting, such as the disector.

The very reality of neuronal loss has been recently challenged [61]. Extra-cellular tangles are, however, definite evidence of neuronal death. The neuronal loss appears to be massive in the entorhinal cortex and cannot be only explained by the density of the neurofibrillary tangles [62]. In the supramarginal gyrus, the loss was found significant only in the late stages of the disease (when the density of neurofibrillary tangles was over 5/mm^2). It then reached the value of several million neurons in the parietal cortex [63].

Tangle formation is, indisputably, one of the causes of neuronal death. Several studies, based on the observation that the amyloid peptide induces apoptosis in cell cultures, have looked for evidence of programmed cell death. The number of neurones positive for *in situ* end-labelling (ISEL) is increased in the patients, but the meaning of that observation has been discussed—since the morphology of apoptotic nuclei is often lacking. ISEL might be related to DNA fragility, rather than to apoptosis [64]. Immunohistochemistry of proteins involved in cell death has also not provided unambiguous evidence of apoptosis [65].

SYNAPSES

The concentration of synaptophysin, located within small presynaptic vesicles, is decreased in the cerebral cortex in correlation with intellectual status [66–

70]. The concentration of chromogranin A located in large dense core vesicles appears, on the contrary, to increase [71]. Observations with electron microscopy have shown that the synapses decrease in number but are enlarged, the total apposition length remaining unchanged [72–75]. It has been shown more recently that presynaptic *membrane* components (synaptotagmin, SNAP-25, and syntaxin 1/HPC-1) are little affected (10% the value of the controls) compared to the vesicular components (synaptobrevin and synaptophysin—30% of the controls) [76]. SNAP-25 immunohistochemistry tends, indeed, to reveal a much smaller synaptic loss than synaptophysin [77, 78]. All the mentioned synaptic markers are presynaptic and depend on the metabolism of cell bodies that are sometimes located far away: it is thus difficult to determine whether the pre-synaptic alterations appear early [79] or late [80] in the cascade of pathological events, and if it is a major [68] or a minor correlate [81] of dementia. It has been shown that the decrease in synaptophysin immunoreactivity was not linked to the presence of Aβ deposits [82] and that it could, on the contrary, be related, in the dentate gyrus system, to the density of neurofibrillary tangles in the entorhinal cortex [67].

TOPOGRAPHY OF THE LESIONS

Aβ and tau-positive lesions have a different distribution.

DISTRIBUTION OF Aβ

Aβ peptide is deposited over large areas of the brain: the cerebral cortex (diffuse and focal deposits) and, to a lesser degree, the white matter, the striatum and the cerebellar cortex (only diffuse deposits). The deposits are diffuse except in the cortex, where cored plaques (i.e. focal deposits) may be abundant. The first area in which Aβ precipitates has not been identified: Braak and Braak have described an antero-basal to postero-lateral progression [83]. Both the frontal and the occipital cortices have been considered most affected, while the hippocampus appears relatively spared. Within the cortex, the upper layers are more severely involved. The deposits are sometimes located around the dendritic tree [84], sometimes strikingly perivascular, an observation that has fostered the hypothesis of its vascular origin [85], nowadays disputed [86].

DISTRIBUTION OF NEUROFIBRILLARY ALTERATIONS

The cortical areas may be ranked in a hierarchical order, such that the involvement of a given area is observed only if the areas of a lower rank are also involved [87, 88]. The parallel between the architectonic maps and the topography of the lesions is striking [89] ('Alzheimer's disease knows neuroanatomy!'). At least three main hypotheses have been proposed to explain that particular distribution:

1. The 'sensitivity' hypothesis: some areas are more prone to respond to the (still unknown) noxious agent, various explanations being in turn proposed to explain those differences in sensitivity (e.g. differences in myelination [90] or in capacity of remodelling [91] or in neurofilament characteristics [26]).
2. The 'inactivity' hypothesis suggests that some neurons, when inactive, develop neurofibrillary tangles [92].
3. The 'connectivity' hypothesis, finally, states that the neurofibrillary pathology propagates through connections [93–96], 'invading' first the limbic, then the associative and finally the primary sensory areas. A set of data support that hypothesis: within involved cortical areas or nuclei, certain layers [97] or subnuclei [98] are selectively lesioned—generally those that are connected with already affected regions. Additional lesions disturb the usual progression of the neurofibrillary pathology: in a disconnected piece of cortex, no neurofibrillary alteration could be seen—although numerous Aβ peptide deposits were present [99]. The senile plaques of the dentate gyrus are located in the upper part of the molecular layer, where axons of the entorhinal neurons end. When those neurons die, the destruction of the axons 'denervates' the senile plaques and leaves a band of spongiosis [99]. The laminar spongiosis seen in layer II of the isocortex in some cases might also be related to disconnection.

Whatever the cause of the differences in the prevalence of the neurofibrillary tangles in the various areas, they are helpful in staging the cases: the presence of neurofibrillary tangles in the hippocampus alone suggests a less severe involvement than tangles in the hippocampus *and* in an associative area. Such a staging has been formalized by Braak and Braak [83] and appears to be particularly reproducible [100]. Large discrepancies from the hierarchical scheme of Braak and Braak seem to be rare [101]. Focal onset of Alzheimer's disease (particularly progressive aphasia) is documented [102]. These cases are intriguing since they could constitute important exceptions to the hierarchical scheme. However, no case of Alzheimer's disease with isocortical neurofibrillary tangles but without hippocampal involvement has ever been documented, to the best of our knowledge.

COMPARISON OF THE DISTRIBUTION OF Aβ AND TAU PATHOLOGY

Three situations may be found according to the cases and the areas: some samples may contain neurofibrillary tangles alone, Aβ deposits alone or both. The first situation is met in little-affected, generally old patients: only neurofibrillary tangles are present in the limbic area—the isocortex and the limbic system being free of Aβ deposits. That distribution of the lesions has been referred to in the literature under the name 'tangle-predominant form of Alzheimer's disease' [103, 104]. The ApoE4 phenotype is underrepresented in that population of patients [105].

Aβ deposits are found alone in some exceptional *cases*: most often, neurofibrillary tangles are present at least in the hippocampus. However, it is quite common to find in some *samples* large amounts of Aβ deposits in the absence of neurofibrillary tangles. We have checked those 'tangle-free areas'—a total of 59 samples in a cohort of 26 cases. Thirteen of those samples (22% of the total number) contained a few neuropil threads. Those neuropil threads could thus be the first signs of tau pathology and precede the accumulation of PHF in the cell bodies. Dystrophic neurites, labelled by anti-APP and anti-ubiquitin antibodies, are also found in tangle-free areas, evidence that they represent an early stage of plaque formation.

CLINICOPATHOLOGIC CORRELATIONS

Large areas of the cortices may contain high numbers of Aβ diffuse deposits, even in normal or little-affected cases [39]; on the contrary, the neurofibrillary pathology involves the cerebral cortex in a hierarchical order. Qualitatively, the clinical deficit corresponds to the areas where neurofibrillary tangles are present [106–108]. Even a small number of tangles in an isocortical area is highly significant; probably because they are late markers of cortical pathology [87, 88].

CHRONOLOGICAL SEQUENCES OF THE LESIONS

The neuropathological course of AD is still partly unknown: human neuropathology permits only a cross-sectional view, except for some isolated cases that have been studied by both biopsy and post mortem [109, 110]. A large survey made on a series of autopsies collected in general hospitals and forensic pathology departments has given some hints concerning the prevalence of Braak stages in the general population [111]. Although the selection of the cases is obviously biased, three conclusions [112] may tentatively be drawn from that study: (a) the prevalence of the first stages (so-called entorhinal) is much higher than previously thought; at 47 years of age, half the population was affected in that cohort; but (b) there was a gap of nearly 40 years between the entorhinal and limbic stages; (c) finally, the neurofibrillary lesions precede the amyloid deposits for more than 25 years. Concerning the last point, opposite conclusions have been drawn from the study of trisomy 21 cases: in that pathology, diffuse deposits are said to precede neurofibrillary tangles; they were indeed isolated in one case [113]. However, in all the 11 other cases with lesions, tangles were seen at least in the amygdaloid body or in the hippocampus. On the whole the 'amyloid only' cases appear to be rare.

CONCLUSIONS

Alzheimer's disease involves a complex series of events that finally lead to dementia. At the present state of our knowledge, the Aβ deposit is at one end and the diffusion of the neurofibrillary tangles within the cortical area at the other. What is the link between Aβ and tau pathologies? The senile plaque, which includes both pathologies, might well hold the secret!

ACKNOWLEDGEMENTS

This work was supported by INSERM (4106 and 4360) and Association Claude Bernard.

REFERENCES*

1. Itoh Y et al. Scanning electron microscopical study of the neurofibrillary tangles of Alzheimer's disease. Acta Neuropathol (Berl) 1997; 94: 78–86.
2. Pollanen MS, Markiewicz P, Goh MC. Paired helical filaments are twisted ribbons composed of two parallel and aligned components: image reconstruction and modeling of filament structure using atomic force microscopy. J Neuropathol Exp Neurol 1997; 56: 79–85.
3. Ruben GC, Iqbal K, Grundke-Iqbal I. Helical ribbon morphology in neurofibrillary tangles of paired helical filaments. In: Iqbal K et al. (eds) Research Advances in Alzheimer's Disease and Related Disorders. Chichester: Wiley, 1995; 477–85.
4. Braak H et al. Occurrence of neuropil threads in the senile human brain and in Alzheimer's disease. A third location of paired helical filaments outside of neurofilament tangles and neuritic plaques. Neurosci Lett 1986; 65: 351–5.
5. Duyckaerts C et al. Fiber disorganization in the neocortex of patients with senile dementia of the Alzheimer type. Neuropath Appl Neurobiol 1989; 15: 233–47.
6. Kowall NW, Kosik KS. Axonal disruption and aberrant localization of tau protein characterize the neuropil pathology of Alzheimer's disease. Ann Neurol 1987; 22: 639–43.
7. Ohtsubo K et al. Curly fibers are tau-positive strands in the pre- and post-synaptic neurites, consisting of paired helical filaments: observations by the freeze-etch and replica method. Acta Neuropathol (Berl) 1990; 81: 111–15.

* Because the limited amount of space, we have been forced to limit the number of references.

8. Perry G et al. Neuropil threads of Alzheimer's disease show a marked alteration of the normal cytoskeleton. J Neurosci 1991; 11: 1748–55.
9. Terry RD, Gonatas JK, Weiss M. Ultrastructural studies in Alzheimer presenile dementia. Am J Pathol 1964; 44: 269–97.
10. Glenner GG. Amyloid deposits and amyloidosis. The β-fibrilloses. N Engl J Med 1980; 302: 1283–92, 1333–43.
11. Scholz W. Studien zur Pathologie der Hirngefässe II. Die drusige Entartung der Hirnarterien und Capillaren. Z Gesamte Neurol Psychiatr 1938; 162: 694–715.
12. Brion JP et al. Mise en évidence immunologique de la protéine tau au niveau des lésions de dégénérescence neurofibrillaire de la maladie d'Alzheimer. Arch Biol (Brux) 1985; 95: 229–35.
13. Kosik KS, Joachim CL, Selkoe DJ. Microtubule-associated protein tau is a major component of paired helical filaments in Alzheimer disease. Proc Natl Acad Sci USA 1986; 83: 4044–8.
14. Delacourte A, Defossez A. Alzheimer's disease: tau proteins, the promoting factors of microtubule assembly are major components of paired helical filaments. J Neurol Sci 1986; 76: 173–86.
15. Grundke-Iqbal I et al. Abnormal phosphorylation of the microtubule associated protein (tau) in Alzheimer cytoskeletal pathology. Proc Natl Acad Sci USA 1986; 83: 4913–17.
16. Matsuo ES et al. Biopsy-derived adult human tau is phosphorylated at many of the same sites as Alzheimer's disease paired helical filament tau. Neuron 1994; 13: 989–1002.
17. Braak E, Braak H, Mandelkow E-M. A sequence of cytoskeleton changes related to the formation of neurofibrillary tangles and neuropil threads. Acta Neuropathol (Berlin) 1994; 87: 554–67.
18. Braak E, Braak H. Alzheimer's disease: transiently developing dendritic changes in pyramidal cells of sector CA1 of the Ammon's horn. Acta Neuropathol 1997; 93: 323–5.
19. Schmidt ML, Murray JM, Trojanowski JQ. Continuity of neuropil threads with tangle-bearing and tangle-free neurons in Alzheimer disease cortex. Mol Chem Neuropath 1993; 18: 299–312.
20. Cummings BJ et al. Beta-amyloid deposition and other measures of neuropathology predict cognitive status in Alzheimer's disease. Neurobiol Aging 1996; 17: 921–33.
21. Lowe J et al. Ubiquitin is common factor in intermediate filament inclusion bodies of diverse type in man, including those of Parkinson's disease, Pick's disease and Alzheimer's disease, as well as Rosenthall fibres in cerebellar astrocytomas, cytoplasmic bodies in muscle, and Mallory bodies in alcoholic liver disease. J Pathol 1988; 155: 9–15.
22. Bancher C et al. Abnormal phosphorylation of tau precedes ubiquitination in neurofibrillary pathology of Alzheimer's disease. Brain Res 1991; 539: 11–18.
23. Schwab C et al. Amyloid P immunoreactivity precedes C4d deposition on extracellular neurofibrillary tangles. Acta Neuropathol (Berl) 1997; 93: 87–92.
24. Vickers JC et al. Alterations in neurofilament protein immunoreactivity in human hippocampal neurons related to normal aging and Alzheimer's disease. Neuroscience 1994; 62: 1–13.
25. de la Monte SM, Wands JR. Diagnostic utility of quantitating neurofilament-immunoreactive Alzheimer's disease lesions. J Histochem Cytochem 1994; 42: 1625–34.

26. Hof PR, Cox K, Morrison JH. Quantitative analysis of a vulnerable subset of pyramidal neurons in Alzheimer's disease: I. Superior frontal and inferior temporal cortex. J Comp Neurol 1990; 301: 44–54.

27. Schmidt ML, Lee VM-Y, Trojanowski JQ. Comparative epitope analysis of neuronal cytoskeletal proteins in Alzheimer's disease senile plaque neurites and neuropil threads. Lab Invest 1991; 64: 352–7.

28. Dickson DW. The pathogenesis of senile plaques. J Neuropathol Exp Neurol 1997; 56: 321–39.

29. He Y et al. Two distinct ubiquitin immunoreactive senile plaques in Alzheimer's disease: relationship with the intellectual status in 29 cases. Acta Neuropathol 1993; 86: 109–16.

30. Probst A et al. Senile plaque neurites fail to demonstrate anti-paired helical filament and anti-microtubule-associated protein tau immunoreactive proteins in the absence of neurofibrillary tangles in the neocortex. Acta Neuropathol 1989; 77: 430–36.

31. Guillozet AL et al. Butyrylcholinesterase in the life cycle of amyloid plaques. Ann Neurol 1997; 42: 909–18.

32. Walker LC et al. Multiple transmitter systems contribute neurites to individual senile plaques. J Neuropathol Exp Neurol 1988; 47: 138–44.

33. Masliah E et al. Localization of amyloid precursor protein in GAP43-immunoreactive aberrant sprouting neurites in Alzheimer's disease. Brain Res 1992; 574: 312–16.

34. Iwatsubo T et al. Visualization of Aβ42(43) and Aβ40 in senile plaques with end-specific Aβ monoclonals: evidence that an initially deposited species is Aβ42(43). Neuron 1994; 13: 45–53.

35. Wisniewski HM, Wegiel J, Kotula L. Some neuropathological aspects of Alzheimer's disease and its relevance to other disciplines. Neuropathol Appl Neurobiol 1996; 22: 3–11.

36. Barelli H, et al. Characterization of new polyclonal antibodies specific for 40 and 42 amino acid-long amyloid beta peptides: their use to examine the cell biology of presenilins and the immunohistochemistry of sporadic Alzheimer's disease and cerebral amyloid angiopathy cases. Mol Med 1997; 3: 695–707.

37. Tagliavini F et al. Preamyloid deposits in the cerebral cortex of patients with Alzheimer's disease and nondemented individuals. Neurosci Lett 1988; 93: 191–6.

38. Delaère P et al. Subtypes and differential laminar distributions of βA4 deposits in Alzheimer's disease: relationship with the intellectual status of 26 cases. Acta Neuropathol 1991; 81: 328–35.

39. Delaère P et al. Large amounts of neocortical βA4 deposits without Alzheimer changes in a non-demented case. Neurosci Lett 1990; 116: 87–93.

40. Dickson DW et al. Identification of normal and pathological aging in prospectively studied non-demented elderly humans. Neurobiol Aging 1991; 13: 179–89.

41. Mochizuki A et al. Amyloid load and neural elements in Alzheimer's disease and non-demented individuals with high amyloid plaque density. Exp Neurol 1996; 142: 89–102.

42. Schmidt ML et al. Monoclonal antibodies to a 100-kd protein reveal abundant Aβ-negative plaques throughout gray matter of Alzheimer's disease brains. Am J Pathol 1997; 151: 69–80.

43. Uchihara T et al. Inconstant apolipoprotein E (ApoE)-like immunoreactivity in amyloid β-protein deposits: relationship with APOE genotype in aging brain and Alzheimer's disease. Acta Neuropathol (Berlin) 1996; 92: 180–85.

44. Uchihara T et al. Widespread immunoreactivity of presenilin in neurons of normal and Alzheimer's disease brains: double-labeling immunohistochemical study. Acta Neuropathol (Berlin) 1996; 92: 325–30.
45. Dickson TC, Saunders HL, Vickers JC. Relationship between apolipoprotein E and the amyloid deposits and dystrophic neurites of Alzheimer's disease. Neuropathol Appl Neurobiol 1997; 23: 483–91.
46. Igeta Y et al. Apolipoprotein E accumulates with the progression of β-deposition in transgenic mice. J Neuropathol Exp Neurol 1997; 46: 1228–35.
47. Wisniewski T, Frangione B. Apolipoprotein E. A pathological chaperone protein in patients with cerebral and systemic amyloid. Neurosci Lett 1992; 135: 235–8.
48. McGeer PL et al. Microglia in degenerative neurological diseases. Glia 1993; 7: 84–92.
49. Eikelenboom P, Veerhuis R. The role of complement and activated microglia in the pathogenesis of Alzheimer's disease. Neurobiol Aging 1996; 17: 673–80.
50. McGeer PL et al. Complement activation in amyloid plaques in Alzheimer's dementia. Neurosci Lett 1989; 107: 341–6.
51. DiPatre PL, Gelman BB. Microglial cell activation in aging and Alzheimer disease: partial linkage with neurofibrillary tangle burden in the hippocampus. J Neuropathol Exp Neurol 1997; 56: 143–9.
52. Wegiel J, Wisniewski HM. The complex of microglia cells and amyloid star in three-dimensional reconstruction. Acta Neuropathol 1990; 81: 116–24.
53. Verbeek MM et al. Accumulation of intercellular adhesion molecule-1 in senile plaques in brain tissue of patients with Alzheimer's disease. Am J Pathol 1994; 144: 104–16.
54. Buee L et al. Immunohistochemical identification of thrombospondin in normal human brain and in Alzheimer's disease. Am J Pathol 1992; 141: 783–8.
55. Snow AD et al. Heparan sulfate proteoglycan in diffuse plaques of hippocampus but not of cerebellum in Alzheimer's disease brain. Am J Pathol 1994; 144: 337–47.
56. Cras P et al. Senile plaque neurites in Alzheimer disease accumulate amyloid precursor protein. Proc Natl Acad Sci USA 1991; 88: 7552–6.
57. McGeer PL et al. Immunohistochemical localization of β-amyloid precursor protein sequences in Alzheimer and normal brain tissue by light and electron microscopy. Neurosci Res 1992; 31: 428–42.
58. Wisniewski T et al. Presenilin-1 is associated with Alzheimer's disease amyloid. Am J Pathol 1997; 151: 601–10.
59. Hauw J-J, Duyckaerts C, Partdrige M. Neuropathological aspects of brain aging and SDAT. In: Modern Trends in Aging Research. Colloque Inserm-Eurage. John Libbey Eurotext Ltd, (1986); 435–42.
60. Duyckaerts C et al. Neuronal loss and neuronal atrophy. Computer simulation in connection with Alzheimer's disease. Brain Res 1989; 504: 94–100.
61. Regeur L et al. No global neocortical nerve cell loss in brains from patients with senile dementia of Alzheimer's type. Neurobiol Aging 1994; 15: 347–52.
62. Gomez-Isla T et al. Profound loss of layer II entorhinal cortex neurons occurs in very mild Alzheimer's disease. J Neurosci 1996; 16: 4491–500.
63. Grignon Y et al. Cytoarchitectonic alterations in the supramarginal gyrus of late onset Alzheimer's disease. Acta Neuropathol 1998; 95: 395–406.
64. Stadelmann C et al. Alzheimer disease: DNA fragmentation indicates increased neuronal vulnerability, but not apoptosis. J Neuropathol Exp Neurol 1998; 57: 456–64.
65. Nagy ZS, Esiri MM. Apoptosis-related protein expression in the hippocampus in Alzheimer's disease. Neurobiol Aging 1997; 18: 565–71.

66. Masliah E et al. Immunohistochemical quantification of the synapse-related protein synaptophysin in Alzheimer disease. Neurosci Lett 1989; 103: 234–9.
67. Hamos JE, DeGennaro LJ, Drachman DA. Synaptic loss in Alzheimer's disease and other dementias. Neurology 1989; 39: 355–61.
68. Terry RD et al. Physical basis of cognitive alterations in Alzheimer's disease: synapse loss is the major correlate of cognitive impairment. Ann Neurol 1991; 30: 572–80.
69. Zhan SS, Beyreuther K, Schmitt HP. Quantitative assessment of the synaptophysin immuno-reactivity in the cortical neuropil in various neurodegenerative disorders with dementia. Dementia 1993; 4: 66–74.
70. Bancher C et al. Correlations between mental state and quantitative neuropathology in the Vienna Longitudinal Study on Dementia. Eur Arch Psychiat Clin Neurosci 1996; 246: 137–46.
71. Lassmann H et al. Synaptic pathology in Alzheimer's disease: immunological data for markers of synaptic and large dense-core vesicles. Neuroscience 1992; 46: 1–8.
72. Scheff SW, DeKosky ST, Price DA. Quantitative assessment of cortical synaptic density in Alzheimer's disease. Neurobiol Aging 1990; 11: 29–37.
73. DeKosky ST, Scheff SW. Synapse loss in frontal cortex biopsies in Alzheimer's disease: correlation with cognitive severity. Ann Neurol 1990; 27: 457–64.
74. Scheff SW, Price DA. Synapse loss in the temporal lobe in Alzheimer's disease. Ann Neurol 1993; 33: 190–99.
75. Bertoni-Freddari C et al. Deterioration threshold of synaptic morphology in aging and senile dementia of Alzheimer's type. Anal Quant Cytol Histol 1996; 18: 209–13.
76. Shimohama S et al. Differential involvement of synaptic vesicle and presynaptic plasma membrane proteins in Alzheimer's disease. Biochem Biophys Res Commun 1997; 236: 239–42.
77. Clinton J et al. Differential synaptic loss in the cortex in Alzheimer's disease: a study using archival material. NeuroReport 1994; 5: 497–500.
78. Dessi F et al. Accumulation of SNAP-25 immunoreactive material in axons of Alzheimer's disease. NeuroReport 1997; 8: 3685–9.
79. Heinonen O et al. Loss of synaptophysin-like immunoreactivity in the hippocampal formation is an early phemomenon in Alzheimer's disease. Neuroscience 1995; 64: 375–84.
80. Lassmann H. Patterns of synaptic and nerve cell pathology in Alzheimer's disease. Behav Brain Res 1996; 78: 9–14.
81. Dickson DW et al. Correlations of synaptic and pathological markers with cognition of the elderly. Neurobiol Aging 1995; 16: 285–304.
82. Masliah E et al. Diffuse plaques do not accentuate synapse loss in Alzheimer's disease. Am J Pathol 1990; 137: 1293–7.
83. Braak H, Braak E. Neuropathological staging of Alzheimer-related changes. Acta Neuropathol (Berlin), 1991; 82: 239–59.
84. Probst A et al. Deposition of β/A4 protein along neuronal plasma membranes in diffuse senile plaques. Acta Neuropathol 1991; 83: 21–9.
85. Miyakawa T et al. The relationship between senile plaques and cerebral blood vessels in Alzheimer's disease and senile dementia. Virchows Arch 1982; 40: 121–9.
86. Kawai M, Cras P, Perry G. Serial reconstruction of β-protein amyloid plaques: relationship to microvessels and size distribution. Brain Res 1992; 592: 278–82.
87. Duyckaerts C et al. Modeling the relation between neurofibrillary tangles and intellectual status. Neurobiol Aging 1997; 18: 267–73.

88. Duyckaerts C et al. Progression of Alzheimer histopathological changes. Acta Neurol Belg 1998; 98.
89. Arnold SE et al. The topographical and neuroanatomical distribution of neurofibrillary tangles and neuritic plaques in the cerebral cortex of patients with Alzheimer's disease. Cerebral Cortex 1991; 1: 103–16.
90. Braak H, Braak E. Development of Alzheimer-related neurofibrillary changes in the neocortex inversely recapitulates cortical myelogenesis. Acta Neuropathol (Berl) 1996; 92: 197–201.
91. Arendt T et al. Cortical distribution of neurofibrillary tangles in Alzheimer's disease matches the pattern of neurons that retain their capacity of plastic remodelling in the adult brain. Neuroscience 1998; 83: 991–1002.
92. Swaab DF, Salehi A. The pathogenesis of Alzheimer disease: an alternative to the amyloid hypothesis. J Neuropathol Exp Neurol 1997; 56: 216.
93. Duyckaerts C, Delaère P, Hauw J-J. Alzheimer's disease and neuroanatomy: hypotheses and proposals. In: Boller F et al. (eds) Heterogeneity of Alzheimer's disease. Springer-Verlag: Berlin, 1992; 144–55.
94. Delacoste MC, White CL. The role of connectivity in Alzheimer's disease pathogenesis. A review and model system. Neurobiol Aging 1993; 14: 1–16.
95. Su JH, Deng G, Cotman CW. Transneuronal degeneration in the spread of Alzheimer's disease pathology: immunohistochemical evidence for the transmission of tau hyperphosphorylation. Neurobiol Dis 1997; 4: 365–75.
96. Hyman BT, Duyckaerts CD, Christen Y. Connections, Cognition and Alzheimer Disease. Research and Perspective in Alzheimer's disease. Berlin: Springer-Verlag, 1997.
97. Duyckaerts C et al. Laminar distribution of neocortical plaques in senile dementia of the Alzheimer type. Acta Neuropathol (Berl) 1986; 70: 249–56.
98. Hyman BT, van Hoesen GW, Damasio AR. Memory-related neural systems in Alzheimer's disease: an anatomical study. Neurology 1990; 40: 1721–30.
99. Duyckaerts C et al. Dissociation of Alzheimer type pathology in a disconnected piece of cortex. Acta Neuropathol 1997; 93: 501–7.
100. Nagy Z et al. Staging of Alzheimer-type pathology: an interrater–intrarater study. Dement Geriatr Cogn Disord 1997; 8: 248–51.
101. Gertz HJ et al. Examination of the validity of the hierarchical model of neuropathological staging in normal aging and Alzheimer's disease. Acta Neuropathol (Berl) 1998; 95: 154–8.
102. Pogacar S, Williams RS. Alzheimer's disease presenting as slowly progressive aphasia. RI Med J 1984; 67.
103. Bancher C, Jellinger KA. Neurofibrillary tangle predominant form of senile dementia of Alzheimer type: a rare subtype in very old subjects. Acta Neuropathol (Berl) 1994; 84: 565–70.
104. Jellinger KA, Bancher C. Senile dementia with tangles (tangle predominant form of senile dementia). Brain Pathol 1998; 8: 367–76.
105. Bancher C et al. Low prevalence of apolipoprotein E epsilon 4 allele in the neurofibrillary tangle predominant form of senile dementia. Acta Neuropathol (Berl) 1997; 94: 403–9.
106. Nielson KA, Cummings BJ, Cotman CW. Constructional apraxia in Alzheimer's disease correlates with neuritic neuropathology in occipital cortex. Brain Res 1996; 741: 284–93.
107. Giannakopoulos P et al. Pathologic correlates of apraxia in Alzheimer disease. Arch Neurol 1998, 55: 689–95.
108. Liu Y et al. Pathological correlates of extrapyramidal signs in Alzheimer's disease. Ann Neurol 1997; 41: 368–74.

109. Mann DMA et al. The progression of the pathological changes of Alzheimer's disease in frontal and temporal neocortex both at biopsy and autopsy. Neuropathol Appl Neurobiol 1988; 14: 177–95.
110. Di Patre PL et al. Progression of Alzheimer disease changes in patients evaluated at biopsy and autopsy (abstr). J Neuropath Exp Neurol 1998; 57: 508.
111. Braak H, Braak E. Frequency of stages of Alzheimer-related lesions in different age categories. Neurobiol Aging 1997; 18: 351–7.
112. Duyckaerts C, Hauw J-J. Prevalence, incidence and duration of Braak's stages in the general population: can we know? Neurobiol Aging 1997; 18: 362–9.
113. Mann DMA, Esiri MM. The pattern of acquisition of plaques and tangles in the brains of patients under 50 years of age with Down's syndrome. J Neurol Sci 1989; 89: 169–79.

Address for correspondence:
C. Duyckaerts,
Laboratoire de Neuropathologie R. Escourolle,
Hôpital de la Salpêtrière, 47 Blvd de l'Hôpital,
75651 Paris Cedex 13, France
Tel: (33) 1 42 16 18 91; fax: (33) 1 44 23 98 28;
e-mail: charles.duyckaerts@psl.ap-hop-paris.fr

17 Neuropathologic Links Between Alzheimer's Disease and Vascular Disease

D. LARRY SPARKS

Ten years ago we discovered what we believed to be neuropathologic evidence of a link between Alzheimer's disease and heart disease [1]. The data indicated that senile plaques (SP) were two to three times more prevalent in non-demented individuals with critical coronary artery disease (cCAD) than age-matched non-demented non-heart disease controls (non-HD). Determined by gross and microscopic inspection, cCAD was defined as greater than 75% stenosis of any one of the four main epicardial arteries. This was based on forensic protocol, where in the absence of any other findings, the cause of an individual's death can be ascribed to cCAD if this level of arterial stenosis is demonstrable. These studies have since been confirmed by Soneira and Scott [2].

We have found that SP in cCAD subjects were indistinguishable from those SP found in AD. The regional distribution of SP in cCAD was remarkably similar to that found in AD, and the numerical densities of SP in many of the cCAD subjects were diagnostic of AD using the established criteria of 1990 [3]. The youngest cCAD individual to date with cerebral SP is 28 years of age. Protracted disease was not the cause of SP production in cCAD, as many of the non-HD subjects died after prolonged illnesses. In many of the cases, cCAD and hypertension were occult disease, in that the patient was unaware of his/her condition.

In the same year two clinico-pathologic studies suggested a link between myocardial infarction (MI) in women and dementia among the very old [4], and between MI, cardiovascular disease and AD [5]. Since cCAD is a risk factor for MI, this further suggests a link between heart disease and AD.

Early on it was realized that chronicity of coronary artery disease was required. We found that individuals dying of acute thrombic occlusion of an epicardial artery resulting in death did not have increased prevalence of SP.

Alzheimer's Disease and Related Disorders
Edited by K. Iqbal, D.F. Swaab, B. Winblad and H.M. Wisniewski
© 1999 John Wiley & Sons Ltd

Because high serum cholesterol level is a known risk factor for cCAD, we hypothesized that high serum cholesterol would induce AD-like histopathology. We confirmed this hypothesis when we discovered that dietary cholesterol induced intraneuronal and some extraneuronal accumulation of β-amyloid immunoreactive material (IRM) in the brains of rabbits [6]. A follow-up study in cholesterol-fed rabbits suggested that if cholesterol was removed from the diet there was clearance of the β-amyloid IRM from the brain [7].

Meanwhile, the epidemiologic evidence continued to accumulate. That same year, Breteler et al. [8] suggested a relationship between cardiovascular disease and cognitive impairment among the elderly, and Jarvik et al. [9] suggested a link between total cholesterol levels, apolipoprotein E genotype and AD.

In further studies [10] we investigated two new human populations. One new group was comprised of non-demented subjects with hypertension, and the other was comprised of those non-demented subjects with both cCAD and hypertension that were drawn from the earlier cCAD group. We found that non-demented hypertensive subjects exhibited an increased prevalence and density of neurofibrillary tangles (NFT) in their brains in addition to SP. In analogous findings, Prince et al. [11] reported a nearly significant relationship between AD and systolic hypertension, and Skoog et al. [12] reported that the severity of previous hypertension was related to the severity of dementia occurring 15 years later. Most recently, the investigators of the Honolulu–Asian Aging Study have also identified a relationship between hypertension and the presence of NFT in the brain (personal communication, H. Pretrovitch).

Based on these observations we have performed a variety of investigations undertaken to determine whether there is neuropathologic overlap between AD, heart disease and the cholesterol-fed rabbit. A compilation of the results from these studies is depicted in Table 1 and delineated below.

Intraneuronal β-amyloid immunoreactive material (IRM) has been noted in AD, hypertension and cCAD [7], similar to the pattern observed in cholesterol-fed rabbit brain [6, 13]. The number of neurons expressing β-amyloid IRM in rabbit brain was proportional to the time the rabbit was on the cholesterol diet (Table 1). We have shown with specific antibodies (Figure 1) and with Western blots that the intraneuronal β-amyloid IRM observed in both man and rabbit is predominantly the C-100 fragment of the β-amyloid precursor protein (β-APP).

It is well established that parenchymal SP in AD are immunoreactive with β-amyloid antibodies, and we have shown that SP in cCAD and hypertension are also immunoreactive with β-amyloid antibodies [14]. In the cholesterol-fed rabbit the prevalence of deposited parenchymal β-amyloid IRM was proportional to the time on the experimental diet [13].

Identical to AD, SP in hypertension and cCAD are silver-positive (Beilschowsky method) and are thioflavin-S-positive [1, 14]. In contrast, the extracellular deposits of β-amyloid IRM in the brains of cholesterol-fed rabbits are neither thioflavin-S- or silver-positive (Table 1).

Table 1. Neuropathological links between Alzheimer's disease, vascular disorders and an animal model of human vascular disease

	Alzheimer's disease	Hyper-tension	CAD	Cholesterol rabbit
β-amyloid				
Intraneuronal (antibody)	Yes	Yes	Yes	Yes ∝ time
Parenchymal (antibody)	Yes	Yes	Yes	Yes ∝ time
Thioflavin-S (senile plaque)	Yes	Yes	Yes	No
Silver positive (senile plaque)	Yes	Yes	Yes	No
NFT (silver and PHF-1)	Yes	Yes	No*	No
Alz-50				
Neurons	Yes	Yes	Yes	No
Threads	Yes	Yes	Yes	No
Neurites	Yes	Yes	Yes	No
Apo-E				
Neuronal IR	Yes	Yes	Yes	Yes ∝ time
Senile plaque IR	Yes	Yes	Yes	No
Genotype (4 allele)	Yes	Yes	Yes	N/A
Genotype α senile plaque density	No	Yes	Yes	N/A
Cholesterol				
Circulating	Yes/No	Ukn	Yes	Yes
Brain	Yes/No	Ukn	Yes	Yes
HSPG				
Senile plaque IR	Yes	Yes	Yes	No
Cathepsin-D				
Neuronal IR	Yes	Yes	Yes	Yes ∝ time
Senile plaque IR	Yes	Yes	Yes	No
Microgliosis	Yes	Yes	Yes	Yes ∝ time
Apoptosis	Yes	Yes	Yes	Yes
Free radical markers				
Neuronal SOD-1 IR	Yes	Yes	Yes	Yes ∝ time
Senile plaque SOD-1 IR	Yes	Yes	Yes	No
Circulating SOD-1 activity	Yes	Yes	Yes	Yes
Brain SOD-1 activity	Yes	Ukn	Ukn	Yes
Circulating TBARS/MDA	Yes/No	Yes	Yes	Yes
Brain TBARS/MDA	Yes	Ukn	Ukn	Ukn
New data—free radical markers				
Vascular SOD-1 IR	Yes	Yes	Yes	Yes ∝ time
Perivascular SOD-1 IR	Yes	Yes	Yes	Yes ∝ time

ApoE = apolipoprotein E; IR = immunoreactivity; HSPG = heparin sulfate proteoglycan; TBARS = thibarbituric acid reactive species; MDA = maliondialdehyde; SOD-1 = Cu/Zn superoxide dismutase; Unk = unknown; * = NFT occurring, but without enhanced prevalence, are silver and PHF-1 positive; Yes/No = both change and no change have been recorded; Yes ∝ time = severity of change is proportional to increasing time.

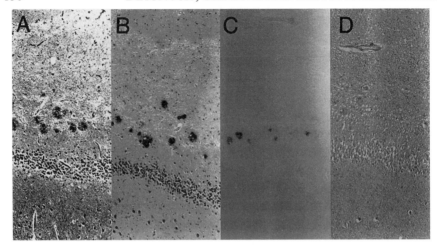

Figure 1. Adjacent 8 μm sections from a 67 year-old cCAD subject stained by the Bielschowsky method (A) and immunohistochemically reacted with N-terminal β-amyloid antibody (B), C-terminal 42 β-amyloid antibody (C) and C-terminal 40 β-amyloid antibody (D). (A) A line of senile plaques (SP) runs parallel to fascia dentata in cCAD, similar to findings in most AD patients. (B) Using N-terminal β-amyloid antibody, the line of SP seen in A are immunoreactive, as are cells in the hilus and of the fascia dentata. (C) Using C-terminal 42 β-amyloid antibody, the line of SP seen in A are immunoreactive, but the cells of the hilus and of the fascia dentata are not. (D) Using C-terminal 40 β-amyloid antibody, no features are immunoreactive. This suggests that intraneuronal β-amyloid immunoreactive material is probably the C-100 fragment of β-APP

Cytoskeletal alterations are identifiable in AD and heart disease brain using Alz-50 antibody (Table 1). This antibody highlights neurons, neuropil threads and neurites in the AD brain, as well as the brains of individuals with hypertension and/or cCAD [10, 14]. In contrast, no Alz-50 immunoreactive features are observed in the brains of cholesterol-fed rabbits.

Apolipoprotein E (ApoE) has been implicated in AD. We have found that there is enhanced neuronal expression of ApoE immunoreactivity in AD, hypertension and cCAD [15] and the increased level of neuronal immunoreactivity induced by cholesterol in rabbits is proportional to the time on the experimental diet [16]. Essentially all SP in AD, hypertension and cCAD are immunoreactive with ApoE antibody [15], but extracellular deposits of β-amyloid IRM in the cholesterol-fed rabbit brain lack ApoE immunoreactivity. Genetically, it is well accepted that there is increased frequency of the ApoE-ε4 allele in AD, and it has been shown that there is increased ApoE-ε4 allele frequency in hypertension and cCAD [17]. Similar analysis in rabbits is not applicable, as the animal has only a single ApoE genotype.

Circulating levels of cholesterol have been reported to be both decreased and increased in AD [9, 18, 19], but most recent data favor a relationship between elevated serum cholesterol and AD [20–22]. Although there is contradictory data, we have found increased levels of cholesterol in the AD brain [15]. Similar increments of cerebral cholesterol levels have been found in cCAD [15] and the cholesterol-fed rabbit [13].

As has been shown in AD with heparan sulfate proteoglycan (HSPG) antibodies [23, 24], SP are HSPG-immunoreactive in cCAD and hypertension [25], and there are alterations in the cerebrovasculature of heart disease subjects, which include vascular irregularities, discontinuities and string vessels. Similar HSPG-immunoreactive features are not found in the cholesterol-fed rabbit brain.

Because cathepsin D could be the enzyme responsible for liberating the N-terminal end of β-amyloid (β-secretase), we investigated the chemical activity and the immunolocalization of cathepsin D in controls, heart disease subjects and AD patients [26]. We found that SP were immunoreactive with cathepsin D antibody in non-HD controls, heart disease and AD, and thus indistinguishable. The numbers of immunoreactive neurons were increased in AD and heart disease, and paralleled the enzymatic activity of cathepsin D. Among cholesterol-fed rabbits there was increased neuronal cathepsin-D immunoreactivity with longer time on the diet, but it occurred after accumulation of β-amyloid IRM [13].

There is increased microgliosis in cCAD and cholesterol-fed rabbits [7, 27]. Our unpublished data suggests a significant activation of microglia in hypertensive individuals. Microgliosis is associated with SP formation in AD.

Apoptosis is a mechanism of neurodegeneration shown to occur in AD and proposed to contribute to the etiology of the disorder. We have morphologically identified apoptosis in AD, Down's syndrome, hypertension, cCAD [25] and in the cholesterol-fed rabbit [27].

We have demonstrated that there is increased neuronal Cu/Zn superoxide dismutase (SOD-1) immunoreactivity and that SP are SOD-immunoreactive in AD and heart disease [15]. Dietary cholesterol also causes increased numbers of SOD-1-immunoreactive neurons in the rabbit brain, proportional to increasing time on the experimental diet [13], but extracellular deposits of β-amyloid IRM are not SOD-1-immunoreactive.

Increased SOD-1 activity accompanies elevated cholesterol levels in AD blood [28], as it does in cCAD, hypertension and the cholesterol-fed rabbit [13]. The activity of SOD-1 is increased in the brains of cholesterol-fed rabbits [13], and both SOD-1 activity and the free radical marker TBARS levels are elevated in the AD brain [29–31]. Increased circulating concentrations of TBARS are recognized in AD, cCAD, hypertension and the cholesterol-fed rabbit. A clue to the mechanism by which free radicals may enter the brain of cholesterol-fed rabbits comes from studies in the aorta. As free radical levels increase in the blood of cholesterol-fed rabbits, there is increasing endothelial damage and upregulation of SOD-1 in vessel walls and perivascular tissue proportional to the concentration of circulating free radicals [32]. Based on this, it was hypothesized that there may be functional flow of free radical activity from the blood to the brain.

Re-evaluation of sections stained with Cu/Zn SOD antibody [13, 15] in both rabbits (Figures 2 and 3) and humans (Figures 4 and 5) has revealed that there are 'halos' of SOD immunoreactivity surrounding vessels in the brains of AD patients, heart disease subjects and cholesterol-fed rabbits. Similar features were not found in age-matched human controls or in rabbits fed a control diet. Such vessels appear to have significantly enhanced SOD immunoreactivity themselves. This would clearly tend to support the contention that there may be backlog of free radicals exiting the CNS or there is a functional flow of free radicals from the blood, through the vasculature into the CNS.

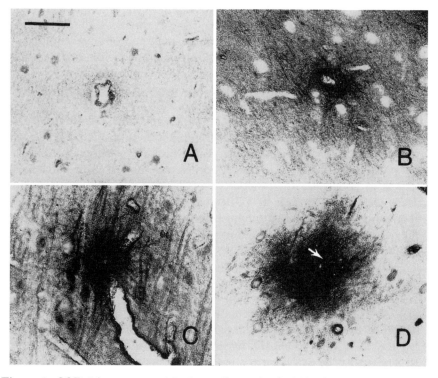

Figure 2. SOD-1 immunoreactivity in small vessels of rabbits fed cholesterol or control diet. 8 µm paraffin sections of frontal pole were simultaneously immunoreacted with Cu/Zn SOD antibody utilizing standard ABC methods. (A) Small vessels in rabbits fed control diet 8 weeks showed no enhanced SOD-1 immunoreactivity. (B) Small vessels in the rabbits fed a 2% cholesterol diet for 4 weeks showed perivascular 'halos' of SOD-1 immunoreactivity. (C) and (D) Progressively severe deposition of SOD-1 immunoreactivity was associated with longer time on the experimental 2% cholesterol diet (C, 6 weeks; D, 8 weeks). The white arrow points out the vessel in D, the lumen of which is barely visible. Calibration bar = 50 µm

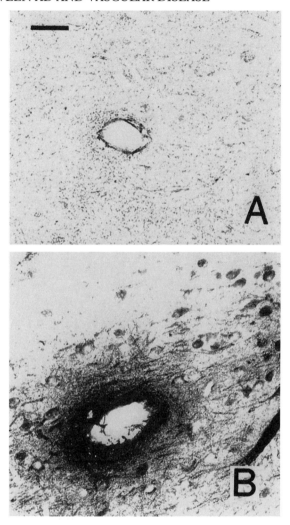

Figure 3. SOD-1 immunoreactive in large vessels of rabbits fed cholesterol or control diet. 8 μm paraffin sections of frontal pole were simultaneously immunoreacted with CU/Zn SOD antibody utilizing standard ABC methods. (A) Large vessels in rabbits fed control diet 8 weeks showed no enhanced SOD-1 immunoreactivity. (B) Large vessels in the rabbits fed a 2% cholesterol diet for 8 weeks showed perivascular 'halos' of SOD-1 immunoreactivity. Progressively severe deposition of SOD-1 immunoreactivity was associated with longer time on the experimental 2% cholesterol diet. Calibration bar = 50 μm

The current studies indicate that there is yet another neuropathologic index which is identical in AD, CAD, hypertension and the cholesterol-fed rabbit, one which may be related to the mechanism of apoptotic neurodegeneration occurring in each condition. These studies indicate that there is cerebral

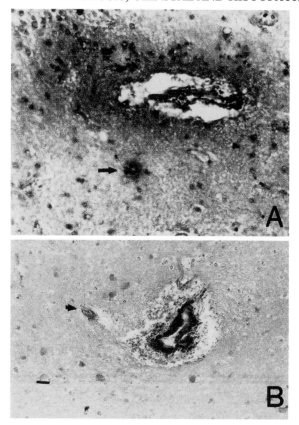

Figure 4. SOD-1 immunoreactivity of large and small vessels in Alzheimer's disease and control brains. 8 μm paraffin sections of hippocampus/parahippocampal gyrus were simultaneously immunoreacted with Cu/Zn SOD antibody utilizing ABC methods. (A) Peri-vascular 'halos' of SOD-1 immunoreactivity are apparent in both small (arrow) and large vessels from this 74 year-old male AD patient. (B) No such peri-vascular 'halo' of SOD-1 immunoreactivity is observed in association with either small (arrow) or large vessels in this 71 year-old non-demented non-heart disease control. Maintenance levels of SOD-1 may produce some immunoreactivity in the control vessels. Calibration bar = 25 μm

upregulation of vascular SOD-1 immunoreactivity consistent with trans-vascular flow of free radical activity from the circulation to the parenchyma. This trans-vascular flow of free radical activity may induce the peri-vascular 'halos' of SOD-1 immunoreactivity around both small and large cerebral vessels in AD, CAD, hypertension and the cholesterol-fed rabbit.

It is possible that increased circulating levels of free radicals cause attenuation of free radical clearance from the brain, accumulations in the vasculature and functional trans-vascular flow into the parenchyma, culminating in enhanced neuronal expression of the free radical scavenger enzyme SOD-1.

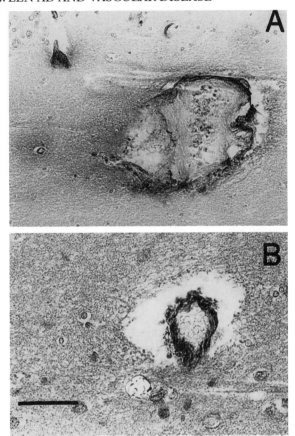

Figure 5. SOD-1 immunoreactivity of large and small vessels in hypertensive and control subjects. 8 μm paraffin sections of hippocampus/parahippocampal gyrus were simultaneously immunoreacted with Cu/Zn SOD antibody utilizing standard ABC methods. (A) Peri-vascular 'halos' of SOD-1 immunoreactivity are apparent in both small and large vessels from this 63 year-old non-demented hypertensive individual with a post-mortem interval of 6 h. This individual was classified as a Braak stage III+ or incipient AD. (B) No such perivascular 'halo' of SOD-1 immunoreactivity is observed in association with the large vessel in this 61 year-old non-demented non-heart disease control. Calibration bar = 50 μm

This free radical burden, identified by increased neuronal SOD-1 activity, may participate in, or could initiate, the apoptotic cell death demonstrable in AD, CAD, hypertension and the cholesterol-fed rabbit. Based on these data it is probable that AD, CAD and hypertension are neuropathologically linked vascular disorders.

REFERENCES

1. Sparks DL et al. Cortical senile plaques in coronary artery disease, aging and Alzheimer's disease. Neurobiol Aging 1990; 11: 601–7.
2. Soneira CF, Scott TM. Severe cardiovascular disease and Alzheimer's disease: senile plaque formation in cortical areas. Clin Anat 1996; 9: 118–27.
3. Khachaturian Z. Diagnosis of Alzheimer's disease. Arch Neurol 1985; 42: 1097–105.
4. Aronson MK et al. Women, myocardial infarction, and dementia in the very old. Neurology 1990; 40: 1102–6.
5. Martins C et al. Effect of age and dementia on the prevalence of cardiovascular disease. Age 1990; 13: 9–11.
6. Sparks DL et al. Induction of Alzheimer-like β-amyloid immunoreactivity in the brains of rabbits with dietary cholesterol. Exp Neurol 1994; 126: 88–94.
7. Sparks DL. Intraneuronal β-amyloid immunoreactivity in the CNS. Neurobiol Aging 1996; 17: 291–9.
8. Breteler MM et al. Cardiovascular disease and distribution of cognitive function in elderly people: the Rotterdam study. Br Med J 1994; 308: 1604–8.
9. Jarvik GP et al. Interactions of apolipoprotein E genotype, total cholesterol level, age, sex in prediction of Alzheimer's disease: a case-control study. Neurology 1995; 45: 1092–6.
10. Sparks DL et al. Increased density of neurofibrillary tangles (NFT) in non-demented individuals with hypertension. J Neurological Sci 1995; 131: 162–9.
11. Prince M et al. Risk factor for Alzheimer's disease and dementia: a case-control study based on the MRC elderly hypertension trial. Neurology 1994; 44: 97–104.
12. Skoog I et al. 15-Year longitudinal study of blood pressure and dementia. Lancet 1996; 347: 1141–5.
13. Sparks DL. Dietary cholesterol induces Alzheimer-like β-amyloid immunoreactivity in rabbit brain. Nutr Metab Cardiovasc Dis 1997; 7: 255–66.
14. Sparks DL et al. Temporal sequence of plaque formation in the cerebral cortex of non-demented individuals. J Neuropath Exp Neurol 1993; 52: 135–42.
15. Sparks DL. Coronary artery disease, hypertension, ApoE, and cholesterol: a link to Alzheimer's disease? Ann NY Acad Sci 1997; 826: 128–46.
16. Sparks DL et al. Increased density of cortical apolipoprotein E immunoreactive neurons in rabbit brain after dietary administration of cholesterol. Neurosci Lett 1995; 187: 142–4.
17. Sparks DL et al. Increased density of senile plaques (SP), but not neurofibrillary tangles (NFT), in non-demented individuals with the apolipoprotein E4 genotype: comparison to confirmed Alzheimer's disease patients. J Neurol Sci 1996; 138: 97–104.
18. Lehtonen A, Luutonen S. High-density lipoprotein cholesterol levels of very old people in the diagnosis of dementia. Age Aging 1986; 15: 267–70.
19. Mahieux F et al. Isoform 4 of apolipoprotein E and Alzheimer disease. Specificity and clinical study. Rev Neurol (Paris) 1995; 151: 231–9.
20. Grant WB. Dietary links to Alzheimer's disease. Alzheimer's Dis Rev 1997; 2: 42–55.
21. Kalmijn S et al. Dietary fat intake and the risk of incident dementia in the Rotterdam study. Ann Neurol 1997; 42: 776–82.
22. Notkola I-L et al. Serum total cholesterol, apolipoprotein ε4 allele, and Alzheimer's disease. Neuroepidemiology 1998; 17: 14–20.

23. Snow AD et al. Heparan sulfate proteoglycan in diffuse plaques of hippocampus but not of cerebellum in Alzheimer's disease brain. Am J Pathol 1994; 144: 337–47.

24. Perlmutter LS. Microvascular pathology and vascular basement membrane components in Alzheimer's disease. Mol Neurobiol 1994; 9: 33–40.

25. Sparks DL. Vascular related and mediated alterations in Alzheimer's disease. In: Morrison J, Peters A (eds) Cerebral Cortex. New York: Raven Press, 1998 (in press).

26. Haas U, Sparks DL. Cathepsin D: activity and immunocytochemical localization in Alzheimer's disease and aging. Mol Chem Neuropathol 1996; 29: 1–14.

27. Streit WJ, Sparks DL. Activation of microglia in the brains of humans with heart disease and hypercholesterolemic rabbits. J Mol Med 1997; 75: 130–38.

28. Ceballos-Picot I et al. Peripheral antioxidant enzyme activities and selenium in elderly subjects and in dementia of Alzheimer's type—place of the extracellular glutathione peroxidase. Free Radic Biol Med 1996; 20: 579–87.

29. Richardson JS. Free radicals in the genesis of Alzheimer's disease. Ann NY Acad Sci 1993; 695: 73–6.

30. Lovell MA et al. Elevated thiobarbituric acid-reactive substances and antioxidant enzyme activity in the brain in Alzheimer's disease. Neurology 1995; 45: 1594–601.

31. McIntosh LJ et al. Increased susceptibility of Alzheimer's disease temporal cortex to oxygen free radical-mediated processes. Free Radic Biol Med 1997; 23: 183–90.

32. Sharma RC et al. Immunolocalization of native antioxidant scavenger enzymes in early hypertensive and atherosclerotic arteries. Arterioscler Thromb 1992; 12: 403–15.

Address for correspondence:
D. Larry Sparks,
Sun Health Research Institute,
Sun City, AZ 85351, USA

18 Cerebral Microvascular Breakdown in Alzheimer's Disease and in Experimental Cerebral Hypoperfusion

ESZTER FARKAS, GINEKE I. DE JONG,
ROB A.I. DE VOS, ERNST N.H. JANSEN STEUR AND
PAUL G.M. LUITEN

INTRODUCTION

Cerebral capillaries represent a major interface between the general circulation and the central nervous system and are responsible for sufficient and selective nutrient transport to the brain. Structural damage or dysfunctioning carrier systems of such an active barrier leads to compromised nutrient trafficking. Subsequently, a decreased nutrient availability in the neural tissue may contribute to hampered neuronal metabolism and hence to cognitive disturbances. Besides decreased endothelial glucose transporter levels [1], abnormal morphological changes in the capillary walls can account for a lower efficiency of transport in aging and Alzheimer's disease (AD).

Damage to brain microvessels can be manifested in noticeable light microscopical pathology, including twisting, tortuous appearance, fragmentation and atrophy of the vessels, as observed in the neocortex of AD patients [2]. Furthermore, the abnormalities described above relate to depositions and vacuoles in the capillary basement membrane (BM) which were also found to be associated with dementia [3, 4, 5]. Cerebral hypoperfusion has been proposed to be either the consequence of capillary damage [6] or the trigger of microvascular pathology [5]. We have gathered here supporting evidence for the latter hypothesis, and demonstrate that chronic cerebral hypoperfusion in rats evokes pathological microvascular alterations which are also present in post-mortem AD brains.

Alzheimer's Disease and Related Disorders
Edited by K. Iqbal, D.F. Swaab, B. Winblad and H.M. Wisniewski
© 1999 John Wiley & Sons Ltd

POST-MORTEM HUMAN BRAIN

Electron microscopy, due to the high resolution it provides, proves to be the method of choice to investigate the morphological alterations occurring in cerebral capillary walls. We have analyzed samples from the cingulate cortex of five AD patients and five age-matched control subjects to highlight potentially relevant, dementia-related pathological changes in the condition of the BM and pericytes. We classified the degenerative features into two major categories: (a) capillary deposits, which are defined as local thickenings of the basement membrane, with or without deposited collagen fibrils (fibrosis); and (b) pericytic degeneration. Approximately 100 capillaries per case were screened throughout the cortical depth. The proportion of damaged microvessels exhibiting one of the above defined characteristics was expressed as percentages of the total number of capillaries encountered. Significance was tested by the non-parametric Mann–Whitney U test. The data show that the percentage of capillaries with deposits was significantly increased in AD brains compared to age-matched controls (Figures 1A, B, 2A). Pericytic degradation seemed to develop independent of dementia and the same level of degeneration could be detected in both AD and control samples (Figure 2A).

The trigger to induce such cerebral capillary abnormalities in AD has not been defined; however, hypoperfusion appears to be one possible candidate. It has been shown, for example, that the regional cerebral blood flow in neocortical areas of AD patients is specifically reduced and correlates with the degree of mental decline [7, 8]. To test a possible relationship between reduced cerebral blood flow, capillary degeneration and its functional consequences,

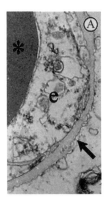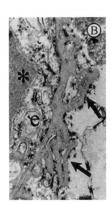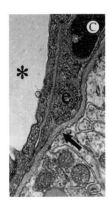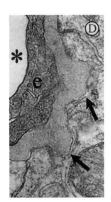

Figure 1. Photographs of human and rat cerebral capillaries (*capillary lumen, with or without erythrocytes; arrows, capillary basement membrane; e, endothelial cytoplasm). (A) Normal human cerebral capillary. (B) Basement membrane duplication and deposits in an AD patient. (C) The normal appearance of a rat cerebral capillary. (D) Basement membrane thickening in rat hippocampus after 2VO

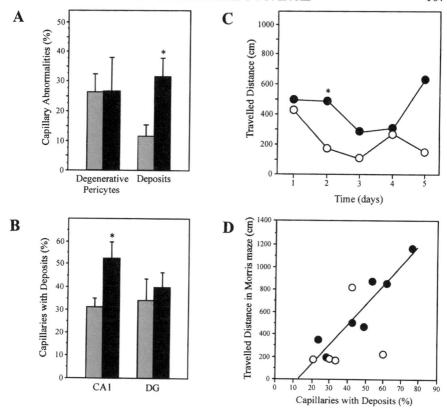

Figure 2. (A) Mean values ± s.e.m. of the percentage of capillaries with either pericytic degeneration or basement membrane (BM) deposits in the cingulate cortex of AD patients (black bars) and age-matched controls (light bars) (*p < 0.02). (B) Mean values ± s.e.m. of the percentage of capillaries with BM deposits in the hippocampus CA1 and DG in sham-operated (light bars) and 2VO (black bars) rats 1 year after surgery (*p < 0.05). (C) The median distance rats traveled before reaching the escape platform in the Morris water maze 1 year after 2VO surgery for five sham-operated (open circles) and seven 2VO animals (solid dots; *p < 0.05). (D) Correlation (r = 0.935, p < 0.002) between cognitive performance measured on day 2 of the training session in the water maze (see graph 1C) and the percentage of capillaries with BM deposits in the hippo-campus CA1 after 2VO (sham controls, open circles; 2VO animals, solid dots)

we have applied an animal model to simulate the effects of hypoperfusion on cognitive performance and cerebromicrovascular morphology.

EXPERIMENTAL CEREBRAL HYPOPERFUSION

The impact of chronic hypoperfusion on cerebral microcirculation and cognitive behavior was examined by permanent bilateral occlusion of the common carotid arteries (2VO) in young adult Wistar rats. The 2VO leads to chronic hypoperfusion since cerebral blood flow decreases to 70% of the original flow rate [9]. Young rats that underwent 2VO displayed an impaired spatial memory compared to sham controls when tested in the Morris water maze [10, 11]. One year after surgery, a decline in spatial memory was still present in 2VO rats when compared to sham-operated controls (Figure 2C).

Following behavioral screening, the animals were sacrificed by transcardial perfusion and the brains processed for electron microscopic analysis. The number of aberrant capillaries was quantified using exactly the same procedure as described above for the human post-mortem material. It has been known for a long time that hippocampal neurons, and especially CA1 pyramidal cells, are selectively vulnerable to ischemic insults. In the 2VO rats, the percentage of capillaries with both pericytic degeneration and capillary deposits was significantly increased in the CA1 but not in the dentate gyrus (DG) of the hippocampus (Figures 1C, D, 2B). This indicates that not only neuronal systems but also the capillary bed in the hippocampus CA1 is extremely vulnerable to mild but chronic ischemic conditions.

It is also common knowledge that the hippocampus is one of the regions where AD pathology, such as plaques and tangles, start to occur [12]. In our animal model we established the correlation between the cognitive performance of rats and capillary morphology. It appeared that in the hippocampus CA1 (but not the DG) a highly significant correlation existed between the occurrence of capillary deposits (but not pericytic degeneration) with the distance a rat traveled before reaching the escape platform in the water maze on day two (Figure 2D). In other words, those rats which possessed significantly fewer capillary deposits in the hippocampus CA1 performed best in a spatial memory task.

De la Torre and co-workers [4] reported that rats with chronic permanent bilateral carotid occlusion (2VO) demonstrated similar features to human dementia, such as spatial memory dysfunction, neuronal damage to the hippocampus and increased immunoreaction to glial fibrillary acidic protein (GFAP). In addition, Kalaria et al. [13] described increased APP accumulation due to parietal ischemia which was imposed by 2VO in rats. Taking these data together, the rat 2VO model appears to be a useful tool for mimicking cerebral hypoperfusion-related pathological and neurological alterations in human dementia, specifically in AD.

CONCLUSIONS

The present findings demonstrate that our observations on human capillary pathology of AD patients, in line with previous studies [3, 5], can be evoked by 2VO in rats, and that chronic cerebral hypoperfusion may very well account for such vascular abnormalities. Furthermore, the correlation that was established between the ratio of capillaries with damaged walls and the degree of spatial memory dysfunction supports the hypothesis that impaired cerebral microcirculation may be an important factor in the development of AD [6]. Our data also indicate that the observed BM depositions probably represent the major microvascular factor eventually contributing to cognitive impairment, as opposed to pericytic aberrations. There was no difference in the degree of pericytic degeneration between human control and AD samples, and a correlation between this structural phenomenon and learning skills in the rat model could not be established, either.

We conclude that, in addition to the neuronal tissue [10], the cerebral capillary network is also vulnerable to chronic hypoperfusion and reacts predominantly by the accumulation of deposits in the BM in response to insufficient blood flow. The distorted microvessel walls, in turn, are directly correlated to dysfunctional memory processes and thus may represent a contributing risk factor in the development of the cognitive symptoms of AD.

REFERENCES

1. Horwood N, Davies DC. Immunolabelling of hippocampal microvessel glucose transporter protein is reduced in Alzheimer's disease. Virchows Arch 1994; 425(1): 69–72.
2. Buée L, Hof PR, Delacourte A. Brain microvascular changes in Alzheimer's disease and other dementias. Ann NY Acad Sci 1997; 826: 7–24.
3. Perlmutter LS, Chui HC. Microangiopathy, the vascular basement membrane and Alzheimer's disease. Brain Res Bull 1990; 24: 677–86.
4. de la Torre JC, Fortin T, Park GAS, Butler KS, Kozlowski P, Pappas BA, de Socarraz H, Saunders JK, Richard MT. Chronic cerebrovascular insufficiency induces dementia-like deficits in aged rats. Brain Res 1992; 582: 186–95.
5. De Jong GI, De Vos RIA, Jansen Steur ENH, Luiten PGM. Cerebrovascular hypoperfusion: a risk factor for Alzheimer's disease? Animal model and postmortem human studies. Ann NY Acad Sci 1997; 826: 56–74.
6. de la Torre JC, Mussivand T. Can disturbed brain microcirculation cause Alzheimer's disease? Neurol Res 1993; 15: 146–53.
7. Eberling JL, Jagust WJ, Reed BR, Baker MG. Reduced temporal lobe blood flow in Alzheimer's disease. Neurobiol Aging 1992; 13: 483–91.
8. Ibanez V, Pietrini P, Alexander GE, Furey ML, Teichberg D, Rajapakse JC, Rapoport SI, Schapiro MB, Horwitz B. Regional glucose metabolic abnormalities are not the result of atrophy in Alzheimer's disease. Neurology 1998; 50(6): 1585–93.
9. Tsuchiya M, Sako K, Yura S, Yonemasu Y. Cerebral blood flow and histopathological changes following permanent bilateral carotid artery ligation in Wistar rats. Exp Brain Res 1992; 89(1): 87–92.
10. Pappas BA, de la Torre JC, Davidson CM, Keyes MT, Fortin T. Chronic reduction of cerebral blood flow in the adult rat: late-emerging CA1 cell loss and memory dysfunction. Brain Res, 708, 50–58.
11. De Jong GI, Farkas E, Plass J, Keyser JN, de la Torre JC, Luiten PGM. Cerebral hypoperfusion yields capillary damage in hippocampus CA1 that is correlated to spatial memory impairment (accepted in Neuroscience).

12. Braak H, Braak E. Neuropathological staging of Alzheimer-related changes. Acta Neuropathol 1991; 82: 239–59.
13. Kalaria RN, Bhatti SU, Lust WD, Perry G. The amyloid precursor protein in ischemic brain injury and chronic hypoperfusion. Ann NY Acad Sci 1993; 695: 190–93.

Address for correspondence:
    Eszter Farkas,
    Dept Animal Physiology,
    PO Box 14,
    9750 AA Haren, The Netherlands
    Tel: 31 50 3632363; fax: 31 50 3635202; e-mail: farkase@biol.rug.nl

19 Brain Region Differences in Fibrillization of Aβ Proteins and the Role of Microglia in Transformation of Diffuse into Neuritic Plaques

H.M. WISNIEWSKI, M. SADOWSKI, J. WEGIEL,
A. GOLABEK AND E. KIDA

INTRODUCTION

The common use of thioflavin-S and Congo red to detect fibrillar Aβ and anti-Aβ antibodies and silver staining techniques to detect both fibrillar and non-fibrillar accumulation of Aβ allowed classification of Aβ deposits into two characteristic categories: (a) diffuse, non-fibrillar, or benign plaques; and (b) neuritic, senile, fibrillar or malignant plaques. Fibrillar and non-fibrillar deposits of Aβ also occur in meningeal and predominantly cortical vessels affected by amyloid angiopathy. Studies of the effect of *in vitro* fibrillization and the presence within plaques of the various Aβ peptides showed that 1–42 and 1–40 isomers polymerize readily (1–42 more than 1–40). However, the 17–42 peptide, also called p3 and showing the strongest reactivity in cerebellar diffuse plaques, is less prone to fibrillize [1]. It also was shown that *in vitro* amyloid-associated proteins, such as ApoE, J and A1; α_1-antichymotrypsin; heparin sulfate proteoglycan; serum; and various cations promote or inhibit Aβ fibrillization [2].

ApoE also affects amyloid load in Alzheimer disease (AD) and ApoE ε4 allele dosage correlates with an increase in Aβ 1–40 immunoreactive plaques [3]. ApoE knock-out mice with human amyloid precursor protein (APP) mutation revealed a lack of thioflavin-positive Aβ plaques even after 22 months [4]. Normally, the APP mutation causes mice to develop fibrillized amyloid plaques starting at 4–5 months. Studies of the diffuse non-fibrillized and neuritic-fibrillized plaques revealed that extensive neuropil pathology is associated with fibrillization of the β-peptide. Also, extensive necrosis of the

Alzheimer's Disease and Related Disorders
Edited by K. Iqbal, D.F. Swaab, B. Winblad and H.M. Wisniewski
© 1999 John Wiley & Sons Ltd

smooth muscle cells in vascular amyloidosis is associated with formation of fibrillar amyloid deposits [5]. Because non-fibrillized Aβ deposits appear to be tolerated well by the tissue at the site of these deposits, understanding the conditions that keep the β-peptide in non-fibrillized form and the conditions leading to fibrillization of the β-protein is of critical importance in developing treatment strategies for AD. From our studies and others, it is known that diffuse non-fibrillized plaques are present in young adults with Down's syndrome (DS), aged dogs, and the cerebellum of persons with AD [6]. We recently found diffuse, lake-like Aβ deposits in the parvopyramidal layer of the presubiculum in AD that show no evidence of fibrillization [7]. The purpose of this report is to use immunocytochemical methods to determine the local conditions that inhibit or lead to fibrillization of Aβ protein in AD and DS.

MATERIAL AND METHODS

Formalin-fixed and paraffin-embedded tissue sections from the hippocampus and temporal neocortex, basal ganglia, cerebellum and brain stem collected from 10 AD patients aged 57–89 years and 10 DS cases aged 12–65 years were immunostained by using the avidin–biotin method and diamino-benzidine in the presence of hydrogen peroxide as a chromogen. The following antibodies were applied: monoclonal antibody (mAb) 4G8, recognizing amino acid residues 17–24 of Aβ peptide; mAb 6E10 raised to amino acids 1–17 of Aβ peptide; polyclonal antibody (pAb) RAS 163, recognizing the end-terminal amino acid of Aβ40; pAb Ras 165, recognizing the end-terminal amino acid of Aβ42; pAb to ApoE; mAb to ApoJ; pAb to ACT; mAb 22C11, recognizing an epitope located between amino acid residues 60–81 of APP; pAb raised to amino acid residues 673–695 of APP; and pAb, recognizing the Kunitz domain of APP. Sections also were stained routinely with thioflavin S and Congo red. Small tissue sections from the neocortex, cerebellar molecular layer, neostriatum and midbrain containing exclusively diffuse plaques were excised from the paraffin blocks, deparaffinized and processed routinely for LR White. Ultrathin sections were immunostained by using mAb 4G8 and protein A gold-labeled (10 nm gold particles) and were examined in a Hitachi 7000 electron microscope.

RESULTS

The immunocytochemical composition of diffuse plaques in the brain regions examined varied distinctly (Table 1). There also were differences in the occurrence of APP-positive dystrophic neurites within diffuse plaques in various brain regions studied; they were the most common in the cerebral cortex and were virtually absent or only observed sporadically in the neostriatum and brain stem. Immunoelectron microscopy examination showed that diffuse plaques in all brain regions examined contained Aβ-positive fibrillar material (Figure 1 A, B). However, the amount of Aβ-positive fibrils was distinctly lower than in neuritic plaques. The amount of Aβ-positive fibrils was the highest in the cerebral cortex and the lowest in the neostriatum.

The progression of amyloidogenesis in the brain region studied is the mildest in the broad areas of the presubiculum occupied by lake-like diffuse plaques (Figure 2) in the cerebellar molecular layer and in the neostriatum; moderate in the brain stem; and severe in the cerebral cortex, including the hippocampus. Extensive fibrillization of the diffuse plaques and their transformation into neuritic plaques was always associated with activation of microglia and astrocytes. Neurofibrillary pathology parallels to a certain degree the above-mentioned pattern, because neurofibrillary tangles are absent in the cerebellar cortex, are rare in the neostriatum and the presubiculum, but numerous in the cerebral cortex and in some brain stem nuclei. In DS individuals 25 years of age and younger, all Aβ plaques were thioflavin-S-negative.

Table 1. Immunoreactivity of diffuse plaques in various brain regions to Aβ and selected amyloid-associated proteins

	mAb 4G8	mAb 6E10	pAb to Ab42	pAb to Ab40	ApoE	ApoJ	ACT
Cerebral cortex	+++	++	+++	+	++	+	+
Presubiculum	+++	+++	+++	+—	—	—	—
Cerebellar molecular layer	+++	+	+++	—	++	—	—
Neostriatum	+++	+++	+++	—	—	—	—
Brain stem	+++	+++	+++	—	—	—	—

+++ All plaques positive; ++ numerous plaques positive; + few plaques positive; +— only individual plaques positive; — absent.

DISCUSSION

Our study discloses that thioflavin-S and Congo red stains are not sufficiently sensitive to detect the small amounts of Aβ-positive fibrils that are present in diffuse plaques. The fact that already-diffuse plaques contain Aβ in a fibrillar form is consistent with the results of *in vitro* studies, which provided evidence that the process of Aβ fibril formation occurs spontaneously and in the absence of any other additional compounds. Thus, an important question remains as to why in certain brain areas the process of amyloidogenesis is relatively mild and arrests at the stage of diffuse plaques mostly, whereas in other brain areas it progresses and results in severe tissue destruction.

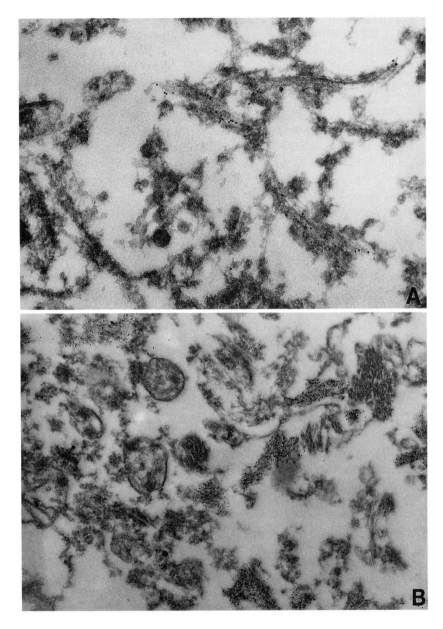

Figure 1. Aβ-positive fibrillar material in lake-like diffuse plaques in the neocortex of a 21 year-old DS case (A) and in the cerebellar molecular layer of an AD case (B). Original magnifications × 30 000 (A) and × 20 000 (B)

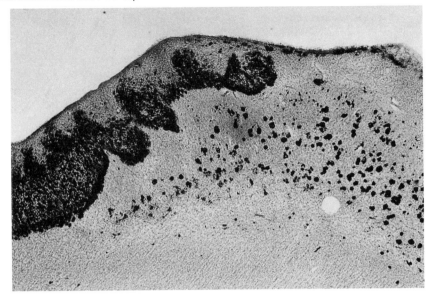

Figure 2. Diffuse lake-like plaque in the parvocellular layer of the presubiculum

Undoubtedly, amyloid-associated proteins, and especially ApoE, may affect this process significantly, either by interacting directly with released Aβ or through their effect on the biology of neurons. Another limiting factor may be the amount of Aβ released locally. However, on the basis of our findings, it is tempting to postulate that only a certain population of neurons in the human brain is susceptible to Aβ toxicity. Studies in cell culture conditions showed that all cell types examined so far, except for smooth muscle cells, are more vulnerable to the presence of Aβ peptides in a fibrillized than in a soluble form. Nevertheless, whether particular types of neurons differ in their vulnerability to Aβ has not yet been addressed. Thus, following our hypothesis, even a small number of extracellular fibrillar Aβ deposits might induce injury of a selected population of vulnerable neurons, triggering a cascade of events that results in additional release of Aβ peptide by damaged cells, with subsequent mobilization of the glial cells in their vicinity (Figure 3). This scenario is supported by recent studies showing that it is a fibrillized Aβ peptide that induces neuronal loss, tau protein alterations and gliosis when applied to the neocortex of aged primates [8]. Thus, it appears that it may be predominantly the type of neuron exposed to Aβ action and the factor(s) related to the aging process that may significantly determine the rate, evolution and severity of β-amyloidosis in the human brain. However, it remains uncertain whether the progressive, selective neuronal degeneration in the AD brain caused by Aβ is initiated by extracellular fibrillar Aβ deposits or by intracellular accumulation of insoluble Aβ1–42. The latter possibility is suggested by recent studies of Lee and colleagues [9].

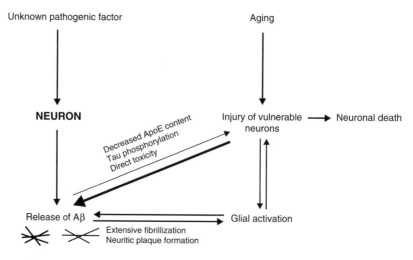

Figure 3. Schematic presentation of pathogenetic events involved in progression of β-amyloidosis

Our data also indicate that the progression of Aβ fibrillization and the transformation of diffuse plaques into neuritic plaques are strongly associated with the activation of microglial cells. The involvement of microglia in amyloid formation was demonstrated by our electron microscopic studies of serially-cut sections of classical and primitive neuritic plaques. These studies showed the presence of amyloid fibers attached to or within altered endoplasmic reticulum and in deep multiple infoldings of microglial cytoplasmic membranes [10]. Histochemical electron microscopy studies of neuritic plaques showed that the nucleoside diphosphatase, the membrane marker of microglial cells, also is present in newly made amyloid [11]. Because a close association between the microglial membranes and amyloid visualized by the electron micrographs might reflect phagocytic, not secretory, activities of the microglial cells, we carried out studies on phagocytosis of amyloid fibers by microglia and macrophages [12, 13]. These studies showed phagocytosed amyloid fibrils in the lysosomal compartments of both microglial cells and macrophages, that is, in intracellular compartments very different from those associated with the presence of amyloid fibrils in microglia in the AD brain. Because activated microglia are also the source of Aβ, amyloid-associated proteins and cytokines, they also may initiate neuropil reaction, leading to neuritic plaque formation. In summary, our studies indicate that some diffuse plaques are transformed into neuritic plaques and stress the role of microglial cells in this phenomenon. These cells may be involved in this process directly through interactions with Aβ, but because of the release of cytokines, they could also be responsible for progressive neuropil degeneration. The cause of microglial activation in some diffuse plaques is not known, but it could be Aβ or some as-yet undetected changes in the synapses involved in the release and accumulation of Aβ.

In conclusion, we have shown brain-region differences in diffuse plaque composition, which might be caused by differences in BPP processing and deposition of Aβ or by different resolution/degradation of deposited Aβ; different vulnerabilities of neurons and neuropil to Aβ accumulation; topographic differences in the distribution of amyloid-associated proteins; and microglia as a source of neuropil fibrillar amyloid and cause of transformation of some diffuse into neuritic plaques.

ACKNOWLEDGEMENTS

This work was supported in part by funds from the New York State Office of Mental Retardation and Developmental Disabilities, a grant from the National Institutes of Health, National Institute on Aging, No. PO1 AG04220, and the fund for the Center for Trace Element Studies and Environmental Neurotoxicology.

REFERENCES

1. Lalowski M, Golabek A, Lemere CA, Selkoe DS, Wisniewski HM, Beavis RC, Frangione B, Wisniewski T. The 'non-amyloidogenic' p3 fragment (amyloid β17–42) is a major constituent of Down's syndrome cerebellar preamyloid. J Biol Chem 1996; 271: 33623–31.
2. Wisniewski T, Castano E, Golabek A, Vogel T, Frangione B. Acceleration of Alzheimer fibril formation by apolipoprotein E *in vitro*. Am J Pathol 1994; 145: 1030–35.
3. Gearing M, Mori H, Mirra SS. Aβ peptide length and apolipoprotein E genotype in Alzheimer's disease. Ann Neurol 1996; 39: 395–9.
4. Bales KR, Verina T, Dodel RC, Du Y, Alstiel L, Bender M, St George-Hyslop P, Johnstone EM, Little SP, Cummins DJ, Piccardo P, Ghetti B, Paul SM. Lack of apolipoprotein E dramatically reduces amyloid β-peptide deposition. Nature Genet 1997; 17: 263–4.
5. Wisniewski HM, Wegiel J, Wang KC, Lach B. Ultrastructural studies of the cells forming amyloid in the cortical vessel wall in Alzheimer's disease. Acta Neuropathol 1992; 84: 117–27.
6. Kida E, Wisniewski KE, Wisniewski HM. Early amyloid-β deposits show different immunoreactivity to the amino- and carboxy-terminal regions of β-peptide in Alzheimer's disease and Down's syndrome brain. Neurosci Lett 1995; 193: 105–8.
7. Wisniewski HM, Sadowski M, Jakubowska-Sadowska K, Tarnawski M, Wegiel J. Diffuse, lake-like amyloid-β deposits in the parvopyramidal layer of the presubiculum in Alzheimer disease. J Neuropathol Exp Neurol 1998; 57: 674–83.
8. Geula CH, Wu Ch-K, Saroff D, Lorenzo A, Yuan M, Yanker BA. Aging renders the brain vulnerable to amyloid β-protein neurotoxicity. Nature Med 1998; 4: 827–31.

9. Skovronsky DM, Doms RW, Lee VM-Y. Detection of a novel intraneuronal pool of insoluble amyloid β protein that accumulates with time in culture. J Cell Biol 1998; 141: 1031–9.

10. Wisniewski HM, Wegiel J, Wang KC, Kujawa M, Lach B. Ultrastructural studies of the cells forming amyloid fibers in classical plaques. Can J Neurol Sci 1989; 16: 535–42.

11. Wisniewski HM, Vorbrodt AW, Epstein MH. Nucleoside diphosphatase (NDPase) activity associated with human β-protein amyloid fibers. Acta Neuropathol 1991; 81: 366–70.

12. Wisniewski HM, Barcikowska M, Kida E. Phagocytosis of β/A₄ amyloid fibrils of the neuritic neocortical plaques. Acta Neuropathol 1991; 81: 588–90.

13. Frackowiak J, Wisniewski HM, Wegiel J, Merz GS, Iqbal K, Wang KC. Ultrastructure of the microglia that phagocytose amyloid and the microglia that produce β-amyloid fibrils. Acta Neuropathol 1992; 84: 225–33.

Address for correspondence:
  H.M. Wisniewski,
  New York State Institute for Basic Research in Developmental
    Disabilities,
  1050 Forest Hill Road,
  Staten Island, New York 10314, USA

20 Abnormally Phosphorylated Tau Protein in Neurons and Glial Cells of Aged Baboons

CHRISTIAN SCHULTZ, ESTIFANOS GHEBREMEDHIN,
IRENA SASSIN, EVA BRAAK AND HEIKO BRAAK

INTRODUCTION

The formation of abnormally phosphorylated, microtubule-associated tau protein is a hallmark of a variety of human degenerative brain diseases. Although the deposition of abnormal tau was once thought to be a neuron-specific process, microglial cells were recently demonstrated to be a major target of tau-positive changes as well [1]. A large number of tau-positive glial inclusions has been described in argyrophilic grain disease (AGD [2, 3]), progressive supranuclear palsy (PSP), Pick's disease (PID) and corticobasal degeneration (CBD [1]). To a lesser extent, glial inclusions are also seen in Alzheimer's disease (AD [4]).

At this point, the molecular mechanisms of abnormal tau phosphorylation in neurons and glial cells are not completely understood. In this context it would be desirable to procure an animal model demonstrating both neuronal and glial cytoskeletal pathology.

This study highlights a previously unreported dense accumulation of abnormal tau in aged non-human primates. The cytoskeletal abnormalities were identified in the brains of baboons (*Papio hamadryas*). Interestingly, both neuronal and glial inclusions were observed.

MATERIALS AND METHODS

The brains of four baboons (*Papio hamadryas*) were examined. The animals had been raised and housed in zoos in Germany. The estimated ages and gender of the animals were: 20 years (female); 24 years (female); 26 years (male); and 30 years (male). All brains were fixed in a 10% aqueous solution of formaldehyde. Series of coronal sections were cut at 100 μm using a

Alzheimer's Disease and Related Disorders
Edited by K. Iqbal, D.F. Swaab, B. Winblad and H.M. Wisniewski
© 1999 John Wiley & Sons Ltd

freezing microtome. Argyrophilic pathology was demonstrated using the modified Gallyas iodide technique [5, 6]. Hyperphosphorylated tau was labeled using the antibody AT8 (Innogenetics, Ghent, Belgium) which detects the abnormally phosphorylated tau epitopes serine 202 and threonine 205 [7]. Sections were incubated with AT8 (1:2000, 4 °C, 40–44 h) and immunoreactions were visualized with the ABC-complex (Vectastain) and 3,3-diaminobenzidine-tetra-HCL/H_2O_2 (DAB, D5637, Sigma).

RESULTS

GENERAL REMARKS

The brains of two baboons, aged 20 and 24 years, respectively, were almost devoid of cytoskeletal changes with the exception of single tau-positive inclusions. By contrast, pronounced AT8-immunoreactive (IR) cytoskeletal changes were identified in the remaining two animals, aged 26 and 30 years (Figure 1). The abnormal tau protein often was distributed diffusely throughout entire cells, extending even into their distal processes (Figure 1C, D). This Golgi-like staining pattern facilitated classification of affected cell types. In both affected animals the inclusions were found not only in neurons but also in glial cells. The brunt of the cytoskeletal changes was born by limbic brain structures, such as the hippocampus and amygdala. By contrast, only sparse changes were noted in neocortical regions and in diencephalic and mesencephalic components of the basal ganglia.

NEURONAL CHANGES

An accumulation of abnormal tau was seen in specific subsets of limbic neurons. Both affected animals exhibited AT8-IR inclusions in pyramidal neurons of the first Ammon's horn sector (CA1, Figure 1C) and in neurons of the amygdala (Figure 1D). In the 30 year-old baboon, a striking lamina-specific pathology was observed in the fascia dentata (Figure 1A). In particular, a pronounced accumulation of abnormal tau was demonstrated in the granule cells (Figure 1B). The density of such AT8-IR inclusions in the granule cells tended to increase from the superficial granule cell layers to the deeper granule cell layers. This differential vulnerability of the granule cells was confirmed

---

Figure 1 (opposite). Cytoskeletal pathology in the baboon labeled by AT8-immunostaining (A–D) and Gallyas silver staining (E–H). (A) Hippocampal formation of a 30 year-old baboon. A moderate pathology is seen in the first and third sector of the Ammon's horn (CA1 and CA3). This pathology is even more pronounced in CA4, whereas CA2 is almost devoid of changes. The strikingly lamina-specific pathology of the fascia dentata (F.D.) is also shown at higher magnification in (B). (B) Layer-specific pathology in the fascia dentata. Tau-positive oligodendrocytes (arrows) are

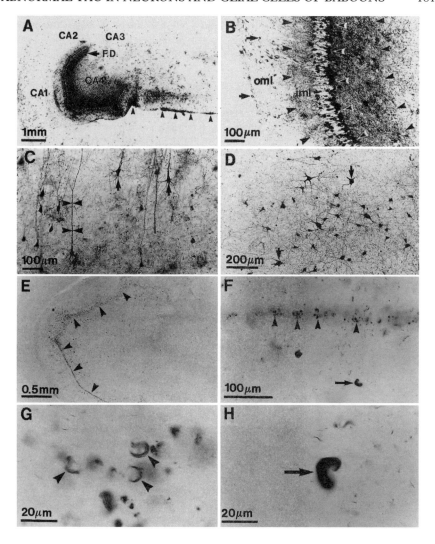

seen in the outer molecular layer (oml; see also Figure 2D). Both the inner molecular layer (iml) and the plexiform layer of the fascia dentata contain altered neuropil structures (black arrowheads). Note the dense accumulation of altered granule cells (G), which is particularly pronounced in the deeper granule cell layers (black on white arrowheads). (C) Diffuse deposition of abnormal tau in pyramidal neurons of CA1 (arrows). Abnormal tau is deposited even in the apical dendrites of CA1 neurons (arrowheads). (D) Diffusely labeled neurons of the amygdala (arrows) of a 26 year-old baboon. (E) Gallyas-positive neurofibrillary tangles (NFTs) in the granule cell layer (arrowheads). (F) Accumulation of NFTs in the deeper granule cells (arrowheads). Larger NFTs are also seen in the hilus/CA4 region (arrow; also shown in H). (G) The NFTs of the granule cells are characterized by crescent-shaped perinuclear deposits of fibrillary material (arrowheads). (H) Large NFT in the hilus (arrow) using the Gallyas technique. A conspicuous accumulation of argyrophilic neurofibrillary tangles (NFTs) was noted in the granule cells (Figure 1E), preferentially affecting deeper cell layers (Figure 1F, G). Occasionally, Gallyas-positive NFTs were also detected in large neurons of the hilus (Figure 1H) and in pyramidal neurons of CA1.

ASTROGLIAL CHANGES

The astroglial origin of additional inclusions in both affected animals was strongly suggested by their characteristic morphology and distribution (Figure 2A, B). Some distinctive inclusions were contained in stellate cell bodies, giving rise to numerous radiating processes. Such inclusions were seen chiefly in subpial, perivascular and subependymal locations. Some of the astroglia-like inclusions exhibited multiple processes abutting upon the walls of blood vessels with endfeet. Additional changes were identified in processes of the glial limiting membrane (Figure 2A). Such changes were distributed along the surface of the hippocampal sulcus (Figure 1A), the tuber cinereum, basal

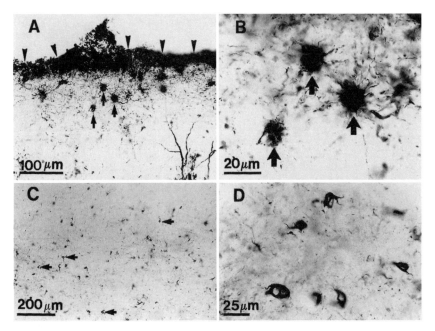

Figure 2. Abnormal tau in glial cells of a 30 year-old baboon (AT8-immunostaining). (A) Subpial tau-positive astrocytes (arrows; also shown in B) and a network of altered processes in the glial limiting membrane (arrowheads). (B) The abnormal tau protein is found in cell bodies and processes of astrocytes. (C) Cytoskeletal changes in the white matter changes of the perforant path consisting of interfascicular fibers and oligodendroglial coiled bodies (arrows). (D) Coiled bodies in the outer molecular layer of the fascia dentata (see also Figure 1B)

forebrain and cerebral peduncle. A portion of the altered processes within the glial limiting membrane emanated from subpial thorn-shaped astrocytes clustered immediately beneath the altered glial limiting membrane (Figure 2B). Using the Gallyas silver staining technique, similar changes of the glial limiting membrane were detected. The distribution of such argyrophilic changes closely corresponded to that demonstrated by AT8 immunostaining.

OLIGODENDROGLIAL CHANGES

Both affected animals exhibited additional white matter changes in the form of small-to-medium-sized AT8-IR cellular inclusions (Figure 2C). These inclusions occurred as curved AT8-IR deposits which often were coiled around a nucleus resembling that of oligodendroglia (Figure 2D). Similar inclusions were also detected using the Gallyas technique. Morphologically, this lesional type was indistinguishable from oligodendroglial coiled bodies described previously in the human brain [8, 9]. The coiled bodies in the baboons were consistently accompanied by thread-like interfascicular fibers. Coiled bodies and interfascicular fibers were mainly seen in limbic fiber tracts, including the perforant path (Figure 2C), alveus and fornix.

DISCUSSION

This study reveals the formation of abnormally phosphorylated tau protein in brains of aged baboons (*Papio hamadryas*). This surprising finding runs counter to the long-standing assumption that aged non-human primates are virtually resistant to formation of abnormal tau. Previous studies on other non-human primate species, such as rhesus monkeys [10, 11, 12], chimpanzees [12] and orang-utans [10, 13], indeed failed to reveal similar cytoskeletal abnormalities. Tau-positive inclusions were previously identified in a few non-primate species, such as sheep [14, 15] and bears [16]. However, these changes were detected only in neurons, not in glial cells. Accordingly, the baboon offers unique opportunities for more comprehensive investigations of both neuronal and glial cytoskeletal changes.

Only a fraction of the AT8-IR cytoskeletal changes in the baboons could be demonstrated using the Gallyas technique. Nonetheless, the argyrophilia of some inclusions is noteworthy and indicates an advanced aggregation of abnormal tau to insoluble fibrillary material.

Some distinctive cellular inclusions in the baboons were considered to be of astroglial origin. Conspicuous changes were seen in the glial limiting membrane mainly comprised of a network of altered processes. This particular subpial pathology frequently was seen in the absence of obvious neuronal inclusions and probably reflects primary astroglial involvement rather than changes developing secondary to neuronal pathology.

The glial pathology in the baboons was not restricted to astrocytes. Additional glial inclusions were contained in small to medium-sized cells with morphological features of oligodendrocytes. These inclusions were indistinguishable from oligodendroglial coiled bodies originally described in the human brain [8, 9].

The changes in baboons need to be compared to specific human brain disorders featuring both neuronal and abundant glial pathology, such as PSP, CBD and PID. The distribution of the changes in the baboons, however, differs from that encountered in these human disorders. The subthalamic nucleus and the substantia nigra, for example, are common targets of PSP, CBD and PID [17], whereas these structures were devoid of changes in the baboons. Therefore, the changes in the baboon cannot be viewed as a potential model of PSP, CBD or PID. Rather, the distribution of cytoskeletal abnormalities in baboons resembles that previously reported in humans afflicted with AGD [2, 18]. In particular, an accumulation of coiled bodies in limbic fiber tracts, such as the perforant path and fornix, has been reported to occur in AGD [2, 3]. The aged baboon thus may be used to explore pathogenetic and functional implications of AGD-related changes afflicting the human brain.

In summary, this study extends the range of pathological changes which can be examined in both the human and non-human brain. The baboon may provide an important *in vivo* model to understand some of the fundamental cellular mechanisms involved in tau hyperphosphorylation of human neurons and glial cells. Such understanding is crucially important for developing treatment modes aimed at preventing or arresting abnormal tau phosphorylation.

ACKNOWLEDGEMENTS

This study was supported by the DFG and the BMBF. The authors thank Dr Schmahl, Munich, for providing brain material and Mrs A. Biczysko, Mrs I. Szasz and Mrs U. Trautmann for their technical assistance.

REFERENCES

1. Chin SS-M, Goldman J. Glial inclusions in CNS degenerative diseases. J Neuropathol Exp Neurol 1996; 55: 499–508.
2. Braak H, Braak E. Argyrophilic grain disease. Frequency of occurrence in different age categories and neuropathological diagnostic criteria. J Neurol Transm 1998; 105: 801–19.
3. Schultz C, Koppers D, Sassin I, Braak E, Braak H. Cytoskeletal alterations in the human tuberal hypothalamus related to argyrophilic grain disease. Acta Neuropathol 1998; 96: 596–602.

4. Papasozomenos SC. Tau protein immunoreactivity in dementia of the Alzheimer-type: II. Electron microscopy and pathogenetic implications. Lab Invest 1989; 60: 375–89.
5. Gallyas F. Silver staining of Alzheimer's neurofibrillary changes by means of physical development. Acta Morphol Acad Sci Hung 1971; 19: 1–8.
6. Braak H, Braak E. Demonstration of amyloid deposits and neurofibrillary changes in whole brain sections. Brain Pathol 1991; 1: 213–16.
7. Goedert M, Jakes R, Vanmechelen E. Monoclonal antibody AT8 recognizes tau protein phosphorylated at both serine 202 and threonine 205. Neurosci Lett 1995; 189: 167–70.
8. Braak H, Braak E. Cortical and subcortical argyrophilic grains characterise a disease associated with adult onset dementia. Neurpathol Appl Neurobiol 1989; 15: 13–26.
9. Yamada T, McGeer PL. Oligodendroglial microtubular masses: an abnormality observed in some human neurodegenerative diseases. Neurosci Lett 1990; 120: 163–6.
10. Selkoe DJ, Bell DS, Podlinski MB, Price DL, Cork LC. Conservation of brain amyloid proteins in aged mammals and humans with Alzheimer's disease. Science 1987; 235: 873–7.
11. Poduri A, Gearing M, Rebeck GW, Mirra SS, Tigges J, Hyman BT. Apolipoprotein E4 and β-amyloid in senile plaques and cerebral blood vessels of aged rhesus monkeys. Am J Pathol 1994; 144: 1183–7.
12. Gearing M, Rebeck GW, Hyman BT, Tigges J, Mirra SS. Neuropathology and apolipoprotein E profile of aged chimpanzees: implications for Alzheimer's disease. Proc Natl Acad Sci USA 1994; 91: 9382–6.
13. Gearing M, Tigges J, Mori H, Mirra SS. β-Amyloid (Aβ) deposition in the brains of aged orangutans. Neurobiol Aging 1997; 18: 139–46.
14. Nelson PT, Greenberg SG, Saper CB. Neurofibrillary tangles in the cerebral cortex of sheep. Neurosci Lett 1994; 170: 187–90.
15. Braak H, Braak E, Strothjohann M. Abnormally phosphorylated tau protein related to the formation of neurofibrillary tangles and neuropil threads in the cerebral cortex of sheep and goat. Neurosci Lett 1994; 171: 1–4.
16. Cork LC, Powers RE, Selkoe D, Davies P, Geyer JJ, Price DL. Neurofibrillary tangles and senile plaques in aged bears. J Neuropathol Exp Neurol 1988; 47: 629–41.
17. Feany MB, Dickson DW. Neurodegenerative disorders with extensive tau pathology: a comparative study and review. Ann Neurol 1996; 40: 139–48.
18. Jellinger KA. Dementia with grains (argyrophilic grain disease). Brain Pathol 1998; 8: 377–86.

Address for correspondence:
Christian Schultz MD,
Department of Anatomy, J.W. Goethe-University,
Theodor-Stern Kai-7, 60590 Frankfurt/Main, Germany
Tel: +49 69 6301 6912; fax: +49 69 6301 6425;
e-mail: Schultz@em.uni-frankfurt.de

21 Paired Helical Filaments Have a Wide Range of Widths with Similar Helical Periods

GEORGE C. RUBEN, JIAN-ZHI WANG,
INGE GRUNDKE-IQBAL AND KHALID IQBAL

If paired helical filaments (PHF) had a regular morphology, then the associations responsible for the regularity could be pharmacologically blocked to disrupt or prevent their assembly as well as Alzheimer's disease (AD) intra-neuronal neurofibrillary tangle formation. If PHF are not regular filaments, then unique or critical filament associations would have to be found for the approach to be successful.

It has been shown that PHF are composed of six tau isoforms [1] that are hyperphosphorylated with 5–9 phosphate groups [2]. The surplus phosphates neutralize positively charged lysines or arginines, making the AD P-tau and the PHF hydrophobic [3]. Enzymatic dephosphorylation of AD P-tau and PHF can restore tau's normal ability to stimulate microtubule formation [4].

Transmission electron microscopy (TEM) observation of filaments in thin-sectioned AD brain tissue was the basis of the paired helical filament (PHF) structure proposed by Kidd [5]. He suggested that the PHF are composed of two ~10 nm cylindrical filaments that twist around each other and form side by side wide regions of 20–25 nm and thin region cross-overs of ~10 nm, with a helical turn period of ~80 nm. This PHF model has been a continuous source of controversy since it was proposed in 1963, although other thin sectioning work has confirmed this structure [6]. Freeze-dried vertically Pt-C replicated PHF have been reported as helical ribbons [7, 8]. Atomic force microscopy (AFM) investigations of PHF have confirmed the original PHF structure [9], have confirmed the helical ribbon structure [10], and recently have described PHF as a pair of aligned helical ribbons [11]. PHF composed of more than two subfilaments (see ref. in [7]) have been reported.

All of these PHF studies have relied on TEM or AFM structural observations using a relatively small population of filaments, which makes generalization risky. To counter this problem, we studied large populations of PHF

Alzheimer's Disease and Related Disorders
Edited by K. Iqbal, D.F. Swaab, B. Winblad and H.M. Wisniewski
© 1999 John Wiley & Sons Ltd

isolated by the long method of Iqbal et al. [12] that were either unsonicated or were sonicated for 1 min using TEM and 2% phosphotungstate (pH 6.8) negative staining on ~10 nm thick carbon films [13]. Negatively stained PHF preparations were photographed with a JEM 100cx at 100 kV at Schertzer focus at ~140 nm underfocus. Phase objects like the PHF were imaged at ~0.7 nm resolution at × 56 000 and × 90 500. These negatives were printed at a × 2.5 enlargement and measured at magnification of × 10 with a recticle with fine spacings of 0.1 mm. The recticle method was used to measure the wide regions, W, and the thin regions, T, of the PHF. The helical turn period, L, was measured with a precision ruler to a few tenths of a millimeter. Measurements were segregated by filament and remained linked to a micrograph number and a data set. The L, W and T measurements were separately summed and divided by the number of mesurements for each PHF. Each PHF is thus represented by average L, W and T values. In Figure 1 the frequency of wide region sizes is recorded for unsonicated and for sonicated PHF, since PHF are usually isolated using one of these treatments. The wide regions of the sonicated PHF shift to larger sizes. The average unsonicated W is 16.8 ± 1.8 nm ($\pm$ SD; n = 44) and the sonicated W is 21.1 ± 2.5 nm (n = 94) (difference > 99.9% confidence level).

In Figure 2 the frequency of thin region sizes is recorded for the unsonicated and the sonicated PHF. The thin regions for the sonicated PHF also shift to larger sizes. The average unsonicated T is 6.4 ± 0.8 nm ($\pm$ SD; n = 44) and the sonicated T averages 8.5 ± 1.3 nm (n = 94) (difference > 99.9% confidence level).

In Figure 3 the frequency of turn period sizes is recorded for unsonicated and for sonicated PHF. The average turn periods of these two preparations are not significantly different and are 77.6 ± 6.1 nm ($\pm$ SD; n = 44) and 80.5 ± 9.3 nm (n = 94), respectively.

In Figure 4 each unsonicated PHF's T vs. W values are plotted and each unsonicated PHF is represented by a circular point. The sonicated T vs. W values are also plotted and each filament is represented by a solid square. Although the unsonicated and sonicated T vs. W values overlap slightly, the majority of the unsonicated values are smaller sizes and the sonicated squares are the larger T and W values. For the PHF model [5] we would expect T = 10 nm and W = 20–25 nm in Figure 4 to be a few points surrounded by a scatter of points. Instead we have a hypothetical line of points with scatter above and below with T varying greatly from 5.5 to 12.5 nm and W varying from 12.5 to 26 nm. This suggests that the filaments in Figure 4 are not a single size but are a family of AD helical filaments.

In the unsonicated PHF preparation, ~2.1 nm filaments were found rafted side by side. These ~2.1 nm tau polymer filaments have previously been found in AD tangles [14, 15]. Two classes of cylindrical filaments, CF, were also found. In Figure 5, CF were unmodulated and modulated with periodic thin regions, CF-PT. The thin regions had an average repeat period of 77.2 ± 7.7 nm

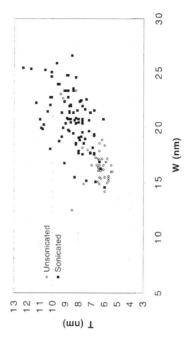

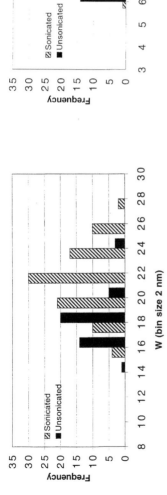

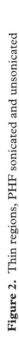

Figure 1. Wide regions, PHF sonicated and unsonicated

Figure 2. Thin regions, PHF sonicated and unsonicated

Figure 3. Turn period, PHF sonicated and unsonicated

Figure 4. T vs. W, PHF sonicated and unsonicated

(± SD; n = 31) indistinguishable from the turn period, L, of the PHF. With sonication CF diameters increased from 11.2 ± 2.3 nm (± SD) to 15.3 ± 2.4 nm, while the CF-PT mostly disappeared. The groove between the two ~10 nm PHF filaments in their wide regions should be distinguishable by negative staining, but the wide regions generally appear continuous. The narrow regions sometimes appear to be a twisted ribbon on edge for the widest PHF [8], whereas the thin regions more often appear to be narrow cylindrical connectors between two wide regions. This characterization suggests that these right-hand helical tangle filaments of variable width and ~80 nm turn periods are best described as AD helical filaments and not PHF.

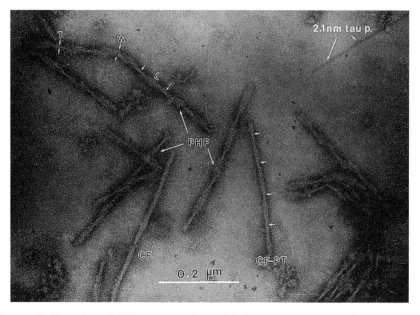

Figure 5. Unsonicated PHF preparation. This image contains all of the filaments described in the text. The thin region, T, the wide region, W, and the helical turn period, L, are labeled on a PHF. A cylindrical filament, CF, is at the lower left. A modulated cylindrical filament with periodic thin regions is at the center of the image and a small number (2–3) of thin (~2.1 nm) filaments rafted together are shown in the upper right

ACKNOWLEDGEMENTS

Support was provided by NIH Grants AG11054, AG05892 and NS18105. G.C.R. thanks TB Roos for statistical work, GeoM Co. for support, and Dartmouth Rippel Electron Microscope Facility for use of the JEM 100CX TEM.

REFERENCES

1. Grundke-Iqbal I, Iqbal K, Quinlan M, Tung Y-C, Zaidi MS, Wisniewski HM. MAP tau: a component of Alzheimer PHF. J Biol Chem 1986: 261: 6084–9; Grundke-Iqbal I, Iqbal K, Tung YC, Quinlan M, Wisniewski HM, Binder LI. Abnormal phosphorylation of the MAP tau in Alzheimer cytoskeletal pathology. Proc Natl Acad Sci USA 1986; 83: 4913–17; Goedert M, Spillantini MG, Cairns NJ, Crowther RA. Tau proteins of Alzheimer paired helical filaments: abnormal phosphorylation of all six brain isoforms. Neuron 1992; 8: 159–68.
2. Köpke E, Tung Y-C, Shaikh S, Alonso A del C, Iqbal K, Grundke-Iqbal I. MAP tau: abnormal phosphorylation of a non-PHF pool in AD. J Biol Chem 1993; 268: 24374–84.
3. Ruben GC, Ciardelli TL, Grundke-Iqbal I, Iqbal K. Alzheimer disease hyperphosphorylated tau aggregates hydrophobically. Synapse 1997; 27: 208–29.
4. Alonso A del C, Zaidi T, Grundke-Iqbal I, Iqbal K. Role of abnormally phosphorylated tau in the breakdown of microtubules in AD. Proc Natl Acad Sci USA 1994; 91: 5562–6.
5. Kidd M. PHF in electron microscopy of Alzheimer's disease. Nature 1963; 197: 192–3.
6. Wisniewski HM, Narang HK, Terry RD. Neurofibrillary tangles of PHF. J Neurol Sci 1976; 27: 173–81.
7. Ruben GC, Iqbal K, Grundke-Iqbal I, Johnson JE Jr. The organization of the MAP tau in Alzheimer PHF. Brain Res 1993; 602: 1–13.
8. Ruben GC, Novák M, Edwards PC, Iqbal K. Alzheimer PHF, untreated and pronase digested, studied by vertical Pt-C replication and high resolution TEM. Brain Res 1995; 675: 1–12.
9. Ikonomovic MD, Armstrong DM, Yen SH, Obcemea C, Vidic B. AFM of PHF isolated from the autopsied brains of patients with Alzheimer's disease and immunolabeled against MAP tau. Am J Pathol 1995: 147: 516–28.
10. Pollanen MS, Markiewicz P, Bergron C, Goh MC. Twisted ribbon structure of PHF revealed by AFM. Am J Pathol 1994; 144: 869–73.
11. Pollanen MS, Markiewicz P, Goh MC. PHF are twisted ribbons conposed of two parallel and aligned components: image reconstruction and modeling of filament structure using AFM. J Neuropathol Exp Neurol 1997; 56: 79–85.
12. Iqbal K, Zaidi T, Thompson CH, Merz PA, Wisniewski HM. Alzheimer PHF: Bulk isolation, solubility and protein composition. Acta Neuropathol (Berlin) 1984; 62: 167–77.
13. Ruben GC, Harris ED Jr, Nagase H. Electron microscope studies of free and proteinase-bound duck ovostatins (ovomacroglobins): model of ovostatin structure and its transformation upon proteolysis. J Biol Chem 1988; 263: 2861–9.
14. Ruben GC, Iqbal K, Grundke-Iqbal I, Wisniewski HM, Ciardelli TL, Johnson JE Jr. The MAP tau forms a triple-stranded left-hand helical polymer. J Biol Chem 1991; 266; 22019–27.
15. Ruben GC, Iqbal K, Wisniewski HM, Johnson JE Jr, Grundke-Iqbal I. Alzheimer neurofibrillary tangles contain 2.1 nm filaments structurally identical to the MAP

tau: a high resolution TEM study of tangles and senile plaque core amyloid. Brain Res 1992; 590: 164–79.

Address for correspondence:
    George C. Ruben,
    Dept. Biological Sciences,
    Dartmouth College,
    Hanover, NH 03766, USA

22 Cerebrospinal Fluid Aspartate Aminotransferase Activity Is Increased in Alzheimer's Disease

T. TAPIOLA, M. LEHTOVIRTA, T. PIRTTILÄ,
I. ALAFUZOFF, P. RIEKKINEN SR AND H. SOININEN

INTRODUCTION

At present, there is no diagnostic biochemical marker for Alzheimer's disease (AD), and the definite diagnosis of AD is currently based on histopathological examination of the brain [1]. Diagnosing probable AD in clinical evaluation provides an accuracy of 80–90% at centers specializing in the evaluation of dementia [2, 3, 4]. A biomarker of AD would be very valuable in confirmation of the clinical diagnosis or in monitoring the progression of the disease and therapeutic responses.

An ideal biochemical marker should have high sensitivity to identify all AD patients, and high specificity to differentiate AD from other dementias. It should also be able to identify presymptomatic cases of AD and reflect the neuropathology of AD. Cerebrospinal fluid (CSF) analyses, such as quantification of β-amyloid [5, 6] and tau protein [7, 8, 9], are promising approaches for the ante-mortem diagnosis of AD. However, searches for new markers and clinical–pathological correlation studies, as well as epidemiological studies of promising biomarkers, are needed to define the usefulness of CSF markers in clinical practice. Recently, Riemenscheider and colleagues [10] reported a specificity of 83% for combined CSF aspartate aminotransferase (AST) activity and tau measurements in the diagnosis of AD and suggested that AST could be useful in distinguishing AD from other dementias. Therefore, we wanted to further analyze the diagnostic value of AST activity measurements in a large number of patients with dementia, including definite AD patients.

Alzheimer's Disease and Related Disorders
Edited by K. Iqbal, D.F. Swaab, B. Winblad and H.M. Wisniewski
© 1999 John Wiley & Sons Ltd

MATERIALS AND METHODS

The study included three groups of dementia patients (patients with AD, vascular dementia (VaD) or other dementia) and two control groups (patients with other neurological diseases, such as amyotrophic lateral sclerosis or polyneuropathy, and patients with psychosomatic disorders). Patients' demographics are shown in Table 1. The demented patients underwent extensive clinical neurological examination, including Mini-Mental State Examination (MMSE) [11], neuropsychological tests, EEG, brain CT or MRI, CSF analysis, and routine laboratory tests. The diagnosis of probable AD was made according to the NINCDS–ADRDA criteria [2], and the diagnoses of other dementias were based on the guidelines of DSM-IV [12]. In addition, the AD diagnosis of 23 patients was confirmed using the neuropathologic criteria of CERAD [1]. In these cases the mean ± SD interval between lumbar puncture and autopsy was 23 ± 14 months. Determination of apolipoprotein E (apoE) genotype was performed as previously described [13]. The study was approved by the local ethics committee of the University of Kuopio and Kuopio University Hospital, and informed consent for participation in the study was obtained from all subjects and caregivers of demented patients.

Lumbar CSF samples were obtained using a standardized protocol and stored at −70 °C until assay. A colorimetric determination kit for transaminases (Sigma Diagnostics, St. Louis, MO, USA) was used for the quantification of the AST activity in CSF. The reaction was performed according to the manufacturer's protocol, with the exception that the total volume was reduced to 610 µl. The absorbances were read at 490 nm using a photometer (Microplate Reader, Model 550, Bio-Rad laboratories, CA, USA).

The data were analyzed by using SPSS for Windows V.6.0.1 software (SPSS Inc., Chicago, IL, USA). The one-way ANOVA with Bonferroni *post*

Table 1. Clinical characteristics of the patients

	N	F/M	Age	Duration	MMSE
Alzheimer's disease	60	44/16	76 ± 9	5.1 ± 3.9	12 ± 9.6
Vascular dementia	20	12/8	76 ± 6	1.8 ± 1.2	20 ± 4.7
Other dementias	29	16/13	68 ± 10	2.8 ± 2.4	19 ± 5.9
Frontal dementia	7	5/2	70 ± 7	1.7 ± 0.8	21 ± 1.7
Lewy body dementia	5	3/2	74 ± 6	1.6 ± 0.9	17 ± 7.6
Unspecified dementia	15	7/8	64 ± 11	3.9 ± 3.0	20 ± 7.2
Parkinson's disease with dementia	2	1/1	77 ± 4	1.0	22 ± 4.9
Other neurological diseases	27	10/17	61 ± 11	—	—
Controls	33	20/13	59 ± 7	—	—

Results are mean values ± SD.

hoc analysis was used to compare differences in means. Correlations were calculated using a two-tailed Pearson's correlation test. The statistical significance was set at $p < 0.05$.

RESULTS

There were no correlations between age and CSF AST activity in any of the groups. The mean $\pm$ SD AST activity in CSF was increased in patients with AD (8.1 ± 1.8 U/l) (Figure 1) compared to patients with psychosomatic disorders (2.6 ± 1.4 U/l; one-way ANOVA $F(4,164) = 50.22$, $p < 0.0001$) or patients with other neurological diseases (6.5 ± 1.7 U/l; $p < 0.01$). However, there was a considerable overlap of values in these groups. Instead, no significant differences were observed in AST values between patients with AD and VaD (7.6 ± 2.0 U/l) or other dementias (unclassified dementia 7.4 ± 2.7 U/l; Lewy body dementia 7.9 ± 1.6 U/l; frontal dementia 6.9 ± 2.3 U/l). VaD and other dementia patients had higher AST values compared to patients with

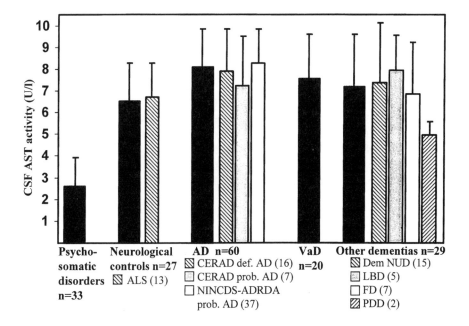

Figure 1. Cerebrospinal fluid aspartate aminotransferase activities (U/l) in Alzheimer's disease, other dementias and control groups. CSF AST was increased in patients with AD compared to neurological controls or patients with psychosomatic disorders. Also, patients with vascular dementia or other dementia had increased AST values. Abbreviations: ALS, amyotrophic lateral sclerosis; VaD, vascular dementia; Dem NUD, unspecified dementia; LBD, Lewy body dementia; FD, frontal dementia; PDD, Parkinson's disease with dementia

psychosomatic disorders, but no differences were found when compared to the patients with other neurological diseases (Figure 1). There were no statistically significant differences in AST activity between patients with at least one apoE ε4 allele and patients without ε4 allele in any study group (ε4+/ε4– AD, 8.4/7.6 U/l; VaD 7.9/7.5 U/l; other dementias 7.4/7.1 U/l).

We found no correlations between CSF AST activity and duration of the disease or severity of dementia. CSF AST activity was increased early in the course of AD. The mean ± SD AST value was 8.4 ± 1.7 in patients with disease duration less than one year (n = 13), whereas the value was 7.7 ± 2.0 U/l in histopathologically confirmed AD cases with disease duration 7.7 ± 3.8 years (n = 23). There was no significant difference of AST values between patients with mild dementia (MMSE ≥ 18; AST 8.7 ± 1.5 U/l) and moderate/severe dementia (MMSE < 18; AST 7.8 ± 1.5 U/l).

DISCUSSION

Our results indicate that the AST activity in CSF is increased in dementias and other neurological disorders. Thus, our results do not support the possibility of distinguishing AD from other dementias using AST measurements. We also found that CSF AST activity is increased early in the course of AD. The origin of increased AST activity in CSF is not known. Previous studies have shown that increased activity of AST in CSF is related to degeneration in the central nervous system [14]. Also, impaired glucose metabolism in AD and the use of glucogenic amino acids as an energy source might increase the activity of aminotransferases [10, 15]. Further studies are needed to determine the use of CSF AST as a marker of degeneration or injury of the central nervous system and its value in increasing the sensitivity and specificity when combined with other diagnostic tests for AD.

REFERENCES

1. Mirra SS, Heyman A, McKeel D et al. The Consortium to Establish a Registry for Alzheimer's Disease (CERAD). Part II. Standardization of the neuropathologic assessment of Alzheimer's disease. Neurology 1991; 41: 479–86.
2. Tierney MC, Fisher RH, Lewis AJ et al. The NINCDS–ADRDA Work Group criteria for the clinical diagnosis of probable Alzheimer's disease. Neurology 1988; 38: 359–64.
3. Morris JC, McKeel DW Jr, Fulling K et al. Validation of clinical diagnostic criteria for Alzheimer's disease. Ann Neurol 1988; 24: 17–22.
4. Kosunen O, Soininen H, Paljärvi L et al. Diagnostic accuracy of Alzheimer's disease: a neuropathological study. Acta Neuropathol 1996; 91: 185–93.
5. Motter R, Vigo-Pelfrey C, Kholodenko D et al. Reduction of β-amyloid peptide$_{42}$ in the cerebrospinal fluid of patients with Alzheimer's disease. Ann Neurol 1995; 38: 643–8.

6. Tamaoka A, Sawamura N, Fukushima T et al. Amyloid β-protein 42(43) in cerebrospinal fluid of patients with Alzheimer's disease. J Neurol Sci 1997; 148: 41–45.

7. Trojanowski JQ, Clark CM, Arai H, Lee VM-Y. Elevated levels of tau in cerebrospinal fluid: implications for the antemortem diagnosis of Alzheimer's disease. Alzheimer Dis Rev 1996; 1: 77–83.

8. Galasko D, Clark C, Chang L et al. Assessment of CSF levels of tau protein in mildly demented patients with Alzheimer's disease. Neurology 1997; 48: 632–5.

9. Tapiola T, Lehtovirta M, Ramberg J et al. CSF tau is related to apolipoprotein E genotype in early Alzheimer's disease. Neurology 1998; 50: 169–74.

10. Riemenschneider M, Buch K, Schmolke M et al. Diagnosis of Alzheimer's disease with cerebrospinal fluid tau protein and aspartate aminotransferase. Lancet 1997; 350: 784.

11. Folstein MF, Folstein SE, McHugh PR. 'Mini-mental state.' A practical method for grading the cognitive state of patients for the clinician. J Psychiatr Res 1975; 12: 189–98.

12. American Psychiatric Association. Diagnostic and Statistical Manual of Mental Disorders, 4th edn. Washington, DC: American Psychiatric Association, 1994.

13. Heinonen O, Lehtovirta M, Soininen H et al. Alzheimer pathology of patients carrying apolipoprotein E ε4 allele. Neurobiol Aging 1995; 16: 505–13.

14. Maas AIR. Cerebrospinal fluid enzymes in acute brain injury. 2. Relation of CSF enzyme activity to extent of brain injury. J Neurol Neurosurg Psychiat 1977; 40: 666–74.

15. Hoyer S, Nitsch R. Cerebral excess release of neurotransmitter amino acids subsequent to reduced cerebral glucose metabolism in early-onset dementia of Alzheimer type. J Neural Transm 1989; 75: 227–32.

Address for correspondence:
Hilkka Soininen, MD, PhD,
Department of Neurology, University of Kuopio,
PO Box 1627,
FIN-70211 Kuopio, Finland
Tel: 358 17 173 012; fax: 358 17 173 019

IV   Molecular Pathology

23 Enrichment of Presenilin 1 Peptides in the Membranes of Neuronal Vesicles: Implications for Alzheimer's Disease

SPIROS EFTHIMIOPOULOS,
ANASTASIOS GEORGAKOPOULOS, ERIK FLOOR,
JUNICHI SHIOI, WEN CUI, THOMAS WISNIEWSKI AND
NIKOLAOS K. ROBAKIS

INTRODUCTION

Most of the known familial Alzheimer's disease (FAD) mutations map on presenilin 1 (PS1), a multi-transmembrane-domain protein that appears in several isoforms derived from alternative splicing [1, 2]. Most cellular PS1 is proteolytically cleaved between amino acids 290 and 300 to yield an approximately 30 kDa N-terminal fragment (PS1/NTF) and an 18 kDa C-terminal fragment (PS1/CTF) [3]. PS1 protein exhibits significant homology to *Caenorhabditis elegans* protein SEL-12, which facilitates Notch receptor function [1, 4]. The construction of PS1-deficient transgenic mice suggests that this protein is required for proper formation of the axial skeleton, neurogenesis and neuronal survival [5]. In addition, PS1-expressing neurons seem to be less vulnerable to AD than neurons expressing no PS1, suggesting that PS1 has a neuroprotective function [6]. PS1 is also homologous to *C. elegans* spe-4 protein, which is involved in cytoplasmic trafficking of proteins during spermatogenesis [7].

The mechanism by which these genes cause FAD is only partially understood. The autosomal dominant mode of transmission of the FAD mutations is consistent with a gain-of-function or dominant-negative mechanism. It has been proposed that the FAD mutations cause AD by increasing production of Aβ1–42 (gain-of-function), which is then deposited in the neuropil as amyloid fibers, where it initiates a cascade of neurotoxic events that lead to neuronal loss (for review, see [8]). These suggestions, however, are

Alzheimer's Disease and Related Disorders
Edited by K. Iqbal, D.F. Swaab, B. Winblad and H.M. Wisniewski
© 1999 John Wiley & Sons Ltd

confounded by reports that frameshift mutations that result in a transcript encoding only a 50 residue N-terminal PS1 are also linked to FAD [9]. This peptide is unlikely to have any function and must represent a loss-of-function mutation. In addition, the increased levels of Aβ1–42 stimulated by certain FAD mutations do not correlate with the age of FAD onset induced by these mutants (for review, see [10]). The amyloid-plaque theory of AD is controversial for additional reasons, including a lack of correlation between the levels of amyloid depositions and several parameters measured in AD, such as degree of dementia, synapse loss, and distribution of cytoskeletal abnormalities. In addition, neuronal death and dystrophic neurites are also observed in areas devoid of amyloid depositions [10, 11]. It should be noted that many amyloid proteins are implicated in a number of diseases, including diabetes, cancer and rheumatoid arthritis; however, these proteins are not usually responsible for initiating the disease, although the amyloid depositions may contribute to the clinical phenotype. A recent report suggests that neuronal cells derived from transgenic mice null for PS1 produce reduced amounts of Aβ [12]. Although it was concluded that PS1 promotes Aβ production directly by modulating γ-secretase activity and APP cleavage, an alternative explanation of the data is that in PS1 –/– cells, APP C-terminal fragments, which are substrates for γ-secretase, fail to be transported to the appropriate subcellular compartment for γ-secretase cleavage. In this case, changes in Aβ production in FAD may in fact be an indicator of such a disturbance in cellular protein transport. This interpretation is consistent with reports that β- and γ-secretase cleavages of APP occur in distinct compartments, and with evidence of a more general disturbance of protein processing in AD, including tau phosphorylation. Although evidence has also been presented that PS2 is involved in apoptosis [13], PS1 showed anti-apoptotic activity in primary neuronal cultures [14].

There is evidence that axoplasmic transport and vesicle biology are disturbed in AD. Nerve terminals in AD brains are often filled with abnormal smooth endoplasmic reticulum (ER) and the Golgi complex of neurons with neurofibrillary tangles (NFTs) is deformed and coalesced in irregular granules, while the Golgi complex of neurons without NFTs is fragmented into disconnected and dispersed elements [15]. Early endosomes of human pyramidal neurons of sporadic AD display a 2.5-fold increase in size relative to the normal average [16], and dystrophic neurites contain high levels of enlarged large dense core vesicles (LDCVs). In addition, abnormal neurites in neuritic plaques (NPs) display increased immunoreactivity for chromogranin A, which is a marker of LDCVs [17]. It has been suggested that this increase in chromogranin was due to accumulation of materials as a consequence of early disturbances in vesicle transport before the development of dystrophic neurites [17]. Here we show that PS1 fragments are present in LDCV and PC12 CCV preparations, suggesting that they have a vesicular function. The potential implications of these observations for AD are discussed.

RESULTS

DETECTION OF FULL-LENGTH AND PS1 FRAGMENTS IN BOVINE CHROMAFFIN AND RAT PC12 CELLS

To examine whether the initial homogenates of bovine adrenal medullary chromaffin granules (CGs) or total extract of rat PC12 cells contained any full-length PS1, we used antibody 97754, directed against PS1 amino acids 1–12. CGs were prepared from bovine adrenal medulla as described [18]. As shown in Figure 1, total PC12 cell extract and crude homogenate of CGs contained both the PS1/NTF of about 30 kDa and the full-length PS1 of about 46 kDa. Immunoreactivity was specific for PS1 antigens because it was completely abolished after preabsorption of the antibody with the corresponding peptide (Figure 1). Although most of the PS1 antigens exist as peptide fragments, our antibody also detected significant amounts of full-length PS1 in the crude extracts.

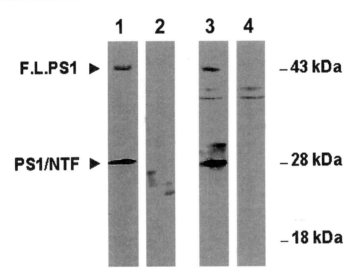

Figure 1. Immunodetection of full-length and N-terminal fragment of PS1 in rat PC12 cells and bovine adrenal medulla CGs. 150 μg protein of either PC12 cell extracts (lanes 1 and 2) or a crude homogenate of bovine adrenal CGs (lanes 3 and 4) were electrophoresed and analyzed by Western blotting using anti-PS1/NTF antibody 97754 (lanes 3 and 2) or this antibody plus peptide used as antigen to prepare the antiserum

THE N- AND C-TERMINAL FRAGMENTS OF PS1 ARE ENRICHED IN DENSE CORE CGs

Bovine adrenal medullary CGs are the functional equivalents of neuronal LDCVs and have been used extensively as a model for neuronal secretion.

Because of their abundance and density properties, CGs can be prepared at high purity from bovine adrenal medulla [18]. Membranes prepared from these purified CGs were greatly enriched relative to the initial crude homogenate of CGs, in both PS1/NTF and PS1/CTF migrating at approximately 30 kDa and 18 kDa, respectively (Figure 2A, B, lanes 1 and 2). The biochemical purity of our preparation was tested using dopamine β-hydroxylase (DBH), a specific marker for CG membrane, and calnexin, a marker of ER membrane. As shown in Figure 2C, our preparation was greatly enriched in DBH while it was almost free of contaminating ER membrane. Transferrin, a marker for endosomal membranes, was also decreased. Densitometric measurements showed that the degree of DBH enrichment was similar to the enrichment observed for both PS1 fragments (Figure 2), suggesting that they are specifically targeted to CG vesicles. Combined, our data indicates that our preparation was greatly enriched in CG membranes, whereas it was essentially free of other contaminating membranes. In contrast to the significant enrichment observed for the PS1 fragments, no full-length PS1 was detected in our preparations of purified CG membranes, suggesting that the full-length protein may not be targeted to these vesicles.

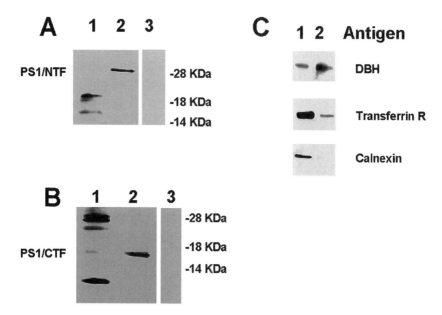

Figure 2. 40 μg of either a crude homogenate (lane 1) or purified (lanes 2 and 3) bovine adrenal medulla CGs were electrophoresed and then analyzed by Western blotting using either anti-PS1/NTF antiserum 97754 (A) or anti-PS1/CTF antiserum 331 (B). Lane 3: staining antibodies were preabsorbed with the corresponding peptides (C): anti-DBH, anti-transferrin receptor (TR), and anti-calnexin were used to examine the quality and enrichment of the CG

PS1 PROTEOLYTIC FRAGMENTS ARE ENRICHED IN LDCVs BUT NOT IN SCCSVs

Our CG data suggested that PS1 fragments may also be targeted to neuronal LDCVs, which are similar to CGs and transport peptides and neurotransmitters. LDCVs were purified along with somatodendritic clathrin-coated vesicles (SCCSVs) from whole rat brain homogenates by a combination of Nycodenz density gradient centrifugation and size exclusion chromatography on a Sephacryl S-1000 column [19]. Figure 3 shows that although the SCCSV preparation was greatly enriched in synaptophysin, which is abundant in these vesicles, no significant levels of PS1 proteolytic fragments were detected, suggesting that these fragments are not targeted to the SCCSVs. The LDCV preparation obtained from the Sephacryl column [19] was significantly enriched relative to the initial homogenate in secretogranin I, a specific lumenal marker for LDCV vesicles (Figure 3). Membranes from these vesicles were not enriched in calnexin, indicating that they are not significantly contaminated with ER membranes (data not shown). As shown in Figure 3, lane 2, our LDCV membrane preparations were enriched in both PS1/NTF and PS1/CTF. Combined with our results with CGs, these data suggest that both the N- and C-terminal fragments of PS1 are targeted to neuronal LDCVs.

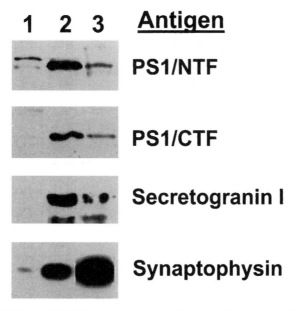

Figure 3. LDCVs and SCCSVs were prepared from whole rat brain. Equal amounts of membrane protein of the initial brain homogenate (lane 1), the LDCV preparation (lane 2), or the SCCSV preparation (lane 3), were analyzed and PS1/CTF and PS1/NTF were examined as in Figure 2. Antibodies against marker proteins for LDCVs and SCCSVs were used to probe the purity of the vesicular preparation. The detection of low levels of secretogranin in the SCCSV preparation (lane 3) indicates the presence of small amounts of contaminating LDCVs

THE PS1 PROTEOLYTIC FRAGMENTS ARE NOT ENRICHED IN NTCCVs

NTCCVs were prepared as previously described [20]. Figure 4 shows that the NTCCV-membrane preparation is enriched relative to the initial homogenate in clathrin, which is a marker for the NTCCV membranes. In addition, these membranes were enriched in synaptophysin (data not shown), which is known to be internalized via NTCCVs [20]. Combined, the data on the marker proteins show that our preparation is greatly enriched in NTCCV. It can be seen in Figure 4 (lane 2), however, that the NTCCV membranes were not enriched in either the PS1/NTF or the PS1/CTF relative to the initial homogenate (lane 1), indicating that these fragments are not targeted to NTCCVs.

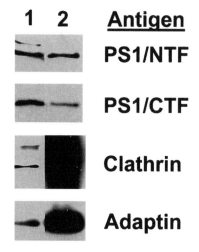

Figure 4. NTCCVs were prepared from whole rat brain. Equal amounts of membranes of the initial homogenate (lane 1) and the NTCCV preparation (lane 2) were analyzed. The presence of PS1/CTF and PS1/NTF was examined, as in Figure 2. Antibodies against proteins clathrin and adaptin, markers for clathrin-coated vesicles, were used to demonstrate the enrichment of our preparation in NTCCVs

THE N- AND C-TERMINAL FRAGMENTS OF PS1 ARE ENRICHED IN PC12 CCVs

The nerve terminal endosomes of neurons are involved in the recycling of presynaptic membrane and synaptic proteins, whereas the somatodendritic endosomes are found in somatodendritic compartments, where they carry out housekeeping functions, such as recycling of transferrin receptor, which is excluded from nerve terminals (for review, see [21]). Because no reliable protocol exists for the preparation of SDCCVs from brain homogenates, we prepared CCVs from undifferentiated PC12 cells. These vesicles are relatively easy to obtain and are used as models of SDCCVs [22]. Figure 5 shows that, as expected, the PC12 CCV preparation was greatly enriched relative to the initial homogenate in clathrin, which is a marker for CCV membranes, and in transferrin receptor, which is an endosomal marker for somatodendritic CCV membranes absent from NTCCVs [22]. The PC12 CCV membranes were not enriched in calnexin, which is an ER marker, indicating that these membranes are not significantly contaminated with ER membranes (data not shown). It can be seen in Figure 5 that both the PS1/NTF and PS1/CTF were significantly enriched in PC12 CCV membrane, indicating that these fragments are specifically targeted to the PC12 CCVs.

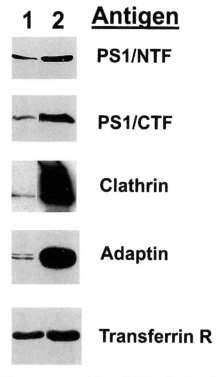

Figure 5. PC12 CCVs were prepared from PC12 cells. Equal amounts of membrane protein of the initial homogenate (lane 1) and the PC12 CCV preparation (lane 2) were analyzed by Western blot. Antibodies against marker proteins were used to demonstrate the purity of the vesicular preparation

DISCUSSION

We examined the distribution of PS1 peptides in adrenal medullary CGs and in rat brain and PC12 neuronal vesicles, including the SCCSVs and LDCVs of the regulated secretory pathway and the SDCCVs and NTCCVs of the endocytic neuronal pathway. The specific enrichment of both N- and C-terminal PS1 fragments in the membranes of LDCVs and CGs, even though these materials were prepared from different sources and by different protocols, indicates that these fragments constitute integral parts of these membranes and may play a role in LDCV-mediated secretion of neuropeptides and neurotransmitters at synaptic sites. Moreover, the presence of PS1 fragments in these vesicles suggests that, as a result of the LDCV–plasma membrane fusion during the LDCV-mediated secretion, these peptides may transiently be expressed on the plasma membrane of presynaptic terminals. Rat brain preparations of SCCSVs or NTCCVs were not enriched in the PS1 fragments, suggesting that PS1 peptides are not targeted to these vesicles. In contrast, these fragments were present in PC12 CCVs, suggesting that PS1 peptides are specifically targeted to neuronal somatodendritic vesicles, in agreement with previous reports [23] that PS1 antigens are expressed in the somatodendritic compartment of neurons. These data suggest that PS1 proteolytic fragments are expressed on the somatodendritic surface of neurons. We did not detect full-length PS1 in any of these vesicular preparations, suggesting that full-length peptide is cleaved in the ER/Golgi complex to yield N- and C-terminal fragments which are then targeted to specific vesicular populations (Figure 6).

The targeting of the PS1 proteolytic fragments to specific neuronal vesicles indicates that they regulate vesicular function. The hypothesis that PS1 plays a role in vesicle and protein transport is further supported by its homology to *C. elegans* protein Spe-4, which is involved in protein trafficking [7]. Although the specific vesicular function of these fragments is currently obscure, our data

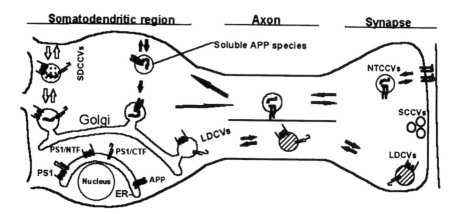

Figure 6. Diagrammatic representation of the vesicular localization of PS1 fragments and APP in neuronal cells. PS1 and APP proteins, marked in the Figure, are co-localized in the ER/Golgi complex but then follow different vesicular routes. Both proteins, however, may also co-localize in SDCCVs, where they can arrive via different routes (see Discussion)

raises the possibility that the PS1 FAD-linked mutations contribute to AD by interfering either with the targeting of the PS1 fragments to various vesicular systems or with specific vesicular function(s) of these fragments. It was recently reported [12] that C-terminal APP fragments, which are substrates for γ-secretase, accumulate in neurons lacking PS1 (PS1-/-). This observation suggests that these fragments may not be transported to the appropriate subcellular compartment for γ-secretase cleavage, thus inhibiting Aβ production. This suggestion is consistent with a role of PS1 in cellular protein trafficking, indicated by its presence in transport vesicles.

Recently it was reported that PS1 and APP proteins interact directly [24] and this interaction was used to explain the increase in the Aβ1–42/1–40 ratio induced by certain PS1 FAD mutants. APP proteins are transported to axon terminals [25], and from there they are internalized via NTCCVs and transported retrogradely to the somatodendritic compartment of neurons [26] (Figure 6). Our data showing that PS1 proteolytic fragments are not enriched in NTCCVs indicate that these fragments do not follow the axonal route of APP but are targeted from the Golgi directly to somatodendritic vesicles (Figure 6). This suggestion is further supported by the high PS1 reactivity in the somatodendritic neuronal area and the low PS1 reactivity in axons [23]. Combined, these observations suggest that APP and PS1 may interact on the somatodendritic neuronal surface and/or in the somatodendritic endocytic vesicles, rather than on the axons or in presynaptic terminals. The two proteins may also interact during their transport from the ER to Golgi. However, evidence has also been presented that PS1 and APP do not interact directly [27]. The expression of PS1 fragments in neuronal vesicles raises the possibility that the PS1 mutations precipitate the AD neuropathology by directly interfering with the function of these fragments in neuronal vesicular trafficking and/or function. This could also affect APP processing, as well as the integrity of the neuronal cytoskeleton. Mutations in several transmembrane proteins, including proteolipid protein [28] and cystic fibrosis protein [29], have been shown to precipitate neurological disorders by interfering with cellular and vesicular protein transport. Cystic fibrosis is caused by a loss of function of the CTRF protein, caused by at least 200 mutations spanning almost the entire length of the protein. Each of these mutations affects a different biological property of this protein, including protein processing, loss of regulation and loss of Cl-conduction [29], all of which ultimately result in a loss-of-protein function. Thus, multiple mutations can cause the same disease phenotype by affecting multiple properties of a protein. Our data that PS1 fragments are localized in vesicular membranes suggest that they have a function associated with the biology of vesicles, e.g. vesicle budding, vesicle fusion or vesicle trafficking. Combined, these observations suggest that some of the PS1 FAD mutations may cause neurodegeneration by affecting the vesicular function or transport of these fragments.

ACKNOWLEDGEMENTS

We thank Drs F. Brodsky, A. Helenius, W. Huttner, R. John, I.S. Trowbridge, J. Hardy and E. Ungenwickell for the antibodies. This work was supported by the Alzheimer's Association and NIA grants AG08200 and AG05138 to N.K.R.

ABSTRACT

Alzheimer's disease (AD) is caused by heterogeneous genetic and probably environmental factors. Although the etiology of the disease is still not clear, several lines of evidence indicate that the integrity and number of cellular organelles that sustain neuronal vesicular axoplasmic transport, including ER, Golgi, endosomes and LDCVs are compromised in AD. These observations suggest that those factors that compromise neuronal vesicular transport may also be causally involved in the development of AD. This hypothesis, while it does not disregard the pathological significance and consequences of NFTs and NPs, emphasizes the need to search for abnormalities in neuronal protein transport upstream of the formation of NFTs and NPs. Presenilin 1 (PS1) is an integral membrane protein of unknown function. Most of this protein is cleaved post-translationally to yield an N-terminal fragment and a C-terminal fragment. Many PS1 mutants have been linked to the development of FAD. We obtained evidence that PS1 proteolytic fragments are enriched in LDCVs, CGs, and SDCCV preparations, suggesting that this protein is expressed in these vesicles and may play a role in vesicular function. These observations raise the possibility that PS1 FAD mutations interfere with the vesicular function of the PS1 fragments and cause AD, according to a model where multiple mutations of a protein induce the same disease phenotype by affecting multiple properties of the protein.

REFERENCES

1. Sherrington R, Rogaev EI, Liang Y, Rogaeva EA, Levesque G, Ikeda M, Chi H, Lin C, Li G, Holman K, Tsuda T, Mar L, Foncin JF, Bruni AC, Montesi MP, Sorbi S, Rainero I, Pinessi L, Nee L, Chumakov I, Pollen D, Brookes A, Saseau P, Polinsky RJ, Wasco W, Da Silva HAR, Haines JL, Pericak-Vance MA, Tanzi RE, Roses AD, Fraser PE, Rommens JM, St George-Hyslop PH. Cloning of a gene bearing missense mutations in early-onset familial Alzheimer's disease. Nature 1995; 375: 754–8.
2. Doan A, Thinakaran G, Borchelt DR, Slunt HH, Ratovitsky T, Podlisny M, Selkoe DJ, Seeger M, Gandy SE, Price DL, Sisodia SS. Protein topology of presenilin 1. Neuron 1996; 17: 1023–30.

3. Thinakaran G, Borchelt DR, Lee MK, Slunt HH, Spitzer L, Kim G, Ratovitsky T, Davenport F, Nordstedt C, Seeger M, Hardy J, Levey AI, Gandy SE, Jenkins NA, Copeland NG, Price DL, Sisodia SS. Endoproteolysis of presenilin 1 and accumulation of processed derivatives *in vivo*. Neuron 1996; 17: 181–90.
4. Levitan D, Greenwald I. Facilitation of lin-12 mediated signalling by sel-12, a *Caenorhabditis elegans* S182 Alzheimer's disease gene. Nature 1995; 377: 351–4.
5. Shen J, Bronson RT, Chen DF, Xia W, Selkoe DJ, Tonegawa S. Skeletal and CNS defects in presenilin-1-deficient mice. Cell 1997; 89: 629–39.
6. Giannakopoulos P, Bouras C, Kovari E, Shioi J, Tezapsidis N, Hof PR, Robakis NK. Presenilin-1-immunoreactive neurons are preserved in late-onset Alzheimer's disease. Am J Pathol 1997; 150: 429–36.
7. L'Hernault SWL, Arduengo PM. Mutation of a putative sperm membrane protein in *Caenorhabditis elegans* prevents sperm differentiation but not its associated meiotic divisions. J Cell Biol 1992; 119: 55.
8. Hardy J. Framing β-amyloid. Nature Genet 1992; 1: 233–4.
9. Tysoe C, Whittaker J, Xuereb J, Cairns NJ, Cruts M, Van Broeckhoven C, Wilcock G, Rubinsztein DC. A presenilin-1 truncating mutation is present in two cases with autopsy-confirmed early-onset Alzheimer disease. Am J Hum Genet 1998; 62: 70–76.
10. Neve RL, Robakis NK. Alzheimer's disease: a re-examination of the amyloid hypothesis. Trends Neurosci 1998; 21: 15–19.
11. Terry RD. The pathogenesis of Alzheimer disease: an alternative to the amyloid hypothesis. J Neuropathol Exp Neurol 1996; 55: 1023–5.
12. De Strooper B, Saftig P, Craessaerts K, Vanderstichele H, Guhde G, Annaert W, Von Figura K, Van Leuven F. Deficiency of presenilin-1 inhibits the normal cleavage of amyloid precursor protein. Nature 1998; 391: 387–90.
13. Wolozin B, Iwasaki K, Vito P, Ganjei JK, Lacana E, Sunderland T, Zhao B, Kusiak JW, Wasco W, D'Adamio L. Participation of presenilin 2 in apoptosis: enhanced basal activity conferred by an Alzheimer mutation. Science 1996; 274: 1710–13.
14. Bursztajn S. De Souza R, McPhie DL, Berman SA, Shioi J, Robakis NK, Neve RL. Overexpression in neurons of human presenilin-1 or presenilin-2. Familial Alzheimer disease mutant does not enhance apoptosis. J Neurosci 18: 9790–99.
15. Stieber A, Mourelatos Z, Gonatas NK. In Alzheimer's disease the Golgi apparatus of a population of neurons without neurofibrillary tangles is fragmented and atrophic. Am J Pathol 1996; 148: 415–26.
16. Cataldo AM, Barnett JL, Pieroni C, Nixon RA. Increased neuronal endocytosis and protease delivery to early endosomes in sporadic Alzheimer's disease: neuropathologic evidence for a mechanism of increased β-amyloidogenesis. J Neurosci 17: 6142–51.
17. Brion JP, Couck AM, Bruce M, Anderton B, Durand JF. Synaptophysin and chromogranin A immunoreactivities in senile plaques of Alzheimer's disease. Brain Res 1991; 539: 143–50.
18. Vassilacopoulou D, Ripellino JA, Tezapsidis N, Hook VYH, Robakis NK. Full-length and truncated Alzheimer amyloid precursors in chromaffin granules: solubilization of membrane amyloid precursor is mediated by an enzymatic mechanism. J Neurochem 1995; 64: 2140–46.
19. Floor E, Leventhal PS, Wang Y, Meng L, Chen W. Dynamic storage of dopamine in rat brain synaptic vesicles *in vitro*. J Neurochem 1995; 64: 689–99.
20. Maycox PR, Link E, Reetz A, Morris SA, Jahn R. Clathrin-coated vesicles in nervous tissues are involved primarily in synaptic vesicle recycling. J Cell Biol 1992; 118: 1379–88.

21. Kelly RB. A question of endosomes. Nature 1993; 364: 487–8.
22. Nordstedt C, Caporaso GL, Thyberg J, Gandy SE, Greengard P. Identification of the Alzheimer β/A4 amyloid precursor protein in clathrin-coated vesicles purified from PC12 cells. J Biol Chem 1993; 268: 608–12.
23. Elder GA, Tezapsidis N, Carter J, Shioi J, Bouras C, Li HC, Johnston JM, Efthimiopoulos S, Friedrich VL Jr, Robakis NK. Identification and neuron specific expression of the S182/presenilin 1 protein in human and rodent brains. J Neurosci Res 1996; 45: 308–20.
24. Weidemann A, Paliga K, Durrwang U, Czech C, Evin G, Masters CL, Beyreuther K. Formation of stable complexes between two Alzheimer's disease gene products: presenilin-2 and β-amyloid precursor protein. Nature Med 1997; 3: 328–32.
25. Ferreira A, Caceres A, Kosik KS. Intraneuronal compartments of the amyloid precursor protein. J Neurosci 1993; 13: 3112–23.
26. Marquez-Sterling NR, Lo ACY, Sisodia SS, Koo EH. Trafficking of cell surface β-amyloid precursor protein: evidence that a sorting intermediate participates in synaptic vesicle recyling. J Neurosci 1997; 17: 140–51.
27. Thinakaran G, Harris CL, Ratovitski T, Regard CM, Bouton ML, Davenport F, Slunt HH, Price DL, Borchlet DR, Sisodia SS. A common pathway for processing of presenilins (PS1 and PS2). 27th Annual Meeting of Society for Neuroscience, 25–30 October 1997, New Orleans, LA, Abstr 117.2.
28. Gow A, Lazzarini RA. A cellular mechanism governing the severity of Pelizaeus–Merzbacher disease. Nature Genet 1996; 13: 422–8.
29. Welsh MJ, Smith AE. Molecular mechanisms of CFTR chloride channel dysfunction in cystic fibrosis. Cell 1993; 73: 1251–4.

Address for correspondence:
Dr Spiros Efthimiopoulos,
Departments of Psychiatry and Neurobiology,
Mount Sinai School of Medicine,
One Gustave Levy Place, Box 1229,
New York, NY 10029, USA
Tel: (212) 241 8370; fax: (212) 831 1947;
e-mail: efthis01@doc.mssm.edu

24 The 18–20 kDa C-Terminal Fragment of Presenilin-1 Is the Major *In Vivo* Substrate for Proteases of the Caspase Family

JÜRGEN GRÜNBERG, JOCHEN WALTER AND
CHRISTIAN HAASS

INTRODUCTION

Mutations in the presenilin (PS) genes are linked to early onset familial Alzheimer's disease (FAD). The two homologous PS proteins are expressed as 45–50 kDa proteins upon over-expression in cultured cells or transgenic mice [1–5]. It appears that endogenous full-length PS is present in very small amounts, whereas robust amounts of proteolytic products of the PS proteins were detected [1, 2]. Proteolytic processing of PS-1 and PS-2 results in the accumulation of two fragments, a ~30 kDa N-terminal fragment (NTF) and a ~20 kDa C-terminal fragment (CTF) [1, 2, 5, 6]. Proteolytic processing of PS-1 is known to occur within the domain encoded by exon 10, since the naturally occurring FAD-associated Δexon10 mutation [7] abolishes proteolytic processing [1]. Proteolytic cleavage within that domain is highly regulated and only small amounts of these fragments are produced, even after over-expression of PS in transfected cells or transgenic mice [1]. However, these fragments appear to be very stable and therefore accumulate *in vivo* in cultured cells and all tissues analyzed [1, 2].

Besides the ~30 kDa NTF and ~20 kDa CTF, additional proteolytic fragments are detected in a variety of tissues and cell lines (Haass and Grünberg, unpublished data). Podlisny et al. [2] described the detection of a 10–14 kDa C-terminal fragment as well as several alternative NTFs. In fully differentiated neurons, a substantial increase of a larger NTF [8, 9] and a smaller CTF was observed [8].

We have now characterized the proteolytic mechanism involved in the generation of the alternative fragments in detail. We found that the alternative cleavage occurs between aspartate 345 and serine 346 of PS-1,

Alzheimer's Disease and Related Disorders
Edited by K. Iqbal, D.F. Swaab, B. Winblad and H.M. Wisniewski
© 1999 John Wiley & Sons Ltd

C-terminal to the originally described cleavage in the domain encoded by exon 10 [1, 2]. Over-expression of caspase 3 (CPP32), a protease of the caspase superfamily, caused an increased alternative cleavage, whereas inhibition of caspases completely blocked the generation of alternative fragments but not the generation of the conventional fragments. By inhibition of *de novo* protein synthesis in untransfected cells, we demonstrate that the conventional C-terminal fragment of PS-1 is a substrate for caspase-like proteases as well. Therefore, full-length and the conventional C-terminal fragment of PS-1 can serve as potential death substrates. Due to the fact that very little full-length PS-1 is expressed *in vivo*, the much more abundant C-terminal fragment and not the full-length precursor is the major *in vivo* substrate for the alternative cleavage of PS-1 by proteases of the caspase superfamily.

MATERIALS AND METHODS

CELL CULTURE

All cell lines were cultured in Dulbecco's minimal essential medium supplemented with 10% FCS. Transient transfections were carried out using DOTAP (Boehringer-Mannheim). All cDNA constructs used are encoding the VRSQ motif [10].

ANTIBODIES

The polyclonal antibodies 2953, 3027 and 4627 used in this study were described previously [2, 8, 11, 12]. The polyclonal antibody 4627 is raised to PS-1$_{457-467}$ [2, 11].

IMMUNOPRECIPITATION

Cells were lysed in STEN buffer (50 mM Tris–HCl, pH 7.6; 150 mM NaCl; 2 mM EDTA; 0.2% NP-40) containing 1% Triton X-100 and 1% SDS for 20 min at 4 °C, 48 h after transfection. The lysates were centrifuged at 15 000 rpm at 4 °C for 20 min. Supernatants were carefully removed and transferred to new Eppendorf tubes. For immunoprecipitation, the SDS concentration was diluted to 0.1% with STEN lysis buffer. The immunoprecipitations were carried out as described by Haass et al. [13], except that the immunoprecipitates were heated to 42 °C for 15 min in sample buffer containing 8 M urea before they were separated on 10–20% Tris/Tricine polyacrylamide gels [14]. Immunoblotting was carried out as described previously [13]. Proteins were transferred to PVDF membranes (Millipore) at 400 mA for 1 h at 4 °C in 1 × electrophoresis buffer without SDS.

SITE-DIRECTED MUTAGENESIS

In vitro mutagenesis of aspartate 345 to asparagine was carried out by PCR. The nucleotide sequence of the oligonucleotides used is available upon request. The resulting fragments were cloned into the *Eco*R1/*Bam*H1 site of pSG5 (Stratagene). The cDNAs were sequenced to prove successful mutagenesis.

INHIBITION OF PROTEIN SYNTHESIS AND
STAUROSPORINE-INDUCED APOPTOSIS

Untransfected COS-7 cells were incubated in the presence of cycloheximide (Biomol; 20 µg/ml) either with or without staurosporine (Biomol; 1 µM) for 15 h. Inhibition of protein biosynthesis was controlled by determining the incorporation of ^{35}S-methionine during incubation with cycloheximide. Cells were collected by centrifugation at $800 \times g$ for 5 min after scraping from culture dishes and lysed in a buffer containing 1% SDS and 1% Triton X-100. Lysates were centrifuged at $14\,000 \times g$ for 10 min and proteolytic fragments of PS-1 were isolated and detected as described above.

RESULTS AND DISCUSSION

IDENTIFICATION OF ALTERNATIVE CLEAVAGE PRODUCTS
OF PS-1

COS-7 cells were transfected with the wild-type (wt) PS-1 cDNA or with a cDNA construct encoding PS-1Δexon10 [7]. The cell lysates were immunoprecipitated with an antibody to the large loop of PS-1 (antibody 3027) [12] and the precipitates were separated on a 10–20% Tris/Tricine gel, transferred to PVDF membranes, and analyzed with the same antibody. We detected the previously described [1] 18–20 kDa C-terminal fragments (CTF$_{18-20}$; Figure 1A) which are not over-expressed upon transfection as expected [1]. In addition to this fragment we reproducibly obtained a smaller fragment of approximately 10 kDa upon transfection of both cDNAs (Figure 1A; CTF$_{10}$). In contrast to CTF$_{18-20}$, CTF$_{10}$ was strongly augmented in transfected cells as compared to untransfected cells (Figure 1A). The identity of the novel PS-1 fragment is proved by its augmentation after over-expression of PS-1, as well as by an expected molecular weight shift upon expression of a C-terminal deleted recombinant PS-1 molecule (data not shown). Since over-expression of wt PS-1 and PS-1Δexon10 (which does not undergo conventional processing) gave rise to the generation of CTF$_{10}$, this fragment can be generated by proteolytic cleavage of the full-length protein.

In addition to the novel CTF$_{10}$, we also detected an alternative NTF of higher molecular weight (NTF$_{H}$; 34 kDa) as the conventional fragment

216

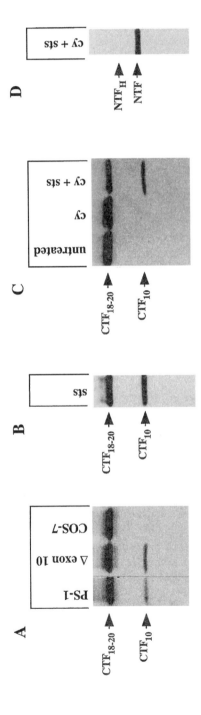

Figure 1. Identification of an alternative proteolytic processing pathway for PS-1. (A) COS-7 cells transfected with the PS-1 or PS-1Δexon10 cDNAs or untransfected COS-7 cells were lysed in a buffer containing Triton X-100 and SDS. CTFs of PS-1 and PS-1Δexon10 were immunoprecipitated with antibody 3027 to the large loop of PS-1. Precipitated CTFs were detected by immunoblotting using the same antibody. The alternative CTF_{10} was strongly augmented upon over-expression. Expression of PS-1Δexon10 leads to the production of CTF_{10}, which demonstrates that this fragment can be generated from full-length PS-1. As a control, endogenous PS-1 was immunoprecipitated from untransfected COS-7 cells. CTF_{18-20} observed in cells transfected with the PS-1Δexon10 cDNA represents the endogenous fragment in a fraction of cells not expressing the *trans* gene. (B) Induction of apoptosis by treatment of untransfected cells with staurosporine (sts) leads to enhanced generation of CTF_{10} (cf. A, lane COS-7). (C) After inhibition of *de novo* synthesis of PS-1 by cycloheximide (cy), staurosporine(sts)-induced apoptosis still allows the generation of large amounts of CTF_{10}, demonstrating caspase-mediated cleavage of CTF_{18-20}. Total cell lysates from untreated cells, cells treated with cycloheximide (cy) alone (note that this has no influence on the accumulation of CTF_{18-20}) and cycloheximide plus staurosporine (cy + sts) were immunoprecipitated as described above. Reproduced with permission from reference [18], © 1998 American Chemical Society

(30 kDa) (data not shown). In contrast to the conventional 30 kDa NTF, the 34 kDa NTF_H is also recognized by antibody 3027 (raised to the large loop), indicating that this peptide is generated by an alternative cleavage C-terminal to the conventional cleavage site [8]. The detection of CTF_{10} together with NTF_H strongly supports the notion that full-length PS-1 can serve as a substrate for alternative cleavage.

Recently it was reported that PS proteins might participate in apoptosis [15–17]. We therefore induced apoptosis by treating COS-7 cells with staurosporine. Indeed, stimulation of apoptosis results in the enhanced production of CTF_{10} (Figure 1B). Since proteases of the caspase superfamily are activated during apoptosis, we treated cells with staurosporine and highly selective caspase inhibitors. Inhibition of caspase activity blocked the generation of CTF_{10} [18]. Furthermore, over-expression of the caspase CPP32 results in the enhanced generation of CTF_{10} [18]. The involvement of caspases in the generation of CTF_{10} is also supported by mutagenesis of the critical aspartates required for substrate recognition of caspases. Mutagenesis of the aspartate at the P_1 position of the cleavage site is known to result in the inhibition of caspase cleavage [19, 20]. When the aspartate at position 345 of PS-1 was mutated to asparagine, caspase-mediated cleavage was efficiently blocked [18]. Very similar results were obtained for PS-2 [21, 22]. Taken together, these results strongly indicate that caspases are involved in an alternative cleavage of PS-1 and PS-2. However, it seems unlikely that caspase 3 (CPP32) is the protease which cleaves PS-1 directly, since the sequence of the PS-1 cleavage site (AQRD) is not homologous to the consensus sequence of caspase 3 (CPP32; DXXD) [23]. We therefore suggest that another member of the caspase cascade, which is activated by over-expressed caspase 3 (CPP32), is involved in alternative cleavage. Members of the caspase superfamily are activated by sequential proteolytic cleavage. Finally, a member of the caspase family or other proteases are cleaving their 'death substrates' such as lamin, actin, poly(ADP)ribose polymerase, rho-GDI, SREBP, and DNA-dependent protein kinase, which then results in the morphological changes typical for programmed cell death [23]. Based on our results, PS-1 therefore represents a novel death substrate most likely for one of the proteases of the caspase superfamily (Figure 2, left panel).

$CTF_{18–20}$ IS THE MAJOR *IN VIVO* SUBSTRATE FOR THE ALTERNATIVE CLEAVAGE

Since very little full-length PS-1 can be detected *in vivo* [1, 2, 11, 12, 24], we analyzed whether the endogenous $CTF_{18–20}$ can serve as a substrate for the caspase cleavage as well. For this purpose we used untransfected COS-7 cells and induced apoptosis with staurosporine [18]. *De novo* synthesis of endogenous PS-1 was inhibited by incubating cells with cycloheximide. As shown

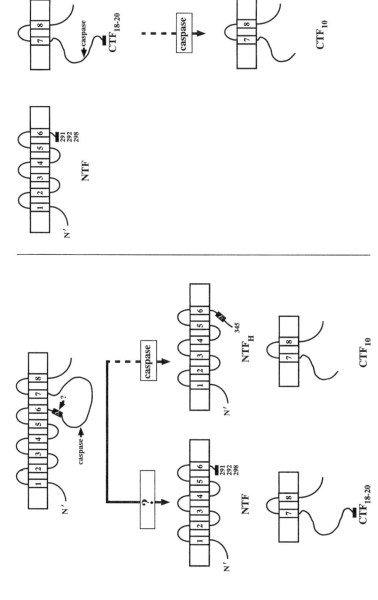

Figure 2. Schematic summary of proteolytic processing of PS-1. PS-1 is proteolytically processed by the conventional cleavage within exon 10. The caspase-mediated cleavage occurs between aspartate 345 and serine 346 and generates CTF_{10} and NTF_H upon cleavage of full-length PS-1 in transfected cells (left panel). Without over-expression of PS-1, CTF_{18-20} is the major substrate for caspase-mediated cleavage (in that case no NTF_H is generated; right panel). Δ = domain encoded by exon 10. Arrows indicate the cleavage sites of the two processing pathways. Reproduced with permission from reference [18], © 1998 American Chemical Society

in Figure 1C, CTF_{10} is still produced during co-incubation of cells with cycloheximide and staurosporine. Moreover, the reduced levels of CTF_{18-20} and the correspondingly increased levels of CTF_{10} demonstrate a precursor product relationship. If CTF_{18-20} is the *in vivo* substrate for caspase-mediated cleavage, one should not detect NTF_H in untransfected cells upon stimulation of apoptosis. We therefore isolated N-terminal PS-1 fragments from cells incubated with staurosporine and cycloheximide. This resulted in the identification of robust amounts of the conventional PS-1 NTF, while no NTF_H could be observed [18]. These data demonstrate that CTF_{18-20} and not full-length PS-1 is the major *in vivo* substrate for the caspase-mediated cleavage. This is further supported by the fact that *in vivo* very little full-length PS-1 can be detected, whereas the conventional fragments (NTF and CTF_{18-20}) accumulate at high levels [1, 2, 11, 12, 24].

Although the biological function of caspase-mediated cleavage of PS proteins is not yet clear, we want to point out that we recently found that caspase cleavage of PS-2 is regulated *in vivo* by phosphorylation at a serine adjacent to the critical aspartate (Walter and Haass, unpublished data). Moreover, phosphorylation of the PS-2 CTF not only prevents caspase cleavage, but also retards the progression of apoptosis. Therefore, caspase cleavage can be required to remove the anti-apoptotic PS-2 CTF.

ACKNOWLEDGEMENTS

We would like to thank Dr P. St George-Hyslop for the PS-1 cDNA. This work was supported by a grant from the Fritz Thyssen Foundation and Boehringer Ingelheim KG (to C.H.).

REFERENCES

1. Thinakaran G et al. Neuron 1996; 17: 181–90.
2. Podlisny M et al. Neurobiol Dis 1997; 3: 325–37.
3. Cook DG et al. Proc Natl Acad Sci USA 1996; 93: 9223–8.
4. Kovacs DM et al. Nature Med 1996; 2: 224–9.
5. Mercken M et al. FEBS Lett 1996; 389: 297–303.
6. Tomita T et al. Proc Natl Acad Sci USA 1997; 94: 2025–30.
7. Pérez-Tur J et al. NeuroReport 1995; 7: 297–301.
8. Capell A et al. J Neurochem 1997; 69: 2432–40.
9. Hartmann H et al. J Biol Chem 1997; 272: 14505–8.
10. Sherrington R et al. Nature 1995; 375: 754–60.
11. Walter J et al. Mol Med 1996; 2: 673–91.
12. Walter J et al. Proc Natl Acad Sci USA 1997; 94: 5349–54.
13. Haass C, Hung AY, Selkoe DJ. J Neuroscience 1991; 11: 3783–93.
14. Haass C et al. Nature 1992; 359: 322–5.
15. Vito P, Lacana L, D'Adamio L. Science 1996; 271: 521–5.
16. Vito P et al. J. Biol Chem 1996; 271: 31025–8.

17. Wolozin B et al. Science 1996; 274: 1710–31.
18. Grünberg J et al. Biochemistry 1998; 37: 2263–70.
19. Thornberry NA et al. Nature 1992; 356: 768–74.
20. Thornberry NA et al. Biochemistry 1994; 33: 3934–9.
21. Loetscher H et al. J Biol Chem 1997; 272: 20655–9.
22. Kim T-W et al. Science 1997; 277: 373–6.
23. Jacobson MD, Weil M, Raff MC. Cell 1997; 88: 347–54.
24. De Strooper B et al. J Biol Chem 1997; 272: 3590–98.

Address for correspondence:
    Jürgen Grünberg,
    Central Institute of Mental Health,
    Department of Molecular Biology, J5,
    68159 Mannheim, Germany
    Tel: 49 621 1703 885; fax: 49 621 23429

25 Biological Effects of Astrocyte-secreted Apoe/Lipoproteins: Role of LRP

DAVID M. HOLTZMAN, MARY JO LaDU,
LINDA VAN ELDIK, GUOJUN BU, SHAN WU,
SHILEN PATEL, ANNE M. FAGAN AND YULING SUN

INTRODUCTION

ApoE is a well-characterized 299 amino acid protein that participates in the regulation of plasma lipid metabolism [1]. In humans, apoE has three major protein isoforms: E2 (cys^{112}, cys^{158}); E3 (cys^{112}, arg^{158}); and E4 (arg^{112}, arg^{158}) that are encoded by a single gene on chromosome 19. Genetic studies have shown that apoE4 is a risk factor for AD as well as for poor outcome following certain injuries to the central nervous system (CNS) [2–4]. These studies and others suggest that apoE may play an important role in the CNS under certain disease conditions.

Within the CNS, as in the plasma, apoE is found in lipoprotein particles [5, 6]. However, apoE in the CSF, unlike in the plasma, is present almost exclusively in HDL-like particles and is derived from within the blood–brain barrier [6, 7]. Within the CNS, apoE is produced and secreted predominantly by non-neuronal glial cells, astrocytes and microglia [8–10]. Thus, it will be important to further characterize the apoE/lipoproteins produced by these cells within the brain in order to understand their role and function under normal and disease conditions.

Utilizing neuronal cell lines, we and others have previously shown that apoE3-enriched plasma lipoproteins can enhance neurite outgrowth, whereas apoE4 either decreased neurite outgrowth or had no effect [11–14]. The apoE receptor known as LRP, which is expressed at high levels in neurons [15–17], was required for these effects [12–14]. These and other findings suggested the hypothesis that isoform-specific differences in the ability of apoE/lipoproteins to promote structural recovery in the damaged CNS may account for why apoE4 is associated with an increased risk of AD and poor outcome following

Alzheimer's Disease and Related Disorders
Edited by K. Iqbal, D.F. Swaab, B. Winblad and H.M. Wisniewski
© 1999 John Wiley & Sons Ltd

brain injury. In order to further test this hypothesis, as well as to understand other potential functional functions of astrocyte-secreted apoE, we have (a) studied the effects of astrocyte-secreted apoE on neurite outgrowth, and (b) examined the composition and structure of apoE-secreted lipoproteins from rats, wild-type mice, apoE knockout (KO) (–/–) mice and apoE3 and E4 transgenic mice.

RESULTS AND DISCUSSION

To begin to define the biological functions of different human apoE isoforms produced in the brain, we generated transgenic mice in which human apoE3 and E4 are expressed under the control of the astrocyte-specific glial fibrillary acid protein (GFAP) promoter [18]. Founder animals were then bred back to apoE (–/–) mice for several generations, such that they expressed human apoE only by astrocytes in the absence of endogenous mouse apoE. Immunohistochemical studies revealed that human apoE protein is found within astrocytes and the neuropil throughout development and into the adult period in different transgenic lines (Figure 1).

The level of expression and the regulation of human apoE protein in response to brain injury in different transgenic lines was very similar to that seen in both the normal mouse and human brain. We found that, when astrocytes were cultured from GFAP-apoE transgenic animals, they secreted apoE into the culture media in HDL-like particles [18]. In order to determine whether the astrocyte-secreted apoE influenced neurite outgrowth, primary hippocampal neurons from E17 mouse hippocampus were grown in the presence of (but not in direct contact with) GFAP-apoE3, GFAP-apoE4 and apoE (–/–) astrocytes. There was neurite outgrowth under all conditions; however, there was significantly greater neurite outgrowth in the presence of apoE3-secreting astrocytes (Figure 2). Furthermore, the receptor-associated protein (RAP), as well as anti-LRP IgG, were able to block the neurite-enhancing effect of apoE3, suggesting that in some way LRP is required for this effect. It remains important to determine whether these isoform-specific differences are due to differences in LRP binding, LRP-mediated endocytosis of cholesterol/lipid, apoE-mediated cholesterol/phospholipid utilization, or differences in a yet-to-be-determined LRP signaling pathway. In addition, it will be interesting to determine whether similar differential effects occur in different *in vivo* paradigms in which there is neuronal/structural injury and subsequent plasticity.

While the effects of astrocyte-secreted human apoE3 on neurite outgrowth are similar to those seen with apoE3-enriched plasma lipoproteins, there are several other possible functions and interactions of apoE in the normal and diseased brain and, in regard to this, we are just beginning to explore the structure, composition and function of astrocyte-produced apoE. As a further

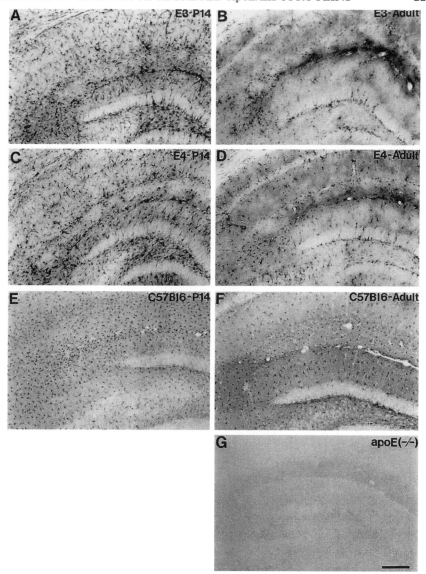

Figure 1. ApoE immunoreactivity is present in the brain of GFAP-apoE3 and GFAP-apoE4 mice. GFAP-apoE3 line 37 (A, B) and GFAP-E4 line 22 (C, D) mice on a mouse apoE (–/–) background were immunostained with a goat-anti-apoE antibody. There was strong staining of cells, which by morphology appear to be astrocytes in the hippocampus in both P14 (A, C) and adult (B, D) mice. In addition to staining in glial cell bodies and their processes, apoE-IR also appears to be present in the neuropil. Qualitatively similar apoE-IR is seen in cells that appear to be glial in C57B16 apoE (+/+) mice in both P14 (E) and adult animals (F). ApoE-IR is not observed in the hippocampus of an apoE (–/–) adult mouse (G). Scale bar, 130 μM. Reproduced with permission from reference [18]

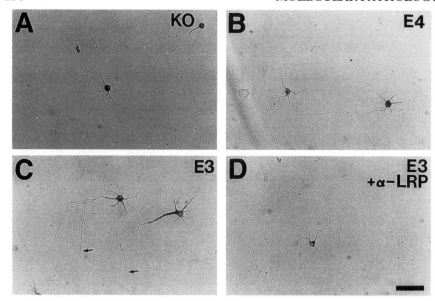

Figure 2. Neurite outgrowth from E19 primary hippocampal neurons is increased when neurons are cultured in the presence of media derived from GFAP-apoE3-secreting astrocytes. E19 primary hippocampal neurons (C57B16) were plated onto poly-D-lysine-coated coverslips and after attachment were incubated in the presence (but not in direct contact with) confluent astrocyte monolayers derived from the forebrain of P1 GFAP-apoE3 line 2 (C, D), GFAP-E4 line 22 (B), or apoE knockout (KO) (–/–) (A) littermate pups. After 44 h in culture, neurites, here identified by MAP-2-IR but also identified by phase-contrast microscopy, were on average longer in the presence of the apoE3-secreting astrocytes than in the presence of apoE4 or apoE (–/–) astrocytes. The increase in neurite outgrowth seen in the presence of apoE3 was blocked by anti-LRP IgG (D). The tips of two axons are identified with arrows in (C). Reproduced with permission from reference [18]

step toward understanding the origin and function of CNS lipoproteins, we have characterized lipoprotein particles from human CSF and compared them to lipoproteins derived from primary cultures of rat astrocytes [19]. As determined by lipid and apolipoprotein profiles, we found that both CSF lipoproteins and nascent rat astrocyte particles were both HDL-like in size and contain cholesterol and phospholipid; however, astrocyte particles have little core lipid (Figure 3). The presence of esterified cholesterol in the CSF particles was consistent with the observation that CSF particles were spherical in shape, as has been seen by others [5, 6, 20]. In contrast, we found that rat astrocyte lipoprotein particles were primarily discoidal in shape (Figure 4).

With regard to apolipoprotein content, CSF lipoproteins were heterogeneous with apoE, the most abundant apolipoprotein, localized to the largest particles, apoAI and apoAII localized to progressively smaller particles,

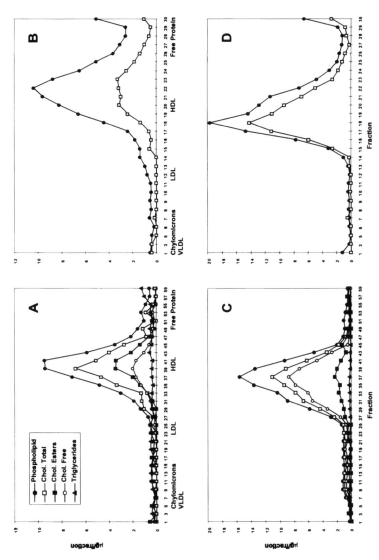

Figure 3. Lipid distribution in human CSF (A and B) and serum-free conditioned media from primary rat astrocytes (C and D) fractionated by size (A and C) and density (B and D). 50 ml of either CSF (A and B) or astrocyte-conditioned media (C and D) were concentrated to 1 ml and then fractionated by gel-filtration chromatography, using tandem Superose 6 columns (A and C), or by single-spin equilibrium ultracentrifugation, using 3–20% sodium bromide gradients (B and D). The resulting fractions were analyzed for lipid, which is expressed at μg/fraction. Reproduced with permission from reference [19]

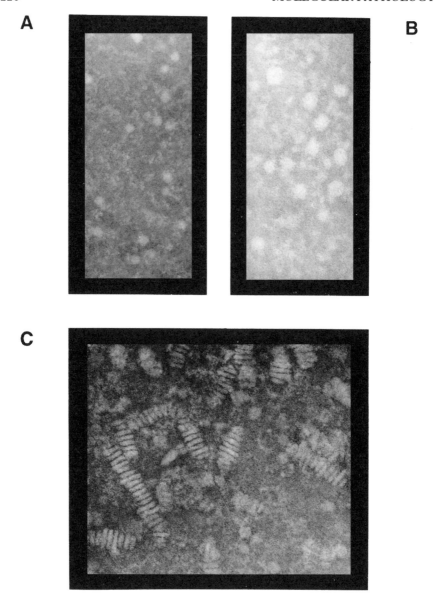

Figure 4. Negative-stained electron micrographs of lipoproteins from human CSF and rat astrocyte-conditioned media. Lipoproteins were isolated by gel-filtration chromatography and a concentrated aliquot (0.5 mg protein/ml) from fractions 37/38 (A) and 43/44 (B) of CSF and 37/38 (C) of astrocyte media was placed on a carbon-coated electron microscopy grid and negatively stained with 2% phosphotungstic acid. In (A), there are small spherical HDL-like particles and in (B) there are larger spherical HDL-like particles. In (C), there is a stack of discoidal particles from rat astrocyte-conditioned media. Reproduced with permission from reference [19]

and apoJ distributed evenly across particle size. The differences between lipoproteins secreted by astrocytes and present in CSF suggest that, in addition to delivery of their constituents to cells, lipoprotein particles secreted in brain by astrocytes may have the potential to participate in cholesterol clearance, developing a core of esterified cholesterol before reaching the CSF. Recent work by Rebeck and colleagues suggests that CSF lipoproteins can in fact efflux cholesterol *in vitro* [21]. Our recent data also suggests that this could be the case *in vivo*. We compared the brains of wild-type mice to those of apoE (−/−) mice following unilateral entorhinal cortex lesions, which removes ~85% of the afferent input to the outer molecular layer of the dentate gyrus [22]. It was found that, while cholesterol- and lipid-laden axonal debris was present in both wild-type mice and apoE (−/−) mice over several days, after 17 days the wild-type mice had cleared the debris. In contrast, there was a persistence of degeneration products in the apoE −/− animals. In preliminary studies, we have found that this debris appears to persist for as long as 30 days following the lesion (D. Holtzman and S. Patel, unpublished observations). This suggests that apoE secreted by CNS glia may play a role in the clearance of cholesterol-laden neurodegeneration products following brain injury through cholesterol efflux and re-delivery to other cells, as has been previously postulated [23]. It will be interesting to determine the clearance mechanisms utilized to remove and scavenge CNS lipoprotein particles containing apoE and apoJ and the receptor systems involved.

Since the primary and secondary structure of apolipoproteins determines the kind of lipoprotein particle in which they reside, we have been characterizing lipoprotein particles secreted by wild-type mouse astrocytes and astrocytes derived from GFAP-apoE3 and GFAP-apoE4 transgenic mice [18]. In preliminary studies we have found that, similar to rat astrocytes, wild-type mouse astrocytes also secrete HDL-like lipoprotein particles which contain apoE, apoJ, cholesterol and phospholipid. These particles, like rat astrocytes, are cholesteryl-ester-poor. It appears that while the lipoprotein particles secreted by the GFAP-apoE astrocytes are similar in size, they may be slightly smaller and contain less lipid, despite having similar amounts of apoE protein (M.J. LaDu, D. Holtzman, A.M. Fagan, unpublished observations). Whether there are differences between astrocyte-secreted lipoproteins containing apoE3 vs. apoE4 is currently being characterized. Finally, we have recently noted that apoE (−/−) astrocytes continue to secrete an amount of apoJ similar to that secreted by wild-type and GFAP-apoE astrocytes; however, they no longer secrete easily detectable phospholipid and cholesterol (M.J. LaDu, D. Holtzman, A.M. Fagan, unpublished observations). It also suggests that differences found between apoE (−/−) mice and mice expressing apoE may arise not only from the lack of apoE but also from a large decrease in the level of CNS-derived lipoprotein particles. Further experiments to test this possibility are under way.

CONCLUSIONS

The ε4 allele of apolipoprotein E (apoE) is associated with an increased risk of Alzheimer's disease (AD) and poor outcome following certain injuries to the central nervous system (CNS). In the CNS, apoE is expressed by glia, predominantly astrocytes. In order to define the potential biological functions of apoE-containing lipoproteins produced within the brain, we have analyzed the composition, structure, and function of astrocyte-secreted apoE. As we found previously with apoE3-enriched plasma lipoproteins, astrocyte-secreted apoE3 but not apoE4 increased neurite outgrowth from primary hippocampal neurons and this stimulation was dependent on the low-density lipoprotein receptor-related protein (LRP). We felt it was likely, however, that astrocyte-derived apoE would have a different composition and may thus differ functionally in other ways from plasma-derived apoE/lipoproteins. We found that cultured rat astrocytes secrete apoE in an HDL-like particle which is cholesteryl-ester-poor and disk-like in shape. Astrocytes derived from wild-type mice, as well as GFAP-apoE3 and apoE4 transgenic mice, secrete apoE in HDL-like particles which also contain cholesterol and phospholipid and are cholesteryl-ester-poor. Recent studies suggest that astrocyte-derived lipoprotein particles are likely to participate in cholesterol efflux as well as cholesterol delivery. Further exploration of the effects of astrocyte-derived apoE and isoform-specific differences in composition, interactions and function may provide new insights into AD pathogenesis.

ACKNOWLEDGEMENTS

This work was supported by NIH grants AG13956 (to D.M.H.) and AG05681 (to G.B. and D.M.H.) and Alzheimer's Association Grant RG3-96-26 (to D.M.H.).

REFERENCES

1. Mahley RW. Apolipoprotein E: cholesterol transport protein with expanding role in cell biology. Science 1988; 240: 622–30.
2. Strittmatter WJ, Saunders AM, Schemechel D et al. Apolipoprotein E: high avidity binding to β-amyloid and increased frequency of type 4 allele in late-onset familial Alzheimer disease. Proc Natl Acad Sci USA 1993; 90: 1977–81.
3. Corder EH, Saunders AM, Strittmatter WJ et al. Gene dose of apolipoprotein E type 4 allele and the risk of Alzheimer's disease in late onset families. Science 1993; 261: 921–3.
4. Roses AD. Apolipoprotein E, a gene with complex biological interactions in the aging brain. Neurobiol Dis 1997; 4: 170–86.

5. Roheim PS, Carey M, Forte T, Vega GL. Apolipoproteins in human cerebrospinal fluid. Proc Natl Acad Sci USA 1979; 76: 4646–9.

6. Pitas RE, Boyles JK, Lee SH et al. Lipoproteins and their receptors in the central nervous system. J Biol Chem 1987; 262: 14352–60.

7. Linton MF, Gish R, Hubl ST et al. Phenotypes of apolipoprotein B and apolipoprotein E after liver transplantation. J Clin Invest 1991; 88: 270–81.

8. Boyles JK, Pitas RE, Wilson E et al. Apolipoprotein E associated with astrocytic glia of the central nervous system and with non-myelinating glia of the peripheral nervous system. J Clin Invest 1985; 76: 1501–13.

9. Pitas RE, Boyles JK, Lee SH et al. Astrocytes synthesize apolipoprotein E and metabolize apolipoprotein E-containing lipoproteins. Biochim Bipohys Acta 1987; 917: 148–61.

10. Stone DJ, Rozovsky I, Morgan TE et al. Astrocytes and microglia respond to estrogen with increased apoE mRNA *in vivo* and *in vitro*. Exp Neurol 1997; 143: 313–18.

11. Nathan BP, Bellosta S, Sanan DA et al. Differential effects of apolipoproteins E3 and E4 on neuronal growth *in vitro*. Science 1994; 264: 850–52.

12. Holtzman DM, Pitas RE, Kilbridge J et al. LRP mediates apolipoprotein E-dependent neurite outgrowth in a CNS-derived neuronal cell line. Proc Natl Acad Sci USA 1995; 92: 9480–84.

13. Bellosta S, Nathan BP, Orth M et al. Stable expression and secretion of apolipoproteins E3 and E4 in mouse neuroblastoma cells produces differential effects on neurite outgrowth. J Biol Chem 1995; 270: 27063–71.

14. Fagan AM, Bu G, Sun Y et al. Apolipoprotein E-containing high density lipoprotein promotes neurite outgrowth and is a ligand for the low density lipoprotein receptor-related protein. J Biol Chem 1996; 271: 30121–5.

15. Rebeck GW, Reiter JS, Strickland DK, Hyman BT. Apolipoprotein E in sporadic Alzheimer's disease: allelic variation and receptor interactions. Neuron 1993; 11: 575–80.

16. Bu G, Maksymovitch EA, Nerbonne JM, Schwartz AL. Expression and function of the low density lipoprotein receptor-related protein (LRP) in mammalian central neurons. J Biol Chem 1994; 269: 18521–8.

17. Moestrup SK, Gliemann J, Pallesen G. Distribution of the α2-macroglobulin receptor/low density lipoprotein receptor-related protein in human tissues. Cell Tiss Res 1992; 269: 375–82.

18. Sun Y, Wu S, Bu G et al. GFAP-apoE transgenic mice: astrocyte specific expression and differing biological effects of astrocyte-secreted apoE3 and apoE4 lipoproteins. J Neurosci 1998; 18: 3261–72.

19. LaDu MJ, Gilligan SM, Lukens SR et al. Nascent astrocyte particles differ from lipoproteins in CSF. J Neurochem 1998; 70: 2070–81.

20. Borghini I, Barja F, Pometta D, James RW. Characterizations of subpopulations of lipoprotein particles isolated from human cerebrospinal fluid. Biochem Biophys Acta 1995; 1255: 192–200.

21. Rebeck GW, Alonzo NC, Berezovska O et al. Structure and functions of human cerebrospinal fluid lipoproteins from individuals of different APOE genotypes. Exp Neurol 1998; 149: 175–82.

22. Fagan AM, Murphy BA, Patel SN et al. Evidence for normal aging of the septo-hippocampal cholinergic system in apoE (–/–) mice but impaired clearance of axonal degeneration products following injury. Exp Neurol 1998; 151: 314–25.

23. Poirer J. Apolipoprotein E in animal models of CNS injury and Alzheimer's disease. Trends Neurol Sci 1994; 17: 525–30.

Address for correspondence:
David M. Holtzman,
Department of Neurology,
Washington University School of Medicine, 660 S. Euclid Ave.,
    Box 8111,
St. Louis, MO 63110, USA
e-mail: holtzman@neuro.wustl.edu

26 Characterization of Protein Kinases Phosphorylating the β-Amyloid Precursor Protein within Its Ectodomain and Identification of *In Vivo* Phosphorylation Sites

ALICE SCHINDZIELORZ, JÜRGEN GRÜNBERG,
CHRISTIAN HAASS AND JOCHEN WALTER

INTRODUCTION

The β-amyloid precursor protein (β-APP) is a transmembrane protein which is phosphorylated on serine residues within its ectodomain [1–3]. After proteolytic processing of β-APP by α-secretase or β-secretase, the phosphorylated ectodomain is secreted into the cellular environment. Recently, two different cellular locations were identified where β-APP can be phosphorylated *in vivo* [3]. Ectodomain phosphorylation can occur in late Golgi compartments, most likely secretory vesicles. In addition, cell surface-located β-APP can be phosphorylated by ecto-protein kinases. The *in vivo* phosphorylation sites within the ectodomain were mapped to serine residues 198 and 206 by mutation analysis. These serine residues are located within recognition motifs for casein kinases (CKs). Analyzing the co-substrate usage of ecto-protein kinases phosphorylating cell surface-located β-APP, we demonstrate that β-APP is phosphorylated *in vivo* by a CK-2 like ecto-protein kinase, which can use GTP and ATP as co-substrate. In addition, β-APP can be phosphorylated *in vitro* by purified CK-2. However, other protein kinase(s) which cannot use GTP are also involved in ectodomain phosphorylation of β-APP.

Alzheimer's Disease and Related Disorders
Edited by K. Iqbal, D.F. Swaab, B. Winblad and H.M. Wisniewski
© 1999 John Wiley & Sons Ltd

METHODS

CELL CULTURE, METABOLIC LABELING AND *IN VIVO* PHOSPHORYLATION

Kidney 293 cells were metabolically labeled with 15 µCi [^{35}S]-methionine or 1.5 mCi [^{32}P]-orthophosphate for 3 h in methionine-free or sodium phosphate-free Dulbecco's minimal essential medium (DMEM). Phosphorylation of cell surface proteins was carried out as described previously [3].

IMMUNOPRECIPITATION, ANTIBODIES AND ELECTROPHORESIS

Immunoprecipitations were carried out as described [4, 5]. The following antibodies were used. Antibody C7 was raised to the last 20 amino acids of β-APP and recognizes full-length β-APP [6]. Antibody B5, which recognizes all forms of APP$_S$, was raised to a fusion protein containing amino acids 444–592 of β-APP$_{695}$ [7]. Antibody 1736 (raised to β-APP 595–611) specifically identifies APP$_S$ cleaved by α-secretase [8].

PHOSPHOPEPTIDE MAPPING BY TRYPTIC DIGESTION

In vivo-[^{32}P]-phosphorylated β-APP was isolated by immunoprecipitation and SDS–PAGE, and transferred to nitrocellulose membrane. Digestion of radiolabeled β-APP was carried out for 24 h at 37 °C with 0.5 µg/µl trypsin (Boehringer-Mannheim, sequencing grade). The tryptic digest was separated on Tris/Tricine gradient gels (10–20%; Novex) and radiolabeled peptides visualized by autoradiography.

MATRIX-ASSISTED LASER DESORPTION/IONIZATION–MASS SPECTROMETRY (MALDI–MS)

Approximately 10 µg of unlabeled β-APP together with a trace of [^{32}P]-labeled β-APP were digested with trypsin and the resulting peptides separated on 10–20% Tris/Tricine gels, as described. Radiolabeled peptide bands were cut out from the gel, extracted twice for 10 min with 100 µl 0.1% aqueous trifluoroacetic acid followed by 100 µl of 60% acetonitrile. The combined supernatants were subjected to a 5 mm micro pre-column (LC Packings) packed with Poros R2 (PerSeptive Biosystems). The peptides were eluted in 10 µl with a step gradient of 80% acetonitrile/0.1% trifluoracetic acid. Molecular masses (isotopic average) of the eluted peptides were determined by a Vision 2000 (Finnigan) mass spectrometer equipped with a nitrogen laser and operated in reflection mode at an accelerating voltage of 5000. 1 µl of the peptide solution was crystallized in matrices consisting of 1% 2,4-dihydroxybenzoic acid in 0.1% aqueous trifluoracetic acid. All peptide spectra were externally calibrated by using the monoisotopic masses of sodium (MW 23.0) and fullerene C70 (MW 840.0).

Peptides were identified by computer-assisted analysis using the SWISSPROT sequence data bank and the special program package HUSAR (developed at the Department of Molecular Biophysics, German Cancer Research Center, Heidelberg).

RESULTS AND DISCUSSION

MAPPING OF PHOSPHORYLATION SITES WITHIN THE ECTODOMAIN OF β-APP

In order to identify the site(s) of β-APP phosphorylation, we first performed tryptic peptide mapping of *in vivo* phosphorylated β-APP molecules. Kidney 293 cells stably transfected with wild-type β-APP695 or cDNA constructs deleting large portions of the N-terminal half (AX construct [1]; Figure 1A) or the C-terminal half (XB construct [1]) were labeled with [^{32}P]-orthophosphate or [^{35}S]-methionine. Secreted forms of the respective β-APP molecules were immunoprecipitated with antibody 1736. In agreement with data published by Hung and Selkoe [1], we found that phosphorylation occurs within the N-terminal portion of β-APP since no phosphate incorporation occurred in cells expressing the N-terminal deletion construct (Figure 1B). Phosphorylated β-APP$_S$ wt as well as the phosphorylated C-terminal deleted β-APP (XB) were digested with trypsin and the digestion products were separated on a 10–20% Tris/Tricine gel. A single phosphorylated peptide of approximately 4.8 kDa was detected for both full-length β-APP and XB constructs (Figure 1C). Computer-assisted analysis of the potentially generated tryptic peptides revealed that the radiolabeled peptide could represent solely the amino acid sequence from 181–224 of β-APP$_{695}$. To prove this in more detail, the radiolabeled ~4.8 kDa peptide was eluted from Tris–Tricine gel and subjected to MALDI–MS (see Materials and Methods). Three monoisotopic masses of 2286.5, 3673.5 and 4877.3 (±10) were detected in the eluate. The masses of 2286.5 and 3673.5 could not be matched to tryptic peptides of β-APP and presumably represent peptides of autocatalytically-cleaved trypsin, migrating close to the phosphorylated β-APP tryptic peptide. In contrast, the mass of 4877.3 matches to the sequence of amino acids 181–224 of β-APP695 in a double phosphorylated form (4714.7 DA + 160 Da). Since the amino acid sequence of this peptide contains four serine residues, we searched for putative phosphor acceptor sites. Serine residues 198 and 206 were identified within an acidic sequence of this peptide, representing potential phosphorylation sites for CK-2 and CK-1, respectively (Figure 2A). These

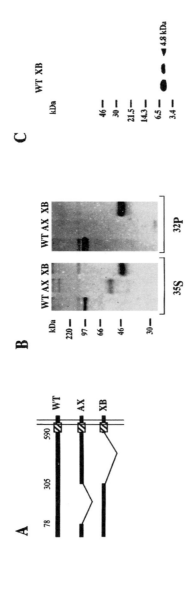

Figure 1. Identification of the phosphorylation sites of β-APP within its ectodomain. (A) Schematic of wild-type β-APP (WT) and the AX and XB construct, missing large portions of the N-terminal and the C-terminal half of the β-APP ectodomain. The Aβ domain is represented by a striped bar, vertical lines represent cellular membranes. The numbers above denote amino acid residues with the restriction sites used to generate the constructs indicated [1]. (B) Kidney 293 cells stably transfected with wild-type (WT) β-APP695, AX or XB were labeled with [35S]-methionine (35S) and [32P]-orthophosphate (32P), respectively, and conditioned media were immunoprecipitated with antibody 1736. Radiolabeled proteins were visualized by autoradiography after separation by SDS–PAGE. (C) Phosphor-peptide map of radiolabeled, secreted forms of wild-type (WT) β-APP or XB. Proteins were digested with trypsin, as described in Materials and Methods. The resulting tryptic peptides were separated on a 10–20% Tris/Tricine gel and analyzed by autoradiography. The position of the phosphorylated 4.8 kDa peptide is marked by an arrowhead

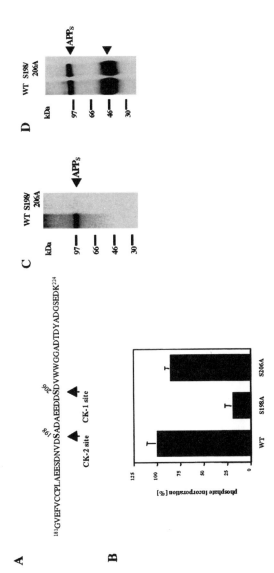

Figure 2. (A) Amino acid sequence of the phosphorylated tryptic peptide (amino acids 181–224), which was identified by mass spectrometry and computer-assisted analysis (see Methods). The serine residues representing potential phosphorylation sites of CK-1 (Ser206) and CK-2 (Ser198A) are shown in bold letters. (B) Quantification of *in vivo* phosphorylation of wild-type β-APP (WT) and β-APP carrying serine-to-alanine mutations at positions 198 (S198A) and 206 (S206A). Kidney 293 cells stably expressing wild-type or mutated forms of β-APP (S198A, S206A) were labeled with [35S]-methionine or [32P]-orthophosphate for 2 h. Quantification of protein expression and phosphate incorporation in the different forms of β-APP were carried out by phospho-imaging. Bars represent means ± SE of three independent experiments. (C, D) *In vivo* phosphorylation of the S198/206A double mutation. Cells stably expressing wt β-APP or the double mutation were labeled with 32P-orthophospate. β-APP was immunoprecipitated and transferred to PVDF membrane. Radiolabeled protein was visualized by autoradiography (C) and total β-APP (labeled arrowheads) was detected by immunostaining the same membrane (D). The unlabeled arrowhead indicates the position of the Ig heavy chain used for immunoprecipitation

serines were mutagenized to alanines and the corresponding cDNA constructs stably transfected into kidney 293 cells. Single cell clones were metabolically labeled with [^{32}P]-orthophosphate or [^{35}S]-methionine and secreted β-APP$_S$ was immunoprecipitated. As shown in Figure 2B, phosphorylation of β-APP containing the Ser198Ala mutation was reduced by about ~80%, while that of the Ser206Ala mutation was reduced by about 15%. Analysis of the corresponding double mutation S198/206A revealed that ectodomain phosphorylation is almost completely blocked (Figure 2B). Taken together, these data demonstrate that both serines represent *in vivo* phosphorylation sites.

PHOSPHORYLATION OF β-APP CAN OCCUR AT THE CELL SURFACE BY ECTO-CASEIN KINASE-2

Because β-APP is also present at the cell surface, we examined whether membrane-bound β-APP can be a substrate for ecto-protein kinases. Intact kidney cells, transfected with wild-type β-APP cDNA, were incubated in the presence of 1 μM [γ-^{32}P]ATP or 1 μM [γ-^{32}P]GTP in the cell supernatant, allowing specific detection of ecto-protein kinase activity [9]. As shown in Figure 3, cell surface-bound full-length β-APP was phosphorylated by ecto-protein kinase activities using both ATP and GTP as co-substrates. The usage of GTP as co-substrate is a unique feature of protein kinase CK-2 [10], indicating that ecto CK-2 is involved in cell surface phosphorylation. The phosphorylation of β-APP with 1 μM [γ-^{32}P]GTP can be suppressed by addition of unlabeled ATP or GTP (Figure 3). This is consistent with the known feature of CK-2, using ATP and GTP as co-substrate to similar extents [10]. In contrast, β-APP phosphorylation with 1 μM [γ-^{32}P]ATP is completely suppressed by unlabeled ATP but not by unlabeled GTP (Figure 3) demonstrating that besides a CK-2-like protein kinase, other protein kinase(s) are involved in cell surface phosphorylation of β-APP, which cannot use GTP as co-substrate. These data indicate that at least two different ecto-protein kinases are involved in cell surface phosphorylation of β-APP, and that one kinase shares characteristics of CK-2. We therefore tested whether β-APP can be phosphorylated *in vitro* by purified CK-2. Conditioned cell-free supernatants of kidney 293 cells containing secreted forms of β-APP were incubated with 1 μM [γ-^{32}P]ATP in the presence or absence of exogenous CK-2. Both APP$_S$ derived from proteolytic processing of the full-length protein and that from the β-APP α-stop mutant are phosphorylated by purified CK-2 *in vitro* (Figure 4).

Together with our previous study [3], our data demonstrate that β-APP is phosphorylated *in vivo* on serine residues 198 and 206, as proved by phosphopeptide mapping, site-directed mutagenesis and mass spectrometry. Ser198 is followed by acidic amino acid residues and therefore represents a putative phosphorylation site for CK-2 [10], while Ser206 is preceded by an acidic domain and represents a CK-1 phosphorylation site [10, 11]. However,

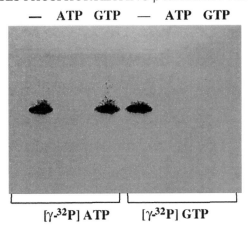

Figure 3. Cell surface phosphorylation of β-APP by ecto-protein kinase activity. Cell surface proteins of kidney 293 cells stably transfected with wt β-APP cDNA (wt) were phosphorylated in the presence of either 1 μM [γ-³²P]ATP or [γ-³²P]GTP for 30 min at 37 °C. 1 mM of unlabeled ATP or GDP was added to the cell supernatants during the phosphorylation reaction, as indicated. Full-length β-APP was immunoprecipitated from cell lysates and detected by autoradiography after separation by SDS–PAGE

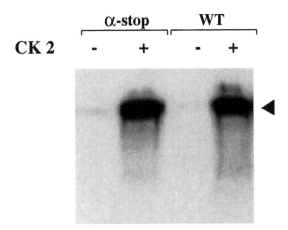

Figure 4. Secreted β-APP is phosphorylated by purified CK-2 *in vitro*. Conditioned cell-free supernatants from stably transfected kidney 293 cells were incubated with 1 μM [γ-³²P]ATP in the presence or absence of 10 ng purified CK-2 for 15 min. Subsequently, 1 mM of unlabeled ATP was added, β-APP was immunoprecipitated and analyzed by autoradiography. Both secreted β-APP (APP$_S$), derived either from processed full-length β-APP or from the β-APP α-stop mutant, are phosphorylated by CK-2

individual mutations of Ser198 and Ser206 differently affected the phosphate incorporation. The Ser198Ala mutation resulted in a reduction of phosphorylation of about 80%, while the Ser206Ala mutation reduced phosphorylation by about 15%. This might be explained by sequential phosphorylation events, in which the first phosphorylation at Ser198 facilitates the subsequent phosphorylation at Ser206 by acidifying this domain. A similar process has been described involving protein kinases A and CK-1 [12, 13].

We also demonstrate that at least two different ecto-protein kinases are involved in the phosphorylation of cell surface-located β-APP. One of them was characterized as a CK-2-like activity. The presence of a CK-2 type ecto-protein kinase was reported previously [14]. However, the additional protein kinase(s) which phosphorylate β-APP remain to be characterized in detail. Initial experiments revealed that CK-1 can also phosphorylate β-APP *in vitro* (data not shown), and we currently investigate whether CK-1 is also involved in the *in vivo* phosphorylation. The functional consequences of this complex regulation of β-APP ectodomain phosphorylation are unknown so far. However, the identified *in vivo* phosphorylation sites of β-APP are located close to known binding sites for copper and zinc ions [15, 16]. It is now of great interest to investigate whether ectodomain phosphorylation regulates the binding of β-APP ligands. One might also speculate that extracellular function(s) of β-APP, e.g. the modulation of neuronal excitability by APP_S [17], could be regulated by selective ectodomain phosphorylation.

ACKNOWLEDGEMENTS

We thank Drs A.Y. Hung and D.J. Selkoe for providing the AX and XB constructs of β-APP and antibodies C7 and 1736. We also than Dr D. Schenk for antibody B5 and Drs A. Krehan and W. Pyerin for purified CK-2. We gratefully acknowledge Dr H. Langen for mass spectrometry. This work was supported by a grant of the Deutsche Forschungsgemeinschaft (HA-1737/2/1) to C.H.

REFERENCES

1. Hung A, Selkoe DJ. Selective ectodomain phosphorylation of β-amyloid precursor protein. EMBO J 1994; 13: 534–42.
2. Knops J, Gandy SE, Greenberg P, Lieberburg I, Sinha S. Serine phosphorylation of the secreted extracellular domain. Biochem Biophys Res Commun 1993; 197: 380–85.
3. Walter J, Capell A, Hung AY, Langen H, Schnölzer M, Thinakaran G, Sisodia SS, Selkoe DJ, Haass C. Ectodomain phosphorylation of β-amyloid precursor protein at two distinct cellular locations. J Biol Chem 1997; 272: 1896–1903.
4. Haass C, Hung AY, Selkoe DJ. Processing of β-amyloid precursor protein in microglia and astrocytes favors an internal locatlization over constitutive secretion. J Neurosci 11: 3783–93.

5. Weidemann A, König G, Bunke D, Fischer P, Salbaum JM, Masters C, Beyreuther K. Identification, biogenesis, and localization of precursors of Alzheimer's disease A4 amyloid protein. Cell 1989; 57: 115–26.
6. Podlisny M, Tolan D, Selkoe DJ. Homology of the β-amyloid precursor protein in monkey and human supports a primate model for β-amyloidosis in Alzheimer's disease. Am J Pathol 1991; 138: 1423–35.
7. Oltersdorf T, Ward PJ, Henriksson T, Beattie EC, Neve R, Lieberburg I, Fritz LC. The Alzheimer amyloid precursor protein. Identification of a stable intermediate in the biosynthetic/degradative pathway. J Biol Chem 1990; 265: 4492–7.
8. Haass C, Koo E, Mellon A, Hung AY, Selkoe DJ. Targeting of cell-surface β-amyloid precursor protein to lysosomes: alternative processing into amyloid-bearing fragments. Nature 1992; 357: 500–503.
9. Kübler D, Pyerin W, Kinzel V. Assays of cell surface protein kinase: importance of selecting cytophilic substrates. J Biol Chem 1982; 257: 322–9.
10. Tuazon PT, Traugh JA. Casein kinase I and II—multipotential serine protein kinases: structure, function, and regulation. Adv Second Messenger Phosphoprot Res 1991; 23: 123–63.
11. Marin O, Meggio F, Pinna LA. Design and synthesis of two new peptide substrates for the specific and sensitive detection of casein kinases-1 and -2. Biochem Biophys Res Comm 1994; 198: 898–905.
12. Flotow H, Roach PJ. Synergistic phosphorylation of rabbit muscle glycogen synthase by cyclic AMP-dependent protein kinase and casein kinase I. J Biol Chem 1989; 264: 9126–8.
13. Flotow H, Roach PJ. Role of acidic residues as substrate determinants for casein kinase I. J Biol Chem 1991; 266: 3724–7.
14. Walter J, Schnölzer M, Pyerin W, Kinzel V, Kübler D. Substrate-induced release of ecto-protein kinase yields CK-1 and CK-2 in tandem. J Biol Chem 1996; 271: 111–19.
15. Bush AI, Multhaup G, Moir RD, Williamson TG, Small DH, Rumble D, Pollwein P, Beyreuther K, Masters CL. A novel zinc(II) binding site modulates the functin of the βA4 amyloid precursor protein of Alzheimer's disease. J Biol Chem 1993; 268: 16109–19112.
16. Hesse L, Beher D, Masters CL, Multhaup G. The beta A4 amyloid precursor protein binding to copper. FEBS Lett 1994; 349: 109–16.
17. Furukawa K, Barger SW, Blalock EM, Mattson MP. Activation of K^+ channels and suppression of neuronal activity by secreted β-amyloid precursor protein. Nature 1996; 379: 74–8.

Address for correspondence:
  Jochen Walter,
  Central Institute of Mental Health,
  Department of Molecular Biology, J5, 68159 Mannheim, Germany
  Tel: +49-621-1703-886; fax: +49-621-23429;
  e-mail: walter@as200.zi-mannheim.de

27 Identification of Monocyte Chemoattractant Protein-1 and CCR2 in Senile Plaques of Alzheimer's Disease

KOKO ISHIZUKA, TAKEMI KIMURA,
RURIKO IGATA-YI, SHOICHI KATSURAGI,
JUNICHI TAKAMATSU, HISAYUKI NOMIYAMA AND
TAIHEI MIYAKAWA

INTRODUCTION

Senile plaques (SP) of Alzheimer's disease (AD) consist mainly of β-amyloid protein (βAP), which may be formed by proteolytic processing of the amyloid precursor protein (APP) in the endosomal–lysosomal system [1, 2]. Some inflammatory factors, such as cytokines, complement proteins and acute phase reactants, have been reported as present in SP [3, 4]. Several epidemiological studies have shown that patients taking anti-inflammatory drugs have a decreased risk of developing AD [5, 6]. Therefore, inflammatory mechanisms may contribute to SP formation.

Monocyte chemoattractant protein-1 (MCP-1) is a member of the chemokine family, whose physiological function is mediated by binding to its receptor (CCR2) [7]. MCP-1 exhibits its principal specificity toward monocytes [8]. In the central nervous system (CNS), MCP-1 occurs in astrocytes [9] and microglia [10]. Since it has been demonstrated that MCP-1 is expressed and produced in the brain with experimental allergic encephalomyelitis [11] and experimental autoimmune encephalomyelitis [12], MCP-1 may be associated with inflammatory processes in the CNS. As inflammatory processes might be involved in SP formation, it seems reasonable to expect a role of MCP-1 and CCR2 in their formation. Thus, to investigate the expression of MCP-1 and CCR2 in SP, we examined the brains of five patients with AD immunohistochemically.

Alzheimer's Disease and Related Disorders
Edited by K. Iqbal, D.F. Swaab, B. Winblad and H.M. Wisniewski
© 1999 John Wiley & Sons Ltd

SUBJECTS AND METHODS

Brain tissue samples were obtained at autopsy from five patients with Alzheimer's disease (AD), aged 60–85 years. These patients were diagnosed according to DSM-IIIR [13] and the neuropathological criteria of AD [14].

For immunohistochemical staining, we used a mouse monoclonal anti-MCP-1 antibody (1:50, Biomedicals) and a mouse monoclonal anti-CCR2 antibody (1:100, R & D). To detect SP, neurofibrillary tangles and microglia, we also used a mouse monoclonal anti-βAP antibody (1:200, Dako), a mouse monoclonal anti-tau antibody (1:1000, Sigma) and a rabbit polyclonal anti-ferritin antibody (1:100, Dako).

Serial 5 μm-thick paraffin-embedded sections were prepared from the medial temporal area (the hippocampus and the parahippocampal gyrus) of the formalin-fixed brain. The immunohistochemical staining was performed as follows. After deparaffinization and immersion in 0.3% H_2O_2 in methanol, and pretreatment with concentrated formic acid for 5 min, tissue sections were incubated with each antibody at 4 °C overnight. Sections were incubated with 1.5 μg/ml biotinylated goat anti-mouse IgG antibody (Vector) or 1.5 μg/ml biotinylated goat anti-rabbit IgG antibody (Vector) for 30 min, followed by incubation with avidin–biotin complex (Vector). Visualization was achieved using diaminobenzidine. Meyer's hematoxylin was added as a counterstain. For double-immunostaining, the sections were subjected to alkaline phosphatase reaction, followed by avidin–biotin complex reaction. Control sections were incubated with non-immune mouse IgG or rabbit IgG instead of each antibody.

RESULTS

SP and neurofibrillary tangles were present in all tissue samples examined. SP are generally divided into diffuse plaques, primitive plaques and classic plaques [15]. In this study, immunostaining of serial sections showed the presence of MCP-1 immunoreaction in most of primitive and classic plaques (Plate IE, H), but little immunoreactivity was seen in diffuse plaques (Plate IB). Control preparations using non-immune mouse IgG revealed no immunoreactivity in all plaques (Plate IC, F, I). CCR2 immunoreaction was also present in some of the SP which were positive for MCP-1 (Plate IIA, B). Double-immunostaining with antibodies against MCP-1 and ferritin, a marker of microglia, demonstrated that most of ferritin-positive microglia in SP were positive for MCP-1, but not all MCP-1 positive regions were stained for ferritin (Plate IJ, K).

DISCUSSION

It was shown that diffuse plaques consisting of non-fibrillar βAP are immature SP, whereas primitive and classic plaques consisting of fibrillar βAP are mature SP [16]. The numbers of primitive and classic plaques, but not diffuse plaques, have been reported to be correlated with cognitive dysfunction [17]. Furthermore, an *in vitro* study showed that fibrillar βAP, but not non-fibrillar βAP, was neurotoxic [18]. Thus, we believe that transformation from immature to mature SP is necessary to induce cognitive dysfunction in AD.

In this study we have shown that MCP-1 is present in primitive, classic plaques and reactive microglia but not in diffuse plaques. At the same time, we have detected CCR2 in certain SP which were positive for MCP-1. Recently, an *in vitro* study revealed that human monocytes produce a significant amount of MCP-1 in response to βAP and that murine microglia stimulated with βAP(23–35) accumulate mRNA encoding JE, a murine counterpart of MCP-1 [10]. Hence, it is suggested that βAP activates microglia to produce MCP-1, which plays a potential role of auto-upregulation using CCR2 for microglia. Therefore, it is suggested that both MCP-1 and CCR2 are related to the maturation of SP.

ACKNOWLEDGEMENTS

We thank Dr Motohiro Takeya for his editorial advice and Mr Toshiyuki Hisano for his excellent technical assistance.

ABSTRACT

Monocyte chemoattractant protein-1 (MCP-1) is a chemotactic factor for human monocyte (microglia) and binds to CCR2 chemokine receptor. Reactive microglia and inflammatory factors were reported to be present in senile plaques in the brain of Alzheimer's disease (AD), suggesting the presence of MCP-1 in senile plaques. To address this issue, we examined five brains of AD immunohistochemically, using specific antibodies for MCP-1 and CCR2. MCP-1 immunoreaction was found in mature senile plaques and reactive microglia but not in immature senile plaques. A CCR2-positive reaction was also present in senile plaques which were stained with anti-MCP-1 antibody. These findings suggest that MCP-1- and CCR2-related inflammatory events contribute to the maturation of senile plaques.

REFERENCES

1. Shoji M, Golde TE, Ghiso J et al. Production of the Alzheimer amyloid β protein by normal proteolytic processing. Science 1992; 258: 126–9.
2. Haass C, Koo EH, Mellon A, Hung AY, Selkoe DJ. Targeting of cell-surface β-amyloid precursor protein to lysosomes: alternative processing into amyloid-bearing fragments. Nature 1992; 357: 500–503.

3. Vandenabeele P, Fiers W. Is amyloidogenesis during Alzheimer's disease due to an IL-1/IL-6-mediated 'acute phase response' in the brain? Immunol Today 1991; 12: 217–19.
4. Griffin WS, Stanley LC, Ling C et al. Brain interleukin 1 and S-100 immunoreactivity are elevated in Down syndrome and Alzheimer disease. Proc Natl Acad Sci USA 1989; 86: 7611–15.
5. Andersen K, Launer LJ, Ott A, Hoes AW, Breteler MM, Hofman A. Do non-steroidal anti-inflammatory drugs decrease the risk for Alzheimer's disease? The Rotterdam Study. Neurology 1995; 45: 1441–5.
6. Rich JB, Rasmusson DX, Folstein MF, Carson KA, Kawas C, Brandt J. Nonsteroidal anti-inflammatory drugs in Alzheimer's disease. Neurology 1995; 45: 51–5.
7. Wong LM, Myers SJ, Tsou CL et al. Organization and differential expression of the human monocyte chemoattractant protein 1 receptor gene. J Biol Chem 1997; 272: 1038–45.
8. Leonard EJ, Yoshimura T. Human monocyte chemoattractant protein-1 (MCP-1). Immunol Today 1990; 11: 97–101.
9. Hurwitz AA, Lyman WD, Berman JW. Tumor necrosis factor alpha and transforming growth factor beta upregulate astrocyte expression of monocyte chemoattractant protein-1. J Neuroimmunol 1995; 57: 193–8.
10. Meda L, Bernasconi S, Bonaiuto C et al. β-amyloid (25–35) peptide and IFN-γ synergistically induce the production of the chemotactic cytokine MCP-1/JE in monocytes and microglial cells. J Immunol 1996; 157: 1213–18.
11. Hulkower K, Brosnan CF, Aquino DA et al. Expression of CSF-1, c-fms, and MCP-1 in the central nervous system of rats with experimental allergic encephalomyelitis. J Immunol 1993; 150: 2525–33.
12. Ransohoff RM, Hamilton TA, Tani M et al. Astrocyte expression of mRNA encoding cytokines IP-10 and JE/MCP-1 in experimental autoimmune encephalomyelitis. FASEB J 1993; 7: 592–600.
13. American Psychiatric Association. Diagnostic and Statistical Manual of Mental Disorders, 3rd edn, Revised. Washington, DC: American Psychiatric Association, 1987.
14. Khachaturian ZS. Diagnosis of Alzheimer's disease. Arch Neurol 1985; 42: 1097–1105.
15. Delaere P, Duyckaerts C, He Y, Piette F, Hauw J-J. Subtypes and differential laminar distributions of β A4 deposits in Alzheimer's disease: relationship with the intellectual status of 26 cases. Acta Neuropathol 1991; 81: 328–35.
16. Hardy J, Allsop D. Amyloid deposition as the central event in the aetiology of Alzheimer's disease. Trends Pharmacol Sci 1991; 12: 383–8.
17. Sparks DL, Liu H, Scheff SW, Coyne CM, Hunsaker JC IIIrd. Temporal sequence of plaque formation in the cerebral cortex of non-demented individuals. J Neuropathol Exp Neurol 1993; 52: 135–42.
18. Yankner BA, Duffy LK, Kirschner DA. Neurotrophic and neurotoxic effects of amyloid beta protein: reversal by tachykinin neuropeptides. Science 1990; 250: 279–82.

Address for correspondence:
Koko Ishizuka,
Department of Neuropsychiatry,
Kumamoto University School of Medicine,
Honjo 1–1–1, Kumamoto 860-8556, Japan
Tel: +81 96 373 5183; fax: +81 96 362 8741

28 Filamentous Tau Protein and α-Synuclein Deposits in Neurodegenerative Diseases

M. GOEDERT, R.A. CROWTHER, R. JAKES,
M. HASEGAWA, M.J. SMITH, J.R. MURRELL, B. GHETTI
AND M.G. SPILLANTINI

INTRODUCTION

Alzheimer's disease and Parkinson's disease are the most common neurodegenerative diseases of the human brain. They are characterized by the presence of ordered filamentous assemblies which gradually develop in a small number of types of nerve cell. In Alzheimer's disease, vulnerable nerve cells develop neurofibrillary tangles, neuropil threads and abnormal neurites, whereas in Parkinson's disease they develop Lewy bodies and Lewy neurites [1, 2]. Alzheimer's disease is characterized by the additional presence of extracellular deposits in the form of amyloid plaques. Over recent years, it has become clear that intraneuronal filamentous deposits of Alzheimer's disease and Parkinson's disease are composed of tau protein and α-synuclein, respectively. Filamentous tau protein deposits are also the defining neuropathological hallmark of a number of other dementing disorders, such as Pick's disease and the group of familial frontotemporal dementias and Parkinsonism linked to chromosome 17 (FTDP-17) [3]. Filamentous α-synuclein deposits in cerebral cortex define dementia with Lewy bodies, a common late-life dementia that exists in a pure form or overlaps with the neuropathological changes of Alzheimer's disease.

The most common neurodegenerative diseases thus share the deposition within some nerve cells of ordered filamentous assemblies. This assembly into insoluble filaments is abnormal, since these proteins normally exist in a soluble, non-filamentous form. It is possible that nerve cells die as the result of the events that lead to filament formation or because of the presence of the filaments themselves.

Alzheimer's Disease and Related Disorders
Edited by K. Iqbal, D.F. Swaab, B. Winblad and H.M. Wisniewski
© 1999 John Wiley & Sons Ltd

TAU PROTEIN IN ALZHEIMER'S DISEASE

The neurofibrillary lesions of Alzheimer's disease are found in nerve cell bodies and apical dendrites as neurofibrillary tangles (NFTs), in distal dendrites as neuropil threads and in the abnormal neurites which are often, but not always, associated with amyloid plaques. Ultrastructurally, these lesions consist of paired helical filaments (PHFs) and the related straight filaments (SFs). About 95% of filaments are in the form of PHFs, with a diameter of 20 nm and a periodicity of 80 nm. The remainder consists of SFs. Both PHFs and SFs are made of microtubule-associated protein tau, in a hyper-phosphorylated state [1].

Tau is a microtubule-associated protein that is involved in microtubule assembly and stabilization. In adult human brain, six tau isoforms are expressed, which are produced by alternative mRNA splicing from a single gene located on the long arm of chromosome 17 [4]. They differ by the presence of three or four tandem repeats located in the C-terminal region, in conjunction with 0, 29 or 58 amino acid inserts located in the N-terminal region. There is also a larger tau isoform, with an additional 254 amino acid insert in the N-terminal region, which is mainly expressed in the peripheral nervous system [5]. The repeat regions of tau and sequences flanking the repeats constitute the microtubule-binding domains, while the function of the amino-terminal region remains unclear [6].

Tau is a phosphoprotein and its mobility on SDS–PAGE is affected by phosphorylation. Tau from PHFs is hyperphosphorylated and abnormally phosphorylated relative to tau from normal adult brain [7]. Thus, PHF-tau runs as three major bands of 60, 64 and 68 kDa and a minor band of 72 kDa [8, 9]. Upon dephosphorylation, six tau bands are seen, which align with the six recombinant brain tau isoforms [10]. Hyperphosphorylation and abnormal phosphorylation are major biochemical characteristics of PHF-tau. They are early events in the development of the neurofibrillary lesions and, as a result, tau is unable to bind to microtubules [11, 12]. A number of protein kinases and protein phosphatases has been implicated in the abnormal phosphoryla-tion of tau, based largely on *in vitro* studies of tau phosphorylation. Recent additions to this growing list include a number of stress-activated protein kinases, chiefly stress-activated protein kinase-3 and stress-activated protein kinase-4 [13]. Relatively little is known about which protein kinases phosphorylate tau in brain. This requires specific protein kinase inhibitors or inactivation of individual protein kinase genes. The use of lithium chloride as a specific inhibitor of glycogen synthase kinase-3 has provided strong evidence that this protein kinase is involved in the phosphorylation of tau in normal brain [14, 15].

Whether hyperphosphorylation and abnormal phosphorylation of tau are sufficient for PHF formation remains unclear. Phosphorylated recombinant tau has consistently failed to assemble into paired helical-like filaments in experiments *in vitro*. By contrast, incubation of recombinant tau with sulphated glycosaminoglycans, such as heparin or heparan sulphate, results in bulk assembly of tau into Alzheimer-like filaments (Figure 1) [16–18]. Tau isoforms with three repeats assemble into twisted paired helical-like filaments, whereas tau isoforms with four repeats assemble into straight filaments. By immunoelectron microscopy, the paired helical-like filaments can be decorated by antibodies directed against the N- and C-termini of tau, but not by an antibody directed against the microtubule-binding repeat region. These results, which indicate that in the filaments the repeat region of tau is inaccessible to the antibody, are identical to those previously obtained with PHFs from Alzheimer's disease brain.

Sulphated glycosaminoglycans also stimulate phosphorylation of tau by a number of protein kinases, prevent the binding of tau to taxol-stabilized microtubules, and disassemble microtubules assembled from tau and tubulin [16, 18, 19]. Moreover, heparan sulphate has been detected in nerve cells in the early stages of neurofibrillary degeneration [16]. Sulphated glycosaminoglycans stimulate tau phosphorylation at lower concentrations than those required for filament formation. The pathological presence of heparan sulphate within the cytoplasm of some nerve cells, perhaps as a result of leakage from membrane-bound compartments, might first lead to increased phosphorylation of tau, resulting in its inability to bind to microtubules. At higher heparan sulphate concentrations tau could then assemble into PHFs and SFs. Formation of tau filaments is also observed after incubation of recombinant tau with RNA [18, 20], which has been shown to be sequestered in the neurofibrillary lesions of Alzheimer's disease [21]. Whether the presence of RNA is an early event remains to be determined. Sulphated glycosaminoglycans and RNA share a repeat sugar backbone and negative charges in the form of sulphates or phosphates. Tau protein is thought to be an extended molecule with little secondary structure, which becomes partially structured upon binding to microtubules. Binding of sulphated glycosaminoglycans or RNA to tau may induce or stabilize a conformation of tau that brings the microtubule-binding repeats of individual molecules into close proximity, creating sites which favour filament formation.

OTHER TAUOPATHIES

Anti-tau antibodies also identify pathology in a number of neurodegenerative disorders other than Alzheimer's disease. As in Alzheimer's disease, these tau lesions stain with available phosphorylation-dependent and phosphorylation-independent anti-tau antibodies. One exception is antibody 12E8, which fails to stain the tau pathology of Pick's disease and argyrophilic grain dementia [22, 23], indicating that Ser262 in tau is not phosphorylated in these lesions. The tau pathology of Alzheimer's disease is almost entirely confined to nerve

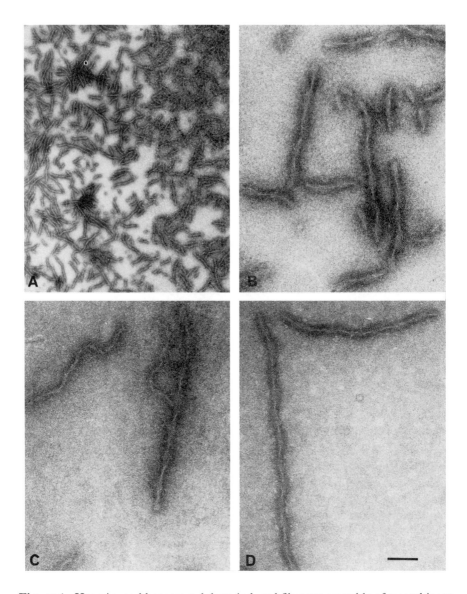

Figure 1. Heparin- and heparan sulphate-induced filament assembly of recombinant htau37 (381-amino acid isoform of human tau). (A) Low-power view of filaments formed after incubation of htau37 with heparin. (B) High-power view of heparin-induced twisted tau filaments. (C) hTau37 Incubated with heparan sulphate. (D) htau37 Incubated with heparan sulphate + 10 μM ZnCl$_2$. Note the presence of paired helical-like filaments in (A–D) and of additional thin, wavy half-twisted filaments in (C). Scale bar (in D), 450 nm for A, 100 nm for B–D. Reproduced with permission from reference [18]

cells. This contrasts with tauopathies, such as corticobasal degeneration and progressive supranuclear palsy, where both nerve cells and glial cells are affected.

Most tauopathies are sporadic diseases, but some are familial and inherited in an autosomal-dominant manner. Over the past few years, FTDP-17 has emerged as a previously unknown group of familial dementing diseases [3]. Their unifying pathological characteristic is the presence of abundant filamentous tau deposits, in the absence of Aβ-amyloid plaques. In some of these families tau deposits are found in both nerve cells and glial cells, whereas in others only nerve cells are affected. Biochemically, the tau filaments fall into at least two groups. They consist either of all six brain tau isoforms, as in Seattle family A [24], or they contain only tau isoforms with four microtubule-binding repeats, as in familial multiple system tauopathy with presenile dementia (MSTD) [25], or they contain predominantly four-repeat tau isoforms, as in Dutch family 1 [26]. In Seattle family A, tau filaments are identical to the PHFs and SFs of Alzheimer's disease, whereas in familial MSTD they have a twisted ribbon-like appearance (Figure 2).

Besides having a filamentous tau pathology in common, the familial frontotemporal dementias also share genetic linkage to chromosome 17q21–22, the same region that contains the tau gene [27–29]. Recently, the first mutations in the tau gene were identified in several of these families [30–32]. Poorkaj et al. have identified two separate exonic mutations in the tau gene in two FTDP-17 families [30]. Hutton et al. have reported six different mutations in the tau gene in 10 FTDP-17 families [31]. Three of these mutations are located in the intron following exon 10, where they disrupt a predicted stem–loop. The other three mutations are found in exons. In familial MSTD, we have identified a G-to-A transition in the nucleotide adjacent to the GT splice-donor site in the intron following exon 10 of the tau gene [32]. It disrupts a predicted stem–loop structure and probably increases binding of U1 snRNA, which may in turn lead to increased splicing of exon 10 (Figure 3). Accordingly, we have observed an abnormal preponderance of four-repeat tau isoforms over three-repeat isoforms in soluble tau from familial MSTD brains [32]. We have also detected a preponderance of transcripts encoding tau isoforms with four repeats over transcripts encoding isoforms with three repeats. Exon trapping experiments have shown that the G-to-A transition leads to an increase in exon 10-containing transcripts (unpublished observations). These findings indicate that an over-production of four-repeat tau isoforms leads eventually to assembly of these isoforms into twisted ribbon-like filaments. In Seattle family A, Poorkaj et al. have shown a Val-to-Met missense mutation at residue 337 in the third microtubule-binding domain of tau [30]. It affects all six tau isoforms, consistent with the presence of all six isoforms in PHFs and SFs. In Dutch family 1, Hutton et al. have shown a Pro-to-Leu missense mutation at residue 301 in the second microtubule-binding domain of tau [31]. It affects only four-repeat tau isoforms, consistent with the

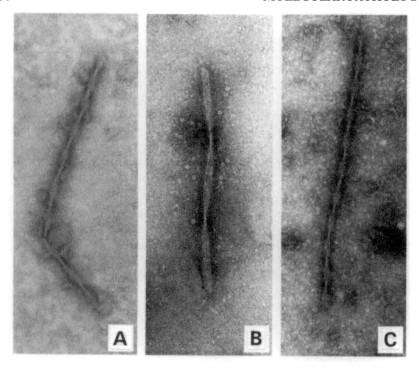

Figure 2. Tau filaments in Seattle family A (A) and familial multiple system tauopathy with presenile dementia (MSTD) (B), two FTDP-17 dementias with mutations in
the tau gene. Comparison with the PHFs of Alzheimer's disease (C). (A) In Seattle
family A, the filaments contain all six tau isoforms in a hyperphosphorylated state and
their morphology is indistinguishable from the PHFs of Alzheimer's disease. Tau
pathology is found in nerve cells and their processes. The tau gene is mutated at codon
337, resulting in a valine-to-methionine substitution in the third microtubule-binding
repeat. (B) In familial MSTD, the filaments contain hyperphosphorylated tau protein
isoforms with four microtubule-binding repeats whose twisted ribbon-like appearance
differs from that of the PHFs of Alzheimer's disease. Tau pathology is found in both
nerve cells and glial cells and their processes. The tau gene is mutated at the nucleotide
adjacent to the exon 10–5' splice-donor site, resulting in an over-production of tau
isoforms with four microtubule-binding repeats. (C) In Alzheimer's disease, PHFs
contain all six tau isoforms in a hyperphosphorylated state. Tau pathology is found in
nerve cells and their processes. No mutations in the tau gene have been reported

presence of predominantly four-repeat tau isoforms in the twisted ribbon-like
filaments.

The functional consequences of the missense mutations in tau remain to be
determined. The mutated proteins may interact less well with microtubules
than does the wild-type protein (Table 1). This may be followed by the
hyperphosphorylation of tau and, through interaction with other cellular factors, by assembly into filaments. Similarly, over-production of four-repeat tau
isoforms resulting from the intronic mutations may result in the inability of a

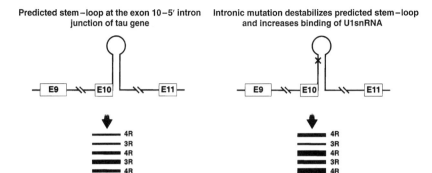

NORMAL BRAIN   **MULTIPLE SYSTEM TAUOPATHY**

Predicted stem–loop at the exon 10–5' intron junction of tau gene   Intronic mutation destabilizes predicted stem–loop and increases binding of U1snRNA

Slight preponderance of three-repeat tau isoforms over four-repeat isoforms   Abnormal ratio of three-repeat to four-repeat tau isoforms
Overproduction of four-repeat isoforms
Excess of unbound four-repeat tau?

Assembly of hyperphosphorylated four-repeat tau isoforms into abnormal filaments in some nerve cells and glial cells

Figure 3. Pathway from the mutation in the tau gene in familial multiple system tauopathy with presenile dementia (MSTD) to tau filament formation. In the wild-type tau gene the presence of a stem–loop structure at the exon 10–5' intron junction is believed to ensure the production of a normal ratio of three-repeat to four-repeat tau isoforms. In familial MSTD, the G-to-A transition in the nucleotide adjacent to the 5' splice-donor site is predicted to destabilize the stem–loop and to lead to increased binding of U1 snRNA. This results in the over-production of four-repeat tau isoforms and their assembly into twisted ribbon-like filaments

proportion of the excess tau to bind to microtubules, leading to its hyperphosphorylation and assembly into filaments. In familial MSTD, tau is hyperphosphorylated at the same sites as in Alzheimer's disease and the tau deposits are immunoreactive for heparan sulphate [25]. The balance between tau protein levels and available binding sites on microtubules appears to be critical for preventing tau from assembling into filaments. This is consistent with transgenic mouse experiments, which showed that the over-production of a four-repeat human tau isoform in nerve cells results in a pathology resembling the pre-tangle pathology of Alzheimer's disease [33]. Thus, a reduced ability to interact with microtubules appears to be the shared primary abnormality in tau protein resulting from the different exonic and intronic mutations in the tau gene. Such initial partial loss of function may be necessary for the later assembly of tau into filaments.

The location of the tau mutations appears to determine the nature of the pathology. Thus, mutations in exon 10 itself or in the intron following exon 10

Table 1. Proposed sequence of events leading from exonic and intronic mutations in the tau gene to neurodegeneration

1. Reduced ability of tau to interact with microtubules
   (partial loss-of-function)

2. Hyperphosphorylation of tau. Interaction with other factors
   (sulphated GAGs, RNA)?

3. Ordered filamentous assemblies
   (gain of toxic function)

4. Degeneration of tau filament-containing nerve cells and glial cells

lead to a filamentous neuronal and glial cell tau pathology, with the filaments consisting predominantly of tau isoforms with four repeats. Mutations outside exon 10 appear to lead to a predominantly neuronal tau pathology, with the filaments consisting of all six tau isoforms. These findings provide a direct link between genetic lesions in tau and its assembly into abnormal filaments, independently of the presence of Aβ amyloid deposits. They suggest that the events leading to tau filament formation, or the presence of the filaments themselves, are sufficient for nerve cell degeneration, not only in FTDP-17 dementias but also in Alzheimer's disease and the other tauopathies.

α-SYNUCLEIN IN LEWY BODY DISEASES

The Lewy body and the Lewy neurite constitute the next most common nerve cell pathologies, after the neurofibrillary lesions of Alzheimer's disease [2]. They are the defining neuropathological features of Parkinson's disease and dementia with Lewy bodies. Ultrastructurally, Lewy bodies and Lewy neurites consist of abnormal filamentous material. Despite the fact that the Lewy body was first described in 1912, its biochemical composition has remained unknown.

In 1997, the discovery of a missense mutation in α-synuclein as a rare cause of familial Parkinson's disease [34] has led us to examine the presence of α-synuclein in Lewy bodies and Lewy neurites in idiopathic Parkinson's disease and in dementia with Lewy bodies [35]. Human α-synuclein is 140 amino acids in length and is abundantly expressed in brain, where it is located in presynaptic nerve terminals [36, 37]. The amino-terminal half of α-synuclein contains imperfect amino acid repeats, with the consensus sequence KTKEGV. The repeats are followed by a hydrophobic middle region and a negatively charged C-terminal region. To stain Lewy bodies and Lewy neurites, we used two antibodies raised against synthetic peptides corresponding to residues 11–34 (PER1) and 116–131 (PER2) of human α-synuclein. PER1 and PER2 gave strong staining of Lewy bodies and Lewy neurites in substantia nigra from Parkinson's disease brain [35]. Both the core and the halo of the

Lewy body were strongly immunoreactive for α-synuclein. Similarly, in dementia with Lewy bodies, PER1 and PER2 stained both brainstem and cortical Lewy bodies, as well as numerous Lewy neurites [35]. Double-staining of the Lewy body pathology for α-synuclein and ubiquitin showed that α-synuclein staining is more extensive than ubiquitin staining [38]. Staining for α-synuclein will therefore probably replace staining for ubiquitin as the preferred means of identifying Lewy bodies and Lewy neurites.

These findings suggest, but do not prove, that α-synuclein is a major component of the abnormal filaments that make up Lewy bodies and Lewy neurites. We investigated this directly by immuno-electron microscopy of sarcosyl-insoluble filaments extracted from the cingulate cortex of patients with dementia with Lewy bodies [38]. Antiserum PER4, which recognizes the C-terminus of α-synuclein, labelled filaments along their entire lengths, indicating that they contain α-synuclein as a major component (Figure 4). The labelled structures had various morphologies, including a 5 nm straight filament and both straight and twisted 10 nm filaments; the 10 nm filaments were more numerous. These appearances would be consistent with a model in which the α-synuclein molecules assembled to form a 5 nm protofilament, two of which could associate to produce a variably twisted filament. These various morphologies suggest that α-synuclein molecules may run parallel with the filament axis. This differs from the packing of tau protein in tau filaments, where individual tau molecules are believed to run mainly perpendicular to the filament axis. Antibody PER1 only ever labelled one filament end [38]. This suggests that the PER1 epitope is buried in the body of the filament and exposed only at one end, and that the filaments are polar structures. In conjunction with the discovery of mutations in α-synuclein in some familial cases of Parkinson's disease [34, 39], these findings suggest that the presence of α-synuclein filaments may be the cause of nerve cell death and that idiopathic Parkinson's disease and dementia with Lewy bodies are α-synucleinopathies.

α-SYNUCLEIN IN MULTIPLE SYSTEM ATROPHY

Multiple system atrophy is a neurodegenerative disorder that comprises olivopontocerebellar atrophy, striatonigral degeneration and Shy–Drager syndrome. Neuropathologically, glial cytoplasmic inclusions (GCIs), which consist of filamentous aggregates, are the defining feature of multiple system atrophy [40]. They are found mostly in the cytoplasm and, to a lesser extent, the nucleus of oligodendrocytes. Inclusions are also observed in the cytoplasm and nucleus of some nerve cells, as well as in neuropil threads. They consist of straight and twisted filaments, with reported diameters of 10–30 nm. GCIs are immunoreactive for ubiquitin and, to a lesser extent, for cytoskeletal proteins, such as tau and tubulin. However, until recently, their biochemical composition was unclear.

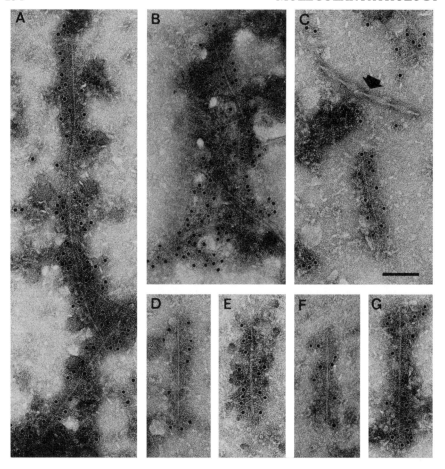

Figure 4. Filaments from cingulate cortex of patients with dementia with Lewy bodies labelled with anti-α-synuclein antibody PER4. (A and B) Small clumps of labelled α-synuclein filaments. (C) A labelled α-synuclein filament and an unlabelled paired helical filament (arrow). The labelled filaments have various morphologies, including 5 nm filament (D); 10 nm filament with dark stain-penetrating centre line (E); twisted filament showing alternating width (F); 10 nm filament with slender 5 nm extensions at ends (G, also C). Scale bar, 100 nm (in C). Reproduced with permission from reference [38]

This has now changed with the discovery that GCIs are strongly immunoreactive for α-synuclein [41, 42] and that filaments from brains of patients with multiple system atrophy are strongly labelled by α-synuclein antibodies [42]. This work indicates that α-synuclein is the major component of these filaments and reveals an unexpected molecular link between multiple system atrophy and Lewy body disorders, such as Parkinson's disease and dementia with Lewy bodies.

CONCLUSION

The past year has brought intraneuronal filamentous inclusions to the forefront. They form in the majority of late-onset neurodegenerative diseases, where they are made of either tau protein or α-synuclein (Table 2). Mutations in the tau gene in some familial forms of frontotemporal dementia and mutations in the α-synuclein gene in some familial forms of Parkinson's disease have provided direct links between genetic lesions and the presence of an intraneuronal filamentous pathology. This relatively simple picture bodes well for the development of therapeutical strategies aimed at preventing assembly into filaments.

Table 2. Intraneuronal filamentous inclusions in neurodegenerative diseases

Disease	Filamentous inclusion	Main component
Alzheimer's disease	Neurofibrillary lesions	Tau protein
Pick's disease	Pick bodies	Tau protein
FTDP-17	Neurofibrillary lesions, glialfibrillary lesions	Tau protein
PSP	Neurofibrillary lesions, glialfibrillary lesions	Tau protein
CBD	Neurofibrillary lesions, glialfibrillary lesions	Tau protein
Parkinson's disease	Lewy bodies, Lewy neurites	α-Synuclein
Dementia with Lewy bodies	Lewy bodies, Lewy neurites	α-Synuclein
Multiple system atrophy	Glial and neuronal inclusions, cytoplasmic and nuclear neuropil threads	α-Synuclein

Abbreviations: FTDP-17, frontotemporal dementia and Parkinsonism linked to chromosome 17; PSP, progressive supranuclear palsy; CBD, corticobasal degeneration.

REFERENCES

1. Goedert M, Trojanowski JQ, Lee VM-Y. The neurofibrillary pathology of Alzheimer's disease. In: Rosenberg RN, Prusiner SB, DiMauro S, Barchi RB (eds) The Molecular and Genetic Basis of Neurological Disease. Boston: Butterworth-Heinemann, 1997; 613–27.
2. Forno LS. Neuropathology of Parkinson's disease. J Neuropathol Exp Neurol 1996; 55: 259–72.
3. Spillantini MG, Bird TD, Ghetti B. Frontotemporal dementia and Parkinsonism linked to chromosome 17: a new group of tauopathies. Brain Pathol 1998; 8: 387–402.

4. Goedert M, Spillantini MG, Jakes R, Rutherford D, Crowther RA. Multiple iso-forms of human microtubule-associated protein tau: sequences and localization in neurofibrillary tangles of Alzheimer's disease. Neuron 1989; 3: 519–26.

5. Goedert M, Spillantini MG, Crowther RA. Cloning of a big tau microtubule-associated protein characteristic of the peripheral nervous system. Proc Natl Acad Sci USA 1992; 89: 1983–7.

6. Goode BL, Feinstein SC. Identification of a novel microtubule binding and assem-bly domain in the developmentally regulated inter-repeat region of tau. J Cell Biol 1994; 124: 769–82.

7. Morishima-Kawashima M, Hasegawa M, Takio K, Suzuki M, Yoshida H, Titani K, Ihara Y. Proline-directed and non-proline-directed phosphorylation of PHF-tau. J Biol Chem 1995; 270: 823–9.

8. Greenberg SG, Davies P. A preparation of Alzheimer paired helical filaments that displays distinct tau proteins by polyacrylamide gel electrophoresis. Proc Natl Acad Sci USA 1990; 87: 5827–31.

9. Lee VM-Y, Balin BJ, Otvos L, Trojanowski JQ. A68—a major subunit of paired helical filaments and derivatized forms of normal tau. Science 1991; 251: 675–8.

10. Goedert M, Spillantini MG, Cairns NJ, Crowther RA. Tau proteins of Alzheimer paired helical filaments: abnormal phosphorylation of all six brain isoforms. Neu-ron 1992; 8: 159–68.

11. Bramblett GT, Goedert M, Jakes R, Merrick SE, Trojanowski JQ, Lee VM-Y. Abnormal tau phosphorylation at Ser396 in Alzheimer's disease recapitulates de-velopment and contributes to reduced microtubule binding. Neuron 1993; 10: 1089–99.

12. Yoshida H, Ihara Y. Tau in paired helical filament is functionally distinct from fetal tau: assembly incompetence of paired helical filament tau. J Neurochem 1993; 61: 1183–6.

13. Goedert M, Hasegawa M, Jakes R, Lawler S, Cuenda A, Cohen P. Phosphoryla-tion of microtubule-associated protein tau by stress-activated protein kinases. FEBS Lett 1997; 409: 57–62.

14. Munoz-Montado JR, Moreno FJ, Avila J, Diaz-Nido J. Lithium inhibits Alz-heimer's disease-like tau protein phosphorylation in neurons. FEBS Lett 1997; 411: 183–8.

15. Hong M, Chen DCR, Klein PS, Lee VM-Y. Lithium-reduced tau phosphorylation by inhibition of glycogen synthase kinase-3. J Biol Chem 1997; 272: 25326–32.

16. Goedert M, Jakes R, Spillantini MG, Hasegawa M, Smith MJ, Crowther RA. Assembly of microtubule-associated protein tau into Alzheimer-like filaments in-duced by sulphated glycosaminoglycans. Nature 1996; 383: 550–53.

17. Pérez M, Valpuesta JM, Medina M, Montejo de Garcini E, Avila J. Polymerization of tau into filaments in the presence of heparin: the minimal sequence required for tau–tau interactions. J Neurochem 1996; 67: 1183–90.

18. Hasegawa M, Crowther RA, Jakes R, Goedert M. Alzheimer-like changes in microtubule-associated protein tau induced by sulfated glycosaminoglycans. Inhi-bition of microtubule binding, stimulation of phosphorylation, and filament as-sembly depend on the degree of sulfation. J Biol Chem 1997; 272: 33118–24.

19. Qi Z, Zhu X, Goedert M, Fujita DJ, Wang JH. Effect of heparin on phosphoryla-tion site specificity of neuronal Cdc2-like kinase. FEBS Lett 1998; 423: 227–30.

20. Kampers T, Friedhoff P, Biernat J, Mandelkow E-M, Mandelkow E. RNA stimu-lates aggregation of microtubule-associated protein tau into Alzheimer-like paired helical filaments. FEBS Lett 1996; 399: 344–9.

21. Ginsberg SD, Crino PB, Lee VM-Y, Eberwine JH, Trojanowski JQ. Sequestration of RNA in Alzheimer's disease neurofibrillary tangles and senile plaques. Ann Neurol 1997; 41: 200–209.
22. Probst A, Tolnay M, Langui D, Goedert M, Spillantini MG. Pick's disease: hyperphosphorylated tau protein segregates to the somatoaxonal compartment. Acta Neuropathol 1996; 92: 588–96.
23. Tolnay M, Spillantini MG, Goedert M, Ulrich J, Langui D, Probst A. Argyrophilic grain disease: widespread hyperphosphorylation of tau in limbic neurons. Acta Neuropathol 1997; 93: 477–84.
24. Spillantini MG, Crowther RA, Goedert M. Comparison of the neurofibrillary pathology in Alzheimer's disease and familial presenile dementia with tangles. Acta Neuropathol 1996; 92: 42–8.
25. Spillantini MG, Goedert M, Crowther RA, Murrell JR, Farlow MR, Ghetti B. Familial multiple system tauopathy with presenile dementia: a disease with abundant neuronal and glial tau filaments. Proc Natl Acad Sci USA 1997; 94: 4113–18.
26. Spillantini MG, Crowther RA, Kamphorst W, Heutink P, van Swieten JC. Tau pathology in two Dutch families with mutations in the microtubule-binding region of tau. Am J Pathol 1998; 153: 1359–63.
27. Wilhelmsen KC, Lynch T, Pavlou E, Higgins M, Nygaard TG. Localization of disinhibition–dementia–Parkinsonism–amyotrophy complex to 17q21–22. Am J Hum Genet 1994; 55: 1159–65.
28. Bird TD, Wijsman EM, Nochlin D, Leehey M, Sumi SM, Payami H, Poorkaj P, Nemens E, Raskind M, Schellenberg GD. Chromosome 17 and hereditary dementia: linkage studies in three non-Alzheimer families and kindreds with late-onset FAD. Neurology 1997; 48: 949–54.
29. Murrell JR, Koller D, Foroud T, Goedert M, Spillantini MG, Edenberg HJ, Farlow MR, Ghetti B. Familial multiple system tauopathy with presenile dementia is localized to chromosome 17. Am J Hum Genet 1997; 61: 1131–8.
30. Poorkaj P, Bird TD, Wijsman E, Nemens E, Garruto RM, Anderson L, Andreadis A, Wiederholt WC, Raskind M, Schellenberg GD. Tau is a candidate gene for chromosome 17 frontotemporal dementia. Ann Neurol 1998; 43: 815–25.
31. Hutton M, Lendon CL, Rizzu P, Baker M, Froelich S, Houlden H, Pickering-Brown S, Chakraverty S, Isaacs A, Grover A, Hackett J, Adamson J, Lincoln S, Dickson D, Davies P, Petersen RC, Stevens M, de Graaff E, Wauters E, van Baren J, Hillebrand M, Joosse M, Kwon JM, Nowotny P, Che LK, Norton J, Morris JC, Reed LA, Trojanowski JQ, Basun H, Lannfelt L, Neystat M, Fahn S, Dark F, Tannenberg T, Dodd PR, Hayward N, Kwok JBJ, Schofield PR, Andreadis A, Snowden J, Craufurd D, Neary D, Owen F, Oostra BA, Hardy J, Goate A, van Swieten J, Mann D, Lynch T, Heutink P. Association of missense and 5'-splice-site mutations in *tau* with the inherited dementia FTDP-17. Nature 1998; 393: 702–5.
32. Spillantini MG, Murrell JR, Goedert M, Farlow MR, Klug A, Ghetti B. Mutation in the tau gene in familial multiple system tauopathy with presenile dementia. Proc Natl Acad Sci USA 1998; 95: 7737–41.
33. Götz J, Probst A, Spillantini MG, Schäfer T, Jakes R, Bürki K, Goedert M. Somatodendritic localization and hyperphosphorylation of tau protein in transgenic mice expressing the longest human brain tau isoform. EMBO J 1995; 14: 1304–13.
34. Polymeropoulos MH, Lavedan C, Leroy E, Ide SE, Dehejia A, Dutra A, Pike B, Root H, Rubenstein J, Boyer R, Stenroos ES, Chandrasekharappa S, Athanassiadou A, Papapetropoulos T, Johnson WG, Lazzarini AM, Duvoisin RC, Di Iorio G, Golbe LI, Nussbaum RL. Mutation in the α-synuclein gene identified in families with Parkinson's disease. Science 1997; 276: 2045–7.

35. Spillantini MG, Schmidt ML, Lee VM-Y, Trojanowski JQ, Jakes R, Goedert M. α-Synuclein in Lewy bodies. Nature 1997; 388: 839–40.
36. Uéda K, Fukushima H, Masliah E, Xia Y, Iwai A, Yoshimoto M, Otero DAC, Kondo J, Ihara Y, Saitoh T. Molecular cloning of cDNA encoding an unrecognized component of amyloid in Alzheimer disease. Proc Natl Acad Sci USA 1993; 90: 11282–6.
37. Jakes R, Spillantini MG, Goedert M. Identification of two distinct synucleins in human brain. FEBS Lett 1994; 345: 27–32.
38. Spillantini MG, Crowther RA, Jakes R, Hasegawa M, Goedert M. α-Synuclein in filamentous inclusions of Lewy bodies from Parkinson's disease and dementia with Lewy bodies. Proc Natl Acad Sci USA 1998; 95: 6469–73.
39. Krüger R, Kuhn W, Müller T, Woitalla D, Graeber M, Kösel S, Przuntek H, Epplen JT, Schöls L, Riess O. Ala30Pro mutation in the gene encoding α-synuclein in Parkinson's disease. Nature Genet 1998; 18: 106–8.
40. Papp MI, Kahn JE, Lantos PL. Glial cytoplasmic inclusions in the CNS of patients with multiple system atrophy. J Neurol Sci 1989; 94: 79–100.
41. Mezey E, Dehejia A, Harta G, Papp MI, Polymeropoulos MH, Brownstein MJ. Alpha synuclein in neurodegenerative disorders: murderer or accomplice? Nature Med 1998; 4: 755–7.
42. Spillantini MG, Crowther RA, Jakes R, Cairns NJ, Lantos PL, Goedert M. Filamentous α-synuclein inclusions link multiple system atrophy with Parkinson's disease and dementia with Lewy bodies. Neurosci Lett 1998; 251: 205–8.

Address for correspondence:
M. Goedert,
MRC Laboratory of Molecular Biology,
Hills Road, Cambridge CB2 2QH, UK
Tel: +44 1223 402036; fax: +44 1223 402197;
e-mail: mg@mrc-lmb.cam.ac.uk

29 Molecular Anatomy of Tau Inclusions with Antibodies to Specifically Recognize Tau Isoforms

S. ARAWAKA, N. SAHARA, G. LEE AND H. MORI

INTRODUCTION

Tau is a microtubule-associated binding protein, occurs in the axonal processes in neurons and is involved in axonal transport, axonal growth and
neural networking. Tau has become more important since it was found to be a
component of Alzheimer's paired helical filaments (PHF) [1–4]. In spite of its
hydrophilicity [5], tau integrated in PHF is highly insoluble and difficult to
solubilize, even in the presence of strong detergents, such as sodium dodecyl
sulfate (SDS) or urea [6]. As its major role is involved in maintaining the
microtubule assembly in order to enable axonal transport, the formation of tau
inclusions follows instability of the microtubules. Such a loss of fundamental
function induces neuronal degeneration, resulting in the neuronal dysfunction
of dementia. Studies on human tau cDNA show the presence of six isoforms
generated by alternative splicing [7–10].

Unlike amyloid β-protein, tau is observed in various neuronal degenerative
disorders besides AD, such as progressive supranuclear palsy (PSP), corticobasal degeneration (CBD) and Pick's disease, among others. Tau isoforms
are expected to be specifically expressed in brains with different diseases.
Delacourte and his colleagues have published information on such isoform-
specific antibodies and have found that some of them are expressed in a
disease-dependent fashion [11]. For instance, biochemical analysis shows tau
bands with Mr 55, 64 and 69 for the AD brain [12–14], with Mr 64 and 69 for
the PSP brain [15–17] and with Mr 55 and 64 for Pick's disease [18–20]. As
these observations were based on SDS gel electrophoresis, their conclusions
are not confirmed because abnormally phosphorylated tau shows retarded
mobility on the gel, like the apparent tau isoforms with higher molecular
weights. In addition, tau is known to undergo phosphorylation [21–23],

Alzheimer's Disease and Related Disorders
Edited by K. Iqbal, D.F. Swaab, B. Winblad and H.M. Wisniewski
© 1999 John Wiley & Sons Ltd

ubiquitination [24], oxidation [25] or glucosylation/glycation [26–28], resulting in changes in electrophoretic mobility. As the previous studies used extra-exon specific antibodies, there was no confirmation of the presence of tau isoforms in the absence of exons. To obtain more concrete evidence for tau expression, we have made five antibodies to distinguish each of six isoforms of human tau and have found that most antibodies can detect some tau-bearing inclusions. Such data will be useful for the diagnosis of various tauopathies and for producing transgenic mice as the fundamental DNA construction information for mimicking pathologies specific to diseases including AD.

MATERIALS AND METHODS

ANTIGEN DESIGNATION

As shown in Figure 1, tau proteins are different in two areas at amino acids 45 and 275, respectively. Six isoforms are distinguishable by the presence or absence of exons 2, 3 or 10. The shortest isoform is calculated to comprise 352 amino acid residues (tau352), while the longest is calculated to comprise 441 amino acid residues (tau441). We designed three different antibodies, against: (a) the amino-junction (AJ) region; (b) exon 2, connected with the shortest backbone sequence (exon 2-junction, E2J); and (c) exon 3 (E3)

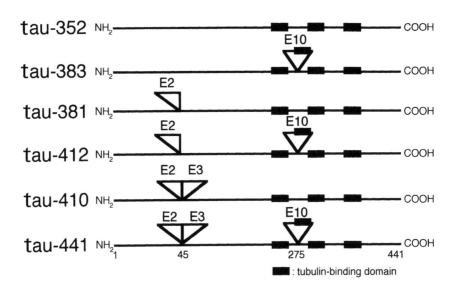

Figure 1. Six isoforms of human tau. Six isoforms are expressed by the alternative splicing of exons 2, 3 and 10. Since exon 3 is always expressed with exon 2, there are four exon 2-containing tau isoforms

sequence. The other antibodies were designed to recognize tau with the three-repeat tubulin-binding domain (RJ) and with the 4-repeat tubulin-binding domain (R2; i.e. the second repeat tubulin-binding domain).

BACTERIAL EXPRESSION OF HUMAN TAU ISOFORM cDNA

Human tau cDNA was integrated into pET bacterial expression vector and transfected. Ampicillin-resistant clones were obtained and IPTG induced to express human tau in *Escherichia coli.*

WESTERN BLOTTING

The bacterial lysates were treated with SDS and applied to 10% poly-acrylamide gel. After electrophoresis, the gels were blotted onto PVDF membranes for CBB protein staining and immunostaining.

IMMUNOHISTOCHEMISTRY

The paraffin-embedded sections of AD brain tissues were deparaffinized with xylene followed by alcohol. After hydration with PBS, the sections were blocked with 20% calf serum in 50 mM Tris–HCl, pH 7.6; 150 mM NaCl (TS buffer). The primary antibodies were incubated overnight and then washed with TS buffer. The biotinylated secondary antibody was used to label the primary antibody. The staining protocol was performed according to the manufacturer's instructions (Vector Co. Ltd, MA, USA).

RESULTS

The antibody (E3) against the exon 3 sequence was found to recognize only tau410 and tau441, but not other isoforms (Figure 2), because these two

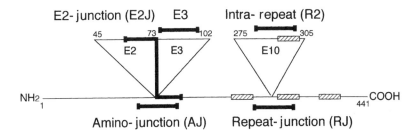

Figure 2. Strategy of antigen peptides for preparing of antibodies to specifically recognize tau isoforms. To prepare the specific antibodies to distinguish tau isoforms, we took the design of synthetic peptides to cover the junction regions of the exons or the sequences of extra-exon 3 or exon 10

isoforms contain exon 3. They stained neurofibrillary tangles (NFT) in paraffin sections of AD brains. The antibody (R2) against exon 10 was also found to recognize three isoforms containing exon 10, tau383, tau412 and tau441 (Figure 2), but not other isoforms. Two antibodies of these, E3 and R2, are relatively easy to prepare since their epitope antigens contain unique sequences and do not cross-react.

Antibody (E2J) made in a sequence-dependent manner against the exon 2 sequence was intended to recognize four tau isoforms, namely tau381, tau412, tau410 and tau441, because exon 2 was shared by these four isoforms (Figure 2). We designed this antigen in order to recognize only tau isoforms with exon 2, but not exon 3 (Figure 1). For this purpose, we made monoclonal antibodies to stain NFT.

The monoclonal antibody AJ was prepared against the junction regions between exon 1 and exon 4, without exons 2 and 3, and found to stain NFT. The other junction-specific monoclonal antibody was prepared against tau with three-repeat tubulin-binding domains. Its epitope was the synthetic peptide covering the carboxyl terminal region of exon 9 and the amino-terminal region of exon 11 lacking exon 10. As already documented, the amino acid sequences of exons 9 and 10 were extremely homologous, the difference being only one amino acid residue. As RJ antibody recognized three-repeat but not four-repeat tau isoforms, it must also recognize the single amino acid-dependent epitope around this junction region.

DISCUSSION

The present study is the first to prepare the full set of antibodies to recognize six tau isoforms in an exon-expression manner and enabled us to examine the disease-dependent gene expression of tau. We expect that these antibodies will be useful for confirmation of the previous clear findings by Delacourte and his colleagues.

We established an ELISA to measure the tau concentration in cerebrospinal fluid (CSF) from normal subjects and AD patients and found the difference between them significant [29]. Such results have been highly consistent and reproducible in many laboratories [30, 31], suggesting the high possibility of a diagnostic indicator. However, we realize that such a high concentration of tau is not specific to AD but is common to various diseases involving dementia, the so-called tauopathies. The dual measurements of tau and Aβ in CSF will be a more potent diagnostic combination for AD [32, 33]. However, we have tried to find more direct information on the tau molecule for the diagnosis of AD and decided to make the present antibodies to distinguish all six tau isoforms.

Extensive examination using the present antibodies will give us further useful information for producing transgenic mice to mimic tauopathies, including

AD and other diseases involving dementia. This is very likely because some preceding studies suggest the disease-specific isoform expression of tau. Moreover, it will be interesting to see whether tau expression in familial cases of tauopathies, such as FTDP-17 [34–36], is similar to sporadic cases, which is important in seeking to understand the molecular mechanism of pathology for AD as well as for general tauopathies.

ACKNOWLEDGEMENTS

This study was supported by Grants-in-Aid for Scientific Research on Priority Areas, from the Ministry of Education, Science and Culture, Japan, to H.M.

ABSTRACT

Tau inclusions are the hallmarks for various diseases with dementia (tauopathies) including Alzheimer's disease. A recent study on Alzheimer's paired helical filaments shows that they are composed of tau isoforms with three repeats while straight tubules are composed of tau isoforms with four repeats, based on a reconstitution experiment using bacterial expressed tau isoforms. This suggests the occurrence of disease-specific isoform expression in tau inclusions.

REFERENCES

1. Ihara Y, Nukina N, Miura R, Ogawara M. J Biochem 1986; 99: 1807–103.
2. Grundke-Iqbal I, Iqbal K, Quinlan M et al. Microtubule-associated protein tau. A component of Alzheimer paired helical filaments. J Biol Chem 1986; 261: 6084–9.
3. Nukina N, Kosik KS, Selkoe DJ. Recognition of Alzheimer paired helical filaments by monoclonal neurofilament antibodies is due to crossreaction with tau protein. Proc Natl Acad Sci USA 1987; 84: 3415–19.
4. Ksiezak-Reding H, Yen SH. Two monoclonal antibodies recognize Alzheimer's neurofibrillary tangles, neurofilament, and microtubule-associated proteins. J Neurochem 1987; 48: 455–62.
5. Lee G, Cowan N, Kirschner M. The primary structure and heterogeneity of tau protein from mouse brain. Science 1988; 239: 285–8.
6. Selkoe DJ, Ihara Y, Salazar FJ. Alzheimer's disease: insolubility of partially purified paired helical filaments in sodium dodecyl sulfate and urea. Science 1982; 215: 1243–5.
7. Goedert M, Wischik CM, Crowther RA et al. Cloning and sequencing of the cDNA encoding a core protein of the paired helical filament of Alzheimer disease: identification as the microtubule-associated protein tau. Proc Natl Acad Sci USA 1988; 85: 4051–5.

8. Goedert M, Spillantini MG, Potier MC et al. Cloning and sequencing of the cDNA encoding an isoform of microtubule-associated protein tau containing four tandem repeats: differential expression of tau protein mRNAs in human brain. EMBO J 1989; 8: 393–9.

9. Mori H, Hamada Y, Kawaguchi M et al. A distinct form of tau is selectively incorporated into Alzheimer's paired helical filaments. Biochem Biophys Res Commun 1989; 159: 1221–6.

10. Goedert M, Spillantini MG, Jakes R et al. Multiple isoforms of human microtubule-associated protein tau: sequences and localization in neurofibrillary tangles of Alzheimer's disease. Neuron 1989; 3: 519–26.

11. Delacourte A, Sergeant N, Wattez A et al. Vulnerable neuronal subsets in Alzheimer's and Pick's disease are distinguished by their tau isoform distribution and phosphorylation. Ann Neurol 1998; 43: 193–204.

12. Delacourte A, Flament S, Dibe EM et al. Pathological proteins tau 45 and 69 are specifically expressed in the somatodendritic domain of the degenerating cortical neurons during Alzheimer's disease: demonstration with a panel of antibodies against tau proteins. Acta Neuropathol 1990; 80: 111–17.

13. Lee VM-Y, Balin BJ, Otvos L et al. A68: a major subunit of paired helical filaments and derivatized forms of normal tau. Science 1991; 251: 675–8.

14. Goedert M, Spillantini MG, Cairns NJ et al. Tau-proteins of Alzheimer paired helical filaments: abnormal phosphorylation of all six brain isoforms. Neuron 1992; 8: 159–68.

15. Schmidt ML, Huang R, Martin JA et al. Neurofibrillary tangles in progressive supranuclear palsy contain the same tau epitopes identified in Alzheimer's PHF tau. Exp Neurol 1996; 55: 534–9.

16. Flament S, Delacourte A, Verny M et al. Abnormal tau proteins in progressive supranuclear palsy: similarities and differences with the neurofibrillary degeneration of the Alzheimer type. Acta Neuropathol 1991; 81: 591–6.

17. Vemersch P, Robitaile Y, Bernier L et al. Biochemical mapping of neurofibrillary degeneration in a case of progressive supranuclear palsy: evidence for general cortical involvement. Acta Neuropathol 1994; 87: 572–7.

18. Buee-Scherrer V, Hof PR, Buee L et al. Hyperphosphorylated tau proteins differentiate corticobasal degeneration and Pick's disease. Acta Neuropathol 1996; 91: 31–359.

19. Delacourte A, Robitaille Y, Sergeant N et al. Specific pathological tau protein variants characterize Pick's disease. J Neuropathol Exp Neurol 1996; 55: 159–68.

20. Feany MB, Mattiace LA, Dickson DW et al. Neuropathologic overlap of progressive supranuclear palsy, Pick's disease and corticobasal degeneration. J Neuropathol Exp Neurol 1996; 55: 53–67.

21. Ishiguro K, Takamatsu M, Tomizawa K et al. Tau protien kinase I converts normal tau protein into A68-like component of paired helical filaments. J Biol Chem 1992; 267: 10897–901.

22. Mandelkow EM, Drewes G, Biernat J et al. Glycogen synthase kinase-3 and the Alzheimer-like state of microtubule-associated protein tau. FEBS Lett 1992; 314: 315–21.

23. Trojanowski JQ, Lee VM-Y. Paired helical filament tau in Alzheimer's disease. The kinase connection. Am J Pathol 1994; 144: 449–53.

24. Mori H, Kondo J, Ihara Y. Ubiquitin is a component of paired helical filaments in Alzheimer's disease. Science 1987; 235: 1641–4.

25. Schweers O, Mandelkow E-M, Biernat J et al. Oxidation of cystein-322 in the repeat domain of microtubule-associated protein tau controls the in vivo assembly of paired helical filaments. Proc Natl Acad Sci USA 1995; 92: 8463–7.

26. Smith MA, Perry G. Oxidative damage in Alzheimer's disease. Nature 1996; 382: 120–1.
27. Ledesma MD, Bonay P, Aviva J. Tau protein from Alzheimer's disease patients is glycated at its tubulin-binding domain. J Neurochem 1995; 65: 1658–64.
28. Alonso AD, Grundke-Iqbal I, Iqbal K. Alzheimer's disease hyperphosphorylated tau sequesters normal tau into tangles of filaments and disassembles microtubules. Nature Med 1996; 2: 783–7.
29. Mori H, Hosoda-K, Matsubara E et al. Tau in cerebrospinal fluids: establishment of the sandwich ELISA with antibody specific to the repeat sequence in tau. Neurosci Lett 1995; 186: 181–3.
30. Jensen M, Basun H, Lannfelt L. Increased cerebrospinal fluid tau in patients with Alzheimer's disease. Neurosci Lett 1995; 186: 189–91.
31. Arai H, Terajima M, Miura M et al. Tau in cerebrospinal fluid: a potential diagnostic marker in Alzheimer's disease. Ann Neurol 1995; 38: 649–52.
32. Motter M, Vigo-Pelfrey C, Kholodenko D et al. Reduction of B-amyloid peptide42 in the cerebral fluid of patients with Alzheimer's disease. Ann Neurol 1995; 38: 643–8.
33. Kanai M, Matsubara E, Isoe K et al. Longitudinal study of cerebrospinal fluid levels of tau, Aβ1–40, Aβ1–42(43) in Alzheimer's Disease: a study in Japan. Ann Neurol 1998; 44: 17–26.
34. Poorkaj P, Bird TD, Wijsman E et al. Tau is a candidate gene for chromosome 17 frontotemporal dementia. Ann Neurol 1998; 43: 815–25.
35. Hutton M, Lendon CL, Rizzu P et al. Association of missense and 5'-splice-site mutations in tau with the inherited dementia FTDP-17. Nature 1998; 393: 702–5.
36. Spillantini MG, Murrell JR, Goedert M et al. Mutation in the tau gene in familial multiple system tauopathy with presenile dementia. Proc Natl Acad Sci USA 1998; 95: 7737–41.

Address for correspondence:
S. Arawaka,
1-4-3 Asahimachi,
Abenoku, Osaka 545-8585, Japan

V Mechanisms of Neurodegeneration

30 Inhibition of Neurofibrillary Degeneration: A Rational and Promising Therapeutic Target

KHALID IQBAL, ALEJANDRA DEL C. ALONSO,
JAVED A. GONDAL, CHENG-XIN GONG,
NILOUFAR HAQUE, SABIHA KHATOON,
AMITABHA SENGUPTA, JIAN-ZHI WANG AND
INGE GRUNDKE-IQBAL

INTRODUCTION

Alzheimer's disease (AD) has polyetiology. Over 90% of the AD cases have the sporadic form of the disease, the cause of which is most likely to be as yet unidentified environmental and or metabolic factors. Of the remaining AD cases that are familial, less than 10%, about one-half, are due to mutations in presenilin-1, presenilin-2 or β-amyloid precursor protein genes (for review, see [1]). Independent of the etiology, i.e. whether genetic or non-genetic, AD is characterized by a specific type of neuronal degeneration, called neurofibrillary degeneration. The neuronal cytoskeleton in AD is progressively disrupted and replaced by bundles of paired helical filaments (PHF), the neurofibrillary tangles [2, 3]. In addition to the neuronal perikaryon, the PHF, the major protein subunit of which is the abnormally hyperphosphorylated microtubule-associated protein tau [4–6], also accumulate in the neuropil as neuropil threads [7] and as dystrophic neurites surrounding wisps or a core of β-amyloid in the neuritic plaques [8, 9]. To date, the exact relationship between the neurofibrillary degeneration and the β-amyloidosis, the two hallmark lesions of AD, is not understood. The bulk of the data suggests that these two lesions can be formed independently of each other and that neither might be the cause of the formation of the other in AD. The number of neurons undergoing neurofibrillary degeneration increases with the progression of the disease and correlates with the degree of dementia (10–14); β-amyloidosis alone, in the absence of neurofibrillary degeneration, does not produce the disease

Alzheimer's Disease and Related Disorders
Edited by K. Iqbal, D.F. Swaab, B. Winblad and H.M. Wisniewski
© 1999 John Wiley & Sons Ltd

clinically. Furthermore, certain mutations in the tau gene segregate with neurodegeneration and dementia in some pedigrees of frontotemporal/ inherited dementias [15–17]. Thus, understanding the molecular mechanism of neurofibrillary degeneration is critical to devising a rational therapeutic treatment of all forms of AD and related conditions that are characterized by tau pathology.

MOLECULAR PATHOLOGY OF ALZHEIMER NEUROFIBRILLARY CHANGES

Neurons with neurofibrillary tangles lack microtubules [18], and microtubule assembly from AD brain cytosol is not observed [19]. PHF are comprised mainly of the microtubule-associated protein (MAP) tau in an abnormally hyperphosphorylated state [4–6]. In addition to PHF there is a pool of cytosolic abnormally phosphorylated tau in the affected neurons [19, 20]. This pool of abnormal tau, seen immunocytochemically as 'stage 0' tangles [21, 22], is most likely the precursor to PHF, since the neurofibrillary tangles have very little turnover, if any, and survive even after the death of the affected neurons as 'ghost' tangles.

In addition to abnormal hyperphosphorylation, the tau in AD brain is also glycosylated [23]. Unlike normal tau, both the AD soluble abnormally phosphorylated tau (AD P-tau) and PHF-tau are immunolabeled by lectins GNA, MAA and DSA, which recognize both the N-glycosidically linked and O-glycosidically linked saccharides. These abnormal taus are labeled weakly or unlabeled by PNA and SNA respectively, which recognize the O-glycosidically linked saccharides. Furthermore, both AD P-tau and PHF-tau can be deglycosylated by endoglycosidase F/N-glycosidase F, which specifically removes only the N-glycosidically linked saccharides from glycoproteins. Furthermore, the deglycosylation of PHF tangles converts them into bundles of straight filaments 2.5 ± 0.5 mm in diameter. All these findings, taken together, suggest that the glycosylation of tau in AD is mainly of the N-glycans type.

Alzheimer neurofibrillary tangles, especially the ghost tangles, are ubiquitinated, whereas neither the AD P-tau nor the stage 'O' tangles are immunolabeled by antibodies to ubiquitin [21, 22, 24]. The levels of conjugated ubiquitin determined by a monoclonal antibody 5–25 raised against isolated tangles, which recognizes the carboxy-terminal region (amino acid residues 64–76) of ubiquitin, are several-fold increased in the neocortex but in neither the cerebral white matter nor the cerebellum of AD cases [25, 26]. This increase in brain ubiquitin correlates strongly with the degree of neurofibrillary changes in the tissue. Thus, it appears that the affected neurons in AD brain do initiate the mechanism to degrade the tangles by the ubiquitin pathway but this attempt is largely unsuccessful.

LEVELS AND NATURE OF THE HYPERPHOSPHORYLATED TAU AND THE PROTEIN KINASES INVOLVED

The AD brain contains as much normal tau as in the normal age-matched control brain. However, in addition to normal tau in AD brain, there is 3–7-fold more abnormally hyperphosphorylated tau [27, 28]. The AD P-tau which can be separated from the normal tau by phosphocellulose chromatography contains 5–9 M phosphate/M protein as compared with a corresponding value of 2–3 M phosphate in the normal protein [20]. Employing phosphorylation-dependent antibodies and by mass spectrometry and amino acid sequencing, to date 21 phosphorylation sites in AD abnormally phosphorylated tau have been identified [29, 30]. Ten of the sites are canonical sites for proline-directed protein kinases (PDPKs) and the rest are the non-PDPK sites, suggesting that both types of kinases are likely to be involved in the abnormal hyperphosphorylation of tau in AD. Tau can be phosphorylated by several PDPKs and non-PDPKs [31–37]. However, in AD the exact role of any of these kinases in the abnormal hyperphosphorylation of tau is not yet understood and to date, the activity of none of these kinases has been found to be upregulated. Thus, the molecular sequence of events that results in abnormal hyperphosphorylation in AD is an extremely complex puzzle. Phosphorylation of tau only on certain specific sites might affect its biological activity, and the remaining sites might either play an important indirect role by way of facilitating phosphorylation of some of the sites involved in the biological activity of tau, or simply make the protein less accessible to processing by proteolysis. Phosphorylation of tau at some sites might be of neither direct nor indirect physiological consequence.

The PDPKs and non-PDPKs might work in certain combinations to generate abnormally hyperphosphorylated tau [38–42]. Both the rate and extent of tau phosphorylation by various protein kinases (A-kinase, CaM Kinase II, C-kinase, CK-1, cdk5 and GSK-3) are dependent on its initial phosphorylation state. For instance, if recombinant tau is prephosphorylated by one of several non-PDPKs (A-kinase, CaM Kinase II, C-kinase), then subsequent phosphorylations catalyzed by PDPKs (cdk5, GSK-3) are stimulated severalfold [38, 40, 41]. The rate and extent to which various tau isoforms are phosphorylated also depend on whether tau contains three or four repeats and zero, one or two N-terminal inserts [39, 40]. Thus, in addition to enzyme level, phosphorylation of tau is regulated at the substrate (tau) level.

IDENTITY OF PROTEIN PHOSPHATASES INVOLVED IN THE ABNORMAL HYPERPHOSPHORYLATION OF TAU

A large number of phosphoprotein phosphatases have been described in mammalian tissues (for review, see ref. [43]). These enzymes can be divided into two broad types, i.e. phosphoseryl/phosphothreonyl–protein phosphatases (PSPs) and phosphotyrosyl protein phosphatases (PTPs). The PSPs have been further subclassified into four subtypes, i.e. PP-1, PP-2A, PP-2B and PP-2C. These phosphatase activities differ in substrate specificity, dependence on divalent cations, and sensitivities to specific inhibitors [43, 44]. To date, only phosphorylation of serines and threonines has been observed in normal tau and AD abnormally hyperphosphorylated tau. Thus, only PSPs are expected to dephosphorylate tau.

Employing phosphorylation-dependent antibodies to tau, site-specific dephosphorylation of the AD P-tau has been investigated [45–49]. AD P-tau can be rapidly dephosphorylated at the abnormal sites Ser 46, Ser 198/Ser 199/Ser 202, Thr 231, Ser 235 and Ser 396/Ser 404 by PP-2B, at all the above sites except Ser 235 by PP-2A, and at only Ser 198/Ser 199/Ser 202, Thr 231 and Ser 396/Ser 404 by PP-1. The activities of all the three phosphatases, i.e. PP-2B, PP-2A and PP-1, towards abnormally phosphorylated tau are markedly increased by the presence of Mn^{2+}. Unlike tau *in vitro* phosphorylated by MAP kinase [50], which is the more preferred substrate to PP-2A$_1$ than PP-2A$_2$, AD abnormal tau is an equally good substrate to both isoforms of PP-2A. Dephosphorylation by PP-2C of the abnormal tau has been detected at none of the above sites [47].

TAU PHOSPHATASE ACTIVITIES IN THE AD BRAIN

The rapid dephosphorylation of AD abnormally phosphorylated tau by alkaline phosphatase [5, 6, 19] and by protein phosphatase (PP)-2A, PP-2B and PP-1 [45–49] *in vitro*, had suggested that the abnormal hyperphosphorylation of tau might in part be the result of a deficiency of the phosphoprotein phosphatase system in the brains of AD patients. To have a direct effect on the regulation of phosphorylation of tau, PP-2A, PP2-B and PP-1 should be present in the affected neurons. Immunocytochemical studies have revealed that these protein phosphatases are present both in granular and pyramidal neurons, including the tangle-bearing neurons [51]. Employing ^{32}P-labeled (with protein kinase A) phosphorylase kinase as substrate and specific inhibitors, it has been shown: (a) that the activities of PP-1, PP-2A, PP-2B and PP-2C can be determined in autopsied (2–7 h) and frozen human brains; and (b) that the activities of PP-1 and PP-2A are decreased in the AD neocortex [52]. Furthermore, studies on site-specific dephosphorylation of AD abnormally phosphorylated tau determined by immunolabeling with phosphorylation-dependent antibodies to tau have revealed: (a) that PP-2A and PP-2B and, to a lesser extent, PP-1 are involved in the dephosphorylation of tau in brain; and (b) that the phosphatase activity towards dephosphorylation of Ser 198/Ser 199/Ser 202, major abnormal phosphorylation sites in the abnormal tau, is decreased by ~30% in the brain of patients with AD [53].

Phosphoseryl/phosphothreonyl protein phosphatases also regulate the activities of several protein kinases. Inhibition of PP-2A and PP-1 activities by okadaic acid in SY5Y neuroblastoma cells stimulates the activities of MAP kinase, cdc2 and cdk5 [54]. Thus, the decrease in the PP-2A and PP-1 activities observed in AD brain might have been responsible for the abnormal hyperphosphorylation of tau, not only by inhibiting the dephosphorylation but also by promoting the phosphorylation reaction.

EFFECT OF DEPHOSPHORYLATION ON THE STRUCTURE AND BIOCHEMISTRY OF NEUROFIBRILLARY TANGLES

The dephosphorylation of neurofibrillary tangles of PHF by the two major tau phosphatases, PP-2A and PP-2B, have been demonstrated to produce marked biochemical, biological and structural alterations [48]. Both PP-2A and PP-2B dephosphorylate PHF-tau at the sites of Ser 198/Ser 199/Ser 202 and only partially dephosphorylate it at Ser 396/Ser 404; in addition, PHF-tau is dephosphorylated at Ser 46 by PP-2A, and Ser 235 by PP-2B. The relative electrophoretic mobility of PHF-tau increases after dephosphorylation by either enzyme. Divalent cations, manganese and magnesium, increase the activities of PP-2A and PP-2B toward PHF-tau. Dephosphorylation by both PP-2B and PP-2A decreases the resistance of PHF-tau to proteolysis by the brain calcium-activated neutral proteases, the calpains. The ability of PHF-tau to promote *in vitro* microtubule assembly is restored after dephosphorylation by PP-2A$_1$ and PP-2B. Microtubules assembled by the dephosphorylated PHF-tau are structurally identical to those assembled by normal tau. Dephosphorylation by both PP-2A$_1$ and PP-2B causes dissociation of the tangles and the PHF; some of the PHF dissociate into straight protofilaments/subfilaments. Approximately 25% of the total tau is released from PHF on dephosphorylation by PP-2A$_1$. These observations have demonstrated that tau in PHF is accessible to dephosphorylation by PP-2A$_1$ and PP-2B, and dephosphorylation makes PHF dissociate, accessible to proteolysis by calpain, and biologically active in promoting the assembly of tubulin into microtubules.

MECHANISM OF NEUROFIBRILLARY DEGENERATION AND THE FORMATION OF NEUROFIBRILLARY TANGLES

Tubulin, the subunit of microtubules, has two GTP binding sites; the α-subunit site is non-exchangeable, whereas the β-subunit site is accessible to the added guanine nucleotides [55, 56]. Binding of GTP to the exchangeable site promotes microtubule assembly. Tau promotes the binding of GTP to tubulin on the exchangeable site and the assembly of tubulin into micro-tubules, and maintains the structure of microtubules [57, 58]. Micro-tubules, in turn, are required for the axonal transport. These functions of tau are regulated by its degree of phosphorylation; hyperphosphorylation of tau depresses the microtubule assembly [59]. The normal brain tau, which is optimally active, has 2–3 M phosphates/M protein. Tau in the AD brain, which is abnormally hyperphosphorylated, contains 5–9 M phosphate/M pro-tein [20]. Tubulin from the AD brain is microtubule assembly-competent. However, microtubules cannot be assembled from AD brain cytosol [19]. This *in vitro* microtubule assembly defect, and the breakdown of the micro-tubule network in the affected neurons *in situ*, are not due to low levels of tau in the AD brain. The levels of tau in the AD cerebral cortex are 4–8-fold higher than that in the corresponding tissue from age-matched control cases. This increase in tau in the AD brain is in the form of abnormally hyper-phosphorylated tau, for there is as much normal tau in the AD brain as in normal control cases [27, 28]. Unlike normal tau, AD abnormally hyper-phosphorylated tau (AD P-tau) does not promote *in vitro* assembly of micro-tubules, bind to microtubules or stabilize their structure [60–62]. The AD P-tau competes with tubulin in binding to normal tau and inhibits the as-sembly of microtubules, and the association of AD P-tau with normal tau results into tangles of ~3.3 nm straight filaments. Unlike normal tau, abnor-mally phosphorylated tau in the AD brain is glycosylated and deglycosyla-tion of AD neurofibrillary tangles by endoglycosidase F/N glycosidase F converts them into tangles of thin straight filaments [23] similar to those formed by the association of AD P-tau and normal tau [61].

In addition to tau, the neuron contains high molecular weight microtubule-associated proteins (HMW-MAPs) MAP1 and MAP2, which also promote microtubule assembly and maintain the structure of microtubules. Like tau, MAP1 and MAP2 associate to AD P-tau and the sequestration of the HMW-MAPs from microtubules by AD P-tau results in the disassembly of micro-tubules [63]. However, the affinity of the binding between AD P-tau and normal tau is higher than that between AD P-tau and the HMW-MAPs. Furthermore, unlike the association between AD P-tau and normal tau, the binding of AD P-tau to MAP1 or MAP2 does not result in the formation of tangles or individual long filaments. This explains the degeneration of many neurites, and consequently the neurons, without any accumulation of PHF in AD brain. HMW-MAPs have not been observed in isolated PHF.

The breakdown of the microtubule network leads to a compromised axonal transport and consequently to loss of synapses and to retrograde degeneration (Figure 1). It is these events which lead to brain atrophy and the dementia syndrome. The neuronal cell bodies, devoid of most of their neurites, are already practically functionally dead prior to their ultimate death. Some of these neurons which contain neurofibrillary tangles leave the latter behind in

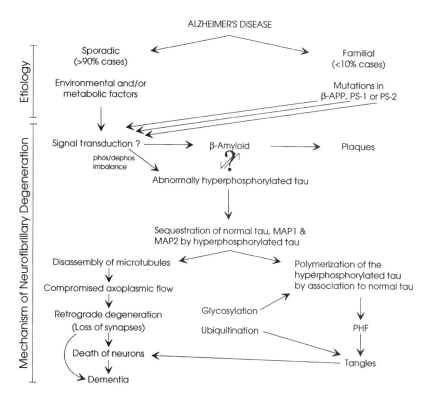

Figure 1. Etiology and mechanism of Alzheimer's disease neurofibrillary degeneration. AD has polyetiology. All of these etiological factors seem to affect a specific signal transduction pathway(s) that, on the one hand, leads to β-amyloid in the extracellular space in brain parenchyma and, on the other hand, produces protein phosphorylation/dephosphorylation imbalance, at least partly by reduction of protein phosphatase activity(s). This imbalance produces abnormal hyperphosphorylation of tau. The abnormal tau sequesters normal microtubule-associated proteins (MAPs) and causes disassembly of microtubules. The breakdown of the microtubule network in the affected neurons compromises axonal transport, leading to retrograde degeneration, which in turn results in dementia. The association between the AD P-tau and normal tau in the presence of glycosylation results in the formation of neurofibrillary tangles. The tangles are ubiquitinated for degradation by the non-lysosomal ubiquitin pathway, but apparently this degradation, if any, is minimal

the extracellular space as 'tombstones'. Unlike the soluble abnormally hyperphosphorylated tau that behaves as a toxic molecule in disrupting the microtubule network, the neurofibrillary tangles are inert structures which increasingly occupy the cell cytoplasm.

The abnormal hyperphosphorylation of tau in the AD brain is, at least in part, due to a downregulation of tau phosphatase activities. Protein phosphatases PP-2A, PP-2B, and to a lesser extent PP-1, can restore not only the normal biological function to AD abnormally hyperphosphorylated tau but also dissociate PHF and release functional tau. Thus, by increasing the activities of one or more of these tau phosphatases, it might be possible to prevent and inhibit neuronal degeneration and consequently both sporadic as well as familial AD.

CSF TAU AND CONJUGATED UBIQUITIN LEVELS AS MARKERS OF ALZHEIMER'S DISEASE

At the rate of ~24 ml/h and a total volume of ~144 ml, the CSF in humans is replaced every 6 h. CSF is thus an excellent indicator of the rate of brain pathology and also the efficacy of the therapeutic drugs that inhibit this pathology.

Studies showing, in AD, large increases in the brain levels of tau [27, 28] and conjugated ubiquitin [26, 64, 65] have led to the examination of the levels of these proteins in the CSF of these patients. The CSF levels of both conjugated ubiquitin [25, 26] and tau (e.g. references [66–68]) are elevated in AD. Although there is increasing evidence for the polyetiology of AD, to date there is no identification of various variants/subgroups of AD. Studies on the CSF molecular markers, i.e. tau, conjugated ubiquitin and $A\beta1$–42, have all shown both wide scatter in the levels of these proteins in AD and as well as overlaps with age-matched normal and neurological controls. These findings suggest that there might be more than one course of AD pathology. Identification of these variants of AD is critical toward developing CSF tests, or for that matter any other laboratory diagnostic tests, of AD. Nevertheless, both CSF tau and conjugated ubiquitin are excellent markers of AD neurodegeneration and it is time for the monitoring of CSF levels of these proteins to be included in examining the rate of the progression of AD pathology, and in testing the efficacy of therapeutic drugs designed to prevent and/or arrest neurodegeneration. Symptomatic drugs such as cholinomimatics or antidepressants should not be expected to alter the CSF levels of these markers.

ACKNOWLEDGEMENTS

We thank Janet Biegelson for secretarial assistance. Autopsied brain specimens were provided by the Brain Tissue Resource Center (PHS grant MH/NS31862), McLean Hospital, Belmont, MA, USA. These studies were supported in part by the New York State Office of Mental Retardation and Developmental Disabilities; National Institutes of Health Grants AG05892, AG08076, NS18105 and TW00507.

REFERENCES

1. Finch C, Tanzi RE. Genetics of Aging. Science 1997; 278: 407–11.
2. Kidd M. Alzheimer's disease: an electron microscopical study. Brain 1964; 87: 307–20.
3. Terry RD, Gonatas NK, Weiss M. Ultrastructural studies in Alzheimer's presenile dementia. Am J Pathol 1964; 44: 269–97.
4. Grundke-Iqbal I, Iqbal K, Quinlan M, Tung Y-C, Zaidi MS, Wisniewski HM. Microtubule-associated protein tau: a component of Alzheimer paired helical filaments. J Biol Chem 1986; 261: 6084–9.
5. Grundke-Iqbal I, Iqbal K, Tung Y-C, Quinlan M, Wisniewski HM, Binder LI. Abnormal phosphorylation of the microtubule associated protein τ (tau) in Alzheimer cytoskeletal pathology. Proc Natl Acad Sci USA 1986; 83: 4913–17.
6. Iqbal K, Grundke-Iqbal I, Smith AJ, George L, Tung Y-C, Zaidi T. Identification and localization of a tau peptide to paired helical filaments of Alzheimer disease. Proc Natl Acad Sci USA 1989; 86: 5646–50.
7. Braak H, Braak E, Grundke-Iqbal I, Iqbal K. Occurrence of neuropil threads in the senile human brain and in Alzheimer's disease: a third location of paired helical filaments outside of neurofibrillary tangles and neuritic plaques. Neurosci Lett 1986; 65: 351–5.
8. Wisniewski HM, Terry RD. Morphology of the aging brain, human and animal. Progr Brain Res 1973; 40: 184–6.
9. Glenner GG, Wong CW. Alzheimer's disease and Down's syndrome: sharing of a unique cerebrovascular amyloid fibril protein. Biochem Biophys Res Commun 1984; 122: 1131–5.
10. Tomlinson BE, Blessed G, Roth M. Observations on the brains of demented old people. J Neurol Sci 1970; 11: 205–42.
11. Alafuzoff I, Iqbal K, Friden H, Adolfsson R, Winblad B. Histopathological criteria for progressive dementia disorders: clinical–pathological correlation and classification by multivariate data analysis. Acta Neuropathol (Berl) 1987; 74: 209–25.
12. Arigada PA, Growdon JH, Hedley-White ET, Hyman BT. Neurofibrillary tangles but not senile plaques parallel duration and severity of Alzheimer's disease. Neurology 1992; 42: 631–9.
13. Dickson DW, Crystal HA, Mattiace LA, Masur DM, Blau AD, Davies P, Yen S-H, Aronson M. Identification of normal and pathological aging in prospectively studied non-demented elderly humans. Neurobiol Aging 1991; 13: 179–89.
14. Barcikowska M, Wisniewski HM, Bancher C, Grundke-Iqbal I. About the presence of paired helical filaments in dystrophic neurites participating in the plaque formation. Acta Neuropathol 1989; 78: 225–31.
15. Poorkaj P, Bird TD, Wijsman E, Nemens E, Garruto RM, Anderson L, Andreadis A, Wiederholt WC, Raskind M, Schellenberg GD. Tau is a candidade gene for chromosome 17 frontotemporal dementia. Ann Neurol 1998: 815–25.
16. Hutton M et al. Association of missense and 5'-splice-site mutations in tau with the inherited dementia FTDP-17. Nature 1998; 393: 702–5.
17. Spillantini MG, Murrell JR, Goedert M, Farlow MR, Klug A, Ghetti B. Mutation in the tau gene in familial multiple system tauopathy with presenile dementia. Proc Natl Acad Sci USA 1998; 95: 7737–41.
18. Terry RD, Wisniewski HM (eds). Ultrastructure of senile dementia and of experimental analogs. In: Aging and the Brain: Advances in Behavioral Biology, Vol 3. New York: Plenum, 1972; 89–116.
19. Iqbal K, Grundke-Iqbal I, Zaidi T, Merz PA, Wen GY, Shaikh SS, Wisniewski HM, Alafuzoff I, Winblad B. Defective brain microtubule assembly in Alzheimer's disease. Lancet 1986; 2: 421–6.

20. Köpke E, Tung Y-C, Shaika S, Alonso A del C, Iqbal K, Grundke-Iqbal I. Microtubule associated protein tau: abnormal phosphorylation of a non-paired helical filament pool in Alzheimer disease. J Biol Chem 1993; 268: 24374–83.
21. Bancher C, Brunner C, Lassmann H, Budka H, Jellinger K, Wiche G, Seitelberger F, Grundke-Iqbal I, Iqbal K, Wisniewski HM. Accumulation of abnormally phosphorylated tau precedes the formation of neurofibrillary tangles in Alzheimer's disease. Brain Res 1989; 477: 90–99.
22. Bancher C, Grundke-Iqbal I, Iqbal K, Fried VA, Smith HT, Wisniewski HM. Abnormal phosphorylation of tau precedes ubiquitination in neurofibrillary pathology of Alzheimer disease. Brain Res 1991; 539: 11–18.
23. Wang J-Z, Grundke-Iqbal I, Iqbal K. Glycosylation of microtubule-associated protein tau: an abnormal post-translational modification in Alzheimer's disease. Nature Med 1996; 2: 871–5.
24. Grundke-Iqbal I, Vorbrodt AW, Iqbal K, Tung Y-C, Wang GP, Wisniewski HM. Microtubule-associated polypeptides tau are altered in Alzheimer paired helical filaments. Mol Brain Res 1988; 4: 43–52.
25. Wang GP, Iqbal K, Bucht G, Winblad B, Wisniewski HM, Grundke-Iqbal I. Alzheimer's disease: paired helical filament immunoreactivity in cerebrospinal fluid. Acta Neuropathol (Berl) 1991; 82: 6–12.
26. Kudo T, Iqbal K, Ravid R, Swaab DF, Grundke-Iqbal I. Alzheimer disease: correlation of cerebrospinal fluid and brain ubiquitin levels. Brain Res 1994; 639: 1–7.
27. Khatoon S, Grundke-Iqbal I, Iqbal K. Brain levels of microtubule-associated protein tau are elevated in Alzheimer's disease: a radioimmuno-slot-blot assay for nanograms of the protein. J Neurochem 1992; 59: 750–3.
28. Khatoon S, Grundke-Iqbal I, Iqbal K. Levels of normal and abnormally phosphorylated tau in different cellular and regional compartments of Alzheimer disease and control brains. FEBS Lett 1994; 351: 80–84.
29. Morishima-Kawashima M, Hasegawa M, Takio K, Suzuki M, Yoshida H, Watanabe A, Titani K, Ihara Y. Hyperphosphorylation of tau in PHF. Neurobiol Aging 1995; 16: 365–80.
30. Iqbal K, Grundke-Iqbal I. Alzheimer abnormally phosphorylated tau is more hyperphosphorylated than the fetal tau and causes the disruption of microtubules. Neurobiol Aging 1995; 16: 375–9.
31. Ishiguro K, Takamatsu M, Tomizawa K, Omori A, Takahashi M, Arioka M, Uchida T, Imahori K. Tau protein kinase I converts normal tau protein into A68-like component of paired helical filaments. J Biol Chem 1992; 267: 10897–901.
32. Baudier J, Cole D. Phosphorylation of tau proteins to a state like that in Alzheimer's brain is catalyzed by a calcium/calmodulin-dependent kinase and modulated by phospholipids. J Biol Chem 1987; 262: 17577–83.
33. Roder HM, Ingram VM. Two novel kinases phosphorylate tau and KSP site of heavy neurofilament subunits in high stoichiometric ratios. J Neurosci 1991; 11: 3325–43.
34. Drewes G, Lichtenberg-Kraag B, Döring F, Mandelkow E-M, Biernat J, Goris J, Doree M, Mandelkow E. Mitogen activated protein (MAP) kinase transforms tau protein into an Alzheimer-like state. EMBO J 1992; 11: 2131–8.
35. Ledesma MD, Correas I, Avila J, Diaz-Nido J. Implication of brain cdc2 and MAP2 kinases in the phosphorylation of tau protein in Alzheimer's disease. FEBS Lett 1992; 308, 218–24.
36. Litersky JM, Johnson GVW. Phosphorylation by cAMP-dependent protein kinase inhibits the degradation of tau by calpain. J Biol Chem 1992; 267: 1563–8.
37. Singh TJ, Grundke-Iqbal I, McDonald B, Iqbal K. Comparison of the phosphorylation of microtubule associated protein tau by non-proline dependent protein kinases. Mol Cell Biochem 1994; 131: 181–9.

38. Singh TJ, Haque N, Grundke-Iqbal I, Iqbal K. Rapid Alzheimer-like phosphorylation of tau by the synergetic actions of non-proline-dependent protein kinases and GSK-3. FEBS Lett 1995; 358: 267–72.

39. Singh TJ, Grundke-Iqbal I, Iqbal K. Differential phosphorylation of human tau isoforms containing three repeats by several protein kinases. Arch Biochem Biophys 1996; 328: 43–50.

40. Singh TJ, Grundke-Iqbal I, Wu Q, Chauhan V, Novák M, Kontzekova E, Iqbal K. Protein kinase C and calcium/calmodulin dependent protein kinase II phosphorylates three-repeat and four-repeat tau isoforms at different rates. Mol Cell Biochem 1997; 168: 141–8.

41. Sengupta A, Wu Q, Grundke-Iqbal I, Iqbal K, Singh TJ. Potentiation of GSK-3-catalyzed Alzheimer-like phosphorylation of human tau by cdk5. J Mol Cell Biochem 1997; 167: 99–105.

42. Sengupta A, Kabat J, Novák M, Wu Q, Grundke-Iqbal I, Iqbal K. Phosphorylation of tau at both Thr 231 and Ser 262 is required for maximal inhibition of its binding to microtubules. Arch Biochem Biophys 1998; 357: 299–309.

43. Cohen P. The structure and regulation of protein phosphatases. Ann Rev Biochem 1989; 58: 453–508.

44. Ingebritsen TS, Cohen P. The protein phosphatases involved in cellular regulation. Classification and substrate specificities. Eur J Biochem 1983; 132: 255–61.

45. Gong C-X, Singh TJ, Grundke-Iqbal I, Iqbal K. Alzheimer disease abnormally phosphorylated tau is dephosphorylated by protein phosphatase 2B (calcineurin). J Neurochem 1994; 62: 803–6.

46. Gong C-X, Grundke-Iqbal I, Iqbal K. Dephosphorylation of Alzheimer disease abnormally phosphorylated tau by protein phosphatase-2A. Neurosci 1994; 61: 765–72.

47. Gong C-X, Grundke-Iqbal I, Damuni Z, Iqbal K. Dephosphorylation of microtubule-associated protein tau by protein phosphatase-1 and -2C and its implication in Alzheimer disease. FEBS Lett 1994; 341: 94–8.

48. Wang J-Z, Gong C-X, Zaidi T, Grundke-Iqbal I, Iqbal K. Dephosphorylation of Alzheimer paired helical filaments by protein phosphatase-2A and -2B. J Biol Chem 1995; 270: 4854–60.

49. Wang J-Z, Grundke-Iqbal I, Iqbal K. Restoration of biological activity of Alzheimer abnormally phosphorylated τ by dephosphorylation with protein phosphatase-2A, -2B and -1. Mol Brain Res 1996; 38: 200–208.

50. Goedert M, Cohen ES, Jakes R, Cohen P. [^{32}P]MAP kinase phosphorylation sites in microtubule-associated protein tau are dephosphorylated by protein phosphatase 2A$_1$; implications for Alzheimer's disease. FEBS Lett 1992; 312: 95–9.

51. Pei J-J, Sersen E, Iqbal K, Grundke-Iqbal I. Expression of protein phosphatases PP-1, PP-2A, PP-2B and PTP-1B and protein kinases MAP kinase and P34[cdc2] in the hippocampus of patients with Alzheimer disease and normal aged individuals. Brain Res 1994; 655: 70–76.

52. Gong C-X, Singh TJ, Grundke-Iqbal I, Iqbal K. Phosphoprotein phosphatase activities in Alzheimer disease. J Neurochem 1993; 61: 921–7.

53. Gong C-X, Shaikh S, Wang J-Z, Zaidi T, Grundke-Iqbal I, Iqbal K. Phosphatase activity toward abnormally phosphorylated τ: decrease in Alzheimer disease brain. J Neurochem 1995; 65: 732–8.

54. Tanaka T, Zhong J, Iqbal K, Trenkner E, Grundke-Iqbal I. The regulation of phosphorylation of τ in SY5Y neuroblastoma cells: the role of protein phosphatases. FEBS Lett 1998; 426: 248–54.

55. Weisenberg RC, Borisy GC, Taylor EW. The colchicine binding protein of mammalian brain and its relation to microtubules. Biochemistry 1968; 7: 4466–77.

56. Weisenberg RC, Denny WJ, Dickinson PJ. Tubulin-nucleotide interactions during the polymerization and depolymerization of microtubules. Biochemistry 1976; 15: 4248–54.
57. Weingarten MD, Lockwood AH, Hwo S-Y, Kirschner MW. A protein of mammalian brain and its relation to microtubule assembly. Proc Natl Acad Sci USA 1975; 72: 1858–62.
58. Khatoon S, Grundke-Iqbal I, Iqbal K. Guanosine triphosphate binding to β-subunit of tubulin in Alzheimer's disease brain: role of microtubule-associated protein τ. J Neurochem 1995; 64: 777–87.
59. Lindwall G, Cole RD. Phosphorylation affects the ability of tau protein to promote microtubule assembly. J Biol Chem 1984; 259: 5301–5.
60. Alonso A del C, Zaidi T, Grundke-Iqbal I, Iqbal K. Role of abnormally phosphorylated tau in the breakdown of microtubules in Alzheimer disease. Proc Natl Acad Sci USA 1994; 91: 5562–6.
61. Alonso A del C, Grundke-Iqbal I, Iqbal K. Alzheimer's disease hyperphosphorylated tau sequesters normal tau into tangles of filaments and disassembles microtubules. Nature Med 1996; 2: 783–7.
62. Iqbal K, Zaidi T, Bancher C, Grundke-Iqbal I. Alzheimer paired helical filaments: restoration of the biological activity by dephosphorylation. FEBS Lett 1994; 349: 104–8.
63. Alonso A del C, Grundke-Iqbal I, Barra HS, Iqbal K. Abnormal phosphorylation of tau and the mechanism of Alzheimer neurofibrillary degeneration: sequestration of MAP1 and MAP2 and the disassembly of microtubules by the abnormal tau. Proc Natl Acad Sci USA 1997; 94: 298–303.
64. Wang GP, Grundke-Iqbal I, Kascsak RJ, Iqbal K, Wisniewski HM. Alzheimer neurofibrillary tangles: monoclonal antibodies to inherent antigen(s). Acta Neuropathol (Berl) 1984; 62: 268–75.
65. Wang GP, Khatoon S, Iqbal I, Grundke-Iqbal I. Brain ubiquitin is markedly elevated in Alzheimer disease. Brain Res 1991; 566: 146–51.
66. Vandermeeren M, Lubke U, Six J, Cras P. The phosphatase inhibitor okadaic acid induces a phosphorylated paired helical filament tau epitope in human L-A-N-5 neuroblastoma cells. Neurosci Lett 1993; 153: 57–60.
67. Vigo-Pelfrey C, Seubert P, Barbour R, Blomquist C, Lee M, Lee D, Coria F, Chang L, Miller B, Lieberburg I, Schenk D. Elevation of microtubule-associated protein tau in the cerebrospinal fluid of patients with Alzheimer's disease. Neurology 1995; 45: 788–93.
68. Motter R, Vigo-Pelfrey C, Kholodenko D, Barbour R, Johnson-Wood K, Galasko D, Chang L, Miller B, Clark C, Green R, Olson D, Southwick P, Wolfert R, Munroe B, Lieberburg I, Seubert P, Schenk D. Reduction of β-amyloid peptide$_{42}$ in the cerebrospinal fluid of patients with Alzheimer's disease. Ann Neurol 1995; 38: 643–8.

Address for correspondence:
Khalid Iqbal,
New York State Institute for Basic Research
  in Developmental Disabilities,
1050 Forest Hill Road,
Staten Island, NY 10314-6399, USA
Tel: 718-494-5259; fax: 718-494-1080;
e-mail: kiqbal@admin.con2.com

31 Truncation of Tau and Neurodegeneration

M. NOVÁK, G. UGOLINI, L. FASULO, M. VISINTIN,
M. OVEČKA AND A. CATTANEO

INTRODUCTION

Alzheimer's disease (AD) is the major cause of memory impairment and intellectual decline in adult life. Intracellular neurofibrillary structures [1] (neurofibrillary tangles, dystrophic neurites, and neuropil threads) are classic hallmarks of AD. Their common denominator is the presence of paired helical filaments (PHFs) [2]. The number of PHFs in the AD brain shows a strong correlation with the degree of intellectual decline [3, 4]. It is therefore important to understand how PHFs are formed and what the cellular consequences of PHF formation are. PHFs are composed of full-length [5, 6, 7] and truncated [8] forms of the microtubule-associated protein tau, which is also abnormally hyperphosphorylated [9, 10], ubiquitinated [11], glycosylated [12] and glycated [13]. It is currently believed that these pathological post-translational modifications may be responsible for the abnormal assembly of tau into PHFs *in vitro* [14, 15, 16]. Normally, tau protein functions as a microtubule-associated protein with the capacity to form reversible interactions with tubulin [17].

The mechanisms by which tau protein is modified to take part in neurofibrillary pathology in AD are unknown. With the phosphorylation-specific monoclonal antibodies AT8 and PHF1, it has been shown that there is no apparent direct correlation between phosphorylation of tau and ISEL-positive nuclei in AD [18]. However, the participation of hyperphosphorylated tau in neuronal degeneration is well-documented [14]. Thus, there should exist at least another intermediate step between phosphorylation of tau, neuronal degeneration and cell death. Previous work showed that a pronase-resistant core of PHFs [7] is made of a group of six 93–95 amino acids long tau fragments [8, 19]. These were used to produce monoclonal antibody MN423 [20]. The antibody stains all the main neurofibrillary hallmarks of AD, including intracellular granular and fibrillary structures [21] and also labels PHFs

Alzheimer's Disease and Related Disorders
Edited by K. Iqbal, D.F. Swaab, B. Winblad and H.M. Wisniewski
© 1999 John Wiley & Sons Ltd

prior to pronase treatment [8]. MN423 does not stain full-length tau. The molecular mapping of its epitope revealed that MN423 recognizes all and only those tau molecules that terminate at Glu-391. Addition or removal of a single residue at the C-terminus abolishes immunoreactivity. Thus, reactivity with MN423 is diagnostic of a C-terminally exposed GAE peptide and represents a marker for endogenous tau truncation in AD [8, 22]. It has been demonstrated that MN423 does not stain sections from age-matched controls [23]. Truncation of tau in AD is becoming a widely recognized phenomenon [24]. However, the incidence and consequences of tau truncation in AD are not well understood. In order to elucidate further the impact of tau truncation on neuronal cells and neurodegeneration in AD, we have studied:

1. MN423 immunocytochemistry, to investigate whether tau truncation is an early pre-tangle event in AD neurons or whether it is a late proteolytic event occurring after cell death.
2. The over-expression of truncated fragments of human tau in COS cells, to understand the functional cellular consequences of tau truncation.
3. Engineering tau truncation *in vitro* and studying its impact on microtubule assembly and binding of tau to microtubules.
4. The role of tau during apoptosis on a granular cell model.

TRUNCATED TAU IS CO-LOCALIZED WITH FRAGMENTED DNA IN ALZHEIMER'S DISEASE NEURONES

We used MN423 immunocytochemistry to investigate whether tau truncation is an early pre-tangle event in AD neurones or whether it is a late proteolytic event occurring after cell death. *In situ* end-labelling (ISEL) of DNA was used for identification of DNA fragmentation in the nuclei of neurons, the marker commonly accepted as suggestive of cell death [25]. MN423 did not stain sections from age-matched NDC brains [23, 26]. On sections from AD brains, two main patterns of staining were produced by MN423: most sections exhibited granular labelling inside the cell bodies of cortical pyramidal neurones without showing any neurofibrillary tangles (brains 1, 2, 3, 4 and 5 in Table 1). In one case we could observe classical labelling of neurofibrillary pathology hallmarks: neurofibrillary tangles, dystrophic neurites and the neuritic component of senile plaques (brain 1 in Table 1). Despite normally axonal localization of tau, we found that MN423-positive granular aggregations were particularly abundant in the somatodentritic compartment. The observation of this intracellular granular material did not show any correlation with the PMD of brains (being already present with PMD as short as 3.45 h). We did not observe any PMD-related MN423 staining in control brains with PMD spanning from 3.00 to 7.20 h.

Table 1. Co-localization of tau-truncated and DNA fragmentation in AD neurons

Brain number	Case	Diagnosis	Age (years)	PMD (h)	MN423+/ISEL+ (% cells)
1	B139	AD	72	17.00	32 ± 10
2	90/118	AD	77	03.50	69 ± 5
3	90/107	AD	84	03.45	62 ± 12
4	92/021	AD	84	04.00	53 ± 9
5	91/109	AD	68	04.05	ND
6	95/062	NDC	80	04.30	Neg
7	95/043	NDC	75	07.20	Neg
8	92/039	NDC	87	03.00	Neg

PMD, post-mortem delay; CFS, cerebrospinal fluid; ISEL, *in situ* end-labelling of DNA; ND, not determined; MN423+/ISEL+, percentage of MN423-positive cells exhibiting DNA fragmentation in their nuclei in double-labelling experiments (mean ± SD; total number of cells counted: 1000 per sample); Neg, section from NDC brains were only occasionally and weakly stained by MN423 and ISEL staining was virtually absent on adjacent sections.

The presence of DNA fragmentation in neurons was visualized by means of the ISEL technique. In sections from NDC brains, ISEL-positive nuclei were extremely rare or virtually absent. On the contrary, when sections from AD brains were processed with the ISEL technique, numerous nuclei were stained in both the parietal and the frontal cortex. Examination of adjacent sections from brains 1, 2, 3 and 4, stained with MN423 and ISEL, respectively, showed a similar pattern of labelling. Therefore, experiments on the co-localization of these two events were performed. Double labelling of sections from the same brains showed that a high proportion of the nuclei of MN423-positive neurons was stained by ISEL (from a minimum of 32% to a maximum of 69%, Table 1). The study suggests that truncation of tau is an early event in AD. Intense granular staining inside neurons which did not exhibit any neurofibrillary changes was clearly shown (see also [21, 22]); therefore, we suggest that truncation of tau precedes the formation of tangles. To exclude the possibility that tau gets truncated due to long PMD, we used brains with different PMD for our study. The span of delay was from 3.45 h to 17.00 h. The granular staining with MN423 was already present in the AD brain with PMD as short as 3.45 h. However, NDC brains with PMD spanning from 3.00 to 7.20 h did not show any PMD-dependent staining with MN423. This is in accordance with previous results [23]. On the basis of these data it can be concluded that tau truncation, as identified by MN423, is not produced by a post-mortem proteolytic event and does not show any correlation with PMD of the brains studied.

It is well documented that neurons die in AD [18, 27, 28]. DNA fragmentation is a marker for cell death. To assess the impact of tau truncation on neuronal degeneration in AD we employed the ISEL technique, which identifies nuclei with fragmented DNA [25]. In accordance with previous results we found few or no ISEL-positive nuclei in sections from NDC brains [18, 26,

27, 28], while numerous nuclei were labelled in sections from AD brains. Adjacent sections from AD brain tissues showed that the regional patterns of MN423 and ISEL staining were similar. MN423/ISEL double-labelling studies demonstrated that truncation of tau and cell degeneration are correlated. This result further strengthens our working hypothesis that tau truncation precedes cytoskeletal changes related to neurofibrillary pathology and processes leading to cell death. Furthermore, it allows us to speculate that tau truncation itself, or some event leading to it, could trigger the cell death cascade. The scenario that cell death precedes truncation becomes rather unlikely, since a significant sub-population of MN423-positive neurons does not display any sign of DNA fragmentation in their nuclei (Table 1). Nevertheless, a certain number of ISEL-positive nuclei could be found which do not show MN423 immunoreactivity in their nuclei. We believe that this result can be accounted for by the presence of dying glial cells [18, 27], in which truncation of tau has never been shown so far.

EXPRESSION OF A TRUNCATED FORM OF TAU INDUCES APOPTOSIS IN COS CELLS

Previous results showed that tau is endogenously truncated in AD and co-localizes with fragmented DNA in diseased neurons. In order to assess the relevance of this abnormal post-translational modification of tau in cell degeneration occurring during the course of AD, we have expressed various tau fragments (Figure 1) encompassing the PHF core in COS cells. The smaller fragment (dGAE) corresponds to one of the PHF fragments, while the tau 151–391 fragment encompasses the proline-rich regions P1 and P2. The cellular distribution of these proteins in transiently transfected COS cells was studied by indirect immunofluorescence with MN7.51, a generic anti-tau antibody recognizing an epitope in the repeat region of tau [29]. The fragment dGAE, corresponding to one of the core PHF tau fragments, is exclusively found in the soluble pool and fails to associate with cellular microtubules. Morphology of the cells expressing the dGAE is normal [30]. However, tau fragment 151–391, which extends the core tau fragments N-terminally to encompass the proline regions P1 and P2, and which is C-terminally ending with MN423 specific Glu-391, induces heavy morphological changes. Around 50% of the cells are rounded, loosely bound to the dish. Confocal images of COS cells expressing the fragment show positive granules (Figure 2) which are intriguingly similar to those seen with MN423 in degenerating neurons in AD [21, 22, 26]. The dramatic change in morphology of transfected cells with truncated tau is suggestive of cell death. In order to characterize this further, nucleosomal DNA fragmentation was assessed by the terminal deoxynucleotidyl transferase (TdT)-mediated deoxyuridine triphosphate nick end-labelling assay (TUNEL). The percentage of the tau 151–391 fragment expressing cells undergoing apoptotic nuclear change was quantified. The number of TUNEL-positive and morphologically changed cells peaked between 48 and 72 h, when more than 40% of transfected cells underwent apoptosis (Figure 1). Cleavage of the lethal substrate poly (ADP-Ribose) polymerase (PARP) to the 85 kDa [31, 32] fragment in transfected cells further substantiated the conclusion that the expression of the MN423-positive fragment (tau 151–391) induces apoptosis.

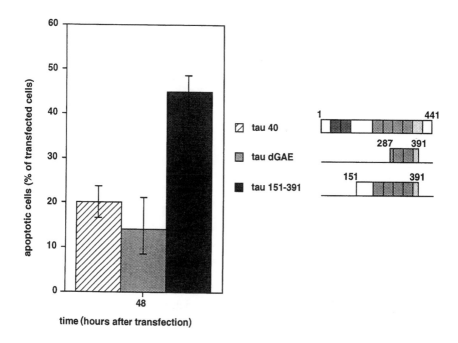

Figure 1. Apoptosis induced by truncated tau (tau dGAE, tau 151–391) in COS cells. The number of transfected COS cells undergoing apoptosis (TUNEL-positive) was evaluated 48 h after the transfection. Average values from two independent transfections are reported; 200 transfected cells were scored for each construct. The longest human tau isoform was used as a control

EFFECT OF TAU TRUNCATION ON THE FUNCTIONAL PROPERTIES OF TAU PROTEIN AS MEASURED BY MICROTUBULE ASSEMBLY AND BINDING ASSAYS *IN VITRO*

In order to gain insight into the functional consequences of tau truncation, we have measured the capacity of various truncated tau fragments (Figure 3) to simulate *in vivo* tau truncation. We found that, despite the presence of microtubule

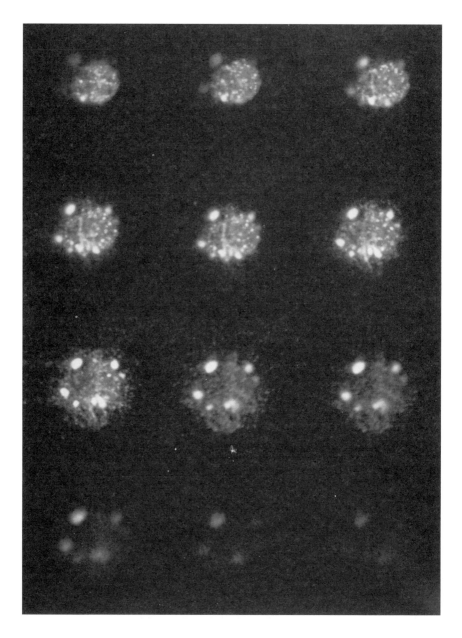

Figure 2. Confocal images of COS cells expressing truncated fragment tau 151–391. Different focal planes of tau 151–391 COS cells stained with pan tau monoclonal antibody MN7.51 show granular intracellular pattern similar to that seen in AD with MN423

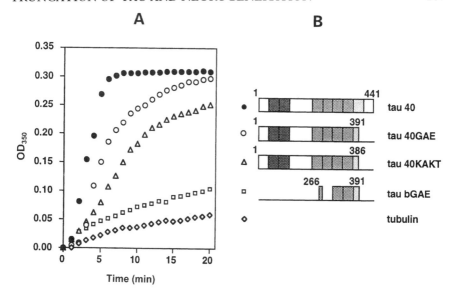

Figure 3. (A) The impact of tau truncation on its functional performance as measured by *in vitro* microtubule assembly assay (MAA). The turbidity of the solution was measured spectrophotometrically and is plotted as a function of time at 37 °C. (B) The scale of tau truncation is schematically outlined. The longest human tau isoform, tau 40, was used as a control

binding domains, the capacity of tau truncated forms to support microtubule assembly (MT) sharply declines with the extent of the truncation (Figure 3).

Another significant marker of the level of the functional efficiency or functional impairment is the strength of the interaction between tau protein and tubulin. Sequential tau truncation, as represented by tau 40GAE, tau 40 KAKT and tau bGAE (full-length tau 40 was used as a control), is causing a sharp increase in Kd values from 1.01 µmol/l for control intact tau 40, to 22.42 µmol/l for tau bGAE (Table 2).

Table 2. Impact of tau truncation on its binding to taxol-stabilized microtubules. The recombinant tau proteins purified to homogeneity was used in microtubule binding assay (MBA) in the following concentrations: 2.5 µM, 5 µM, 7.5 µM, 10 µM, 15 µM and 20 µM. The concentration of loose and bound tau proteins was densitometrically quantified with the help of the NIH-Image programme. Kd and n values were calculated from binding curves

	Kd [µM]	n
Tau 40	1.01	0.51
40GAE	1.41	0.41
40KAKT	1.93	0.43
bGAE	22.42	0.45

TAU PROTEIN IS CLEAVED AND DEPHOSPHORYLATED DURING NEURONAL APOPTOSIS

As described in the first part of this work, we have shown that tau truncation occurs inside AD neurons as an early intracellular event preceding cell death in AD. Apoptosis is an essential, controlled and genetically programmed process of self-destruction and present work shows that apoptosis may play a role in the pathogenesis of AD. Our observations led us to investigate the effect of apoptosis on tau protein, in order to understand if and how tau protein is affected by the apoptosis process itself and what the role of tau protein is in this process. For this study we have used a cerebellar granular cell model [33]. The cells, after lowering the level of potassium and absence of serum, undergo apoptosis [34] within 24–48 h. Western blotting of granular cell extracts with tau 1 showed a dominant 17 kDa band and a ladder of intermediate bands, probably corresponding to incomplete cleavage of tau within 6 h of inducing apoptosis. Since at this time apoptosis is largely reversible [35] and all cells are still alive and morphologically well-preserved [34], tau cleavage is a very early event in this apoptotic process. This characteristic is common to other death substrates [36]. Inhibition of apoptosis using a number of known anti-apoptotic reagents [33] leads to the disappearance of the 17 kDa truncated tau (tau 17). Using a set of well-characterized anti-tau monoclonal antibodies (304, MN7.51, T49), the 17 kDA fragment was located within 242 amino acids between amino acid residues 73 and 315. Loss of the T49 epitope shows that tau 17 is N-terminally truncated as well. Extraction studies revealed that tau 17 is unable to bind microtubules, since quantitatively it has been found in the soluble fraction. It was further observed that apoptosis changes the phosphorylation state of tau [33]. During apoptosis tau phosphorylation epitopes were reduced, particularly those recognized by mAbs 12E8 and AT8 (by 80–90%). mAb PHF1 showed two types of staining; one identifying the smaller band (45–55 kDa) was significantly reduced (80–90%), while the larger one (68 kDa) was nearly intact. These 68 kDa tau forms are not able, like their AD counterparts, to bind the microtubules, since they are not re-covered in the insoluble fraction. The characteristics of the latter forms are similar to those found in AD [6]. The fact that increase in staining with tau 1 is coupled with complete loss of AT8 immunoreactivity further strengthens the results showing sharp decrease in phosphorylation of tau during apoptosis. As we mentioned earlier, tau truncation is an early event during apoptosis. Examination of the sensitivity of this cleavage to different proteases showed that the formation of the 17 kDa fragment could be nearly completely inhibited with calpain inhibitor-leupeptin alone. Protease inhibitors with different specificities were not able to interfere with the production of tau 17 fragment. This suggests that the protease in cerebellar granule cells responsible for the production of tau 17 (17 kDa fragment) is calpain. Further confirmations of this result came from *in vitro* results. Apoptotically-induced cerebellar granule cells were also treated with various caspase inhibitors: YVAD-co (caspase 1); z-DEVD-fmk (caspase 3); or z-VAD-fmk (general caspase) [37]. The most effective was z-VAD-fmk, which reduced the intensity of the 17 kDa band by 80–98%, while z-DEVD-fmk reduced it by 35% and caspase 1 inhibitor YVAD-co had no effect. Experiments with *in vitro* translated tau cleaved with caspase 3 produced similar sized fragments to those seen when apoptotic granules are treated with calpain inhibitors. These results indicate that tau is a substrate for both calpain and caspase 3 and that cleavage with both of these proteases occurs in this model system.

ABSTRACT

Our results suggest that truncation of tau is an early event in AD. We have shown intense granular staining inside neurons which did not exhibit any neurofibrillary changes. Therefore, we suggest that truncation of tau precedes the formation of tangles. The process of tau truncation is independent of post-mortem delay (tested up to 17 h PMD). It is well documented that neurons die in AD. To assess the impact of tau truncation on neuronal degeneration in AD we employed the ISEL technique, which identifies nuclei with fragmented DNA. In accordance with previous results, we found few or no ISEL-positive nuclei in sections from non-demented control brains, while numerous nuclei were labelled in sections from AD brains. MN423/ISEL double-labelling studies demonstrated that truncation of tau and cell degeneration are correlated. This result, together with our latest data from cellular models, further strengthens our working hypothesis that tau truncation precedes cytoskeletal changes related to neurofibrillary pathology. Furthermore, we have shown that tau is an *in vivo* substrate for proteases during apoptosis. Thus, the truncation of tau appears to be not only an early but also, together with hyperphosphorylation, the most deleterious event in neuronal degeneration.

REFERENCES

1. Alzheimer, A. Uber eine eigenartige Erkrankung der Hirnrinde. Allg Z Psychiat 1907; 64: 146–8.
2. Kidd M. Paired helical filaments in electron microscopy of Alzheimer's disease. Nature 1963; 197: 192–3.
3. Blessed G, Tomlinson BE, Roth M. The association between qualitative measures of dementia and senile change in the cerebral grey matter of elderly subjects. Br J Psychiatry 1968; 114: 797–811.
4. Braak H, Braak E. Neuropathological staging of Alzheimer-related changes. Acta Neuropathol 1991: 82: 239–59.
5. Greenberg SG, Davies P. A preparation of Alzheimer paired helical filaments that display distinct tau proteins by polyacrylamide gel electrophoresis. Proc Natl Acad Sci USA 1990; 87: 5827–31.

6. Lee VM-Y, Balin BJ, Otvos L Jr, Trojanowski JQ. A68: a major subunit of paired helical filaments and derivatized forms of normal tau. Science 1991: 251: 675–8.

7. Wischik CM, Novák M, Thogersen HC, Edwards PC, Runswick MJ, Jakes R, Walker JE, Milstein C, Roth M, Klug A. Isolation of a fragment of tau derived from the core of the paired helical filaments of Alzheimer disease. Proc Natl Acad Sci USA 1988; 85: 4506–10.

8. Novák M, Kabat J, Wischik CM. Molecular characterization of the minimal protease resistant tau unit of the Alzheimer's disease paired helical filament. EMBO J 1993; 12: 365–70.

9. Grundke-Iqbal I, Iqbal K, Tung Y-C, Quinlan M, Wisniewski HM, Binder LI. Abnormal phosphorylation of the microtubule associated protein tau in Alzheimer cytoskeletal pathology. Proc Natl Acad Sci USA 1986; 83: 4913–17.

10. Ihara Y, Nukina N, Miura R, Ogawara M. Phosphorylated tau protein is integrated into paired helical filaments in Alzheimer's disease. J Biochem 1986; 99: 1807–10.

11. Mori H, Kondo J, Ihara Y. Ubiquitin is a component of paired helical filaments in Alzheimer's disease. Science 1981; 235: 1641–4.

12. Wang J-Z, Grundke-Iqbal I, Iqbal K. Glycosylation of microtubule-associated protein tau: an abnormal posttranslational modification in Alzheimer's disease. Nature Med 1996; 2: 871–5.

13. Ledesma MD, Bonay P, Colaco C, Avila J. Analysis of microtubule-associated protein tau glycation in paired helical filaments. J Biol Chem 1994; 269: 21614–19.

14. Alonso AC, Grundke-Iqbal I, Iqbal K. Alzheimer's disease hyperphosphorylated tau sequesters normal tau into tangles of filaments and disassembles microtubules. Nature Med 1996; 2: 783–7.

15. Goedert M, Jakes R, Spillantini MG, Hasegawa M, Smith MJ, Crowther RA. Assembly of microtobule-associated protein tau into Alzheimer-like filaments induced by sulphated glycosaminoglycans. Nature 1996; 383: 550–53.

16. Kampers T, Fridhoff P, Biernat J, Mandelkow E-M, Mandelkow E. RNA stimulates aggregation of microtubule-associated protein tau into Alzheimer-like paired helical filaments. FEBS Lett 1996; 399: 344–9.

17. Cleveland CB, Sygowski LA, Scott CW, Sobel EI. Purification of tau, a microtubule associated protein that induces assembly of microtubules from purified tubulin. J Mol Biol 1977; 116: 207–25.

18. Su JH, Anderson AJ, Cummings BJ, Cotman CW. Immunohistochemical evidence for apoptosis in Alzheimer's disease. NeuroReport 1994; 5: 2529–33.

19. Jakes R, Novák M, Davison M, Wischik CM. Identification of 3- and 4-repeat tau isoforms within the PHF in Alzheimer's disease. EMBO J 1991; 10: 2725–9.

20. Novák M, Wischik CM, Edwards PC, Pannell R, Milstein C. Characterization of the first monoclonal antibody against the pronase resistant core of the Alzheimer PHF. Progr Clin Biol Res 1989; 317: 755–61.

21. Bondareff W, Wischik CM, Novák M, Roth M. Sequestration of tau by granulovacuolar degeneration in Alzheimer's disease. Am J Pathol 1991; 139(3), 641–7.

22. Novák M. Truncated tau protein as a new marker for Alzheimer's disease. Acta Virol 1994; 38: 173–89.

23. Mena R, Wischik CM, Novák M, Milstein C, Cuello C. A progressive deposition of paired helical filaments (PHFs) in the brain characterises the evolution of dementia in Alzheimer's disease. An immunocytochemical study with a monoclonal antibody against the PHF core. J Neuropath Exp Neurol 1991; 50: 474–90.

24. Johnson GVW, Seubert P, Cox TM, Motter R, Brown JP, Galasko D. The tau protein in human cerebrospinal fluid in Alzheimer's disease consists of proteolytically derived fragments. J Neurochem 1997; 68: 430–33.

25. Gavrieli Y, Sherman Y, Ben-Saason SA. Identification of programmed cell death *in situ* via specific labeling of nuclear DNA fragmentation. J Cell Biol 1992; 119: 493–501.
26. Ugolini G, Cattaneo A, Novák M. Co-localization of truncated tau and DNA fragmentation in Alzheimer's disease neurones. NeuroReport 1997; 8: 3709–12.
27. Lassmann H, Bancher C, Brietschopf H, Weigiel J, Bobinski M, Jellinger K, Wisniewski HM. Cell death in Alzheimer's disease evaluated by DNA fragmentation *in situ*. Acta Neuropathol 1995; 89: 35–41.
28. Anderson AJ, Su J, Cotman CW. DNA damage and apoptosis in Alzheimer's disease: colocalization with c-Jun immunoreactivity, relationship to brain area, and effect of postmortem delay. J Neurosci 1996; 16: 1710–19.
29. Novák M, Jakes R, Edwards PC, Milstein C, Wischik CM. Difference between the tau protein of Alzheimer paired helical filament core and normal tau revealed by epitope analysis of monoclonal antibodies 423 and 7.51. Proc Natl Acad Sci USA 1991; 88: 5837–41.
30. Fasulo L, Ovečka M, Kabat J, Bradbury A, Novák M, Cattaneo A. Overexpression of Alzheimer's PHF core tau fragments: implications for the tau truncation hypothesis. Alzheimer's Res 1996; 2: 195–200.
31. Tewari M, Quan LT, O'Rourke K, Desnoyers S, Zeng Z, Beidler DR, Poirier GG, Salvesen GS, Dixit VM. Yama/cpp32β, a mammalian homolog of CED-3, is a CrmA-inhibitable protease that cleaves the death substrate poly (ADP)-ribose) polymerase. Cell 1995; 81: 801–9.
32. Fasulo L, Visintin M, Novák M, Cattaneo A. Tau truncation in Alzheimer's disease: expression of a fragment encompassing PHF core tau induces apoptosis in COS cells. Alzheimer's Rep 1998; 1: 25–32.
33. Canu N, Dus L, Barbato Ch, Ciotti MT, Brancolini C, Rinaldi AM, Novák M, Cattaneo A, Bradbury A, Calissano P. Tau cleavage and dephosphorylation during neuronal apoptosis. J Neurosci 1998; 18: 7061–74.
34. D'Mello SR, Galli C, Ciotti MT, Calissano P. Induction of apoptosis in cerebellar granule neurons by low potassium: inhibition of cell death by insulin-growth factor I and cAMP. Proc Natl Acad Sci USA 1993; 90: 10989–93.
35. Galli C, Meucci O, Scorziello A, Werge T, Calissano P, Schettini G. Apoptosis in cerebellar granule cells is blocked by high KCl, forskolin, and IGF-1 through distinct mechanism of action: the involvement of intracellular calcium and RNA synthesis. J Neurosci 1995; 15: 1172–9.
36. Cryns V, Bergeron L, Zhu H, Li H, Yuan J. Specific cleavage of a fodrin during Fas- and tumor necrosis factor-induced apoptosis is mediated by an interleukin-1β-converting enzyme/ced-3 protease distinct from the poly (ADP-ribose) polymerase protease. J Biol Chem 1996; 271: 31277–82.
37. Cohen GM. Caspase: the executioner of apoptosis. Biochem J 1997; 326: 1–16.

Address for correspondence:
Michal M. Novák,
Institute of Neuroimmunology,
Slovak Academy of Sciences,
Dubravska str.9, 842 46 Bratislava, Slovak Republic
e-mail: Nilunova@savba.savba.sk

32 Regulation of Tau Phosphorylation in Normal and Diseased Cells

BRIAN H. ANDERTON, JO BETTS,
WALTER BLACKSTOCK, JEAN-PIERRE BRION,
DANIEL R. DAVIS, GRAHAM GIBB, DIANE P. HANGER,
EFTERPI KARDALINOU, SIMON LOVESTONE,
JANICE PEARCE, C. HUGH REYNOLDS AND
MARIE-THÉRÈSE WEBSTER

Tau in paired helical filaments (PHF-tau) has been shown by sequencing studies to be phosphorylated on at least 25 serines/threonines and there may yet be additional sites to be identified [1, 2]. Many, but not all, of these amino acids are followed in the sequence by a proline residue, making proline-directed kinases putative tau kinases, although it is almost certain that other classes of protein kinases are also physiologically important. However, we have focused on the ability of several proline-directed kinases to phosphorylate tau at sites found to be phosphorylated in PHF-tau. We have also investigated the ability of apolipoprotein E isoforms to modulate tau phosphorylation. These kinases are glycogen synthase kinase-3α and -3β, p44 MAP kinase (ERK1), p42 MAP kinase (ERK2), p38 MAP kinase and p54β c-jun N-terminal kinase (JNK 3).

All of these kinases phosphorylate recombinant tau *in vitro* at numerous sites, reducing the electrophoretic mobility of tau on SDS–PAGE and generating epitopes for a panel of commonly used monoclonal antibodies that recognize PHF-tau [3]. However, there are differences between the abilities of these kinases to phosphorylate tau at particular sites. For example, GSK-3β readily phosphorylates Ser199 *in vitro*, whereas this site is less well phosphorylated by ERK2, JNK 3 and p38 MAP kinase which, on the other hand, phosphorylate Ser202 and Thr205 apparently more efficiently than Ser199. The data are summarized in Table 1.

We have investigated whether apolipoprotein E isoforms modulate the *in vitro* phosphorylation of tau by GSK-3β by phosphopeptide mapping and

Alzheimer's Disease and Related Disorders
Edited by K. Iqbal, D.F. Swaab, B. Winblad and H.M. Wisniewski
© 1999 John Wiley & Sons Ltd

Table 1. Tau phosphorylation sites identified by protein sequencing of foetal rat brain tau, adult rat brain tau and human PHF-tau, and human recombinant tau phosphorylated *in vitro*

Residue (of largest tau isoform)	Foetal rat tau	Adult rat tau	PHF-tau	Identified protein kinases for *in vitro* phosphorylation	Spot number in Figure 1
Thr175			+	MAPK	
Thr181	+	+	+	MAPK	5
Ser184/185			+		
Ser195				GSK	13a
Ser198	+		+		
Ser199	+		+	GSK-3 > MAPK/JNK/ p38 MAPK	13a
Ser202	+	+	+	MAPK/JNK/p38 MAPK > GSK-3 (cdk5 also phosphorylates this site)	15
Ser208			+		
Ser210			+		
Thr212			+	MAPK, GSK-3	3a
Ser214			+	PKA, PKC	
Thr217	+		+	GSK-3	3b
Thr231	+	+	+	GSK-3, cdk5	6
Ser235	+			MAPK, GSK-3, cdk5	6
Ser237			+	PK	
Ser238			+		
Ser262		+	+	GSK-3, PKA, PKC, p110K, PK	2
Ser356			+	GSK-3, PKA, p110K	1
Ser396	+		+	MAPK, GSK-3	13b
Ser400	+		+	GSK-3	13b
Thr403			+		
Ser404	+	+	+	MAPK, GSK-3, cdk5	13b
Ser409	+		+	PKA	
Ser412			+		
Ser413	+		+	GSK-3	
Ser422			+	MAPK	

mass spectrometry. In the presence of apolipoproteins E3 or E4, the phosphopeptide maps were generally not qualitatively different from tau phosphorylated in the absence of any apolipoprotein, but the relative intensities of particular spots on the maps were different (Figure 1). Most notably, Ser262 and Ser356 were relatively more phosphorylated in the presence of apolipoprotein E than in its absence. Furthermore, in the presence of apolipoprotein E2, three new phosphopeptides were observed compared to phosphorylation in the presence of either apolipoprotein E3 or E4, although the sites in tau to which these spots on the maps correspond have yet to be identified. It will be important in future to determine whether apolipoprotein E isoforms differentially modulate tau phosphorylation in cells and *in vivo*.

Although all of these proline-directed kinases readily phosphorylate tau *in vitro*, their abilities to phosphorylate tau in cells is different. We have previously demonstrated that GSK-3α and GSK-3β both phosphorylate tau in non-neuronal COS cells co-transfected with kinase and tau [4]. In this cellular model of tau phosphorylation, tau becomes phosphorylated at numerous sites that are labelled by monoclonal antibodies, including AT8, RT97, 8D8, AT180 and AT270. Tau in these cells also is maximally retarded in

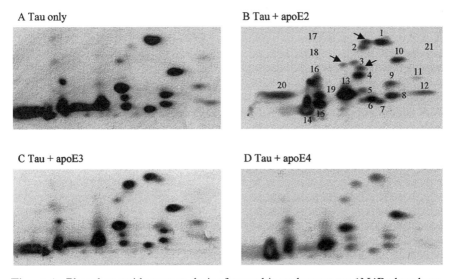

Figure 1. Phosphopeptide map analysis of recombinant human tau 1N4R phosphorylated by GSK3β in the absence (A) or presence of apoE2 (B), apoE3 (C) or apoE4 (D). Additional phosphopeptide spots in the apoE2-treated sample are indicated (arrows). These data demonstrate that all three isoforms of apoE affect *in vitro* phosphorylation of tau by GSK-3β, resulting in changes in the stoichiometry of phosphorylation at certain sites (compare relative intensities of spots 1 and 2 in the presence of any isoform of apoE with the relative intensities in the absence of apoE). In addition, in the presence of apoE2 several new phosphopeptides (arrows) are found that are absent from the control (i.e. no apoE) and from phosphorylation in the presence of apoE3 or apoE4

electrophoretic mobility by GSK-3α and -3β phosphorylation, such that different isoforms migrate in the same positions as the PHF-tau bands known to contain those isoforms [5]. Thus, GSK-3α and -3β both have the required properties to be physiological tau kinases.

We previously also reported that p44 MAP kinase, ERK1, phosphorylates tau in non-neuronal cells but not as extensively as GSK-3α and -3β, since the electrophoretic mobility was less retarded and few, if any, epitopes to known monoclonal antibodies were generated [6]. We have now extended these studies with p44 MAP kinase and have also investigated p38 MAP kinase and JNK 3. In all cases, COS cells were transfected with the cDNA for tau and the above protein kinases. We confirmed that p44 MAP kinase induced a retardation in the electrophoretic mobility of co-transfected tau but that this was less marked than when GSK-3β was expressed with tau (Figure 2). Co-expression of either p38 MAP kinase or JNK 3 with tau failed to induce a reduction in electrophoretic mobility of tau (Figure 2). However, when tau was co-expressed with both p44 MAP kinase and GSK-3β together, there was an additive effect on tau phosphorylation. A similar additive effect was observed in cells co-expressing both p38 MAP kinase and GSK-3β together but not by JNK 3 and GSK-3β together. These results demonstrate that in cells GSK-3β is apparently the most potent tau kinase, followed by p44 MAP kinase and possibly p38 MAP kinase, but that JNK 3 is only a poor kinase, if at all able to phosphorylate tau.

Previously, we showed that either treatment of primary rat cortical neuronal cultures with excitotoxic levels of glutamate, or subjecting the cultures to oxidative stress with hydrogen peroxide, result in a dephosphorylation of tau [7, 8]. Both of these experimental conditions subject the neurons to metabolic stress; the reduction in tau phosphorylation suggests that stress-activated protein kinases, of which p38 MAP kinase and JNK 3 are members, are not physiological tau kinases.

It has recently been demonstrated that lithium inhibits GSK-3 [9, 10]. We and others have therefore investigated the effects of lithium on tau phosphorylation in primary neuronal cultures [11]. The endogenous tau in primary neurons in culture is partially in a hyperphosphorylated state and is reactive with all of the monoclonal antibodies that label PHF-tau. However, treatment of such cultures with lithium reduces the labelling of tau with many of these antibodies (e.g. AT8, AT180, AT270, 8D8), the degree of reduction being dependent upon the lithium concentration, including at concentrations of lithium (1 mM) that are used therapeutically as a mood stabilizer in bipolar disorder. We have obtained indirect but convincing evidence that GSK-3 is inhibited by lithium in these neurons, since lithium induces a rise in cytosolic β-catenin. Increases in cytosolic β-catenin is diagnostic for reduced GSK-3β activity in a variety of cell types, β-catenin being downstream in the wingless/ wnt pathway, and its level regulated by GSK-3β activity. These data are further confirmatory evidence that GSK-3β is a physiological tau kinase.

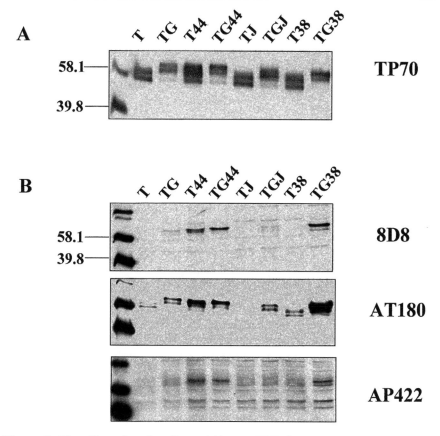

Figure 2. The effect of proline-directed kinases GSK3β (G), p44 MAP kinase [44], p38 MAP kinase [38] and JNK 3 (J) on tau (T) phosphorylation. COS7 cells transiently expressing tau, GSK3β, p44 MAP kinase, p38 MAP kinase, JNK 3 alone or in combination, were treated to activate the indicated kinases. (A) Western blot analysis using the phosphorylation-independent antibody, TP70. GSK3β, and to a lesser extent p44 MAP kinase, can induce a higher mobility shift on tau than p38 MAP kinase or JNK 3. However, when p44 MAP kinase and p38 MAP kinase are co-expressed with GSK3β, the effect on tau phosphorylation was synergistic, whereas co-expressed JNK 3 negatively regulated GSK3β-induced tau phosphorylation. (B) Phosphorylation-dependent tau antibodies show that p44 MAP kinase, in contrast to p38 MAP kinase or JNK 3, phosphorylates tau on similar epitopes to GSK3β. Co-expression of the different MAP kinases with GSK3β and staining with the above antibodies produces similar results to those observed using the TP70 antibody

We have exploited the inhibition of GSK-3 by lithium to investigate phosphorylation of tau by endogenous MAP kinase in neurons. Primary rat cortical neuronal cultures were treated with 25 mM lithium to inhibit endogenous GSK-3 and thus induce a marked reduction in tau phosphorylation, as assessed by its electrophoretic mobility and reactivity with a panel of phosphorylation-sensitive monoclonal antibodies. When these cultures were co-treated with 200 ng/ml EGF to activate maximally MAP kinase, MAP kinase was indeed activated as shown by increased immunoreactivity with an anti-active MAP kinase phosphotyrosine antibody. Under these conditions, there was also a modest increase in labelling of tau by monoclonal antibodies AT180 and AT270 but not AT8, compared to control cultures treated with 25 mM lithium but without EGF co-treatment, suggesting site-specific phosphorylation by MAP kinase in these cells. These results demonstrate that tau can be a substrate for endogenous MAP kinase although tau phosphorylation appears to be dominated by GSK-3.

Phosphorylation of tau by GSK-3β modulates the effects on microtubule organization. We have investigated this functional aspect of phosphorylation in transfected cells using green fluorescent protein-tagged tau (GFP-tau) [11]. In COS cells transfected with GFP-tau, the microtubules were decorated by GFP-tau and were bundled. In cells that were co-transfected with GSK-3β and GFP-tau, binding of GFP-tau to microtubules was reduced and the microtubules exhibit a typical organization. When these cells were treated with lithium to inhibit GSK-3β activity, there was a gradual increase in GFP-tau binding to microtubules and the microtubules became progressively more bundled. This process was reversed on washing out of the lithium. These experiments demonstrate that phosphorylation of tau by GSK-3 modulates the properties of tau with respect to its microtubule binding and bundling.

In summary, although tau is likely to be phosphorylated *in vivo* by several different protein kinases, GSK-3β (and possibly GSK-3α) is a strong candidate as a physiological tau kinase. Future research will need to identify the crucial mechanisms by which turnover of phosphate on tau is regulated and if this regulation is defective in degenerating neurons in Alzheimer's disease and related conditions that also exhibit hyperphosphorylated forms of tau.

ACKNOWLEDGEMENTS

This work was supported by the Wellcome Trust and the UK Alzheimer's Disease Society.

REFERENCES

1. Hanger DP, Betts JC, Loviny TLF, Blackstock WP, Anderton BH. New phosphorylation sites identified in hyperphosphorylated tau (PHF-tau) from Alzheimer's disease brain using nanoelectrospray mass spectrometry. J Neurochem 1998; 71: 2465–76.
2. Morishima-Kawashima M, Hasegawa M, Takio K, Suzuki M, Yoshida H, Titani K, Ihara Y. Proline-directed and non-proline-directed phosphorylation of PHF-tau. J Biol Chem 1995; 270: 823–9.

3. Lovestone S, Reynolds CH. The phosphorylation of tau: a critical stage in neurodevelopment and neurodegenerative processes. Neuroscience 1997; 78: 309–24.
4. Lovestone S, Reynolds CH, Latimer D, Davis DR, Anderton BH, Gallo J-M, Hanger D, Mulot S, Marquardt B, Stabel S, Woodgett JR, Miller CCJ. Alzheimer's disease-like phosphorylation of the microtubule-associated protien tau by glycogen synthase kinase-3 in transfected mammalian cells. Curr Biol 1994; 4: 1077–86.
5. Mulot SFC, Hughes K, Woodgett JR, Anderton BH, Hanger DP. PHF-tau from Alzheimer's brain comprises four species on SDS–PAGE which can be mimicked by *in vitro* phosphorylation of human brain tau by glycogen synthase kinase-3β. FEBS Lett 1994; 349: 359–64.
6. Latimer DA, Gallo J-M, Lovestone S, Miller CCJ, Reynolds CH, Marquardt B, Stabel S, Woodgett JR, Anderton BH. Stimulation of MAP kinase by *v-raf* transformation of fibroblasts fails to induce hyperphosphorylation of transfected tau. FEBS Lett 1995; 365: 42–6.
7. Davis DR, Anderton BH, Brion J-P, Reynolds CH, Hanger DP. Oxidative stress induces dephosphorylation of τ in rat brain primary neuronal cultures. J Neurochem 1997; 68: 1590–97.
8. Davis DR, Brion J-P, Couck A-M, Gallo J-M, Hanger DP, Ladhani K, Lewis C, Miller CCJ, Rupniak T, Smith C, Anderton BH. The phosphorylation state of the microtubule-associated protein tau as affected by glutamate, colchicine and β-amyloid in primary rat cortical neuronal cultures. Biochem J 1995; 309: 941–9.
9. Klein PS, Melton DA. A molecular mechanism for the effect of lithium on development. Proc Natl Acad Sci USA 1996; 93: 8455–9.
10. Stambolic V, Ruel L, Woodgett JR. Lithium inhibits glycogen synthase kinase-3 activity and mimics Wingless signalling in intact cells. Curr Biol 1996; 6: 1664–8.
11. Lovestone S, Davis DR, Webster M-T, Kaech S, Brion J-P, Matus A, Anderton BH. Lithium reduces glycogen synthase kinase-3 induced tau phosphorylation—effects in living cells and in neurons at therapeutic concentrations. Biol Psychiat 1998 (in press).

Address for correspondence:
Brian H. Anderton,
Department of Neuroscience, Institute of Psychiatry,
De Crespigny Park, London SE5 8AF, UK

33 Phosphorylation of Tau Protein in Interphase and Mitosis: Influence on Microtubules and Relationship with PHF-Tau in Alzheimer's Disease

S. ILLENBERGER, Q. ZHENG-FISCHHÖFER,
U. PREUSS, K. STAMER, R. GODEMANN, B. TRINCZEK,
J. BIERNAT, E.-M. MANDELKOW AND E. MANDELKOW

INTRODUCTION

The major function of the neuronal microtubule-associated protein tau is to stabilize axonal microtubules, which provide the basis for axonal transport and neuronal polarity. The hyperphosphorylation of tau and its aggregation into highly insoluble paired helical filaments (PHFs) are hallmarks of the neurofibrillary pathology in AD. PHF-tau isolated from AD brain tissue can no longer bind to microtubules due to its high state of phosphorylation [1]. Phosphorylation has been shown to be the key factor regulating MAP–microtubule interactions [2, 3], but little is known about the mechanisms leading to the increase of tau phosphorylation in AD. In a previous investigation we had shown that tau phosphorylation increases seven-fold during mitosis, concomitant with detachment from microtubules. Part of this phosphorylation can be monitored with diagnostic phosphorylation-dependent antibodies that recognize tau in mitotic cells only [4]. To analyze tau phosphorylation more comprehensively, we have now metabolically radiolabeled CHO cells stably transfected with the longest human tau isoform and LAN5, a human neuroblastoma cell line that expresses tau endogenously. In non-synchronized cultures, the phosphorylation pattern was remarkably similar in both cell lines. Of the total phosphate incorporated, we were able to attribute ~80% to 17 phosphorylation sites, most of which are in SP or TP motifs, except S214 and S262. In cells arrested in mitosis by

Alzheimer's Disease and Related Disorders
Edited by K. Iqbal, D.F. Swaab, B. Winblad and H.M. Wisniewski
© 1999 John Wiley & Sons Ltd

nocodazol, phosphorylation increases mainly in phosphopeptides containing T153, T181, S202/T205, T212/T217, S235 and S214. Most of these represent SP or TP motifs and are compatible with the activation of the cell-cycle kinase cdc2. However, S214 is a prominent non-proline-directed phosphorylation site, enhanced in mitosis, which can be phosphorylated by PKA *in vitro*. Phosphorylation at this site detaches tau from microtubules and prevents microtubule nucleation *in vitro*. This site is also part of the epitope of AT100, a highly specific antibody recognizing PHF-tau only. The epitope is formed by the sequential phosphorylation, first of T212 by GSK-3, then of S214 by PKA, suggesting the concerted action of these kinases in AD [6].

MATERIALS AND METHODS

All materials and methods have recently been published [7]. In brief, the cell lines used in this study were CHO cells stably over-expressing the longest human tau isoform [4] and LAN-5 neuroblastoma cells [8]. A polyclonal anti-tau (DAKO) and monoclonal anti-tubulin antibody DM1A (Sigma) were used for immunofluorescence. Immunofluorescence and metabolic labeling was performed as described [4, 7]. Thin layer electrophoresis/chromatography was essentially carried out as described [9]. The antibody AT100 was kindly provided by E. Van Mechelen (Innogenetics SA, Ghent, Belgium).

RESULTS

IDENTIFICATION OF PHOSPHORYLATION SITES

From our earlier immunocytochemical studies in CHO stably over-expressing tau [4], we knew that tau was phosphorylated in interphase and became more highly phosphorylated during mitosis. To determine the phosphorylation sites we analyzed tau from transfected CHO cells and endogenous tau protein from LAN5 neuroblastoma cells after metabolic labeling with ^{32}P-phosphoric acid. The two patterns were remarkably similar (Figure 1A, B), suggesting a similar balance of kinases and phosphatases with respect to tau protein. With radio-labeled reference, phosphopeptides that had been generated by *in vitro* phosphorylation of recombinant tau with cdc2, CDK5, MAPK, GSK3β, PKA and MARK [7], we identified 17 phosphorylation sites containing ~80% of the total phosphate incorporated. Most of the sites were of the SP or TP type located in the proline-rich domain of the protein. The only non-proline-directed sites were S214 and S262, the latter being the only phosphorylation site identified in the repeat domain (Figure 1C).

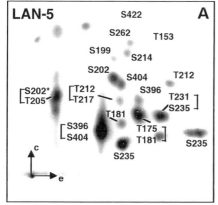

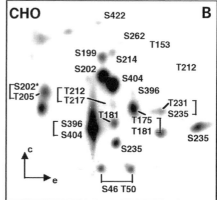

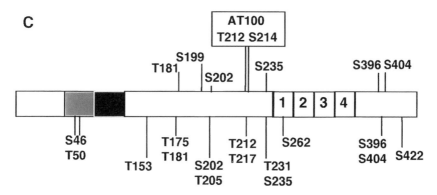

Figure 1. Analysis of tau phosphorylation in LAN-5 and CHO cell lines by 2-D thin layer electrophoresis/chromatography; 1000 cpm were loaded per sample and detected via autoradiography. (A) Tryptic digest of endogenous tau protein immunoprecipitated from LAN-5 cells. (B) Analysis of tau protein immunoprecipitated from stably transfected CHO cells. (C) Bar diagram of the longest human tau isoform showing all *in vivo* phosphorylation sites identified in this study, as well as the phospho-epitope of the PHF-specific antibody AT100 (T212/S214)

A SIGNIFICANT FRACTION OF TAU PROTEIN DETACHES FROM MICROTUBULES DURING MITOSIS

To see whether the increase in tau phosphorylation during mitosis is also accompanied by reduced binding of tau to microtubules, we transfected CHO cells with a GFP–tau fusion protein to be able to monitor living cells. In interphase cells (Figure 2A, left panel), most GFP–tau is bound to microtubules. In contrast, mitotic cells (Figure 2A, right panel) show significant cytosolic fluorescence besides staining of the mitotic spindle. Similar observations were made when CHO cells stably over-expressing the longest human

304

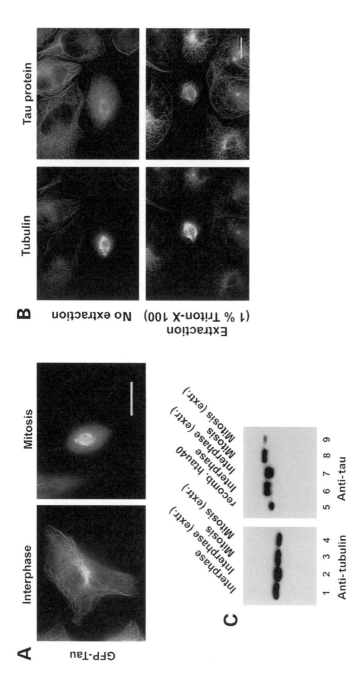

Figure 2. Tau–microtubule interactions during mitosis. (A) Living CHO cell expressing GFP-tau in interphase (left) and metaphase (right). (B) Immunofluorescence analysis of tau-stable CHO cells without (upper panels) and after extraction (low panels) with Triton-X 100. (C) Western blot analysis

tau isoform were fixed with methanol and tau or microtubules were visualized by indirect immunofluorescence (Figure 2B, upper panels). If the cells were treated with 1% Triton-X 100 for 1 min prior to fixation (Figure 2B, lower panel), tau immunofluorescence in interphase cells essentially remained unaffected, whereas in mitotic cells only the cytosolic stain was extracted, so that the mitotic spindle became the only prominent feature in these cells. To obtain an estimate of how much tau protein was extracted from mitotic cells, Western blot analyses were performed on cell extracts from interphase and from nocodazole-treated mitotic cells, either without extraction or after treatment with 1% Triton-X 100. Tubulin levels remained essentially the same, irrespective of cell cycle phase and treatment (Figure 2C, left panel). Extraction, however, had a dramatic effect on mitotic cells, reducing tau to ~22%. Consistent with the immunofluorescence, this is equivalent to the fraction of tau that remains associated with the mitotic spindle.

cdc2 AND PKA ARE CANDIDATE KINASES FOR THE MITOTIC PHOSPHORYLATION OF TAU

Synchronization with nocodazole arrests cells mainly in metaphase [10]. 2D phosphopeptide analysis of nocodazole-treated cells, where metaphase cells were separated from the interphase cells by mechanical shake-off, revealed a major increase in the phosphopeptides (Figure 3) containing T181, S202/T205, T212/T217, S235, S214 and two further putative proline-directed sites (arrows Figure 3B). The phosphorylation pattern most closely resembled that of cdc2 generated *in vitro*, making this cell cycle-dependent kinase a likely candidate for the mitotic phosphorylation of tau. S214 is the major phosphorylation site of PKA *in vitro* [7], consistent with the observation that PKA may be involved in cell cycle progression [11].

THE MITOTIC PHOSPHORYLATION SITE S214 STRONGLY AFFECTS THE TAU–MICROTUBULE INTERACTION

Phosphorylation at proline-directed sites has only moderate effects on the tau–microtubule interaction, in contrast to phosphorylation at S262 in the first repeat phosphorylated by MARK [2, 12, 13]. Since S214 is another non-proline-directed site, we wanted to assess the effect of S214 phosphorylation on microtubule assembly. Under appropriate conditions, PKA, stoichiometrically phosphorylates tau protein only at S214 [7]. Using dark-field video microscopy, we observed that phosphorylation of S214 prevents the nucleation of microtubules (Figure 4, left). In contrast, a tau mutant where S214 had been converted into alanine showed no changes, irrespective of the phosphorylation of other sites by PKA (Figure 4, right). These data argue that the mitotic phosphorylation of S214 is likely to play a role in the observed

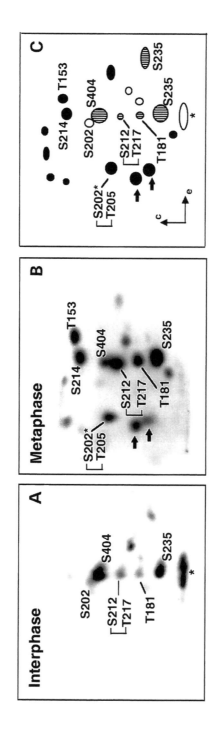

Figure 3. 2-D phosphopeptide analysis of tau-transfected CHO cells in interphase and metaphase after mitotic arrest with 0.4 μg/ml nocodazole (5 h). (A) Interphase. (B) Metaphase. (C) Schematic diagram of phosphopeptides. Open circles represent phosphopeptides present in interphase only, closed circles show mitotic phosphorylation sites, shaded circles are constitutively phosphorylated sites

detachment of tau from microtubules during mitosis and the concomitant increase in MT dynamics.

THE EPITOPE OF THE ALZHEIMER-SPECIFIC ANTIBODY AT100 IS GENERATED BY SEQUENTIAL PHOSPHORYLATION

Many of the antibodies raised against PHF-tau recognize phosphorylated SP or TP motifs. This type of phosphorylation by proline-directed kinases is prominent in AD but occurs to some extent in normal tissue as well [5]. Antibody AT100 is one of the few exceptions, in that it reacts uniquely with PHF-tau. The epitope was shown to depend on a complex reaction [6]: it requires a PHF-like conformation induced by polyanions (such as RNA, poly-Glu or heparin), phosphorylation of T212 by GSK-3, and then phosphorylation of S214 by PKA. Reversing this order fails to induce the epitope. This suggests a specific sequential interaction between tau and the two kinases, which appears to be characteristic of degenerating neurons only.

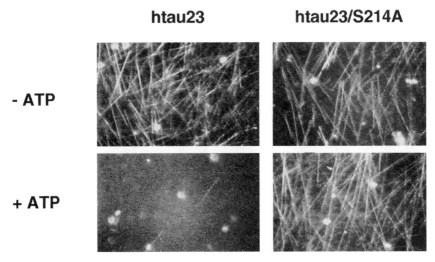

Figure 4. Phosphorylation of tau at S214 by PKA inhibits microtubule assembly. Dark-field video microscopy of microtubules in the presence of 10 µM recombinant tau (left panels) or S214A tau mutant (right panels), each unphosphorylated (upper panels) or prephosphorylated by PKA (lower panels) in the presence of 2 mM ATP

DISCUSSION

There is increasing evidence that mitotic mechanisms may be involved in the abnormal phosphorylation of tau in AD neurons: tau from fetal brain tissue, still undergoing cell division, has an elevated phosphate content and is recognized by diagnostic AD antibodies (reviewed in [14]). In several cell lines the phosphorylation of tau is elevated during mitosis, mimicking PHF-tau [4, 7, 15]. cdc2 Kinase is associated with PHFs [16] and postmitotic neuronal cells undergo apoptosis under conditions where mitosis is re-initiated [17]. Furthermore, there must be a general link between mitosis and apoptosis that seems to converge at the level of cyclin-dependent kinases [18], and apoptosis may indeed be elevated in AD brain tissue [19]. Our results further strengthen the hypothesis that, due to some hitherto un-known insult, postmitotic neurons in the AD brain reactivate some of the cell cycle machinery. Most phosphorylation sites found to be phosphory-lated during the cell cycle are also phosphorylated in PHF-tau [20], consis-tent with the fact that most PHF-antibodies recognize tau in mitotic cells. Furthermore, the MPM2 antibody directed against mitotic epitopes stains PHFs in AD tissue [15].

In contrast to our expectations, based on earlier investigations [2, 3], S262 is not phosphorylated in metaphase. However, since it has been identified as a phosphorylation site in non-synchronized cells (Figure 1), it may well play a role in a different mitotic phase. In comparison with phosphorylation of S262 by MARK (which causes microtubule disruption *in vitro* and *in vivo*), phosphorylated S214 has a smaller effect on the tau–microtubule interaction [3, 7, 13]. Since in prophase microtubule dynamics are highest and tubulin polymer levels are lowest [21], it is tempting to speculate that phosphorylation of S262 by MARK might be involved in the observed drop in tubulin polymer during prophase, but it remains to be shown that MARK activity is cell cycle-regulated. From our data we conclude that in metaphase tau becomes mainly phosphorylated by cdc2 and PKA. In this context it is interesting to note that another regulatory protein of MT dynamics, Op18/stathmin, is also regulated by the same combination of kinases during mitosis [22]. Taken together, the identification of S214 as a prominent phosphorylation site in mitosis, which also detaches tau from microtubules *in vitro*, we have provided another strong hint toward mitotic mechanisms in AD. Finally, phosphorylated S214 has now been identified to be part of the epitope of AT100, an antibody highly specific for PHF-tau [6]. It recognizes phosphorylation at T212 and S214 (see Figure 1), which can be achieved *in vitro* only by sequential phosphorylation by PKA and GSK3β. These results will provide tools to study the question of why the phosphorylation of tau in mitosis and the effects on microtubule dynamics show the striking similarity to that of PHF-tau in degenerating neurons in AD.

REFERENCES

1. Grundke-Iqbal I, Iqbal K, Tung Y, Quinlan M, Wisniewski H, Binder L. Abnormal phosphorylation of the microtubule-associated protein tau in Alzheimer cytoskeletal pathology. Proc Natl Acad Sci USA 1986; 83: 4913–17.
2. Biernat J, Gustke N, Drewes G, Mandelkow E-M, Mandelkow E. Phosphorylation of Ser262 strongly reduces binding of tau-protein to microtubules—distinction between PHF-like immunoreactivity and microtubule-binding. Neuron 1993; 11: 153–63.
3. Drewes G, Ebneth A, Preuss U, Mandelkow E-M, Mandelkow M. MARK, a novel family of protein kinases that phosphorylate microtubule-associated proteins and trigger microtubule disruption. Cell 1997; 89: 297–308.
4. Preuss U, Döring F, Illenberger S, Mandelkow E-M. Cell cycle-dependent phosphorylation and microtubule-binding of tau-protein stably transfected into chinese hamster ovary cells. Mol Biol Cell 1995; 6: 1397–1410.
5. Matsuo ES, Shin RW, Billingsley ML, Vandevoorde A, Oconnor M, Trojanowski JQ, Lee VM-Y. Biopsy-derived adult human brain tau is phosphorylated at many of the same sites as Alzheimer's disease paired helical filament tau. Neuron 1994; 13: 989–1002.
6. Zheng-Fischhöfer Q, Biernat J, Mandelkow E-M, Illenberger S, Godemann R, Mandelkow E. Sequential phosphorylation of tau protein by GSK3β and protein kinase A at Thr212 and Ser214 generates the Alzheimer-specific epitope of antibody AT100 and requires a paired helical filament-like conformation. Eur J Biochem 1998; 252: 542–52.
7. Illenberger S, Zheng-Fischhöfer Q, Preuss U, Stamer K, Baumann K, Trinczek B, Biernat J, Godemann R, Mandelkow E-M, Mandelkow E. The endogenous and cell cycle-dependent phosphorylation of tau protein in living cells: implications for Alzheimer's disease. Mol Biol Cell 1998; 9: 1495–1512.
8. Seeger R, Danon Y, Rayner S, Hoover F. Definition of a Thy-1 determinant on human neuroblastoma, glioma, sarcoma and teratoma cells with a monoclonal antibody. J Immunol 1982; 128: 983–9.
9. Boyle WJ, van der Geer P, Hunter T. Phosphopeptide mapping and phosphoamino acid analysis by two-dimensional separation on thin-layer cellulose plates. Methods Enzymol 1991; 201: 110–49.
10. Jordan M, Thrower D, Wilson L. Effects of vinblastine, podophyllotoxin and nocodazole on mitotic spindles. Implications for the role of microtubule dynamics in mitosis. J Cell Sci 1992; 102: 401–16.
11. Grieco D, Porcellini A, Avvedimento EV, Gottesmann ME. Requirement for cAMP-PKA pathway activation by Mphase promoting factor in the transition from mitosis to interphase. Science 1996; 271: 1718–23.
12. Trinczek B, Biernat J, Baumann K, Mandelkow E-M, Mandelkow E. Domains of tau protein, differential phosphorylation, and dynamic instability of microtubules. Mol Biol Cell 1995; 6: 1887–1902.
13. Drewes G, Trinczek B, Illenberger S, Biernat J, Schmitt-Ulms G, Meyer HE, Mandelkow E-M, Mandelkow E. Microtubule-associated protein/microtubule affinity regulating kinase (p110mark)—a novel protein-kinase that regulates tau–microtubule interactions and dynamic instability by phosphorylation at the Alzheimer-specific site serine-262. J Biol Chem 1985; 270: 7679–88.
14. Friedhoff P, Mandelkow E. Tau protein. In: Kreis Th, Vale R (eds) Guidebook of the Cytoskeletal and Motor Proteins. Oxford: Oxford University Press, 1998 (in press).

15. Vincent I, Rosado M, Davies P. Mitotic mechanisms in Alzheimer's disease? J Cell Biol 1996; 132: 413–25.
16. Vincent I, Jicha G, Rosado M, Dickson DW. Aberrant expression of mitotic cdc2/cyclin b1 kinase in degenerating neurons of Alzheimer's disease brain. J Neurosci 1997; 17: 3588–98.
17. Farinelli SE, Greene LA. Cell cycle blockers mimosine, ciclopirox, and deferoxamine prevent the death of PC12 cells and postmitotic sympathetic neurons after removal of trophic support. J Neurosci 1996; 16: 1150–62.
18. Pandey S, Wang E. Cells en route to apoptosis are characterized by the upregulation of c-fos, c-myc, c-jun, cdc2, and RB phosphorylation, resembling events of early cell-cycle traverse. J Cell Biochem 1995; 58: 135–50.
19. Smale G, Nichols NR, Brady DR, Finch CE, Horton WE. Evidence for apoptotic cell death in Alzheimer's disease. Exp Neurol 1995; 133: 225–30.
20. Morishima-Kawashima M, Hasegawa M, Takio K, Suzuki M, Yoshida H, Titani K, Ihara Y. Proline-directed and non-proline-directed phosphorylation of PHF-tau. J Biol Chem 1995; 270: 823–9.
21. Zhai Y, Borisy GG. Quantitative determination of the proportion of microtubule polymer present during the mitosis interphase transition. J Cell Sci 1994; 107: 881–90.
22. Gradin H, Larsson N, Marklund U, Gullberg M. Regulation of microtubule dynamics by extracellular signals: cAMP-dependent protein kinase switches off the activity of oncoprotein 18 in intact cells. J Cell Biol 1998; 140: 131–41.

Address for correspondence:
S. Illenberger,
Max Planck Research Unit for Structural Molecular Biology,
Notkestr. 85, D-22603 Hamburg, Germany
Tel: +49 40 89982810; fax: +49 40 89716822;
e-mail: mand@mpasmb.desy.de

34 Protein Kinase-A and Glycogen Synthase Kinase-3 in Combination Hyperphosphorylate Tau to an Alzheimer's Disease-like State

JIAN-ZHI WANG, INGE GRUNDKE-IQBAL AND
KHALID IQBAL

INTRODUCTION

In Alzheimer's disease (AD), the neuronal cytoskeleton is disrupted and re-placed by accumulation of tangles of paired helical filaments (PHFs), resulting in retrograde degeneration of the neurons and thereby dementia. The major protein subunit of PHFs is the abnormally phosphorylated and glycosylated microtubule-associated protein tau [1–2]. Two functions have been described for tau based on its ability to interact with tubulin: microtubule assembly-promoting activity *in vitro* [3–4] and microtubule-stabilizing activity *in vivo* [5]. Phosphorylation of tau depresses its ability to promote the *in vitro* assembly of microtubules [6]. AD abnormally phosphorylated tau is not only microtubule-assembly incompetent [7–9] but also inhibits assembly and dis-assembles the preassembled microtubules *in vitro* [10–12]. In the tangle-bearing neurons in the AD brain, the normal cytoskeleton is disrupted and replaced with PHFs. Thus, it is likely that the abnormal hyperphosphorylation of tau in the AD brain leads to the depolymerization of microtubules, impaired axonal transport and neuronal degeneration [12].

The protein kinases involved and the phosphorylation sites responsible for this malfunction of tau are currently not understood. Phosphorylation at ser-262 is re-ported to cause the decreased microtubule binding of tau [13–14]. However, phosphorylation of ser-262 only induces about 40% inhibition in microtubule-binding activity [15], suggesting that phosphorylation of other sites is necessary to completely inhibit its biological activity. The effect of these phosphorylations on the biological activity of tau and the sites phosphorylated are, however, not known.

Alzheimer's Disease and Related Disorders
Edited by K. Iqbal, D.F. Swaab, B. Winblad and H.M. Wisniewski
© 1999 John Wiley & Sons Ltd

Twenty-one phosphorylation sites in PHF-tau have been identified using reactivity with antibodies to various phosphorylation sites and protein sequencing techniques. Among them, 10 sites are on ser/thr-pro motifs and 11 are on non-ser/thr-pro motifs [16–17]. The ser/thr-pro and non-ser/thr-pro sites are probably phosphorylated by proline-dependent protein kinases (PDPKs) and non-PDPKs, respectively. The various PDPKs and non-PDPKs that can phosphorylate tau include MAP kinase [18–19] cdc-2 kinase [20], cdk-2, cdk-5 [21] and GSK-3 [22–24]. The non-PDPKs include A-kinase [25–27], C-kinase [26–29], CaM kinase II [26, 27, 30], CK-1 [26, 27] and CK-2 [26, 31]. The interaction of PDPK and non-PDPK in tau hyperphosphorylation has been reported [27, 32]. However, the effect of these combination phosphorylations on the biological activity of tau and the sites phosphorylated were not mapped. We have investigated the effect of phosphorylation of tau by individual kinase or combination of kinases on the biological activity of tau and mapped the corresponding sites phosphorylated by these kinases (see [33]). In this article we review the details of these studies.

PHOSPHORYLATION OF TAU BY A COMBINATION OF PROTEIN KINASES

Human tau3L was separately incubated in the absence or presence of CK-1 (400 m units/ml), A-kinase (6 µg/ml) and GSK-3 (350 mU/ml) in a reaction mixture containing 1 mg/ml of tau, 7 mM $MgCl_2$, 12 mM 2-mercaptoethanol, 0.5 mM ATP, 20 mM Hepes (pH 7.5). Reaction was initiated by the addition of kinase. After incubation at 30 °C for 2 h, the reaction was stopped by heating at 95 °C for 5 min and denatured kinase removed by centrifugation (10 000 × g for 10 min). The phosphorylated heat-stable tau was also further phosphorylated with GSK-3 for 4 h at 30 °C. In order to determine the stoichiometry of phosphorylation in parallel, tau was phosphorylated using identical conditions as above except with [γ-^{32}P] ATP. In 2 h, the ^{32}P incorporation by CK-1, A-kinase and GSK-3 was determined to be 3.4, 1.1 and 1.2 mol/mol of tau, respectively, and the subsequent ^{32}P incorporation by GSK-3 in 4 h was 1.5 and 3.2 mol/mol in tau prephosphorylated by CK-1 and A-kinase, respectively. The data indicate a synergistic role between PDPKs (such as GSK-3) and non-PDPKs (such as A-kinase and CK-1) in tau phosphorylation.

EFFECT OF PHOSPHORYLATION ON MICROTUBULE BINDING AND ASSEMBLY ACTIVITIES OF TAU

We examined the effect of the phosphorylation of human tau3L by various kinases on its microtubule assembly-promoting and microtubule-binding activities. When acting singly, tau phosphorylated by different kinases inhibited microtubule assembly in the order of A-kinase > GSK-3 > CK-1-phosphorylated tau. A greater inhibition of microtubule assembly was observed when tau was phosphorylated by a combination of CK-1 and GSK-3 or A-kinase and GSK-3. Tau phosphorylated by the latter combination of kinases was most potent in inhibiting microtubule assembly (Figure 1). When viewed by electron microscopy, a large mass of microtubules was seen in the assembly promoted by non-kinase-treated taus, CK-1 phosphorylated tau, GSK-3 phosphorylated tau and A-kinase phosphorylated tau, whereas only an occasional microtubule was seen in the assembly promoted by CK-1 plus GSK-3 and A-kinase plus GSK-3-treated taus. We also examined the binding of tau to taxol-stabilized microtubules. When tau was phosphorylated by CK-1, GSK-3 or A-kinase acting alone, the subsequent binding of the phosphorylated tau to microtubules was decreased by ~10–13%. Like microtubule assembly seen in Figure 1, the strongest inhibition of binding of tau to microtubules was observed when tau was phosphorylated by a combination of CK-1 and GSK-3 (~39%) or A-kinase and GSK-3 (~50%) (Table 1). These data suggest that the maximal inhibition of tau function requires the concerted actions of both PDPKs and non-PDPKs.

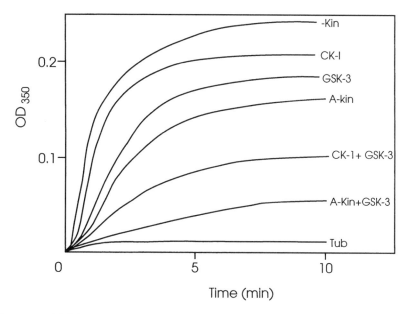

Figure 1. Inhibition of microtubule assembly promoting activity of tau phosphorylated by various kinases. Tau was phosphorylated with individual kinases A-kinase, GSK-3, CK-1 or CK-1 plus GSK-3, A-kinase plus GSK-3 combinations; tau, identically treated but without any kinase, served as a control. Reproduced from reference [33]

Table 1. Binding of different species of phosphorylated tau
to microtubules

Tau phosphorylated by	Tau bound (%)
None	94 ± 5.2
CK-1	87 ± 6.1
GSK-3	86 ± 4.6
A-kinase	81 ± 10.1
CK-1 + GSK-3	61 ± 5.2
A-kinase + GSK-3	50 ± 6.6

Reproduced from reference [33].

ISOLATION AND PURIFICATION OF ^{32}P-LABELED PHOSPHOPEPTIDES OF TAU

As described above, tau phosphorylated by the combination of A-kinase and GSK-3 was most effective in inhibiting microtubule assembly (Figure 1) and inhibition of binding to microtubules (Table 1). Hence, we chose to identify the sites phosphorylated in tau by this combination of kinases. Tau phosphorylated by GSK-3 alone was used as a control. Tau (0.3 mg) was first incubated in the absence or presence of A-kinase and non-radioactive ATP for 2 h. Reaction mixtures were then heated at 95 °C for 5 min to inactivate A-kinase and centrifuged. GSK-3 and [γ-^{32}P]ATP were then added to the tau, which is heat-stable and is recovered in the supernatant, and the incubation continued for another 4 h. Tau was then precipitated with trichloroacetic acid and digested with trypsin. After trypsin digestion, ^{32}P-labeled peptides were isolated by FeCl$_3$ affinity column chromatography. The recovery of ^{32}P peptides was about 97% for tau phosphorylated by a combination of A-kinase and GSK-3, and about 87% for tau phosphorylated by GSK-3 alone. The ^{32}P-labeled peptides eluted from the FeCl$_3$ affinity column were pooled, lyophilized, resuspended in 150 μl of 0.1% TFA and further purified by reverse-phase liquid chromatography (RPLC), using a C$_{18}$ column previously equilibrated in 0.1% TFA. Eight major radioactive peaks which contained phosphorylated tau sequences (labeled I–VIII) could be resolved on RPLC for A-kinase plus GSK-3 preparation. Under identical conditions, four radioactive tau peptides (labeled IX–XII) were seen in GSK-3 control alone.

MAPPING OF TAU SITES PHOSPHORYLATED BY A-KINASE PLUS GSK-3 AND BY GSK-3 ALONE

Analysis of the phosphopeptide peaks by high-voltage electrophoresis on thin-layer silicon plates revealed that peaks I–V and IX contained both p-ser and p-thr, whereas peaks VI–VIII and X–XII contained only p-ser. Amino acid sequence analysis and sequential manual Edman degradation of ^{32}P fractions isolated by RPLC demonstrated that S(p)GYS(p)S(p)PGS(p)PGT(p)PGSR, T(p)PPKS(p)PSSAK, IGS(p)TENLK, IGS(p)LDNITHVPGGGNK, SPV-VSGDTS(p)PR were the parent peptides containing the sites phosphorylated by A-kinase plus GSK-3, whereas T(p)PPS(p)SGEPPK, SPVVS(p) GDTSPR, IGS(p)TENLK and IGS(p)LDNITHVPGGGNK were the peptides that contained sites phosphorylated by GSK-3 alone. Peaks I and II had the same sequence of ser-198 to arg-209; only peptide I contained one more phosphorylation site (ser-202) than peptide II. Peaks III and IV shared the same sequence of ser-195 to arg-209. Peak IV might have been contaminated by a small amount of Peak III, which smeared a little on the RPLC separation; 'tailing' of this type is not uncommon. Peaks V, VI, VII and VIII represented tau fragments of thr-231 to lys-240, Ile-260 to lys-267, ser-396 to arg-406 and Ile-354 to lys-369, respectively. Peaks IX–XII corresponded to the sequences of thr-181 to lys-190, ser-396 to arg-406, Ile-260 to lys-267 and Ile-354 to lys-369, respectively. Alignment of the phosphorylated peptides of ^{32}P-tau by A-kinase plus GSK-3 demonstrated that the corresponding phosphorylated sites were ser-195, ser-198, ser-199, ser-202, thr-205, thr-231, ser-235, ser-262, ser-356 and ser-404 (Figure 2). By the same procedure, it was demonstrated that tau phosphorylated by GSK-3 alone generated sites at thr-181, ser-184, ser-262, ser-356 and ser-400 (Figure 2).

SUMMARY AND CONCLUSIONS

Previously, we have shown that both non-PDPKs and PDPKs phosphorylate tau at some of the same sites as in PHF-tau, as determined by immunoreactivity with phosphorylation-dependent tau antibodies [27, 34]. Furthermore, a prephosphorylation of tau by various non-PDPKs (A-kinase, C-kinase, CK-1 and CaM KII) served to stimulate a subsequent phosphorylation catalyzed by GSK-3. The highest level of such stimulation was obtained with tau 3L, which was prephosphorylated by A-kinase [27]. In the present study, we present further evidence that the interaction of A-kinase with GSK-3 phosphorylates tau at 8 of 21 sites seen in PHF-tau and markedly inhibits its ability to promote *in vitro* assembly and binding to microtubules. Our data demonstrated: (a) that A-kinase and GSK-3 combination induced a two- to three-fold higher incorporation of ^{32}P to tau than by GSK-3 alone; (b) that phosphorylation of tau with the combined kinases led to a most potent inhibition of biological activity of tau; and (c) that the A-kinase and GSK-3 combination was capable of phosphorylating at least 10 sites (ser-195, ser-198, ser-199, ser-202, thr-205, thr-231, ser-235, ser-262, ser-356 and ser-404), whereas GSK-3 alone only phosphorylated five sites (thr-181, ser-184, ser-262, ser-356 and ser-400) under identical conditions. Among the 21

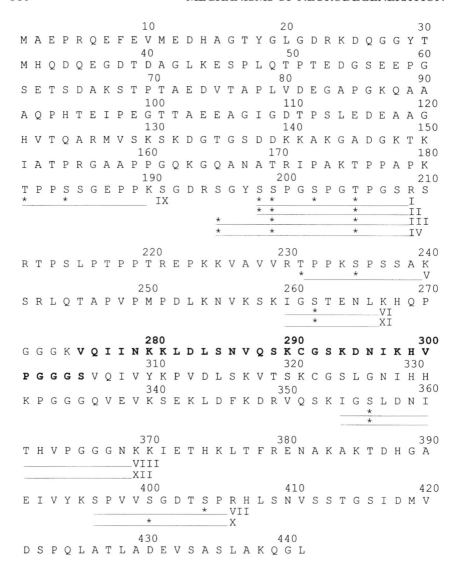

Figure 2. Alignment in tau sequence of the phosphopeptide identified from tau phosphorylated by A-kinase plus GSK-3 (I–VIII) or GSK-3 alone (IX–XII). Reproduced from reference [33]

phosphorylation sites (ser-46, ser-123, ser-198, ser-199, ser-202, thr-205, ser-208, ser-210, ser-212, ser-214, ser-231, ser-235, ser-262, ser-396, ser-400, ser-403, ser-404, ser-409, ser-412, ser-413 and ser-422) found in Alzheimer PHF-tau [17, 35–41], GSK-3 alone only phosphorylated ser-262 and ser-400, whereas an A-kinase and GSK-3 combination phosphorylated

Table 2. Comparison of sites phosphorylated by GSK-3 before and after phosphorylation of tau3L by A-kinase

Kinases	Phosphorylation sites	Tau source	Reference
A-kinase	Ser-214, ser-324, ser-356, ser-409, ser-416	τ3	[43]
GSK-3 (α)	Ser-235, ser-404	Bovine	[44]
GSK-3 (β)	Ser-199, thr-231, ser-396, ser-413	Bovine	[45]
GSK-3 (α + β)	Ser-181, ser-184, ser-262, ser-400	τ3L	Present work
A-kinase + GSK-3	Ser-195, ser-198, ser-199, ser-202, thr-205, thr-231, ser-235, ser-262, ser-356, ser-404	τ3L	

Reproduced from reference [33].

ser-198, ser-199, ser-202, thr-205, thr-231, ser-235, ser-262 and ser-404. These data suggest strongly that the interaction of A-kinase with GSK-3 generates a more AD-like state of tau, indicating that it might be a potential system involved in AD neuronal degeneration.

Phosphorylation of tau at specific sites inhibits the microtubule assembly and reduces the binding of tau to taxol-stabilized microtubules (see Figure 1 and Table 1). Dephosphorylation of PHF-tau restores the biological activity of tau in promoting the assembly of microtubules [7–9]. Recent studies report that ser-262 is a most potent site in regulating the binding of tau to microtubules [13]. Using recombinant tau3L as a substrate and reactivity with an antibody (12E8) to P-ser-262 and P-ser-356, we recently found that phosphorylation at ser-262 reduces only about 40% of microtubule binding as well as causing a slight inhibition of microtubule assembly-promoting activity of tau [15]. In the present study, we further demonstrated that a more effective inhibition was seen when in addition to ser-262, Alzheimer sites ser-198, ser-199, ser-202, thr-205, thr-231, ser-235 and ser-404 were also phosphorylated. It implied that phosphorylation of tau at the above-mentioned sites is involved in theregulation of biological activity of tau.

Phosphorylation of tau by individual kinases has been extensively studied recently. It has been found that a kinase phosphorylates different taus at different rates and sites. Such a differential phosphorylation exists between bovine tau and human tau, even among human tau isoforms ([27, 34, 42]. For instance, A-kinase phosphorylated tau3 at ser-214, ser-324, ser-356, ser-409 and ser-416 [43] whereas it phosphorylated tau4L at ser-262, ser-293, ser-305, ser-324 and ser-356 [14]. Using bovine tau (a mixture of six isoforms) as substrate, it was found that GSK-3α phosphorylated tau at ser-235 and ser-404 [44], while GSK-3β phosphorylated tau at ser-199, thr-231, ser-396 and ser-413 [45]. We have mapped biochemically the sites phosphorylated in human tau3L by GSK-3 and A-kinase plus GSK-3 which have not been reported previously (see Table 2).

In short, the present study revealed that phosphorylation of tau3L by various kinases differentially inhibits the biological activity of tau in microtubule assembly-promoting and microtubule-binding. The most potent-inhibition was seen in the combined phosphorylation of tau by A-kinase and GSK-3. Under these conditions, at least eight AD-like phosphorylation sites (ser-198, ser-199, ser-202, thr-231, ser-235, ser-262 and ser-404) were obtained, while only two of them (ser-262 and ser-400) were seen by GSK-3 alone. The interaction of A-kinase with GSK-3 might be one of the most potent systems responsible for the degeneration of neurons with neurofibrillary/tau pathology in Alzheimer's disease.

ACKNOWLEDGEMENTS

We are grateful to Dr A. Smith for his help in auto amino acid sequence analysis; to Dr T.J. Singh for his help in phosphorylation of tau; to Dr A. Sengupta for providing GSK-3; to the Biomedical Photography Unit for preparation of the figures; to Janet Biegelson for secretarial help. These studies were supported in part by the New York State Office of Mental Retardation and Developmental Disabilities and National Institutes of Health Grants AG05892, AG08076, NS18105 and TW00703.

REFERENCES

1. Grundke-Iqbal I, Iqbal K, Tung Y-C, Quinlan M, Wisniewski HM, Binder LI. Abnormal phosphorylation of the microtubule associated protein τ (tau) in Alzheimer cytoskeletal pathology. Proc Natl Acad Sci USA 1986; 83: 4913–17.
2. Wang J-Z, Grundke-Iqbal I, Iqbal K. Glycosylation of microtubule-associated protein tau: an abnormal posttranslational modification in Alzheimer's disease. Nature Med 1996; 2: 871–5.
3. Cleveland DW, Hwo SY, Kirschner MW. Physical and chemical properties of purified tau factor and the role of tau in microtubule assembly. J Mol Biol 1977; 116: 227–47.
4. Weingarten MD, Lockwood AH, Hwo SY, Kirschner MW. A protein factor essential for microtubule assembly. Proc Natl Acad Sci USA 1975; 72: 1858–62.
5. Drubin DG, Kirschner MW. Tau protein function in living cells. J Cell Biol 1986; 103: 2739–46.
6. Lindwall G, Cole RD. Phosphorylation affects the ability of tau protein to promote microtubule assembly. J Biol Chem 1984; 259: 5301–5.
7. Iqbal K, Zaidi T, Bancher C, Grundke-Iqbal I. Alzheimer paired helical filaments: restoration of the biological activity by dephosphorylation. FEBS Lett 1994; 349: 104–8.
8. Wang J-Z, Gong C-X, Zaidi T, Grundke-Iqbal I, Iqbal K. Dephosphorylation of Alzheimer paired helical filaments by protein phosphatase-2A and -2B. J Biol Chem 1995; 270: 4854–60.

9. Wang J-Z, Grundke-Iqbal I, Iqbal K. Restoration of biological activity of Alzheimer abnormally phosphorylated τ by dephosphorylation with protein phosphatase-2A, -2B and -1. Mol Brain Res 1996; 38: 200–208.

10. Alonso A del C, Zaidi T, Grundke-Iqbal I, Iqbal K. Role of abnormally phosphorylated tau in the breakdown of microtubules in Alzheimer disease. Proc Natl Acad Sci USA 1994; 91: 5562–6.

11. Alonso A del C, Grundke-Iqbal I, Iqbal K. Alzheimer's disease hyperphosphorylated tau sequesters normal tau into tangles of filaments and disassembles microtubules. Nature Med 1996; 2: 783–7.

12. Alonso A del C, Grundke-Iqbal I, Barra HS, Iqbal K. Abnormal phosphorylation of tau and the mechanism of Alzheimer neurofibrillary degeneration: sequestration of MAP1 and MAP2 and the disassembly of microtubules by the abnormal tau. Proc Natl Acad Sci USA 1997; 94: 298–303.

13. Biernat J, Gustke N, Drewes G, Mandelkow E-M, Mandelkow E. Phosphorylation of ser[262] strongly reduces binding of tau to microtubules: distinction between PHF-like immunoreactivity and microtubule binding. Neuron 1993; 11: 153–63.

14. Drewes G, Trinczek B, Illenberger S, Biernat J, Schmitt-Ulms G, Meyer HE, Mandelkow E-M, Mandelkow E. Microtubule-associated protein/microtubule affinity-regulating kinase (P110[mark]). J Biol Chem 1995; 270: 7679–88.

15. Singh TJ, Wang J-Z, Novák M, Kontzekova E, Grundke-Iqbal I, Iqbal K. Calcum/calmodulin-dependent protein kinase II phosphorylates tau at Ser-262 but only partially inhibits its binding to microtubules. FEBS Lett 1996; 387: 345–8.

16. Iqbal K, Grundke-Iqbal I. Alzheimer abnormally phosphorylated tau is more hyperphosphorylated than the fetal tau and causes the disruption of microtubules. Neurobiol Aging 1995; 16: 375–9.

17. Morishima-Kawashima M, Hasegawa M, Takio K, Suzuki M, Yoshida H, Titani K, Ihara Y. Proline-directed and non-proline-directed phosphorylation of PHF-tau. J Biol Chem 1995; 270: 823–9.

18. Drewes G, Lichtenberg-Kraag B, Döring F, Mandelkow E-M, Biernat J, Goris J, Dorée M, Mandelkow E. Mitogen activated protein (MAP) kinase transforms tau protein into an Alzheimer-like state. EMBO J 1992; 11: 2131–8.

19. Goedert M, Cohen ES, Jakes R, Cohen P. P[42] map kinase phosphorylation sites in microtubule-associated protein tau are dephosphorylated by protein phosphatase $2A_1$: implications for Alzheimer's disease. FEBS Lett 1992; 312: 95–9.

20. Vulliet R, Halloran SM, Braun RK, Smith AJ, Lee G. Proline-directed phosphorylation of human tau protein. J Biol Chem 1992; 267: 22570–74.

21. Baurnann K, Mandelkow E-M, Biernat J, Piwnica-Worms H, Mandelkow E. Abnormal Alzheimer-like phosphorylation of tau protein by cyclin-dependent kinase cdk2 and cdk5. FEBS Lett 1993; 336: 417–24.

22. Mandelkow E-M, Drewes G, Biernat J, Gustke N, Lint JV, Vandenheede JR, Mandelkow E. Glycogen synthase kinase-3 and the Alzheimer-like state of microtubule-associated protein tau. FEBS Lett 1992; 314: 315–21.

23. Yang SD, Song JS, Shiah SG. Protein kinase F_A/GSK-3 phosphorylates τ on Ser[235]-Pro and Ser[404]-Pro that are abnormally phosphorylated in Alzheimer's disease brain. J Neurochem 1993; 61: 1742–7.

24. Ishiguro K, Shiratsuchi Sato S, Omori A, Arioka M, Kobayashi S, Uchida T, Imahori K. Glycogen synthase kinase 3β is identical to tau protein kinase I generating several epitopes of paired helical filaments. FEBS Lett 1993; 325: 167–72.

25. Litersky JM, Johnson GVW. Phosphorylation by cAMP-dependent protein kinase inhibits the degradation of tau by calpain. J Biol Chem 1992; 267: 1563–8.

26. Singh TJ, Grundke-Iqbal I, McDonald B, Iqbal K. Comparison of the phosphorylation of microtubule associated protein tau by non-proline dependent protein kinases. Mol Cell Biochem 1994; 131: 181–9.

27. Singh TJ, Zaidi T, Grundke-Iqbal I, Iqbal K. Modulation of GSK-3-catalyzed phosphorylation of microtubule-associated protein tau by non-proline-dependent protein kinases. FEBS Lett 1995; 358: 4–8.
28. Baudier J, Lee SH, Cole RD. Separation of the different microtubule associated tau protein species from bovine brain and their mode II phosphorylation by Ca^{2+}/phospholipid-dependent protein kinase C. J Biol Chem 1987; 262: 17584–90.
29. Correas I, Diaz-Nido J, Avila J. Microtubule-associated protein tau is abnormally phosphorylated by protein kinase C on its tubulin binding domain. J Biol Chem 1992; 267: 15721–8.
30. Baudier J, Cole D. Phosphorylation of tau proteins to a state like that in Alzheimer's brain is catalyzed by a calcium/calmodulin-dependent kinase and modulated by phospholipids. J Biol Chem 1987; 262: 17577–83.
31. Greenwood JA, Scott CW, Spreen RC, Claudia B, Johnson GVW. Casein kinase II preferentially phosphorylates human tau isoforms containing an amino-terminal insert. J Biol Chem 1994; 269: 4373–80.
32. Sengupta A, Wu QL, Grundke-Iqbal I, Iqbal K, Singh TJ. Potentiation of GSK-3-activated Alzheimer-like phosphorylation of human tau by cdk5. Mol Cell Biochem 1997; 167: 99–105.
33. Wang J-Z, Wu QL, Smith A, Grundke-Iqbal I, Iqbal K. τ is phosphorylated by GSK-3 at several sites found in Alzheimer disease and its biological activity markedly inhibited only after it is prephosphorylated by A-kinase. FEBS Lett 1998; 436: 28–34.
34. Sing TJ, Zaidi T, Grundke-Iqbal I, Iqbal K. Non-proline-dependent protein kinases phosphorylate several sites found in tau from Alzheimer disease brain. Mol Cell Biochem 1996; 154: 43–151.
35. Iqbal K, Grundke-Iqbal I, Smith AJ, George L, Tung Y-C, Zaidi T. Identification and localization of a tau peptide to paired helical filaments of Alzheimer disease. Proc Natl Acad Sci USA 1989; 86: 5646–50.
36. Hasegawa M, Morishima-Kawashima M, Takio K, Suzuki M, Titani K, Ihara Y. Protein sequence and mass spectrometric analyses of tau in the Alzheimer's disease brain. J Biol Chem 1992; 267: 17047–54.
37. Lee VM-Y, Balin BJ, Otvos L Jr, Trojanowski JQ. A68: a major subunit of paired helical filaments and derivatized forms of normal tau. Science 1991; 251: 675–8.
38. Biernat J, Mandelkow E-M, Schröter C, Lichtenberg-Kraag B, Steiner B, Berling B, Meyer H, Mercken M, Vandermeeren A, Goedert M, Mandelkow E. The switch of tau protein to an Alzheimer-like state includes the phosphorylation of two serine-proline motifs upstream of the microtubule binding region. EMBO J 1992; 11: 1593–7.
39. Goedert M, Jakes R, Crowther RA, Six J, Lübke U, Vandermeeren M, Cras P, Trojanowski JQ, Lee VM-Y. The abnormal phosphorylation of tau protein at Ser-202 in Alzheimer disease recapitulates phosphorylation during development. Proc Natl Acad Sci USA 1993; 90: 5066–70.
40. Liu WK, Moore WT, Williams RT, Hall FL, Yen SH. Application of synthetic phospho- and unphospho-peptides to identify phosphorylation sites in a subregion of the tau molecule which is modified in Alzheimer's disease. J Neurosci Res 1993; 34: 371–6.
41. Lang E, Szendrei IG, Lee VM-Y, Otvos L Jr. Immunological and conformational characterization of a phosphorylated immunodominant epitope on the paired helical filaments found in Alzheimer's disease. Biochem Biophys Res Comm 1992; 187: 783–90.
42. Singh TJ, Grundke-Iqbal I, Wu QL, Chauhan V, Novák M, Kontzekova E, Iqbal K. Protein kinase C and calcium/calmodulin-dependent protein kinase II phosphorylate three repeat and four repeat tau isoforms at different rates. Mol Cell Biochem 1997; 167: 141–8.

43. Scott CW, Vulliet PR, Caputo CB. Phosphorylation of tau by proline-directed protein kinase (P34^{cdc2}/P58^{cyclinA}) decreases tau-induced microtubule assembly and antibody SMI33 reactivity. Brain Res 1993; 611: 237–42.

44. Yang SD, Song JS, Hsieh YT, Liu HW, Chan WH. Identification of the ATP Mg-dependent protein phosphatases activator (F_A) as a synapsin I kinase that inhibits cross-linking of synapsin I with brain microtubules. J Protein Chem 1992; 11: 539–46.

45. Ishiguro K, Takamatsu M, Tomizawa K, Omori A, Takahashi M, Arioka M, Uchida T, Imahori K. Tau protein kinase I converts normal tau protein into A68-like component of paired helical filaments. J Biol Chem 1992; 267: 10897–901.

Address for correspondence:
   Dr Khalid Iqbal,
   Chemical Neuropathology Laboratory,
   NYS Institute for Basic Research in Developmental Disabilities,
   1050 Forest Hill Road, Staten Island, New York 10314–6399, USA
   Tel: 718 494 5259; fax: 718 494 1080;
   e-mail: <kiqbal@admin.con2.com>

35 Association of Presenilin 1 with Glycogen Synthase Kinase-3β and Its Substrate Tau

A. TAKASHIMA, M. MURAYAMA, O. MURAYAMA, T. HONDA, T. TOMITA AND T. IWATSUBO

INTRODUCTION

The neuropathological diagnosis of Alzheimer's disease (AD) requires the presence of both senile plaques and neurofibrillary tangles (NFT) [1]. Senile plaques are largely composed of amyloid β-protein (Aβ), while NFT are composed of hyperphosphorylated tau organized into paired helical filaments (PHF) [2–4]. Mutations on PS1 cause an early-onset form of AD with an autosomal dominant inheritance pattern [5–8]. The role of PS1 in AD is particularly interesting because it has a strong causal connection with the disease; genetic studies show that mutations for PS1 exhibit 100% penetrance in causing AD [8], but the mechanism itself is still unclear. Mutations in presenilins affect Aβ processing. Recent studies indicate that cell lines, transgenic mice or patients expressing mutant forms of PS1 show a selective increase in production of $A\beta_{1-42}$ [9–11]. Mutations in the presenilins also activate apoptotic pathways and render neurons more vulnerable to stressors, such as Aβ neurotoxicity [12–15]. These findings suggest that mutant PS1 affects both APP processing and apoptosis. To better understand the mechanism underlying PS1 mutation and the development of AD, we investigated PS1 proteins.

RELATIONSHIP BETWEEN PS1 AND Aβ

To investigate the relationship between PS1 mutations and $A\beta_{1-42}$ secretion, we examined the level of Aβ secretion in COS-1 cells doubly transfected with cDNAs encoding β-APP695 and 31 PS1 mutations. The level of each Aβ40 and $A\beta_{1-42}$ in conditioned medium was determined by the two-site ELISAs

Alzheimer's Disease and Related Disorders
Edited by K. Iqbal, D.F. Swaab, B. Winblad and H.M. Wisniewski
© 1999 John Wiley & Sons Ltd

using a combination of monoclonal antibodies BAN77 with BAN27 for Aβ40, and BC05 for $A\beta_{1-42}$. Although Aβ in conditioned media is not detected in PS1 transfection or vector transfection, cells doubly transfected with β-APP695 and PS1 wild-type cDNA or a single transfection of β-APP695 show a detectable amount of Aβ40 and $A\beta_{1-42}$, and in both cases $A\beta_{1-42}$ was approximately 11% of the total released Aβ in the conditioned media, indicating that wild-type PS1 expression did not affect β-APP processing. All PS1 mutations significantly increased the $A\beta_{1-42}$ ratio up to four times more than wild-type, the extent of the increase being dependent upon each PS1 mutation (Figure 1A). If only $A\beta_{1-42}$ secretion were the cause of AD, the age of onset would be dependent on the level of $A\beta_{1-42}$ secretion. However, $A\beta_{1-42}$ processing and onset age are not strictly correlated (Figure 1B). These results suggest that the increased $A\beta_{1-42}$ secretion is a factor for development of AD, but not on its own the cause of onset of AD.

CORRELATION OF PS1, GSK-3β AND TAU

Comparison of PS1 and AD-related proteins in human brains revealed the correlations levels of PS1, tau and GSK-3β.

In order to investigate the interactions of PS1 with tau and GSK-3β *in vivo*, we investigated whether these proteins were associated during immunoprecipitation (Figure 2). PS1 was immunoprecipitated from Triton-X 100 extracts of human brain using a MKAD3.4 affinity column. PS1 was eluted from the column in fractions 1 and 2, using a buffer containing 0.1 M glycine/ HCl (pH 2.5) (Figure 2A); no PS1 was observed in the flow-through or wash (F or W, Figure 2A). The same fractions were then examined using the anti-tau antibody, JM (Figure 2B) and the anti-GSK-3β antibody (Figure 2C). Although most of the tau and GSK-3β reactivity was in the flow-through, a small amount of reactivity for both proteins co-eluted with PS1 (Figure 2B, C). The JM that co-eluted with PS1 showed a set of bands in the 50–70 kDa range characteristic of tau (Figure 2B). The anti-GSK-3β reactivity that co-eluted with PS1 showed a 47 kDa band characteristic of GSK-3β (Figure 2C). Omission of primary antibody from the immunoblots eliminated the bands (Figure 2B, C, lane 4). Pre-absorption of the JM antibody with recombinant human tau eliminated all reactivity (Figure 2D, lane 2). Probing the eluates with three unrelated antibodies, anti-neuron specific enolase (NSE), anti-amyloid protein precursor (APP) and anti-MAP kinase (Figure 2E), produced no reaction in the eluate fraction, indicating that the tau and GSK-3β reactivity that was present represented genuine associations with PS1. Although Xia et al. [16] reported that APP directly bound to PS1, our experiment did not show any immunoreactivity for APP (Figure 2E). Possibly this is because the affinities of PS1 with tau and GSK-3β are higher than that of PS1 with APP.

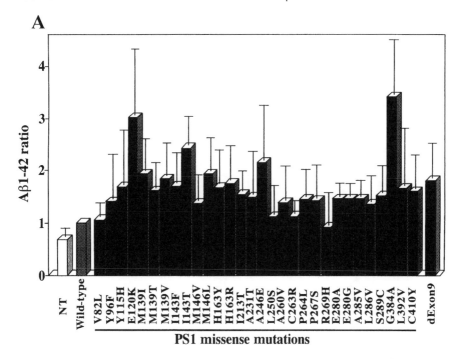

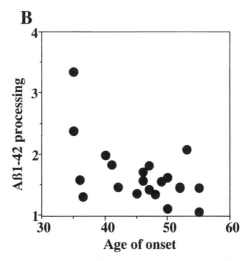

Figure 1. Relationship between $A\beta_{1-42}$ secretion and age of onset in PS1 mutation. (A) The level of each Aβ40 and $A\beta_{1-42}$ in conditioned medium was determined by the two-site ELISAs using a combination of monoclonal antibodies, BAN77 with BAN27, for Aβ40 or BC05 for $A\beta_{1-42}$. $A\beta_{1-42}$ ratio in mutant PS1 was represented as relative to PS1 wild-type. (B) $A\beta_{1-42}$ processing and the corresponding age of onset was plotted and analyzed by linear regression (slope of regression line = −0.04, R^2 = 0.28)

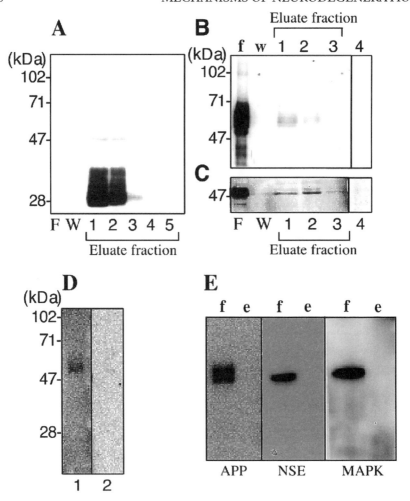

Figure 2. Analysis of PS1 associated tau and GSK-3β in human brain. Triton-X 100 soluble fractions (10 ml) of clinically normal human brain (2 g) was loaded onto a MKAD3.4 immunoaffinity column in order to purify PS1 and associated proteins. (A) Purification profiles show the flow-through fraction (20 µl) (f), the fraction of last wash (20 µl/total 5 ml) by TBS containing 1% Triton-X 100 (w), and purified fraction (20 µl per lane was loaded from total 500 µl eluate). The immunodetection of each fraction using MKAD3.4 (1:5) did not show any reactivity in the flow-through or the wash. Eluate fractions 1 and 2 revealed abundant reactivity, corresponding to the 47 kDa full-length and 28 kDa N-terminal fragment of PS1. JM (1:3000) was used for immunodetection of tau (B) and anti-GSK-3β (1:1000) was used to detect GSK-3β (Transduction Laboratories) (C). Most of the tau and GSK-3β was recovered in the flow-though fractions (20 µl). The JM antibody reacted with bands at 50–70 kDa, while anti-GSK-3β reacted with a band at 47 kDa. Reactivity for both antibodies was recovered in fractions 1 and 2 (20 µl). Only secondary antibody incubation, as negative control, did not show any visible bands in the eluate fraction 1 (20 µl) (lane 4). (D) The JM reactive band in eluate fraction 1 (20 µl) (lane 1) was eliminated by pre-

ANALYSIS OF BINDING SITE

To elucidate the nature of the interaction between PS1, tau and GSK-3β, we generated a number of PS1 cDNA constructs containing varying deletions (Figure 3A, B). N305, N298 and N250 are PS1 constructs that have the C-terminus deleted (Figure 4A). The D290–319 construct contains a deletion corresponding to exon 9 of the PS1 gene and is therefore not cleaved, and the D322–450 construct contains a deletion after the PS1 cleavage site. To determine the site of association of PS1 with tau, we transfected htau40 cDNA and each PS1 deletant cDNA into COS-7 cells. Tau was then immunoprecipitated using anti-human tau antibody, JM, and the subsequent immunoblots were probed using the anti-PS1 antibody, MKAD3.4. All of the PS1 constructs co-immunoprecipitated with tau with the exception of N250 (Figure 3B). This indicates that PS1 directly binds tau protein and the site of interaction is between residues 250 and 298 of PS1. For the next stage, each PS1 deletant cDNA construct was transfected into COS-7 cells, and the endogenous GSK-3β immunoprecipitated. The subsequent immunoblot was probed using MKAD3.4 (Figure 3C). Like tau, all PS1 constructs except N250 co-immunoprecipitated with endogenous GSK-3β, indicating that PS1 interacts with GSK-3β between residues 250 and 298. Thus, tau and GSK-3β both bind to the same region of PS1 residues 250–298. Moreover, the ability of PS1 to bring tau and GSK-3β into close physical proximity suggests that PS1 could play an important role in regulating the phosphorylation of tau by GSK-3β.

EFFECTS OF PS1 MUTANTS ON TAU PHOSPHORYLATION

Since region 250–298 on PS1 is a 'hot spot' for AD mutations, we sought to determine whether the AD-associated mutations in this region of PS1 might affect the interaction of PS1 with GSK-3β or tau. Each of the PS1 constructs containing point mutations in the 250–298 region, C263R and P264L, were co-transfected into COS-7 cells with htau40 cDNA construct. PS1 was immunoprecipitated from the lysates with MKAD3.4 and the immunoblots were probed with either the anti-GSK-3β antibody or the anti-tau antibody JM. Interestingly, each of the PS1 mutations increased the PS1/GSK-3β association by more than three times that of wild-type PS1 association. The mutations did not significantly increase binding to tau. Next, we sought to

absorption with human recombinant tau (lane 2). No reactivity is seen in lane 2. (E) Eluate fraction 1 (e) and the flow-through fraction (f) were incubated with anti-neuron-specific enolase (NSE), anti-amyloid protein precursor (APP) and anti-mitogen activating protein kinase (MAPK). No reactivities are seen in the eluate fraction

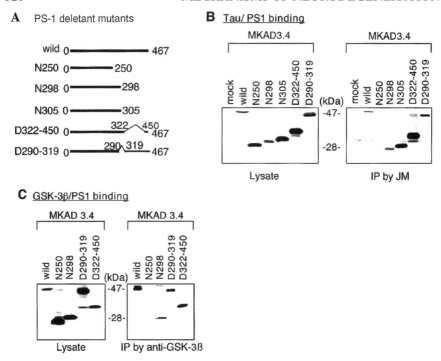

Figure 3. Direct binding of PS1 with tau and GSK3β. (A) Schematic drawing of PS1 deletant mutants. Wild-type PS1 consists of 467 amino acids (wild). The N250, N298 and N305 deletion constructs have the C-terminus of PS1 deleted beyond residues 250, 298 and 305, respectively. The D322-450 and D290-319 deletion constructs contain deletions between residues 322–450 and 290–319, respectively. (B) The expression of each PS1 was analyzed using 1/10 volume of total cell lysate (left panel). The rest of each cell lysate was used for immunoprecipitation by the anti-tau antibody (JM), and analyzed for the formation of immunocomplexes of tau with PS1 deletant mutants (right panel). N298, N305, D322-450 and D290-319 co-precipitated with tau, while N250 did not. (C) The mutant PS1 constructs were transiently transfected with COS-7 cells. The expression of PS1 was analyzed using 1/10 volume of total cell lysate (left panel). The remainder of each cell lysate was used for immunoprecipitation with the rabbit polyclonal anti-GSK-3β antibody (C1), and analyzed for formation of immunocomplexes of endogenous GSK-3β with the PS1 deletion constructs (right panel). N298, N305, D322-450 and D290-319 were recovered in the immunocomplex of GSK-3β, while N250 was not

determine whether the increased GSK-3β-binding activity of the PS1 mutants might affect the tau-directed kinase activity of GSK-3β. Lysates from the PS1/ tau co-transfections were probed with the phospho-tau specific antibody, PS199. The phosphorylation of htau40 was increased in the mutant C263R and P264L PS1 transfections. The results suggest that PS1 mutations may enhance the ability of GSK-3β to phosphorylate tau.

DISCUSSION

The functional consequences of presenilin mutations on the biology of the cell are only beginning to be understood. Expression of mutant presenilins increases production of $A\beta_{1-42}$ in the 31 mutations we investigated. The extent of increased $A\beta_{1-42}$ in each mutant did not coincide with age of onset, suggesting that there might be another mechanism to determine the onset age by each mutation. In this study, PS1 and GSK-3β can be found in association with NFTs in the AD brain, which further suggests that there may be a physiological connection between PS1, GSK-3β and tau. In order to pursue these intriguing connections, we investigated whether PS1 might directly associate with GSK-3β and tau, and have shown that PS1 binds GSK-3β and its substrate, tau. AD-associated mutations in PS1 located in the tau binding region, residues 250–298, increase binding to GSK-3β and its tau-directed kinase activity. This suggests that PS1 may be acting to control the association of GSK-3β with its substrates and, by increasing binding of GSK-3β, mutations in PS1 may enhance the ability of GSK-3β to phosphorylate its targets. Recently we found that PS1 binds to β-catenin, which is also a substrate of

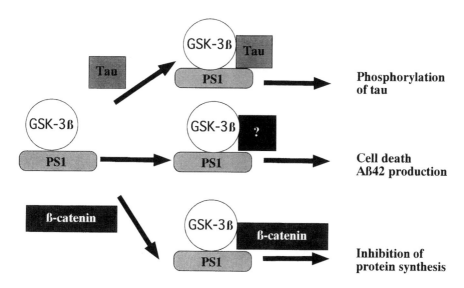

Figure 4. Role of PS1/GSK-3β complex on AD. PS1 may act as a molecular tether, connecting GSK-3β with important substrates. PS1/GSK-3β complex binds to tau, producing phosphorylation. Also, catenin was reported to be a PS1 binding protein, which is a substrate for GSK-3β. PS1/β-catenin binding affects soluble β-catenin level, and reduces the transcription activity of Tcf-4, resulting in the reduction of Tcf-linked protein synthesis. There may be a protein which associates with PS1 and is a substrate for GSK-3β. There may be a GSK-3β substrate protein associated with PS1 connected with apoptosis or $A\beta_{1-42}$

GSK-3β [17, 18]. Moreover, PS1 inhibits the β-catenin-regulated Tcf transcription activity. Probably the enhancing phosphorylation of β-catenin by GSK-3β leads to the degradation of β-catenin via the ubiquitin–proteasome cascade [19]. Thus, PS1 may act as a molecular tether, connecting GSK-3β with important substrates (Figure 4). According to this hypothesis, the PS1/GSK-3β connection may explain the increase of $A\beta_{42}$. Therefore, a protein that is a substrate for GSK-3β may be a factor altering the metabolism of APP to $A\beta_{1-42}$.

ACKNOWLEDGEMENTS

We are grateful to Dr K. Maruyama for providing us with the APP cDNA, Dr K. Ishiguro for providing us with the phosphorylation-dependent tau antibodies, and Dr H. Yamaguchi for providing us with human brain.

REFERENCES

1. Selkoe DJ. The molecular pathology of Alzheimer's disease. Neuron 1991; 6: 487–98.
2. Grundke-Iqbal I, Iqbal K, Quinlan M, Tung Y-C, Zaidi MS, Wisniewski HM. Microtubule-associated protein tau: a component of Alzheimer paired helical filament. J Biol Chem 1986; 261: 6084–9.
3. Grundke-Iqbal I, Iqbal K, Tung Y-C, Quinlan M, Wisniewski HM, Binder LI. Abnormal phosphorylation of the microtubule-associate protein tau in Alzheimer cytoskeletal pathology. Proc Natl Acad Sci USA 1986; 83: 4913–17.
4. Ihara Y, Nukina N, Miura R, Ogawara M. Phosphorylated tau protein is integrated into paired helical filaments in Alzheimer's disease. J Biochem 1986; 99: 1807–10.
5. Selkoe DJ. Amyloid beta-protein and the genetics of Alzheimer's disease. J Biol Chem 1996; 271(31): 18295–8.
6. Selkoe DJ. Alzheimer's disease: genotypes, phenotypes, and treatments. Science 1997; 275(5300): 630–31.
7. Sherrington R, Rogaev EI, Liang Y et al. Cloning of a gene bearing missense mutations in early-onset familial Alzheimer's disease (see comments). Nature 1995; 375(6534): 754–60.
8. Van Broeckhoven C. Presenilins and Alzheimer disease (news). Nature Genet 1995; 11(3): 230–32.
9. Borchelt DR, Thinakaran G, Eckman CB et al. Familial Alzheimer's disease-linked presenilin 1 variants elevate Aβ1–42/1–40 ratio *in vitro* and *in vivo*. Neuron 1996; 175(5): 1005–13.
10. Citron M, Westaway D, Xia W et al. Mutant presenilins of Alzheimer's disease increase production of 42-residue amyloid beta-protein in both transfected cells and transgenic mice (see comments). Nature Med 1997; 3(1): 67–72.
11. Duff K, Eckman C, Zehr C et al. Increased amyloid-beta42(43) in brains of mice expressing mutant presenilin 1. Nature 1996; 383(6602): 710–13.

12. Guo Q, Furukawa K, Sopher BL et al. Alzheimer's PS-1 mutation perturbs calcium homeostasis and sensitizes PC12 cells to death induced by amyloid beta-peptide. NeuroReport 1996; 8(1): 379–83.
13. Guo Q, Sopher BL, Furukawa K et al. Alzheimer's presenilin mutation sensitizes neural cells to apoptosis induced by trophic factor withdrawal and amyloid beta-peptide: involvement of calcium and oxyradicals. J Neurosci 1997; 17(11): 4212–22.
14. Deng G, Pike CJ, Cotman CW. Alzheimer-associated presenilin-2 confers increased sensitivity to apoptosis in PC12 cells. FEBS Lett 1996; 397(1): 50–54.
15. Wolozin B, Iwasaki K, Vito P et al. Participation of presenilin 2 in apoptosis: enhanced basal activity conferred by an Alzheimer mutation. Science 1996; 274(5293): 1710–13.
16. Xia W, Zhang J, Perez R, Koo EH, Selkoe DJ. Interaction between amyloid precursor proteins and presenilins in mammalian cells: implications for the pathogenesis of Alzheimer disease. Proc Natl Acad Sci USA 1997; 94: 8208–13.
17. Korinek VBN, Morin PJ, van Wichen D, de Weger R, Kinzler KW, Vogelstein B, Clevers H. Constitutive transcriptional activation by a beta-catenin–Tcf complex in APC–/– colon carcinoma. Science 1997; 275: 1784–7.
18. Kirpatrick PM. Not just glue: cell–cell junctions as cellular signaling centers. Curr Opin Genet Dev 1995; 5: 56–65.
19. Aberle HBA, Stappert J, Kispert A, Kemler R. β-catenin is a target for the ubiquitin-proteasome pathway. EMBO J 1997; 16(13): 3797–3804.
20. Miller AR, Moon RT. Signal-transduction through β-catenin and specification of cell fate during embryogenesis. Genes Dev 1996; 10: 2527–39.

Address for correspondence:
Akihiko Takashima,
Laboratory for Alzheimer's Disease,
Brain Science Institute, Riken,
2–1 Hirosawa, Wako-shi,
Saitama 351-0198, Japan

36 Function and Dysfunction of Presenilins in Alzheimer's Disease

SANGRAM S. SISODIA, GOPAL THINAKARAN,
DAVID R. BORCHELT, PHILIP C. WONG,
MICHAEL K. LEE AND DONALD L. PRICE

INTRODUCTION

While the vast majority of AD occurs as an age-associated disorder, autosomal dominant inheritance of mutant genes, encoding presenilin 1 (PS) or presenilin 2 (PS2), cause early-onset AD in several families (FAD). These mutant polypeptides cause dysfunction/death of vulnerable populations of nerve cells, with the resulting clinical syndrome of progressive dementia. In this chapter, we briefly discuss the genetics of PS-linked AD and efforts to understand the normal biology of presenilins, and the biology of mutant form of presenilins in cellular and transgenic animal models.

GENETICS OF *PRESENILIN*-LINKED EARLY-ONSET AD

Using positional cloning approaches, Sherrington and colleagues defined a minimal co-segregating region using genetic markers from 14q24.3 in 21 pedigrees with autosomal dominant AD, then isolated a novel cDNA, clone *S182*, encoding a 467 amino acid protein that contained single nucleotide substitutions that resulted in five independent amino acid substitutions in affected members of selected FAD pedigrees [1]. Sequence databases revealed the presence of a gene highly homologous to *PS1*, termed *presenilin 2* (*PS2*), and candidate pathogenic missense mutations in *PS2* were subsequently identified in affected individuals of the VG and an Italian pedigree [2, 3, 4]. Since 1995, over 45 different mutations in *PS1* have been described in over 80 families of various ethnic origins with early-onset FAD, while only two

Alzheimer's Disease and Related Disorders
Edited by K. Iqbal, D.F. Swaab, B. Winblad and H.M. Wisniewski
© 1999 John Wiley & Sons Ltd

mutations in *PS2* have been described in families with variable onset, autosomal dominant FAD (for review, see [5, 6]). Over 75% of the reported FAD mutations in *PS1* occur in single kindreds, thus characterizing them as 'private' mutations. With two notable exceptions, mutations in *PS* are missense substitutions that result in single amino acid changes. One of these exceptions is that in several unrelated pedigrees [7, 8, 9, 10], mutations in *PS1* lead to *PS1* mRNAs lacking sequences encoded by exon 9 of the *PS1* gene (ΔE9); these transcripts encode PS1 with an in-frame deletion of 29 amino acids and an amino acid substitution. The only other exception to the missense mutations is the presence of a single nucleotide deletion at the consensus splice donor sequence in intron 4 in two related individuals with autopsy-confirmed, early-onset AD; one of these cases had a family history of early-onset AD [11]. The resulting mutant transcripts are predicted to encode prematurely truncated PS1 polypeptides.

PS1 AND *PS2* mRNA EXPRESSION AND TOPOLOGY

PS1 and *PS2* mRNA are expressed in a wide variety of peripheral tissues and in brain; *in situ* hybridization studies of mammalian brain reveal expression in many neuronal populations and glia (for review, see [5]). Semi-quantitative reverse transcriptase–polymerase chain reaction (RT–PCR) studies have revealed that *PS1* and *PS2* transcripts are expressed at significantly different levels among tissues and during brain development [12], arguing that the homologous proteins are not functionally redundant.

Secondary structure algorithms predict that PS1 contains between seven [1] and nine transmembrane domains [13] and includes a hydrophilic 'loop' region encompassing amino acids 263–407. Antibody accessibility studies established that the N-terminus, loop and C-terminus of PS1 are orientated towards the cytoplasm [14, 15]. Similarly, the topology of the *Caenorhabditis elegans* presenilin homologs, termed SEL-12 and HOP-1, was determined using a series of SEL-12 β-galactosidase chimeras. These studies showed that SEL-1 and HOP-1 span the membrane eight times, with the N- and C-termini and 'loop' regions being exposed to the cytosol [16, 17].

METABOLISM OF THE PRESENILINS

Biochemical studies indicate that PS1/PS2 are not substrates for sulfation, glycosylation or acylation [15, 18, 19]. However, serine residues in the N-terminus of PS2 and in the cytosolic loop domain of PS1 [15, 19, 20] are *in vivo* substrates for phosphorylation. PS1 phosphorylation is enhanced in response to activation of either protein kinase C or cAMP-dependent protein kinase or to the inhibition of protein phosphatase 1 or 2A [19, 20]. The physiological significance of PS phosphorylation is not currently understood.

Although PS1 is synthesized as a ~42–43 kDa polypeptide, the preponderant PS1-related species that accumulate in cultured mammalian cells and in the brains and systemic tissues of rodents, transgenic mice expressing human PS1 (HuPS1), primates and humans are 27–28 kDa N-terminal (NTF) and ~16–17 kDa C-terminal (CTF) derivatives [19, 21, 22, 12, 23, 24]. Epitope mapping studies indicated that PS1 is cleaved within a region that encompasses amino acids 260–320, a domain in which >50% of identified FAD-linked PS1 mutations occur [21], and radiosequencing analysis revealed heterogeneity at the N-terminus of the CTF with a principal terminus at amino acid 299 [24]. These results are consistent with the demonstration that the FAD-linked PS1 ΔE9 variant, which lacks amino acids 290–319, fails to be cleaved [21]. At present, neither the identity of the protease nor the physiological significance of PS1 proteolysis is known.

Over-expression studies of HuPS1 in brains of transgenic mice revealed that the accumulation of ~27 kDa and ~17 kDa HuPS1-specific NTF and CTF is highly regulated and saturable [21, 25]; levels of PS1 derivatives are remarkably disproportionate to levels of transgene-derived mRNA or full-length HuPS1. The stoichiometry of accumulated ~27 kDa NTF and ~17 kDa CTF is ~1:1 in non-transgenic and transgenic mouse brains; this ratio is independent of the levels of transgene-derived HuPS1 mRNA [21]. The mechanism(s) involved in regulating the levels of accumulated PS1 derivatives have not been fully established, but several important insights have emerged. For example, in transfected cells over-expressing PS1 or PS2, only a small fraction of newly synthesized full-length PS1 and PS2 are converted to fragments, while the remaining full-length polypeptides are rapidly degraded [24, 26, 27]; in cultured cells, over-expressed PS2 is polyubiquinated and degraded by a lactacystin-sensitive, proteosome pathway [27].

In view of the demonstration of a paucity of full-length PS1 and highly regulated accumulation of processed derivatives *in vivo*, it is highly likely that PS1 fragments are the 'functional units' [21]. In mouse N2a cell lines and in the brains of transgenic mice expressing human PS1, accumulation of human PS1 derivatives is accompanied by a compensatory, and highly selective, decrease in the steady-state levels of murine PS1 and PS2 derivatives. Similarly, the levels of murine PS1 derivatives are diminished in cultured cells over-expressing human PS2 [28]. Interestingly, over-expression of the PS1 ΔE9 variant, which fails to be cleaved, also resulted in compromised accumulation of murine PS1/PS2 derivatives; thus, the 'replacement' of murine PS1/PS2 by over-expressed human PS1 independent of endoproteolysis [25, 28]. These results are consistent with a model in which the abundance of PS1 and PS2 derivatives is coordinately regulated by competition for shared, but limiting, cellular factor(s) [28].

The observation that PS1 or PS2 fragments accumulate to 1:1 stoichiometry suggested that the NTFs and CTFs may co-associate, perhaps in higher-order assemblies. Two lines of evidence support the idea that N- and C-terminal PS1 or PS2 derivatives are co-resident: in cultured mammalian cells, these fragments can be specifically cross-linked *in situ*, and the two fragments can be co-immunoprecipitated from mild detergent lysates of cultured cells or mammalian brain [29, 30]. Moreover, gel filtration chromatography, and velocity gradient fractionation of cultured cell lysates prepared with non-ionic detergents, reveal that PS1 N- and C-terminal fragments appear to remain associated in larger SDS and Triton X 100-sensitive complexes of ~100–150 kDa [20, 30]. Interestingly, on glycerol velocity gradients, ΔE9 PS1 molecules sediment at a molecular weight similar to the endogenous proteolytically cleaved fragments, a finding that offers an appealing notion that the uncleaved deletion variant retains the ability to associate with components of the functional complex [30]. The nature of the higher-order complexes containing PS fragments has not been determined. Extending these latter observations, subcellular fractionation of membrane preparations in equilibrium density gradients reveals that, while full-length PS1 and ~50% of the PS1 derivatives are present in fractions that co-localize with ER-resident polypeptides, BiP and GRP 78, the remaining PS1 derivatives are in fractions of low density that bear neither ER, Golgi, trans-Golgi, endosomal nor plasma membrane markers (Kim, Thinakaran and Sisodia, unpublished observations). These biochemical studies have been confirmed using confocal microscopy which indicate that PS1-immunoreactivity co-localizes both with ER markers and currently uncharacterized membranous compartments that are not decorated by a panel of conventional organelle-specific markers.

SUBCELLULAR LOCALIZATION OF PRESENILINS

Immunocytochemical analysis of a variety of cultured non-neuronal cells that transiently over-express full-length PS1 and PS2 revealed that the proteins are localized to similar intracellular membranous compartments, including the endoplasmic reticulum and, to a varying extent, the Golgi complex [15, 18, 19, 31]. In untransfected and stably transfected cells, PS1 immunoreactivity is restricted to the endoplasmic reticulum [14, 19] (Kim, Thinakaran and Sisodia, unpublished observations). Other studies have localized PS to the cell surface [32] and to the nuclear membrane, kinetochores and centrosomes [33]. However, and reflecting ambiguities in the assays used to validate antibody specificity, these two latter studies have not been reproduced in other laboratories.

In cultured rat hippocampal neurons, PS1 is concentrated in somatodendritic compartments, but is also present at lower levels in axons [18]. Light microscopic immunocytochemical studies of rodent [12, 34], primate [35], and human brains [36], using antibodies selective for N-terminal or 'loop' domains of PS1, revealed that PS1 was present in all brain regions, with the strongest labeling in neurons and the neuropil, including axons and dendrites; weaker immunoreactivity was present in glial cells. Subcellular fractionation of monkey cortex revealed PS1 enrichment in non-synaptic vesicle membrane compartments [35]. Notably, immuno-electron microscopy of monkey cortex using an antibody specific for epitopes in the PS1 N-terminus disclosed selective immunoreactivity on cytoplasmic surfaces of smooth membranous organelles in cell bodies of neurons, suggesting localization in the endoplasmic reticulum–Golgi intermediate compartment and less prominent localization in coated transport vesicles [35]. In the neuropil, PS1 immunoreactivity was present in dendritic spines and occasional presynaptic structures. In dendritic spines, PS1-immunoreactive structures had the general appearance of smooth tubular membranes, reminiscent of smooth endoplasmic reticulum; no staining was observed on presynaptic structures, including synaptic vesicles [35].

FUNCTIONS OF PRESENILINS

The first major insight regarding PS function emerged with the discovery of a homologous gene in *C. elegans*, termed *sel-12*; mutant alleles of *sel-12* were uncovered as suppressors of a multivulval phenotype in *C. elegans* mediated by gain-of-function (hypermorphic) alleles of the *C. elegans* Notch homologs *lin-12* and *glp-1* [37]. Notch and LIN-12/GLP-1 are transmembrane receptors required for the specification of cell fate and lateral inhibition during development [38]. The molecular mechanisms by which SEL-12 facilitates signaling mediated by LIN-12 are poorly understood. An egg-laying defect associated with loss of SEL-12 function in *C. elegans* is rescued efficiently by the expression of HuPS1 and HuPS2; the rescue efficiency of HuPS was essentially indistinguishable to transgenic worms that express SEL-12 [39, 40]. Notably, the egg-laying defect was only weakly rescued in transgenic worms that express several human FAD-linked PS1 variants [39, 40], suggesting that PS1 missense variants exhibit reduced function. Interestingly, the PS1ΔE9 variant showed considerable rescue activity relative to other PS1 missense variants. These results indicated that PS1 endoproteolysis is not obligatory for function [39, 40] and fully supported the earlier biochemical studies documenting that the PS1ΔE9 variant exhibits biochemical properties not unlike the constitutively-generated PS1 derivatives.

Although the *C. elegans* experiments provided valuable insights into PS function, the biological function(s) of PS1 and PS2 in mammals during development is not fully understood. Several strategies have been employed to address these issues. Initial *in situ* hybridization studies and RT–PCR approaches in mouse embryos revealed that PS are expressed ubiquitously during mouse embryonic development [12]. However, the general spatial and temporal expression patterns of *PS* mRNA do not directly coincide with the expression patterns of any specific member of the known mammalian *Notch* homologs, results which suggested that during mammalian development, PS1 function is not limited to Notch signaling alone [12]. A number of investigations have utilized yeast two-hybrid approaches to identify attempted to isolate proteins that interact with the N-terminal and 'loop' domains of PS1 and PS2;

the cytosolic domains of PS1 and PS2 are highly divergent (<10% identity in the N-terminal 70 amino acids and between amino acids 305–375 in the loop domain), suggesting that these regions mediate cell- or PS-specific functions via differential interactions with proteins in the cytoplasm. One isolate from a two-hybrid screen was a fragment of δ-catenin [41]; δ-catenin, expressed predominantly in the nervous system, is a member of a larger family of catenins related to a *Drosophila* protein, termed 'armadillo', involved in inductive signaling events during development, and regulation of cell proliferation. It will be of great interest to define the functional relationship(s) between PS1 and δ-catenin in developmental and/or aging processes.

To examine the *in vivo* role of PS1 in mammalian development, mice with a targeted disruption of the *PS1* gene were generated [42, 43]. Most homozygous mutant mice died in late embryogenesis, or immediately after birth. The most striking phenotype observed in PS1 (–/–) embryos was a severe perturbation in the development of the axial skeleton and ribs. The failed development of the axial skeleton in PS1(–/–) animals was traced to defects in somitogenesis; in E8.5 and E9.5 embryos, somites were irregularly shaped and misaligned along the entire length of the neural tube and largely absent at the most caudal regions. Remarkably, the expression of mRNA that encodes Notch1 and Dll1 is reduced considerably in the presomitic mesoderm of PS1(–/–) mice [42]. In addition, all PS1 (–/–) embryos exhibited intra-parenchymal hemorrhages after day 11 of gestation.

In view of the evidence in *C. elegans* which documented that FAD-linked mutant PS failed to completely rescue an egg-laying defect in worms lacking *sel-12*, investigations have tested the ability of an FAD-linked PS1 variant to complement the embryonic lethality and axial skeletal defects in mice lacking PS1. It is now clear that both wild-type and mutant human PS1 transgenes rescue *Notch 1* mRNA expression in the presomitic mesoderm in early embryos [44] and the entire spectrum of developmental deficits in PS1(–/–) mice [44, 45]. Thus, the FAD-linked A246E PS1 variant, and presumably other mutants, retain sufficient normal function during mammalian embryonic development.

THE ROLE OF PS IN Aβ METABOLISM

The mechanisms by which FAD-linked PS1 and PS2 variants cause FAD are not fully understood, but several important insights have emerged. The most provocative insight emerged from studies showing that the ratio of Aβ42(43):Aβ40 in conditioned medium from fibroblasts or other plasma from affected members of pedigrees with PS1/PS2-linked mutations was significantly elevated relative to unaffected family members [46]. These data have been supported by the demonstration that Aβ42 production is elevated in mammalian cells and the brains of transgenic mice expressing mutant PS [47–50]. The observation that every mutant PS in a variety of cell types elevates Aβ42 provoked studies to examine potential genotype–phenotype correlations. Over 50% of PS1 mutations are observed in two major clusters: in a domain including transmembrane domains 1 and 2; and a domain encompassing transmembrane 6 and ~30 residues of the 'loop'. The average age of onset observed for pedigrees with mutations in these clusters is earlier (~40–45 years) than pedigrees with other PS1 mutations (~48 years) [5]. However, an analysis of stable cell lines expressing seven different human PS1 variants has revealed that there is no correlation of the level of AB42(43) production and the age of onset [51], arguing that the age of onset is not determined by Aβ42(43) production alone, but is influenced by additional (or epistatic) genetic modifiers.

Finally, in the brains of transgenic mice co-expressing mutant HuPS1 and APP harboring mutations (K595N, M596L) linked to FAD pedigrees, amyloid deposits are observed much earlier than in mice that express the APP transgene, alone [52, 53]. These data convincingly demonstrate that the FAD-linked HuPS1 acts synergistically with APPswe to accelerate the rate of amyloid deposition. These findings suggest that the principal mechanism by which mutations in PS1 cause disease is through elevating extracellular concentrations of Aβ42 and, thereby, accelerating the deposition of amyloid.

The mechanism(s) by which mutant PS influence Aβ42 production have not been defined. It has been proposed that mutant PS1 acts as a pathological 'chaperone' to facilitate proteolytic cleavage by 'γ-secretase' and this view is supported by the demonstration that full-length PS1 and PS2 form stable heteromeric assemblies with APP in cultured mammalian cells [54, 55]. While attractive, this model is highly implausible, since the *in vivo* stoichiometry of PS1 and APP is ~1:100. Indeed, using a variety of experimental conditions which permit successful cross-linking or co-precipitation of PS NTF and CTF, or co-isolation of APP and a *bona fide* interacting protein, Fe65 [56], interactions between PS1/PS2 and APP have not been detected [29] (C. Haass, personal communication; P. St George-Hyslop, personal communication). Mechanistically, and in view of the remarkable effects of loss of PS1 activity on protein trafficking (see below), it is much more likely that mutant PS1/PS2 promotes co-compartmentalization of putative 'γ-42-secretase(s)' and their substrates (i.e. APP or its potentially amyloidogenic C-terminal derivatives). The most remarkable observations regarding the influence of PS1 on γ-secretase processing recently emerged by analysis of neurons from PS1 knockout mice [57]. These studies revealed that lack of PS1 leads to defects in secretion of Aβ peptides and intracellular accumulation of APP C-terminal fragments (CTFs) bearing varying extents of the Aβ region. These findings were interpreted as proof that PS1 influences intramembranous γ-secretase processing of APP [58]. Considering the abundance of PS1 (see above), it seemed unreasonable that the effect of loss of PS1 function would selectively effect APP metabolism. Supporting this notion, studies have documented that accumulation of a CTF derived from the APP homolog, APLP1, also accumulates in PS1(–/–) neurons [59]. Because the APP and APLP1 transmembrane domains have very limited homology, it is inconceivable that PS1 directly modulates γ-secretase activity. Rather, we envision a broader role for PS1 in directing membrane-bound CTFs derived from APP family members or other transmembrane proteins to appropriate cleavage and/or degradation compartments. The loss of P1 expression also affects the rate of maturation and the biology of other integral membrane glycoproteins. For example, the rate of maturation of the receptor tyrosine kinase, TrkB, and brain derived neurotrophic factor (BDNF)-mediated TrkB autophosphorylation are severely compromised in PS1(−/−) neurons [59]. These data argue that PS1 plays a global role in trafficking and metabolism of proteins in the secretory pathway.

CONCLUSIONS AND FUTURE DIRECTIONS

The discovery that mutations in genes encoding PS1 and PS2 are linked to FAD has ushered in a new and extremely exciting era of research aimed at clarifying the cellular and molecular biology of the PS polypeptides and the relationships of the genetic variants to the pathogenesis of AD.

The first important observation is that the preponderant PS-related polypeptides that accumulate in vivo are N-terminal ~27–30 kDa C-terminal ~17–20 kDa derivatives and that the fragments accumulate in a highly regulated, saturable manner and at equistoichiometric levels. These findings, taken together with reports showing that the derivatives can be co-isolated and co-fractionate on gel filtration columns, velocity and equilibrium gradients, offer compelling support for the notion that the PS1 derivatives are the 'functional units' of PS activity in vivo. What remains unresolved is the manner by which the PS derivatives assemble in the lipid bilayer. Protein topology studies revealed that PS contains eight transmembrane domains; endoproteolytic cleavage within residues 291–298 in the large hydrophilic 'loop' region is predicted to generate an NTF containing six transmembrane domains and a CTF containing two transmembrane domains. The most likely scenario is that the PS1 NTF and CTF associate via interactions between closely located hydrophobic transmembrane domains, but high resolution cryo-electron microscopic approaches will be required to fully define the nature of PS transmembrane domain interactions. It is also essential to define the nature of the apparatus responsible for regulating PS subcellular localization, including the enzyme(s) responsible for PS endoproteolysis, and the limiting cellular factors that associate with, and stabilize, PS derivatives.

It is of considerable interest that FAD-linked mutant PS1 cause selective increases in the extracellular concentrations of highly fibrillogenic Aβ42 peptides. This effect is unlikely to be mediated by interactions between mutant PS1 and APP, but it is conceivable that mutant PS1 promotes co-compartmentalization of putative 'γ-42-secretase(s)' and their substrates (i.e. APP or its potentially amyloidogenic C-terminal derivatives). Supporting this view, it is very clear that trafficking and post-translational processing of membrane proteins is markedly affected in cells lacking PS1. It has also become evident that mutant PS-mediated extracellular elevations of Aβ1–42 peptides in brains of transgenic mice leads to accelerated Aβ deposition. These transgenic mice offer opportunities to generate a series of 'snapshots' of the evolving abnormalities that occur at different stages of disease, and to detect subtle abnormalities and high-resolution investigations of the temporal and spatial relationships in these processes.

Finally, the role of PS during development was established by the demonstration that cerebral hemorrhages, abnormalities in somite segmentation and loss of segment polarity lead to improper patterning of the axial skeleton and spinal ganglia, and reduction in mRNA encoding *Dll1* and *Notch 1* mRNAs in the paraxial mesoderm. Notwithstanding these efforts, little information is available regarding the role of PS1 in facilitating Notch signaling. These issues can be addressed in cell lines derived from PS1 knockout animals, or in genetically tractable organisms such as *C. elegans* or *Drosophila melanogaster*, that express PS homologs. Despite the demonstration that PS1 is essential for mouse embryonic development, the function(s) of PS1 during maturation and aging is not at all clear and future efforts directed at generating transgenic animals in which PS1 genes can be conditionally ablated in a temporal and/or tissue-specific manner will be necessary in order to address these outstanding issues.

ACKNOWLEDGEMENTS

The authors thank Drs Hui Zheng, Lee Martin, Andrew Doan, Seong Kim, Satoshi Naruse, Janine Davis, Sam Gandy, Mary Seeger, Steve Wagner, Allan Levey, Nancy Jenkins, Neil Copeland and Ms Hilda Slunt, Ms Frances Davenport and Ms Tamara Ratovitski for their contributions to some of the work mentioned in this text. Aspects of this work were supported by grants from the US Public Health Service (NIH NS20471, AG05146, AG10491, AG10480, AG14248) as well as the Metropolitan Life Foundation, the Adler Foundation, the Alzheimer's Association, the American Health Assistance Foundation, the Claster Family and the Develbiss Fund.

REFERENCES

1. Sherrington R, Rogaev EI, Liang Y, Rogaeva EA, Levesque G, Ikeda M, Chi H, Lin C, Li G, Holman K, Tsuda T, Mar L, Foncin J-F, Bruni AC, Montesi MP, Sorbi S, Rainero L, Pinessi L, Nee L, Chumakov I, Pollen D, Brookes A, Sanseau P, Polinsky RJ, Wasco W, Da Silva HAR, Haines JL, Pericak-Vance MA, Tanzi RE, Roses AD, Fraser PE, Rommens JM, St George-Hyslop PH. Cloning of a gene bearing missense mutations in early-onset familial Alzheimer's disease. Nature 1995; 375: 754–60.

2. Levy-Lahad E, Wasco W, Poorkaj P, Romano D, Oshima J, Pettingell W, Yu C-E, Jondro P, Schmidt S, Wang K, Crowley A, Fu Y-H, Guenette S, Galas D, Nemens E, Wijsman E, Bird T, Schellenberg G, Tanzi R. Candidate gene for the chromosome 1 familial Alzheimer's disease locus. Science 1995; 269: 973–7.

3. Levy-Lahad E, Wijsman E, Nemens E, Anderson L, Goddard K, Weber J, Bird T, Schellenberg G. A familial Alzheimer's disease locus on chromosome 1. Science 1995; 269: 970–73.

4. Rogaev EI, Sherrington R, Rogaeva EA, Levesque G, Ikeda M, Liang Y, Chi H, Lin C, Holman K, Tsuda T, Mar L, Sorbi S, Nacmias B, Piacentini S, Amaducci L, Chumakov I, Cohen D, Lannfelt L, Fraser PE, Rommens JM, St George-Hyslop PH. Familial Alzheimer's disease in kindreds with missense mutations in a gene on chromosome 1 related to the Alzheimer's disease type 3 gene. Nature 1995; 376: 775–8.

5. Tanzi R, Kovacs D, Kim T-W, Moir R, Guenette S, Wasco V. The gene defects responsible for familial Alzheimer's disease. Neurobiol Dis 1996; 3: 159–68.

6. Hardy J. Amyloid, the presenilins and Alzheimer's disease. Trends Neurosci 1997; 20: 154–9.

7. Pérez-Tur J, Froelich S, Prihar G, Crook R, Baker M, Duff K, Wragg M, Busfield F, Lendon C, Clark R, Roques P, Fuldner R, Johnston J, Cowburn R, Forsell C, Axelman K, Lilius L, Houlden H, Karran E, Roberts G, Rossor M, Adams M, Hardy J, Goate A, Lanfelt L, Hutton M. A mutation in Alzheimer's disease destroying a splice acceptor site in the presenilin-1 gene. NeuroReport 1995; 7: 297–301.

8. Ishii K, Ii K, Hasegawa T, Shoji S, Doi A, Mori H. Increased AB 42(43)-plaque deposition in early-onset familial Alzheimer's disease brains with the deletion of exon 9 and the missense point mutation (H163R) in the PS-1 gene. Neurosci Lett 1997; 228: 17–20.

9. Crook R, Verkkoniemi A, Pérez-Tur J, Mehta N, Baker M, Houlden H, Farrer M, Hutton M, Lincoln S, Hardy J, Gwinn K, Somer M, Paetau A, Kalimo H, Ylikoski R, Poyhonen M, Kucera S, Haltia M. A variant of Alzheimer's disease with spastic paraphrasis and unusual plaques due to deletion of exon 9 of presenilin 1. Nature Med 1998; 4: 1–4.

10. Kwok J, Taddei K, Hallupp M, Fisher C, Brooks W, Broe G, Hardy J, Fulham M, Nicholson G, Stell R, St George-Hyslop P, Fraser P, Kakulas B, Clarnette R, Relkin N, Gandy S, Schofield P, Martins R. Two novel (M233T and R278T) presenilin-1 mutations in early-onset Alzheimer's disease pedigrees and preliminary evidence for association of presenilin-1 mutations with a novel phenotype. NeuroReport 1997; 8: 1537–42.

11. Tysoe C, Whittaker J, Xuereb J, Cairns N, Cruts M, Van Broeckhoven C, Wilcock G, Rubinsztein D. A presenilin-1 truncating mutation is present in two cases with autopsy-confirmed early-onset Alzheimer disease. Am J Hum Genet 1998; 62: 70–76.

12. Lee MK, Slunt HH, Martin LJ, Thinakaran G, Kim G, Gandy SE, Seeger M, Koo E, Price DL, Sisodia SS. Expression of presenilin 1 and 2 (PS1 and PS2) in human and murine tissues. J Neurosci 1996; 16: 7513–25.

13. Slunt HH, Thinakaran G, Lee MK, Sisodia SS. Nucleotide sequence of the chromosome 14-encoded *S182* cDNA and revised secondary structure prediction. Amyloid: Int J Exp Clin Invest 1995; 2: 188–90.

14. Doan A, Thinakaran G, Borchelt DR, Slunt HH, Ratovitsky T, Podlisny M, Selkoe DJ, Seeger M, Gandy SE, Price DL, Sisodia SS. Protein topology of presenilin 1. Neuron 1996; 17: 1023–30.

15. De Strooper B, Beullens M, Contreras B, Levesque L, Craessaerts K, Cordell B, Moechars D, Bollen M, Fraser P, St George-Hyslop P, Vanleuven F. Phosphorylation, subcellular localization, and membrane orientation of the Alzheimer's disease-associated presenilins. J Biol Chem 1997; 272: 3590–98.

16. Li X, Greenwald I. Membrane topology of the *C. elegans* SEL-12 presenilin. Neuron 1996; 17: 1015–21.

17. Li X, Greenwald I. A *Caenorhabditis elegans* presenilin appears to be functionally redundant with SEL-12 presenilin and to facilitate LIN-12 and GLP-1 signaling. Proc Natl Acad Sci USA 1997; 94: 12204–9.

18. Cook DG, Sung JC, Golde TE, Felsenstein KM, Wojczyk BS, Tanzi RE, Trojanowski JQ, Lee VM-Y, Doms RW. Expression and analysis of presenilin 1 in a human neuronal system: localization in cell bodies and dendrites. Proc Natl Acad Sci USA 1996; 93: 9223–8.

19. Walter J, Grünberg J, Capell A, Pesold B, Schindzielorz A, Citron M, Mendla K, St George-Hyslop P, Multhaup G, Selkoe DJ, Haass C. Proteolytic processing of the Alzheimer disease-associated presinilin-1 generates an *in vivo* substrate for protein kinase C. Proc Natl Acad Sci USA 1997; 94: 5349–54.

20. Seeger M, Nordstedt C, Petanceska S, Kovacs DM, Gouras GK, Hahne S, Fraser P, Levesque L, Czernik AJ, St George-Hyslop P, Sisodia SS, Thinakaran G, Tanzi RE, Greengard P, Gandy S. Evidence for phosphorylation and oligomeric assembly of presenilin 1. Proc Natl Acad Sci USA 1997; 94: 5090–94.

21. Thinakaran G, Borchelt DR, Lee MK, Slunt HH, Spitzer L, Kim G, Ratovitski T, Davenport F, Nordstedt C, Seeger M, Hardy J, Levey AI, Gandy SE, Jenkins N, Copeland N, Price DL, Sisodia SS. Endoproteolysis of presenilin 1 and accumulation of processed derivatives *in vivo*. Neuron 1996; 17: 181–90.

22. Mercken M, Takahashi H, Honda T, Sato K, Murayama M, Nakazato Y, Noguchi K, Imahori K, Takashima A. Characterization of human presenilin 1 using N-terminal specific monoclonal antibodies: evidence that Alzheimer mutations affect proteolytic processing. FEBS Lett 1996; 389: 297–303.

23. Hendriks L, Thinakaran G, Harris CL, De Jonghe C, Martin J-J, Sisodia SS, Van Broeckhoven C. Processing of presenilin 1 in brains of Alzheimer's disease patients and controls. NeuroReport 1997; 8: 1717–21.

24. Podlisny MB, Citron M, Amarante P, Sherrington R, Xia W, Zhang J, Diehl T, Levesque G, Fraser P, Haass C, Koo EHM, Seubert P, St George-Hyslop P, Teplow DB, Selkoe DJ. Presenilin proteins undergo heterogeneous endoproteolysis between Thr_{291} and Ala_{299} and occur as stable N- and C-terminal fragments in normal and Alzheimer brain tissue. Neurobiol Dis 1997; 3: 325–37.

25. Lee MK, Borchelt DR, Kim G, Thinakaran G, Slunt HH, Ratovitski T, Martin LJ, Kittur A, Gandy S, Levey AI, Jenkins N, Copeland N, Price DL, Sisodia SS. Hyperaccumulation of FAD-linked presenilin 1 variants *in vivo*. Nature Med 1997; 3: 756–60.

26. Ratovitski T, Slunt HH, Thinakaran G, Price DL, Sisodia SS, Borchelt DR. Endoproteolytic processing and stabilization of wild-type and mutant presenilin. J Biol Chem 1997; 272: 24536–41.

27. Kim T-W, Pettingell WH, Hallmark OG, Moir RD, Wasco W, Tanzi RE. Endoproteolytic cleavage and proteasomal degradation of presenilin 2 in transfected cells. J Biol Chem (1997a) 272: 11006–10.

28. Thinakaran G, Harris CL, Ratovitski T, Davenport F, Slunt HH, Price DL, Borchelt DR, Sisodia SS. Evidence that levels of presenilins (PSI and PS2) are coordinately regulated by competition for limiting cellular factors. J Biol Chem 1997; 272: 28415–22.

29. Thinakaran G, Regard JB, Bouton CML, Harris CL, Sabo S, Price DL, Borchelt DR, Sisodia SS. Stable association of presenilin derivatives and absence of presenilin interactions with APP. Neurobiol Dis 1997; 4: 438–53.

30. Capell A, Grunberg J, Pesold B, Diehlmann A, Citron M, Nixon R, Beyreuther K, Selkoe DJ, Haass C. The proteolytic fragments of the Alzheimer's disease-associated presenilin-1 form heterodimers and occur as a 100–150 kDa molecular mass complex. J Biol Chem 1998; 273: 3205–11.

31. Kovacs DM, Fausett HJ, Page KJ, Kim T-W, Moir RD, Merriam DE, Hollister RD, Hallmark OG, Mancini R, Felsenstein KM, Hyman BT, Tanzi RE, Wasco W. Alzheimer-associated presenilins 1 and 2: neuronal expression in brain and localization to intracellular membranes in mammalian cells. Nature Med 1996; 2: 224–9.

32. Dewji NN, Singer SJ. Cell surface expression of the Alzheimer disease-related presenilin proteins. Proc Natl Acad Sci USA 1997; 94: 9926–31.

33. Li J, Xu M, Zhou H, Ma J, Potter H. Alzheimer presenilins in the nuclear membrane, interphase kinetochores, and centrosomes suggest a role in chromosome segregation. Cell 1997; 90: 917–27.

34. Moussaoui S, Czech C, Pradier L, Blanchard V, Bonici B, Gohin M, Imperato A, Revah F. Immunohistochemical analysis of presenilin-1 expression in the mouse brain. FEBS Lett 1996; 383: 219–22.

35. Lah JJ, Heilman CJ, Nash NR, Rees HD, Yi H, Counts SE, Levey AI. Light and electron microscopic localization of presenilin-1 in primate brain. J Neurosci 1997; 17: 1971–80.

36. Busciglio J, Hartmann H, Lorenzo A, Wong C, Baumann K, Sommer B, Staufenbiel M, Yankner BA. Neuronal localization of presenilin-1 and association with amyloid plaques and neurofibrillary tangles in Alzheimer's disease. J Neurosci 1997; 17: 5101–7.

37. Levitan D, Greenwald I. Facilitation of *lin-12*-mediated signaling by *sel-12*, a *Caenorhabditis elegans* S182 Alzheimer's disease gene. Nature 1995; 377: 351–4.

38. Artavanis-Tsakonas S, Matsuno K, Fortini ME. Notch signaling. Science 1995; 268: 225–32.

39. Baumeister R, Leimer U, Zweckbronner I, Jakubek C, Grünberg J, Haass C. Human presenilin-1, but not familial Alzheimer's disease (FAD) mutants, facilitate *Caenorhabditis elegans* Notch signaling independently of proteolytic processing. Genes & Funct 1997; 1: 149–59.

40. Levitan D, Doyle TG, Brousseau D, Lee MK, Thinakaran G, Slunt HH, Sisodia SS, Greenwald I. Assessment of normal and mutant human presenilin function in *Caenorhabditis elegans*. Proc Natl Acad Sci USA 1996; 93: 14940–44.

41. Zhou J, Liyanage U, Medina M, Ho C, Simmons AD, Lovett M, Koski KS. Presenilin 1 interaction in the brain with a novel member of the armadillo family. NeuroReport 1997; 8: 2085–90.

42. Wong PC, Zheng H, Chen H, Becher MW, Sirinathsinghji DJS, Trumbauer ME, Chen HY, Price DL, Van der Ploeg LHT, Sisodia SS. Presenilin 1 is required for *Notch1* and *Dll1* expression in the paraxial mesoderm. Nature 1997; 387: 288–92.

43. Shen J, Bronson RT, Chen DF, Xia W, Selkoe DJ, Tonegawa S. Skeletal and CNS defects in *presenilin-1*-deficient mice. Cell 1997; 89: 629–39.

44. Davis JA, Chen H, Naruse S, Price DL, Borchelt DR, Sisodia SS, Wong PC. An Alzheimer's disease-linked PS1 variant rescues the developmental abnormalities of *PS1*-deficient embryos. Neuron 1998; 20: 603–9.

45. Qian S, Jiang P, Guan X, Singh G, Trumbauer M, Yu H, Chen H, Van der Ploeg L, Zheng H. Mutant human presenilin 1 protects presenilin 1 null mouse against embryonic lethality and elevates Ab1-42/43 expression. Neuron 1998; 20: 611–17.

46. Scheuner D, Eckman C, Jensen M, Song X, Citron M, Suzuki N, Bird TD, Hardy J, Hutton M, Kukull W, Larson E, Levy-Lahad E, Viitanen M, Peskind E, Poorkaj P, Schellenberg G, Tanzi R, Wasco W, Lannfelt L, Selkoe D, Younkin S. Secreted amyloid β-protein similar to that in the senile plaques of Alzheimer's disease is increased *in vivo* by the presenilin 1 and 2 and *APP* mutations linked to familial Alzheimer's disease. Nature Med 1996; 2: 864–52.

47. Borchelt DR, Thinakaran G, Eckman CB, Lee MK, Davenport F, Ratovitsky T, Prada C-M, Kim G, Seekins S, Yager D, Slunt HH, Wang R, Seeger M, Levey AI, Gandy SE, Copeland NG, Jenkins NA, Price DL, Younkin SG, Sisodia SS. Familial Alzheimer's disease-linked presenilin 1 variants elevate Aβ1–42/1–40 ratio *in vitro* and *in vivo*. Neuron 1996; 17: 1005–13.

48. Duff K, Eckman C, Zehr C, Yu X, Prada C-M, Pérez-Tur J, Hutton M, Buee L, Harigaya Y, Yager D, Morgan D, Gordon MN, Holcomb L, Refolo L, Zenk B, Hardy J, Younkin S. Increased amyloid-β42(43) in brains of mice expressing mutant presenilin 1. Nature 1996; 383: 710–13.

49. Citron M, Westaway D, Xia W, Carlson G, Diehl T, Levesque G, Johnson-Wood K, Lee M, Seubert P, Davis A, Kholodenko D, Motter R, Sherrington R, Perry B, Yao H, Strome R, Lieberburg I, Rommens J, Kim S, Schenk D, Fraser P, St George-Hyslop P, Selkoe DJ. Mutant presenilins of Alzheimer's disease increase production of 42-residue amyloid β-protein in both transfected cells and transgenic mice. Nature Med 1997; 3: 67–72.

50. Tomita T, Maruyama K, Saido TC, Kume H, Shinozaki K, Tokuhiro S, Capell A, Walter J, Gruenberg J, Haass C, Iwatsubo T, Obata K. The presenilin 2 mutation (N141I) linked to familial Alzheimer disease (Volga German families) increases the secretion of amyloid β protein ending at the 42nd (or 43rd) residue. Proc Natl Acad Sci USA 1997; 94: 2025–30.

51. Mehta N, Refolo L, Eckman C, Sanders S, Yager D, Pérez-Tur J, Younkin S, Duff K, Hardy J, Hutton M. Increased AB42(43) from cell lines expressing presenilin 1 mutations. Ann Neurol 1998; 43: 256–8.

52. Borchelt DR, Ratovitski T, Van Lare J, Lee MK, Gonzales VB, Jenkins NA, Copeland NG, Price DL, Sisodia SS. Accelerated amyloid deposition in the brains of transgenic mice co-expressing mutant presenilin 1 and amyloid precursor proteins. Neuron 1997; 19: 939–45.

53. Holcomb L, Gordon MN, McGowan E, Yu X, Benkovic S, Jantzen P, Wright K, Saad I, Mueller R, Morgan D, Sanders S, Zehr C, O'Campo K, Hardy J, Prada C-M, Eckman C, Younkin S, Hsiao K, Duff K. Accelerated Alzheimer-type phenotype in transgenic mice carrying both mutant *amyloid precursor protein* and *presenilin* 1 transgenes. Nature Med 1998; 4: 97–100.

54. Weidemann A, Paliga K, Dürrwang U, Czech C, Evin G, Masters CL, Beyreuther K. Formation of stable complexes between two Alzheimer's disease gene products: presenilin-2 and β-amyloid precursor protein. Nature Med 1997; 3: 328–32.

55. Xia W, Zhang J, Perez R, Koo EH, Selkoe DJ. Interaction between amyloid precursor protein and presenilins in mammalian cells: implications for the pathogenesis of Alzheimer disease. Proc Natl Acad Sci USA 1997; 94: 8208–13.

56. Fiore F, Zambrano N, Minopoli G, Donini V, Duilio A, Russo T. The regions of the FE65 protein homologous to the phosphotyrosine interaction/phosphotyrosine binding domain of Shc bind the intracellular domain of the Alzheimer's amyloid precursor protein. J Biol Chem 1995; 270: 30853–6.

57. De Strooper B, Saftig P, Craessaerts K, Vanderstichele H, Guhde G, Annaert W, Von Figura K, Van Leuven F. Deficiency of presenilin-1 inhibits the normal cleavage of amyloid precursor protein. Nature 1998; 391: 387–90.

58. Haass C, Selkoe D. A technical KO of amyloid-B peptide. Nature 1998; 391: 339–40.

59. Naruse S, Thinakaran G, Luo J-J, Kusiak JW, Tomita T, Iwatsubo T, Qian X, Ginty DD, Price DL, Borchelt DR, Wong PC, Sisodia SS. Effects of PS1 deficiency on membrane protein trafficking in neurons. Neuron (in press).

Address for correspondence:
    S.S. Sisodia,
    Dept. Pharmacological and Physiological Sciences,
    947 E. 58th Street, Abbott 316,
    University of Chicago,
    Chicago, IL 60637, USA

37 Caspase Cleavage Abolishes Molecular Interaction between Presenilin-1 and β-Catenin

G. TESCO, T.-W. KIM AND R.E. TANZI

INTRODUCTION

Missense mutations in presenilin-1 (PS1) and presenilin-2 (PS2) are responsible for roughly 50% of early-onset familial Alzheimer's disease (FAD) [1]. The presenilins are transmembrane proteins localized in the endoplasmic reticulum (ER) and Golgi [2]. To date, over 50 different PS1 mutations have been described and three FAD mutations have been identified in PS2. Both proteins are normally cleaved within the domain encoded by exon 10 [1]. Presenilins can be also degraded by the proteasome following ubiquitination [3]. During staurosporine-induced programmed cell death, presenilins undergo an 'alternative' cleavage mediated by caspases resulting in the production of smaller C-terminal fragments which are Triton-insoluble [4]. To elucidate the biological function of presenilins, efforts have been made to identify molecules that interact with presenilins. Recently it has been shown that the large hydrophilic loop of PS1 physically interacts with β-catenin in non-neuronal cells and with δ-catenin in the brain [5]. β- and δ-catenin are two different members of the catenin family of proteins which are involved in the Wingless pathway and in the regulation of cell–cell adhesion [6]. The aim of this study was to evaluate whether the alternative cleavage of PS1 affects the interaction with β-catenin.

MATERIALS AND METHODS

CELL CULTURE, INDUCTION AND INHIBITION OF CELL DEATH

H4 human neuroglioma cells were cultured in DMEM (high-glucose) containing 10% heat-inactivated FCS, 100 U/ml penicillin, 100 µg/ml streptomycin, 2 mM L-glutamine. For the induction of apoptosis, cells were

Alzheimer's Disease and Related Disorders
Edited by K. Iqbal, D.F. Swaab, B. Winblad and H.M. Wisniewski
© 1999 John Wiley & Sons Ltd

seeded at a density of 5×10^6 cells for each 150 mm Petri dish. After 48 h, the cell layer was washed twice with PBS and the standard media was replaced with serum-free DMEM containing 1 μM staurosporine (STS) (Calbiochem). A time-course experiment was performed: H4 cells were collected at time-points 0, 6, 8, and 16 of STS treatment. Cells were pelleted by centrifugation and washed once with PBS.

WESTERN BLOT ANALYSIS AND IMMUNOPRECIPITATION

Pellets from apoptotic and non-apoptotic cells were detergent extracted on ice using IP buffer (10 mM Tris–HCl, pH 7.4, 150 mM NaCl, 2 mM EDTA, 0.5% Nonidet P-40) plus protease inhibitors. The lysates were centrifuged at $1000 \times g$ for 10 min at 4 °C. The supernatants were collected and used for immunoprecipitation. The pellets were heated at 50 °C for 10 min in sample buffer. For immunoprecipitation with monoclonal antibodies, goat anti-mouse-IgG magnetic beads-conjugated were precoated using 1.5 μg of anti-β-catenin (571-781 Transduction Laboratorier), for each sample. The lysates were incubated with anti-mouse-IgG magnetic beads-conjugated precoated with anti-β-catenin$_{C-100}$ antibody, or with 1 μl of αPS1loop antibody (gift of G. Thinakaran and S. Sisodia), and incubated overnight in the cold room. The samples immunoprecipitated with αPS1loop were further incubated with protein A magnetic beads-conjugated for 2 h in the cold room. Immunoprecipitates were washed twice in IP buffer then collected using a magnetic bead collector and heated at 50 °C for 10 min in sample buffer. Cell lysates from each time-point of the STS time-course experiment were immunoprecipitated with 1.5 μg anti-β-catenin$_{571-781}$ antibody (Transduction Laboratories). Both immunoprecipitates and pellets were subjected to SDS–PAGE using 4–20% gradient Tris/glycine gels under reducing conditions (Novex). Proteins were transferred to polyvinylidene difluoride membrane (Bio-Rad) using a semi-dry electrotransfer system (Hoefer). The blots were blocked with 5% non-fat dry milk in TBST (25 mM Tris, pH 7.4, 137 mM NaCl, 0.15% Tween 20) for 1.5 h, incubated with primary antibodies (anti-β-catenin:horseradish peroxidase-conjugated (HRPO), 1:1000 in 5% non-fat dry milk TBST; αPS1loop, 1:2500 in TBST) for 1 and 1.5 h, respectively, and incubated with secondary antibodies (horseradish peroxidase-conjugated anti-mouse or anti-rabbit antibodies, 1:5000 [Pierce]) in 5% non-fat dry milk TBST for 1 h. Between steps, the blots were washed with TBST for 30 min. The blots were visualized using the ECL or ECL plus Western blot detection system (Amersham).

RESULTS

In this study, we set out to examine whether endogenous forms of PS1–CTF (PS1–C-terminal fragments) interact with β-catenin in H4 human neuroglioma cells and whether caspase-mediated cleavage affects this interaction. Detergent lysates prepared from apoptotic and non-apoptotic H4 cells were subjected to immunoprecipitation (IP) using αPS1loop antiserum (Figure 1A, lanes 2 and 4, respectively). β-catenin co-immunoprecipitated with the endogenous PS1–CTF in normal cells as shown by Western blot analysis of immunoprecipitates using anti-β-catenin antibody (Figure 1A, upper panel, lane 4). In cell lysates from apoptotic cells, β-catenin did not co-immunoprecipitate with PS1 (Figure 1A, upper panel, lane 2), although both the normal PS1–CTF and aCTF were successfully immunoprecipitated, as shown by immunodetection with αPS1loop antiserum (Figure 1A, lower panel, lanes 2 and 4). Since it has previously been shown that during apoptosis [7], β-catenin holoprotein undergoes sequential cleavage by caspases at multiple sites, resulting in the appearance of a ~90 kDa species owing to the removal of a fragment of ~2 kDa from the C-terminus of β-catenin, and that the ~90 kDa species is then further cleaved into a smaller fragment of ~65 kDa, cell lysates from each time-point of the STS treatment time-course experiment were immunoprecipitated with anti-

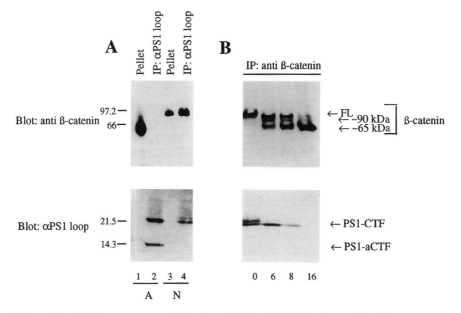

Figure 1. (A) Immuno-coprecipitation of PS1–CTF with β-catenin. Upper panel, Western blot analysis using anti-β-catenin antibody; lower panel, Western blot analysis using αPS1loop antibody. Lanes 1 and 3: pellet from apoptotic and non-apoptotic cells, respectively. Lanes 2 and 4: the detergent extract supernatants from the same cells as lanes 1 and 2, immunoprecipitated with αPS1loop antibody. (B) Co-immuno-precipitation of β-catenin and PS1–CTF during staurosporine treatment time-course experiment. Upper panel, Western blot analysis using anti-β-catenin antibody; lower panel, Western blot analysis using αPS1loop antibody. Cell lysates from each time-point were immunoprecipitated with anti-β-catenin antibody

β-catenin$_{571-781}$ antibody (Figure 1B). Western blot analysis of immuno-precipitates using anti-β-catenin antibody detected β-catenin holoprotein at time-point 0 h, ~90 kDa and ~65 kDa β-catenin species at 6, 8, and 16 h timepoints (Figure 1B, upper panel). At the later time-points the ~65 kDa species of β-catenin became the prevalent species. Immunodetection of the same blot using αPS1loop antibody showed that PS1–CTF co-immunoprecipitated with all β-catenin species at time-points 0, 6 and 8, but PS1–CTF was not detected at time-point 16 (Figure 1B, lower panel). Although the normal PS1–CTF undergoes caspase-mediated cleavage during STS-induced apoptosis, as demonstrated by the decrease in the amount (Figure 1B, lower panel, time-points 0, 6 and 8), the aCTF was not detected. Taken together, these data demonstrate a specific interaction between endogenous β-catenin and the endogenous PS1–CTF in H4 cells and the caspase-mediated abrogation of β-catenin–PS1–CTF during apoptosis.

DISCUSSION

Apoptosis, or programmed cell death, is characterized morphologically by loss of cell volume, membrane blebbing, and chromatin condensation that lead to cellular detachment from the substratum in adherent cells or to a loss of cell–cell contact in suspended cells (for review, see [8]). The initiation of the cell death program includes the proteolytic activation of caspases which, through auto-activation and activation of other caspases, results in the cleavage of a large set of cell death substrates. Caspase-mediated cleavage events promote the 'execution' stage of apoptosis by disrupting several types of interactions (e.g. β-catenin/α-catenin binding [7]). Since β-catenin has been shown to play a role in the Wingless pathway and in cadherin-mediated cell–cell adhesion, diverse physiological functions of β-catenin may be mediated by different molecular interactions. It has previously been reported that caspase-mediated cleavage of β-catenin abrogates its interaction with α-catenin, thereby disrupting actin organization in the apoptotic cell [7]. Alterations in the actin cytoskeleton lead to the loss of cell–cell adhesion and changes in cell shape which are associated with anchorage-related apoptosis, or anoikis [9]. We now show that the β-catenin interacts with endogenous PS1–CTF and that β-catenin–PS1 interaction is abrogated by caspase-mediated cleavage. It is possible that β-catenin–PS1 interaction is also involved in the regulation of cell–cell adhesion or cytoskeleton organization. As caspase-mediated cleavage of β-catenin serves to disrupt cell–cell adhesion in cells programmed to die, it is possible that the abrogation of β-catenin–PS1 binding might contribute to the cellular changes that are essential for the execution of apoptosis. Since it has been shown that during apoptosis there is an increase in the production of aCTF in cells expressing FAD-linked mutant forms of PS1 (Kovaks et al., this volume), it is possible that in Alzheimer's patients with PS1 mutations the β-catenin–PS1–CTF interaction could be adversely affected, leading to cytoskeleton alterations that activate or contribute to the cell death program in the CNS.

ACKNOWLEDGEMENTS

These studies were supported by grants from the NINDS, NIA and Alzheimer's Association (T.L.L. Temple Award). G.T. is a recipient of The John Douglas French Alzheimer's Foundation Fellowship; T.-W.K. is a recipient of Partners Investigators Nesson Award. We thank Dr S. Sisodia and Dr G. Thinakaran for the generous gift of the αPS1loop antibody.

REFERENCES

1. Tanzi RE. The molecular genetics of Alzheimer's disease. In: Martin JB (ed) Scientific American Molecular Neurology. New York: Scientific American, 1998; 55–75.
2. Kovacs DM, Fausett HJ, Page KJ, Kim T-W, Mori RD, Merriam DE, Hollister RD, Hallmark OG, Mancini R, Felsenstein KM, Hyman BT, Tanzi RE, Wasco W. Alzheimer associated presenilins 1 and 2: neuronal expression in brain and localization to intracellular membranes in mammalian cells. Nature Med 1996; 2: 224–9.
3. Kim T-W, Pettingell WH, Hallmark OG, Moir RD, Wasco W, Tanzi RE. Endoproteolytic processing and proteasomal degradation of presenilin 2 in transfected cells. J Biol Chem 1997; 272: 11006–10.
4. Kim T-W, Pettingell WH, Jung Y-K, Kovacs DM, Tanzi RE. Alternative cleavage of Alzheimer-associated presenilins during apoptosis by caspase-3 family protease. Science 1997; 277: 373–6.
5. Zhou J, Liyanage U, Medina M, Ho C, Simmons AD, Lovett M, Kosik KS. Presenilin 1 interacts in brain with a novel member of the Armadillo family. NeuroReport 1997; 8: 1489–94.
6. Barth AI, Näthke IS, Nelson WJ. Cadherin, catenin, and APC protein: interplay between cytoskeletal complexes and signaling pathways. Curr Opin Cell Biol 1997; 9: 683–90.
7. Brancolini C, Lazarevic D, Rodriguez J, Schneider C. Dismantling cell–cell contacts during apoptosis is coupled to a caspase-dependent proteolytic cleavage of β-catenin. J Cell Biol 1997; 139: 759–71.
8. Villa P, Kaufmann SH, Earnshaw WC. Caspases and caspase inhibitors. TIBS 1997; 22: 388–93.
9. Frisch SM, Ruoslahti E. Integrins and anoikis. Curr Opin Cell Biol 1997; 7: 701–6.

Address for correspondence:
  R.E. Tanzi,
  Department of Neurology, Genetics and Aging Unit, Massachusetts
    General Hospital—East,
  149 13th Street, Charlestown, MA 02129, USA
  Tel: 617 726 6845; fax: 617 726 5677;
  e-mail: tanzi@helix.mgh.harvard.edu

38 Role of Presenilin Processing and Caspases for Amyloid β-Peptide Generation and NOTCH signaling

SASCHA RÖHRIG, MANFRED BROCKHAUS,
HARALD STEINER, ANJA CAPELL,
JÜRGEN GRÜNBERG, JOCHEN WALTER, UWE LEIMER,
HANSRUEDI LOETSCHER, NICOLE WITTENBURG,
HELMUT JACOBSEN, RALF BAUMEISTER AND
CHRISTIAN HAASS

INTRODUCTION

Numerous mutations have been identified in the genes encoding the two homologous presenilin proteins PS1 and PS2 [1]. PS proteins undergo proteolytic processing [1, 2], which might be required for their pathological as well as their biological function [3]. In addition to the conventional processing pathway mediated by the unknown presenilinase, a second processing pathway was characterized recently (Figure 1). In this alternative pathway, proteases of the caspase superfamily cleave PS1 and PS2 further C-terminal to the conventional site, which results in the production of smaller C-terminal fragments (CTF) and larger N-terminal fragments (NTF) [4–6]. Moreover, caspase-mediated processing of PS2 might be enhanced in brains from patients with the Volga–German PS2 mutation probably indicating a pathological role of caspases for the generation of the 42 amino acid amyloid β-peptide (Aβ42) [4]. Inhibition of caspases is currently discussed as a novel approach to slow the progression of neurodegenerative disorders such as amyotrophic lateral sclerosis (ALS), Parkinson's disease, trauma, hypoxia–ischemia and Alzheimer's disease (AD) [7]. We therefore analyzed if conventional- and/or caspase-mediated processing is required for amyloidogenesis. In addition we also investigated the role of proteolytic fragments of PS in NOTCH signaling.

Alzheimer's Disease and Related Disorders
Edited by K. Iqbal, D.F. Swaab, B. Winblad and H.M. Wisniewski
© 1999 John Wiley & Sons Ltd

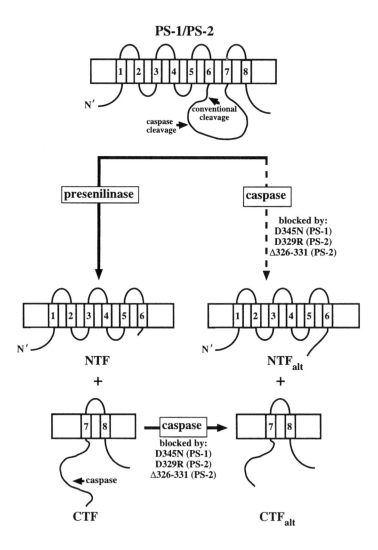

Figure 1. Schematic representation of conventional proteolytic processing (left panel) of PS proteins as well as caspase-mediated processing (right panel). Caspase-mediated cleavage occurs further towards the C-terminal after Asp345 (PS1) or Asp326 and Asp329 (PS2) and can be inhibited by the indicated mutations

METHODS

The methods are described in detail in [6, 8–10].

RESULTS

CASPASE-MEDIATED PROCESSING OF PRESENILINS IS NOT REQUIRED FOR THEIR PATHOLOGICAL FUNCTION IN Aβ42 GENERATION

PS2 proteins are proteolytically cleaved by caspases to yield a C-terminal fragment of 119 amino acids (Ser330–Ile448) [4, 5]. This cleavage is blocked by specific inhibitors of caspases or can be completely inhibited by mutagenesis of the cleavage site [4, 5]. We asked whether interference with caspase-processing of FAD mutant PS2 would prevent pathological Aβ42 generation. PS2-transfected Neuro2a cells (wild-type, wt) and the FAD-associated mutation Met239Val were treated for 48 h with increasing concentrations of the cell-permeable caspase inhibitor z-VAD-FMK and culture supernatants were assayed for Aβ40 and Aβ42 using a highly specific ELISA. We observed neither a consistent decrease in the overall level of Aβ peptides nor a change in the ratio of Aβ42:Aβ40 in the wt PS2 transfectants grown in the presence of z-VAD-fmk (Figure 2A). Moreover, inhibition of caspase-mediated cleavage did not block the pathological effect of the FAD-associated PS2 mutant on Aβ42 generation (Figure 2B).

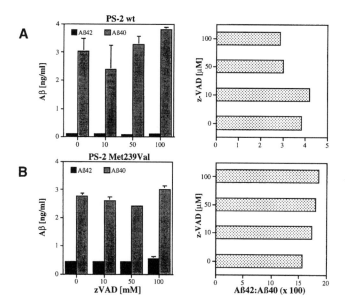

Figure 2. Stably transfected Neuro2a cells were treated for 48 h with increasing concentrations of caspase inhibitor z-VAD-FMK and supernatants were harvested for the Aβ peptide assays. The figures show the concentrations of Aβ42 and Aβ40 in the supernatant (left panel) and their ratios (right panel) for each individual cell line. (A) PS2 wild-type transfected cells. (B) Cells transfected with the PS2 FAD mutant Met239Val

These data therefore suggest that caspase-mediated processing of PS2 is not required for Aβ40 or Aβ42 production. To further prove that Aβ42 formation occurs independently of caspase-mediated processing, we stably transfected Neuro2a cells with PS2 cDNA constructs containing point mutations which inhibit caspase-mediated processing. We expressed the mutation Asp329Arg and the deletion mutation PS2$_{326-331}$. The point mutation completely blocks caspase cleavage at the Asp329/Ser330 bond, whereas the deletion inhibits the minor caspase cleavage after Asp326 as well [5]. These mutations were introduced into the PS2 FAD mutant Asn141Ile (Figure 3). Conditioned media from stably transfected cells were assayed for Aβ42 and Aβ40. As noted previously, the absolute concentrations of the two Aβ peptides varied among the different clones. However, from a comparison of their calculated ratios it became evident that inactivation of the caspase site(s) in PS2 Asn141Ile did not reverse the relative increase in Aβ42, but rather enhanced the amyloidogenic activity of the FAD mutant 2–3-fold (Figure 3). This effect was measured for several individual clones in independent experiments. The increased Aβ42 production might be due to the protection of PS2 from caspase-mediated processing.

Similar results were obtained when caspase cleavage of PS1 was inhibited [8]. Again, PS1 mutations affected pathological generation of Aβ42 independent of caspase-mediated processing.

These data therefore demonstrate that caspase-mediated processing is not required for the pathological activity of PS1 and PS2 in amyloidogenesis. Moreover, a therapeutic approach using caspases as a target might even result in the enhanced generation of Aβ42.

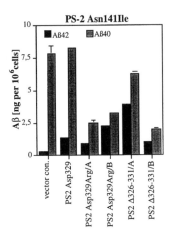 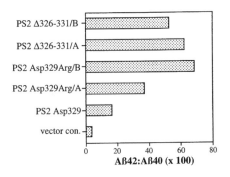

Figure 3. Inhibition of caspase-mediated processing by mutagenizing the critical aspartates does not affect Aβ42 generation. Supernatants were harvested for the Aβ assays after 48 h of culture. The figures show the concentrations of Aβ42 and Aβ40 in the supernatant (left panel) and their ratios for each individual cell line (right panel)

CASPASE-MEDIATED PROCESSING OF PS2 IS NOT REQUIRED FOR ITS PHYSIOLOGICAL FUNCTION IN NOTCH SIGNALING

To further test the physiological function of the engineered presenilin variants with inactivated caspase cleavage sites, we introduced the mutant cDNA constructs into *Caenorhabditis elegans sel-12* (ar171) worms, which lack a functional SEL-12 protein. We and others had previously shown that human PS1 and PS2 can fully rescue the egg-laying defect of *sel-12*-deficient animals [9, 11]. We now used a similar approach to assess the *in vivo* activity of PS mutants defective in caspase cleavage. *sel-12* (ar171) animals cannot lay eggs due to a strong reduction of *sel-12* activity. This defect can be efficiently rescued by expressing PS1 and PS2 wt genes under the control of the *sel-12* promoter [9, 11]. Similarly, the engineered variants PS1 Asp345Asn, PS2 Asp329Arg and PS2 Δ326–331 rescue the *sel-12* egg-laying defect in the same way as PS1 and PS2 wild-type (Table 1). These data therefore demonstrate that both PS proteins are biologically active in the NOTCH signaling pathway of *C. elegans* in the absence of caspase cleavage sites.

Table 1. Rescue of the *sel-12* egg-laying defect by human presenilin derivatives. Wild-type presenilins, as well as mutants that are not cleaved by caspase, rescue the egg-laying defect in *sel-12* mutant worms. Animals injected with the expression vector alone or the PS1 Asp385Asn mutant are not rescued. The latter is a mutation of an Asp residue conserved in all PS1 genes cloned so far and does not affect caspase-mediated cleavage. The lack of biological activity might indicate that we have created an artificial mutation similar to the FAD-associated mutations, which do not rescue the *sel-12* mutant phenotype. Data are collected from at least three independent transgenic lines and 34–80 worms per injected construct

Injected construct	egl$^+$ (%)
PS1 wt	86
PS1 Asp345Asn	86
PS1 Asp385Asn	0
PS2 wt	90
PS2 Asp329Arg	85
PS2 Δ326–331	82
Vector	0

RECOMBINANT N-TERMINAL PS FRAGMENTS ARE NOT SUFFICIENT FOR THE PRODUCTION OF Aβ42

We next expressed artificial PS1 NTFs (NTF$_{292}$) with and without a FAD-associated mutation by introducing a stop codon at the major cleavage site after amino acid 292 [12]. In contrast to endogenous PS fragments, which are highly stable, such recombinant fragments are rapidly degraded. Pulse chase experiments revealed inhibition of the proteasome-blocked degradation of NTF_{292} [10]. Expression of a mutant NTF_{292} containing a FAD-associated mutation is not sufficient for the production of increased amounts of Aβ42, even upon inhibition of the proteasome (Figure 4a). This result suggests that: (a) 'free' proteolytic fragments of PS proteins are unstable and are removed by the proteasome; and (b) 'free' mutant fragments lose their pathological function in Aβ42 generation.

In order to test whether 'free' NTFs not incorporated into the PS complex are sufficient to rescue the *sel-12* mutant phenotype of *C. elegans*, we expressed a cDNA construct with a stop codon inserted shortly after the transmembrane domain 6 in the mutant worm. In contrast to the full-length PS1 cDNA, expression of the recombinant fragment does not rescue the mutant phenotype (Figure 4b). This indicates that the full-length PS protein or its proteolytic processing is required for the biological activity.

As reported previously [13, 14], PS proteins are expressed as a heterodimeric complex, which might represent the functional unit of PS proteins. In order to test whether the recombinant NTF_{292} fails to incorporate into the PS complex and might therefore lose its biological and pathological function, we performed co-immunoprecipitation experiments. We depleted membrane extracts from the PS complex using an antibody to the CTF (antibody 3027). After depletion, cell lysates were re-immunoprecipitated with an antibody raised to the NTF (antibody 2953). Interestingly, when this experiment was carried out in a cell line expressing full-length PS1, no NTF could be isolated after re-immunoprecipitation (Figure 5). In contrast, the same immunoprecipitation of depleted lysates derived from cells stably transfected with the recombinant NTF_{292} led to the detection of large amounts of NTF_{292}, strongly indicating that NTF_{292} is not incorporated into the PS complex.

We therefore conclude from these data that PS fragments which do not participate in complex formation are biologically and pathologically inactive. Both activities appear to require the formation of the heterodimeric PS complex.

CONCLUSIONS

Caspase-mediated processing of presenilins is not required for their pathological function in Aβ42 generation. Therefore, proteases of the caspase family

---

Figure 4 (opposite). (A) Mutant NTF_{298} does not increase the production of Aβ42, even upon its stabilization. K293 cells stably expressing Swedish βAPP and NTF_{298} with and without the Y115H mutation were treated with and without LLnL to inhibit the proteasome. Note that the mutant NTF_{298} (NTF_{298}Y115H) does not induce Aβ42 generation, even upon its stabilization with LLnL. (B) A recombinant NTF highly similar to NTF_{292} fails to rescue the *sel-12* mutant phenotype. Left panel: the

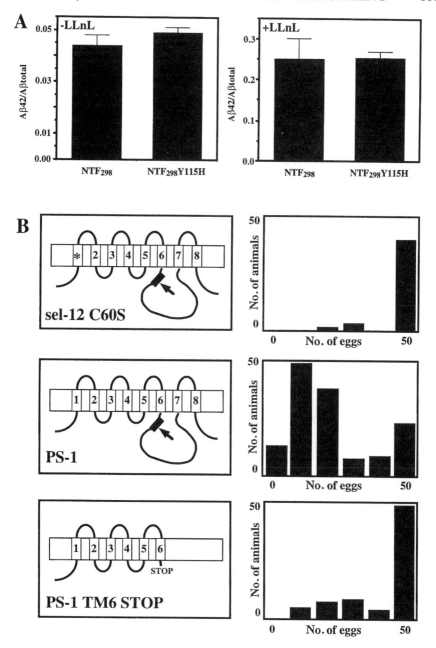

putative structure of the *C. elegans* SEL-12 and human PS proteins. Right panel: steady-state levels of unlaid eggs in *sel-12* (ar131) animals carrying the respective PS construct. Bars represent the number of animals (y axis) with a given number of eggs (x axis). Data shown for SEL-12 (C60S) represent the phenotype of *sel-12* (ar131)

Detection: PS1N

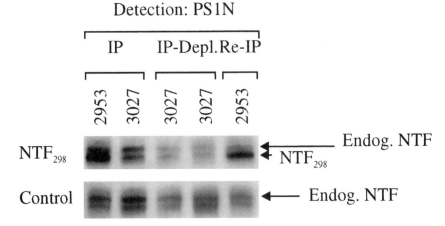

Figure 5. NTF$_{298}$ does not co-immunoprecipitate with the PS1 heterodimeric complex. Untransfected K293 cells (lower panel; control) or K293 cells stably transfected with the NTF$_{298}$ cDNA (upper panel; NTF$_{298}$) were immunoprecipitated with antibodies 2953 or 3027 (first two lanes, IP). Immunoprecipitated fragments were detected with antibody PS1N (14). Immunoprecipitation with antibody 3027 to the large loop of PS1 co-isolates the endogenous NTF (upper and lower panel, second lane [13, 14]). In cells transfected with the NTF$_{298}$ cDNA, an additional band is detected which migrates below the prominent endogenous PS1 NTF. Note that in the immunoprecipitations of cell lysates from the transfected cells using the N-terminal antibody 2953, the lower band is strongly enriched as compared to the immunoprecipitation carried out with the antibody 3027 to the large loop of PS1. This already indicates that NTF$_{298}$ does not co-immunoprecipitate with the heterodimeric complex. Cell lysates were depleted from the PS1 heterodimeric complex by two additional rounds of co-immunoprecipitation using antibody 3027 (IP-Depl.). As shown by the decreasing detection of the co-immunoprecipitated NTF (detected by antibody PS1N), this procedure removes large amounts of the PS1 heterodimeric complex. After depletion, the cell lysate was again immunoprecipitated (Re-IP), but now with an antibody to the N-terminal domain of PS1 (2953). In cells stably expressing NTF$_{298}$, this reveals a prominent band (arrowhead), which migrates below the endogenous NTF (arrow) and thus represents NTF$_{298}$. In untransfected K293 cells, no prominent NTF is revealed, demonstrating that NTF$_{298}$ is not co-immunoprecipitated with the PS1 heterodimeric complex

are unlikely to represent a novel target for drugs supposed to slow the progression of FAD. Moreover, caspase-mediated processing is not required for the physiological activity of PS proteins in *C. elegans*, since inhibition of caspase cleavage does not abolish the biological function of human PS1 and PS2 in NOTCH-signaling. We propose that the formation of a heterodimeric PS complex, probably together with other binding proteins, is essential for the physiological and pathological function of presenilins.

ACKNOWLEDGEMENTS

This work was supported by grants from the Verum Foundation, the Fritz Thyssen Foundation and the Deutsche Forschungsgemeinschaft to C.H. (SFB 317), and to R.B. We thank Dennis Selkoe and Martin Citron for PS-transfected cell lines, and Oliver Hobert and Gary Ruvkun for providing ttx-3:GFP.

REFERENCES

1. Haass C. Presenilins: Genes for life and death. Neuron 1997; 18: 687–90.
2. Thinakaran G, Borchelt DR, Lee MK, Slunt HH, Spitzer L, Kim G, Ratovitsky T, Davenport F, Nordstedt C, Seeger M, Hardy J, Levey AI, Gandy SE, Jenkins NA, Copeland NG, Pric DL, Sisodia SS. Endoproteolysis of presenilin 1 and accumulation of processed derivatives *in vivo*. Neuron 1996; 17: 181–90.
3. Grünberg J, Capell A, Leimer U, Steiner B, Steiner H, Walter J, Haass C. Proteolytic processing of presenilin proteins: degradation or biological activation? Alzheimer's Res 1997; 3: 253–9.
4. Kim T-W, Pettingell WH, Jung Y-K, Kovacs DM, Tanzi RE. Alternative cleavage of Alzheimer-associated presenilins during apoptosis by a caspase-3 family protease. Science 1997; 277: 373–6.
5. Loetscher H, Deuschle U, Brockhaus M, Reinhardt D, Nelboeck P, Mous J, Grünberg J, Haass C, Jacobsen H. Presenilins are processed by caspase-type proteases. J Biol Chem 1997; 272: 20655–9.
6. Grünberg J, Walter J, Loetscher H, Deuschle U, Jacobsen H, Haass C. Alzheimer's disease associated presenilin-1 holoprotein and its 18–20 kDa C-terminal fragment are death substrates for proteases of the caspase family. Biochemistry 1998; 37: 2263–70.
7. Holtzman D, Deshmukh M. Caspases: a treatment target for neurodegenerative diseases? Nature Med 1997; 3: 954–5.
8. Brockhaus M, Loetscher H, Jacobsen H, Baumeister R, Zweckbronner I, Jakubek C, Grünberg J, Haass C. Caspase-mediated cleavage is not required for the activity of presenilins in amyloidogenesis and NOTCH signaling. NeuroReport 1997; 9: 1481–6.
9. Baumeister R, Leimer U, Zweckbronner I, Jakubek C, Grünberg J, Haass C. Human presenilin-1, but not familial Alzheimer's disease (FAD) mutants, facilitate *Caenorhabditis elegans* NOTCH signalling independently of proteolytic processing. Genes Funct 1997; 1: 149–59.
10. Steiner H, Capell A, Pesold B, Citron M, Selkoe D, Romig H, Mendla K, Haass C. Expression of Alzheimer's disease associated presenilin-1 is controlled by multiple proteolytic pathways. J Biol Chem 1998; 273: 32322–31.
11. Levitan D, Doyle T, Brousseau D, Lee M, Thinakaran G, Slunt H, Sisodia S, Greenwald I. Assessment of normal and mutant human presenilin function in *Caenorhabditis elegans*. Proc Natl Acad Sci USA 1996; 93: 14940–44.
12. Podlisny M, Citron M, Amarante P, Sherrington R, Xia W, Zhang J, Diehl T, Levesque G, Fraser P, Haass C, Koo E, Seubert P, St George-Hyslop P, Teplow D, Selkoe D. Presenilins proteins undergo heterogeneous endoproteolysis between Thr291 and Ala299 and occur as stable N- and C-terminal fragments in normal and Alzheimer brain tissue. Neurobiol Dis 1997; 3: 325–37.

13. Thinakaran G, Regard JB, Bouton CML, Harris CL, Sabo S, Price DL, Borchelt DR, Sisodia SS. Stable association of presenilin derivatives and absence of presenilin interactions with APP. Neurobiol Dis (in press).
14. Capell A, Grünberg J, Pesold B, Diehlmann A, Citron M, Nixon R, Beyreuther K, Selkoe DJ, Haass C. The proteolytic fragments of the Alzheimer's disease-associated presenilin-1 form heterodimers and occur as a 100–150 kDa molecular mass complex. J Biol Chem 1998; 273: 3205–11.

Address for correspondence:
 Christian Haass PhD,
 Central Institute of Mental Health, Dept. Molecular Biology,
 J5 68155 Mannheim, Germany
 Tel: 01149 621 1703 884; fax: 01149 621 23429;
 e-mail: Haass@as200.zi-mannheim.de

 Ralf Baumeister PhD,
 Genzentrum, Feodor-Lynen-Str.25, 81377 Munich, Germany
 Tel: 089 7401 7347; fax: 089 7401 7314;
 e-mail: Bmeister@LMB.UNI-Muenchen.de

39 Caspase Activation in Dystrophic Neurites in Alzheimer's Disease and Aged HuAPPsw Transgenic Mice

GREG M. COLE, FUSHENG YANG, P.P. CHEN, S.A. FRAUTSCHY AND K. HSIAO

INTRODUCTION

Loss of synapses exceeds neuron loss in AD and is a better correlate of dementia than other pathological measures [1, 2]. In plaque-forming APP transgenic mouse models for AD, neuron loss has been difficult to quantify [3, 4]. Because cumulative loss is focal, age-related and slow, we sought to develop markers of active neurodegeneration involving loss of neuronal arbor and synapses prior to loss of neuronal cell bodies.

Activation of specific 'caspase' endopeptidase cascades leads to delayed cell death or apoptosis, conventionally characterized by intranucleosomal DNA fragmentation. This is detected as 'laddering' on gels or by DNA end-labeling (TUNEL) *in situ*, which is increased in the AD brain [5, 6]. Initiation of caspase activation has been linked to extranuclear events including trophic factor withdrawal, oxidative damage and mitochondrial release of cytochrome c [7]. Local involvement of these triggers could result in focal caspase activation in synapses, axons or dendrites and thus play a role in dying back prior to the loss of entire neurons. In order to detect caspase activation in distal parts of cells, we made an end-specific antibody for a 32 kDa caspase-cleaved fragment of actin, 'fractin', and demonstrated plaque-associated neuron and microglia labeling in AD brains [8]. We have used confocal double labeling for fractin and cell markers to describe plaque-associated caspase activation in nerve terminals in AD and in the APPsw transgenic mice.

Alzheimer's Disease and Related Disorders
Edited by K. Iqbal, D.F. Swaab, B. Winblad and H.M. Wisniewski
© 1999 John Wiley & Sons Ltd

MATERIALS AND METHODS

Frozen AD cortex and hippocampus, from NIH AD Centers [Drs H. Vinters (UCLA) and Carol Miller (USC)] and 12 and 18 month-old Tg2576 HuAPPsw mice [9] were cryostat-sectioned and immunostained, as previously described, with affinity purified rabbit fractin, an antibody which labels a 32 kDa actin fragment produced by caspase cleavages [8]. Pseudoconfocal double- and triple-labeled immunofluorescent images (Scanalytics) were obtained using rabbit fractin antibody and mouse monoclonal antibody to a cell marker followed by anti-rabbit FITC, anti-mouse rhodamine and then biotin–10G4 anti-Aβ and avidin–Oregon Blue (Molecular Probes).

RESULTS

We have previously described immunohistochemical fractin labeling of plaque-associated neurons, processes and microglia in the AD brain [8]. Figure 1 illustrates punctate fractin labeling in 12 month-old HuAPPsw mouse brains, revealing its association with plaques as in the AD brain. Confocal immunofluorescence triple labeling was used to clarify plaque-associated fractin labeling in the AD brain and aged mice. Insets show the individual staining patterns as they appeared in color (red, green, blue; RGB) and arrows indicate RG overlap (yellow in original color image). As shown in Figure 2, fractin (G) frequently colocalized (arrows) with synaptophysin (R) in plaques identified by Aβ antibody (B) in AD (Figure 2A) and APPsw mouse (Figure 2B–F) but only occasionally with a phosphotau epitope, AT8(R) (Figure 2D). By contrast, MAPII and GFAP showed little, if any, overlap with fractin (not shown). Unlike the AD brain, brains of 12–18 month-old mice showed little or no fractin labeling of entire cells with microglial or neuronal morphology. However, lectin-stained microglia frequently exhibited fractin labeling of isolated puncta (arrows), which often appeared on the edge of, or were engulfed by, microglia (Figure 2C). An anti-nitrotyrosine monoclonal antibody (R) labeled some vessels and many plaque-associated processes in 12 and 18 month-old transgenic mice (Figure 2E), frequently overlapping with fractin (G) (arrows). This is consistent with oxidative damage caused by nitric oxide in the vicinity of plaques. Immunostaining of structures resembling astrocytes and microglia with antibody for the anti-apoptotic protein Bcl-2 were found closely associated with plaques (not shown). Plaque astrocytes labeled with GFAP (R) overlapped partially with Bcl-2 (G) (arrow, Figure 2F). Lectin-labeled microglia also overlapped with Bcl-2 (not shown). Bcl-2 was rarely found in identifiable neurons.

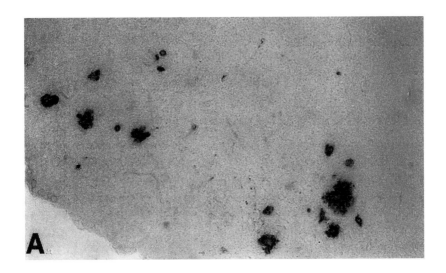

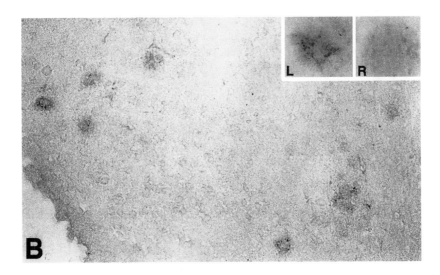

Figure 1. (A) β-amyloid (4G8) plaques in the entorhinal cortex of 12 month-old HuAPPsw mouse and the adjacent section (B), labeled with fractin antibody to caspase-cleaved actin, shows punctate plaque-associated staining (× 250). Inset: L, punctate fractin labeling in individual plaque and R, peptide antigen absorbed blocking of same plaque in adjacent section with hematoxylin counterstain demonstrates specificity of fractin labeling (× 1000)

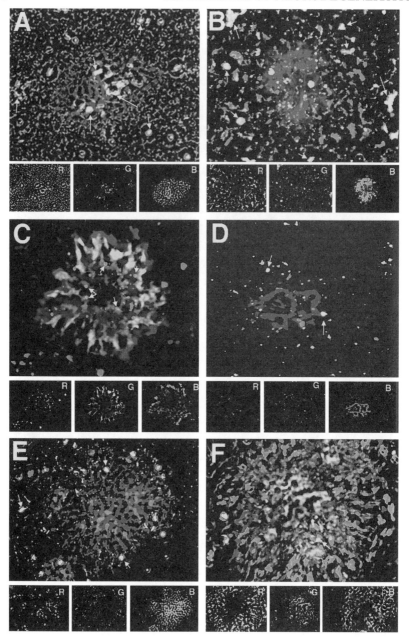

Figure 2. Panels A–F indicate RGB merged images from confocal pseudocolor immunofluorescent triple labeling while insets indicate individual red (R), green (G) or blue (B) channels. Arrows depict examples of R–G overlap (yellow in original color image). (Panels A–B) β-amyloid peptide (B), synaptophysin (R) and fractin (G). (Panel A) Alzheimer's disease cortex. (Panel B) entorhinal cortex, HuAPPsw mouse.

DISCUSSION

These results suggest that plaque-associated caspase activation and cleavage of actin occurs in synaptophysin-positive presynaptic nerve terminals in Alzheimer's disease and in the HuAPPsw mouse. More recent data from confocal and immuno-EM suggests postsynaptic activation as well. Figure 3 illustrates one interpretive model. Activated microglia and reactive astrocytes (not shown) surround plaques in HuAPPsw mice [10], producing reactive oxygen species (ROS) such as nitric oxide and toxic cytokines, which diffuse to surrounding cells and nerve terminals. Aβ complexed to lipoproteins or α-2 macroglobulin can be endocytosed into nerve terminal lysosomes via the lipoprotein-related receptor, LRP. Alternatively, Aβ can directly induce ROS such as hydrogen peroxide [11]. Both sources of ROS result in peroxynitrite- or hydroxyl-mediated mitochondrial damage, leading to focal cytochrome c release and caspase activation. Additional evidence of oxidative damage surrounding HuAPPsw plaques has been reported [12, 13]. Activated caspase cleaves actin, leading to fractin staining in the synapses (Figure 2A, B) and externalization of the inner membrane lipid (PS), the proximal signal for phagocytosis by glia (Figure 2C). Evidence of caspase activation was restricted to nerve terminals which frequently did not contain tau phosphoserine 202 epitopes. Its absence in neuronal cell bodies in 12–18 month-old HuAPPsw mice is consistent with the absence of quantifiable neuron loss [3]. Neuron loss may be prevented by the neuroprotective effects of APP, antioxidant enzymes or anti-apoptotic genes such as Bcl-2, which was elevated in plaques (Figure 2E). However, since we did not find significant neuronal Bcl-2 staining, it is possible that neuron loss may require more extensive tau (e.g. tangle) pathology or activation of other unknown factors.

In regions where fractin labeling was dense, such as the entorhinal cortex, we found highly significant synaptophysin loss in aged HuAPPsw mice (data not shown). Fractin labeling of nerve terminals appears to be an active marker for dying back of neuronal arbor and synapse loss via 'synapoptosis'. As a marker for active synapse loss, fractin labeling may be potentially useful for rapid preclinical trials of neuroprotective agents.

(Panel C) HuAPPsw mouse, biotinylated *Griffonia (Bandeirea) simplicifolia* isolectin B4 (Vector Laboratories, Burlingame, CA), a plant lectin specific for microglia (G) and fractin (R). Arrows show overlap of fractin and microglia, consistent with phagocytosis of fractin-positive terminals. (Panel D) HuAPPsw mouse, red (R) AT8 (Innogenetics, phosphoserine 202 in tau) immunopositive dystrophic neurites around a blue (B) amyloid plaque show occasional overlap with fractin (G). (Panel E) HuAPPsw mouse, red (R) nitrotyrosine and green (G) fractin show overlap in punctate plaque staining. (Panel F) HuAPPsw mouse, Bcl-2 immunolabeling (G) was frequently plaque-associated and showed limited overlap with glial fibrillary acidic protein (R)

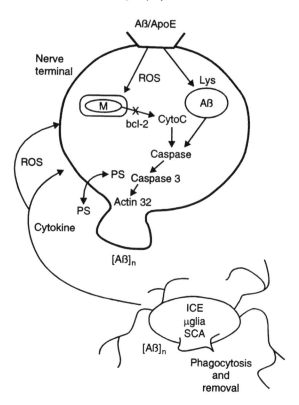

Figure 3. Schematic diagram of 'synapoptosis' illustrating how Aβ may induce reactive oxygen species (ROS) leading to focal mitochondrial damage in nerve terminals, caspase activation and phosphatidyl serine (PS) exposure resulting in phagocytosis by microglia

ACKNOWLEDGEMENTS

We are grateful to Lisa Adams, Walter Beech and Thuy Tran for technical assistance. This work was supported by Grants VA Merit and NIH AG13741 (GMC).

REFERENCES

1. Regeur L, Jensen GB, Pakkenberg H, Evans SM, Pakkenberg B. No global neo-cortical nerve cell loss in brains from patients with senile dementia of Alzheimer's type. Neurobiol Aging 1994; 15: 347–52.
2. Terry RD, Masliah E, Salmon DP, Butters N, DeTeresa R, Hill R, Hansen LA, Katzman R. Physical basis of cognitive alterations in Alzheimer's disease: synapse loss is the major correlate of cognitive impairment. Ann Neurol 1991; 30: 572–80.
3. Irizarry MC, McNamara M, Fedorchak K, Hsiao K, Hyman BT. App$_{sw}$ trans-genic mice develop age-related Aβ deposits and neuropil abnormalities, but no neuronal loss in CA1. J Neuropathol Exp Neurol 1997; 56: 965–73.
4. Irizarry MC, Soriano F, McNamara M, Page KJ, Schenk D, Games D, Hyman BT. Aβ deposition is associated with neuropil changes, but not with overt neuronal loss in the human amyloid precursor protein V717F (PDAPP) transgenic mouse. J Neurosci 1997; 17: 7053–9.
5. Cotman CW, Anderson AJ. A potential role for apoptosis in neurodegeneration and Alzheimer's disease. Mol Neurobiol 1995; 10: 19–45.
6. Lassman H, Bancher C, Breitschopf H, Wegiel J, Bobinski M, Jellinger K, Wisniewski HM. Cell death in Alzheimer's disease evaluated by DNA fragmenta-tion *in situ*. Acta Neuropathol 1995; 89: 35–41.
7. Yang JC, Cortopassi GA. Induction of the mitochondrial permeability transition causes release of the apoptogenic factor cytochrome c. Free Radical Biol Med 1998; 24: 634–41.
8. Yang F, Sun X, Beech W, Teter B, Wu S, Sigel J, Vinters HV, Frautschy SA, Cole GM. Antibody to caspase-cleaved actin detects apoptosis in differentiated neuro-blastoma and neurons and plaque associated neurons and microglia in Alzheimer's disease. Am J Pathol 1998; 152: 379–89.
9. Hsiao K, Chapman P, Nilsen S, Eckman C, Harigaya Y, Younkin S, Yang F, Cole G. Correlative memory deficits, Aβ elevation and amyloid plaques in transgenic mice. Science 1996; 274: 99–102.
10. Frautschy SA, Yang F, Irrizarry M, Hyman B, Saido TC, Hsiao K, Cole GM. Microglial response to amyloid plaques in APPsw transgenic mice. Am J Pathol 1998; 152: 307–17.
11. Behl C, Davis JB, Lesley R, Schubert D. Hydrogen peroxide mediates amyloid β protein toxicity. Cell 1994; 77: 817–27.
12. Pappolla MA, Chyan Y-J, Omar RA, Hsiao K, Perry G, Smith MA, Bozner P. Evidence of oxidative stress and *in vivo* neurotoxicity of β-amyloid in a transgenic mouse model of Alzheimer's disease. Am J Pathol 1998; 152: 871–7.
13. Smith MA, Hirai K, Hsiao K, Papolla MA, Harris PL, Siedlak SL, Tabaton M, Perry G. Amyloid-β deposition is associated with oxidative stress. J Neurochem 1998; 70: 2212–15.

Address for correspondence:
Greg M. Cole,
Sepulveda VAMC GRECC11E,
UCLA Depts. Medicine (SFVP) and Neurology,
16111 Plummer Street, Sepulveda, CA 91343, USA
Tel: 818 891 7711, ext. 9949; fax: 818 895 5835;
e-mail: gmcole@UCLA.edu

40 K$^+$ Efflux Mediated by Delayed Rectifier K$^+$ Channels Contributes to Neuronal Death

SHAN PING YU AND DENNIS W. CHOI

INTRODUCTION

The neurotoxicity of β-amyloid peptide (Aβ), the main component of the senile plaques observed in the brains of patients with Alzheimer's disease, has been suggested to contribute to the pathogenesis of neuronal degeneration in that disease [1], perhaps by inducing programmed cell death [2–7]. Programmed cell death culminating in apoptosis occurs throughout the body in a variety of normal and abnormal conditions [8, 9]. Whatever their type, apoptotic cells share common characteristics: cell body shrinkage, chromatin condensation, cytoplasmic vacuolization, membrane blebbing, and DNA fragmentation [10, 11]. In the last few years, a great deal has been learned about the molecular underpinnings of apoptosis, including the identification of key mediators such as caspases [12–14] and key modulators such as Bcl-2 or Bax [15, 16]. However, relatively little is known about alterations in ion homeostasis associated with apoptosis, beyond changes in intracellular free calcium, [Ca^{2+}]$_i$. Even there, studies have disagreed as to whether [Ca^{2+}]$_i$ is high or low in cells undergoing apoptosis [17–22], or the importance of changes in [Ca^{2+}]$_i$ for cell survival [23, 24].

We have recently focused scrutiny upon another intracellular cation, K$^+$, initially attracted by a general notion that cell body shrinkage would require efflux of this most abundant, osmotically important cation. In the presence of the K$^+$ channel blockers, 4-aminopyridine (4-AP), spateine or quinidine, cytokine deprivation-induced apoptotic shrinkage of human eosinophils was inhibited in a dose-dependent manner [25]. In addition, the selective K$^+$ ionophore, valinomycin, can trigger apoptosis in rodent thymocytes and tumor cell lines [26–28].

We summarize here several observations suggesting that excessive K$^+$ efflux via voltage-gated K$^+$ channels may be a key event in several forms of central

Alzheimer's Disease and Related Disorders
Edited by K. Iqbal, D.F. Swaab, B. Winblad and H.M. Wisniewski
© 1999 John Wiley & Sons Ltd

neuronal programmed cell death, including that induced by toxic exposure to β-amyloid peptide (Aβ) [29, 30].

K+ EFFLUX MEDIATED BY THE DELAYED RECTIFIER K+ CHANNEL, I_K, IS A MEDIATOR OF SOME FORMS OF CORTICAL NEURONAL APOPTOSIS

The non-inactivating outward delayed rectifier current I_K and the transient outward current I_A were the two main voltage-gated K+ currents present in murine cultured cortical neurons (Figure 1A) [31]. We demonstrated that cortical neuronal programmed cell death, induced by either serum deprivation or staurosporine, is associated with a selective enhancement of I_K current (Figure 1B, C), which doubled 3–11 h after insult onset. Inhibiting I_K current by tetraethylammonium (TEA) or raising extracellular K+, but not blocking I_A with 4-AP or applying the inactive control substance, tetramethylammonium (TMA), prevented many neurons from undergoing apoptosis (Figure 2). Both TEA and high K+ increase $[Ca^{2+}]_i$ primarily due to activation of voltage-gated Ca^{2+} channels [32–35]; however, their protective effects persisted even when the Ca^{2+} entry and associated $[Ca^{2+}]_i$ increase were blocked with the broad-spectrum Ca^{2+} channel antagonist, gadolinium (Gd^{3+}, 2–10 μM), or the L-type Ca^{2+} channel antagonist, nifedipine (5 μM).

CHRONIC EXPOSURE TO β-AMYLOID FRAGMENTS ENHANCED DELAYED RECTIFIER K+ CURRENT

Based on the above observations, we considered the hypothesis that an enhancement of outward K+ current might play a similarly important role in the pathogenesis of Aβ-induced neuronal death. In addition, we noted that Aβ fragments increase K+ channel activity in rat cortical astrocytes [36], that the secreted form of the Aβ precursor protein (which includes a partial Aβ sequence) enhances high conductance, charybdotoxin (CTX)-sensitive K+ channels in hippocampal neurons [37], and that Aβ fragments can form non-selective cation channels in natural or artificial membranes [38–43].

Acute incubation with Aβ fragments 25–35 or 1–42 (20 μM for each for 15–30 min) did not alter I_K currents (Figure 3B). However, after 7–11 h exposure to Aβ 25–35 (20 μM) or Aβ 1–42 (10–20 μM), I_K at +40 mV was enhanced by 68% and 81%, respectively (Figure 3, Table 1). Current density was more than doubled (Table 1), arguing against the possibility that the observed increase in I_K was simply explained by sampling larger cells; furthermore, the transient outward current I_A (Figure 3B, Table 1) and the inward rectifier K+

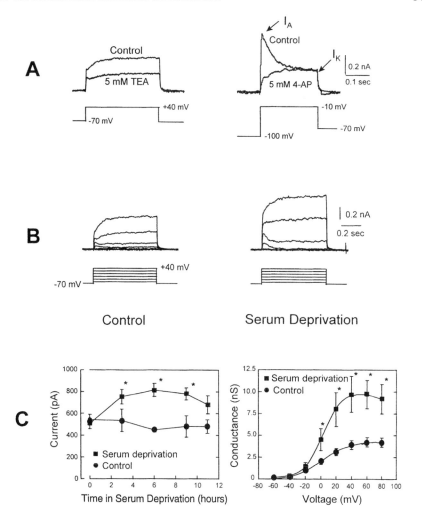

Figure 1. Voltage-gated K+ currents in cultured cortical neurons (DIV 7–12). Cortical cultures were prepared as described previously (31, 60). (A) Normal I_K recorded from neurons in mixed neuronal–glial cultures (left). The current was activated by stepping from a holding potential of −70 mV to +40 mV for 300–600 ms, with leak current subtraction. The non-inactivating outward current was dose-dependently blocked by 1–40 mM bath-applied TEA (effects shown is 5 mM). The transient I_A current was triggered by a 90 mV pulse from a pre-conditional level of −100 mV to −10 mV (right). 4-AP at 5 mM selectively blocked I_A. (B) I_K current recorded at different voltage levels in a control cell (left) and a cell after 6 h serum deprivation (right). During serum deprivation, the same voltage steps triggered much larger currents and outward rectification. (C) Change in I_K with time in control cells, and in cells undergoing apoptosis induced by serum deprivation, n = 5–15 cells at each point (left). Increased K+ conductance via I_K channels after 6 h in serum-free medium (right). * Difference from control at $p < 0.05$ by Student's t test. Modified from reference [31], with permission

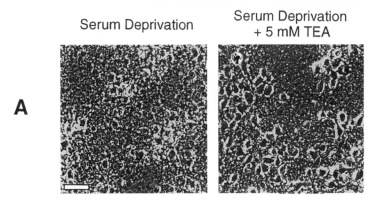

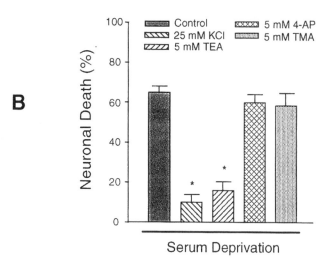

Figure 2. Prevention of apoptosis by the I_K blocker TEA or by raising extracellular K^+. Pure neuronal culture (DIV 7–9) in 24-well plates was used for serum deprivation and mixed culture containing neurons and a glia bed (DIV 10–12) was used for staurosporine exposure (0.1 μM) [13]. NMDA receptor antagonist 1 μM MK-801 and non-NMDA receptor blocker NBQX (5 μM) were added to block glutamate excitotoxicity in serum deprivation experiments. Neuronal death was detected 24 and 48 h after apoptotic insult by LDH release [61]. (A) Phase-contrast micrograph of a pure neuronal culture 48 h after onset of serum deprivation, showing widespread neuronal apoptosis (left). Preservation of neurons in serum-free medium in the presence of 5 mM TEA (right). Bar = 50 μm. (B) Neuronal apoptosis, expressed as a fraction of the total number of neurons, induced by 48 h exposure to serum deprivation, either alone or in the presence of the indicated bath-applied drug, mean ± SEM, n = 4–16 cultures per condition. Cell death was assessed by LDH release or cell counts after staining with 0.4% Trypan blue dye. * Significant difference from the control at p < 0.05 by Student's *t* test, with Bonferroni correction for four comparisons. Modified from reference [31], with permission

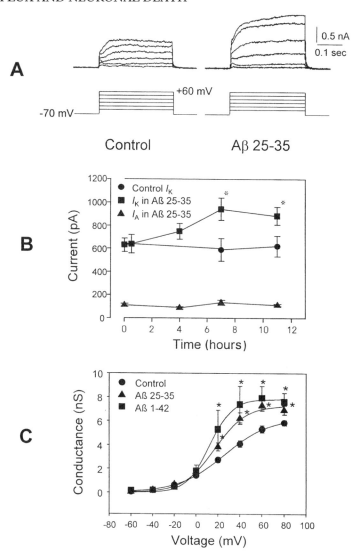

Figure 3. Enhancement of I_K by β-amyloid 25–35 in cortical neurons. Whole-cell I_K current was recorded in cortical neurons of DIV 8–10. (A) I_K triggered by different voltage steps from a holding potential of –70 mV. Representative currents are shown before treatment and after an 11 h exposure to 20 μM Aβ25–35. (B) Time course of I_K enhancement induced by Aβ exposure, I_K in control medium was not changed during same period of time (●). Aβ25–35 exposure did not effect I_A (▲). Each point represents data from 8–19 cells (mean ± SEM). (C) Upmodulation of I_K conductance by Aβ fragments. After 7–11 h in 20 μM Aβ25–35 (▲) or 20 μM Aβ1–42, the I_K activation curves were shifted to the left and the maximal conductance was increased (n = 29 for Aβ25–35 and n = 5 for Aβ1–42, mean ± SEM). ★ Significant difference from control currents (●); (n = 17) at p < 0.05 by Student's t test. Adapted from reference [30], with permission

Table 1. Effects of Aβ fragments on I_K and I_A

	I_K					I_A			
	at +40 mV (pA)	I_K density (pA/pF)	G_{max} (nS)	$V_{1/2}$ (mV)	n	at −20 mV (pA)	G_{max} (nS)	$V_{1/2}$ (mV)	n
Control	562 ± 38	22.5 ± 5.6	6.3 ± 0.1	41.9 ± 2.9	15	110 ± 14	5.8 ± 0.6	16.2 ± 5.5	9
Aβ25–35	942 ± 95*	47.1 ± 4.8*	7.3 ± 0.2*	33.3 ± 2.6*	19	133 ± 22	6.7 ± 0.8	15.8 ± 7.1	8
Aβ1–42	1019 ± 211*	50.6 ± 10.5*	7.8 ± 0.1*	32.8 ± 5.0	6	119 ± 28	6.4 ± 0.4	11.6 ± 3.9	7

Aβ25–35, 20 μM; Aβ1–42, 10–20 μM; both were added into culture medium for 7–11 h before whole-cell patch recordings. I_K at +40 mV was measured as the steady-state current during the last 200 ms of 400–500 ms voltage pulses from a holding potential of −70 mV. I_A at −20 mV was taken as the peak current activated from a conditioning potential of −110 mV. K+ conductance was calculated by the equation: $G = I/(V_{step} - V_{rev})$, where I is the current measured after leak subtraction, V_{step} is the membrane voltage reached by depolarization pulses, and V_{rev} is the reversal potential (−98 mV). Values for G_{max} and $V_{1/2}$ were obtained from fitted curves using the logistic equation: $G = G_{max}/(1 + \exp((V_{1/2} - V)/A))$, where V was membrane potential, $V_{1/2}$ was the potential for half-activation and A was the slope factor. * Indicates difference from respective control parameter at $p < 0.05$ by Student's t test. Mean values are reported with standard error of the mean (SEM).

current (data not shown) were not altered by the Aβ treatment. I_K in sham-washed control neurons remained stable for up to 11 h (Figure 3B). We tested the possibility that Aβ peptides may upregulate the BK channel [37]; however, no outward K+ current sensitive to a 1–3 min bath application of 0.1 μM CTX was seen, either in control neurons (n = 5 cells, p = 0.97), or in neurons exposed for 10 h to 20 μM Aβ1–42 (n = 8, p = 0.13) or 20 μM Aβ25–35 (n = 4, p = 0.57).

The enhancement of I_K induced by Aβ reflected both an increase in maximal conductance and a shift in the voltage for half-activation ($V_{1/2}$) towards hyperpolarized levels (Figure 3C, Table 1). The resting holding current at −70 mV gradually increased during exposure to Aβ25–35 or Aβ1–42. This holding current, although small at −70 mV, increased with membrane depolarization, exhibited outward rectification, and merged with the control current at approximately −100 mV, consistent with mediation by K+ efflux. Furthermore, Aβ enhancement of the resting holding current was absent when K+ in recording pipette was replaced by Cs+ (n = 3).

ATTENUATION OF β-AMYLOID-INDUCED NEURONAL DEATH BY TEA AND 25 mM K+

?If the observed enhancement of I_K played an important role in Aβ-induced neuronal death, we hypothesized that blocking I_K should render neurons resistant to Aβ-induced death. Both Aβ25–35 and Aβ1–42 induced slowly-developed neuronal death; incubation in 20 µM Aβ25–35 or Aβ1–42 for 24 h caused 39 ± 8% and 31 ± 3% neuronal death, respectively (n = 16 and 32 cultures per condition; assayed by lactate dehydrogenase (LDH) release). Morphological features consistent with apoptosis, such as membrane blebbing and cell shrinkage, were observed after 24 h in Aβ peptides, consistent with previous reports [2–7]. Co-application of 5 mM TEA with 20 µM Aβ25–35 or Aβ1–42 produced an attenuation of resultant cell death 24 and 48 h later (Figure 4). The TEA protection was concentration-dependent between 0.1 to 5 mM. In contrast, the TEA analog TMA did not reduce Aβ1–42 toxicity (Figure 4).

Raising extracellular K+ to 25 mM reduced I_K by 27 ± 6% (n = 3) and also reduced the neuronal death induced by 48 h exposure to 20 µM Aβ1–42 (Figure 4). While raising extracellular K+ should also affect I_A, the I_A selective blocker 5 mM 4-AP did not alter Aβ1–42 or Aβ25–35 toxicity (n = 8 cultures for each condition). TEA may, in addition, inhibit Cl⁻ currents in cortical neurons [44]; however, no neuroprotection was observed with the Cl⁻ channel antagonist anthracene-9-carboxylic acid (ACA, 500 µM; n = 8 control or

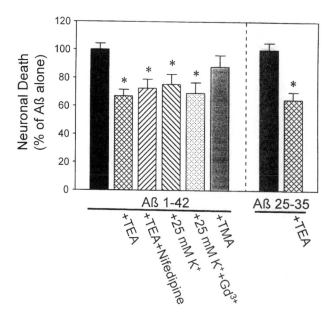

Figure 4. Attenuation of β-amyloid toxicity by TEA and 25 mM K+. Aβ-induced neuronal death was attenuated by TEA and high K+ medium with or without a Ca²⁺ channel antagonist. Neuronal death, induced by exposure to 20 µM Aβ1–42 or Aβ25–35 for 48 h alone (= 100%), or in the presence of the indicated treatments, 5 mM TEA or TMA, 5 µM nifedipine or Gd³⁺, or 25 mM K+ (n = 12–16 cultures per condition, mean + SEM), as assessed by LDH release into the medium. * Significant differences from Aβ alone at p < 0.05 by Student's *t* test, with Bonferroni correction for five comparisons in the case of Aβ1–42. Modified from reference [30], with permission

drug-treated cultures). Addition of 5 μM Gd^{3+} or 5 μM nifedipine did not
eliminate the neuroprotective effect of TEA or 25 mM K$^+$ on Aβ1–42 toxicity
(Figure 4).

K$^+$ CHANNEL EXPRESSION AND INDUCTION OF APOPTOSIS

To test further the hypothesis that excessive K$^+$ efflux is a key event in neuronal apoptosis, we have recently examined whether the over-expression of
cloned K$^+$ channels would induce enhanced vulnerability to apoptosis. To
begin testing this hypothesis, we used the human embryonic kidney cell line
HEK293 cells previously utilized for K$^+$ channel transfection [45, 46]. An
unexpected confounding factor was the detection of an endogenous outward
I_K-like current in native HEK293 cells [47]. However, HEK293 cells stably
transfected with Kv2.1 channels (*shah* family of delayed rectifier channels),
exhibited higher levels of apoptosis after 24–48 h exposure to 20 μM C$_2$-
ceramide than native HEK cells.

DISCUSSION

Our studies support the novel hypothesis that an enhancement of the delayed
rectifier current I_K participates in the pathogenesis of neuronal death induced
by exposure to the Aβ fragments 25–35 or 1–42 or certain other apoptotic
insults. Both the identity of the K$^+$ channel(s) undergoing enhancement and
the conditions capable of triggering the enhancement exhibited specificity.
Recent studies have suggested that exposure to Aβ may lead to the impairment
of the Na$^+$/K$^+$-ATPase due to membrane lipid peroxidation [48], an event
that could further magnify the intracellular K$^+$ loss initiated by enhanced K$^+$
efflux via I_K channels. Of note is the finding that Aβ induced a persistent
outward K$^+$ current at membrane potentials positive to -100 mV, reflecting a
shift in the I_K I–V relationship to hyperpolarized potentials, a finding that
suggests that exposure to Aβ may increase K$^+$ efflux even around the resting
membrane potential and thus perhaps alter resting membrane excitability.

Raising extracellular K$^+$ or adding TEA has been previously found to be neuroprotective against β-amyloid neurotoxicity in primary hippocampal cell cultures
[49] and the SN56 cholinergic septal cell line [50], although in each case neuroprotective effects were attributed to a consequent elevation of [Ca^{2+}]$_i$, which
may inhibit apoptosis [32–35]. Here, we demonstrated that the ability of both
TEA and elevated extracellular K$^+$ to protect neurons against β-amyloid-induced
cortical neuronal death persisted even when [Ca^{2+}]$_i$ was kept at resting levels,
suggesting that these drugs can block β-amyloid-induced neuronal death independent of effects on [Ca^{2+}]$_i$—we hypothesize by reducing K$^+$ efflux.

Further studies will be needed to delineate the mechanisms by which I_K can be upmodulated by exposure to Aβ peptide and other apoptotic insults. The several-hour latency between onset of Aβ exposure and alterations in I_K raise the possibility that several intermediate steps may be involved, although alternatively a slow direct interaction between Aβ and I_K channels, for example involving further peptide aggregation, can be entertained. Further study will also be needed to delineate how an upmodulation in I_K current, presumably leading to loss of intracellular K+, might promote neuronal apoptosis. Intracellular K+ may suppress programmed cell death in macrophages, monocytes, and thymocytes by inhibiting the activation of caspase-3 (51–55). Hyperosmotic KCl has also been suggested to block caspase-3 activation in HeLa cells by preventing loss of intracellular K+ [56]. Alternatively, the possibility of a critical apoptosis-promoting effect of intracellular K+ loss on endonuclease activation has also been recently raised [57].

Potassium channel blockers have already been brought into short-term clinical trials in Alzheimer's disease patients, motivated by the possibility of improving acetylcholine release [58, 59]. While limiting side effects of such treatments, especially on the cardiovascular system, represents a challenge, present data provide an additional rationale for exploring the possibility that attenuating outward K+ currents, particularly the I_K current, might benefit patients with Alzheimer's disease.

REFERENCES

1. Hardy JA, Higgins GA. Alzheimer's disease: the amyloid cascade hypothesis. Science 1992; 256: 184–5.
2. Forloni G, Chiesa R, Smiroldo S, Verga L, Salmona M, Tagliavini F, Angeretti N. Apoptosis mediated neurotoxicity induced by chronic application of β amyloid fragment 25–35. NeuroReport 1993; 4: 523–6.
3. Loo DT, Copani A, Pike CJ, Whittemore ER, Walencewicz AJ, Cotman CW. Apoptosis is induced by β-amyloid in cultured central nervous system neurons. Proc Natl Acad Sci USA 1993; 90: 7951–5.
4. Johnson EM Jr. Possible role of neuronal apoptosis in Alzheimer's disease. Neurobiol Aging 1994; 15: S187–9.
5. Su JH, Anderson AJ, Cummings BJ, Cotman CW. Immunohistochemical evidence for apoptosis in Alzheimer's disease. NeuroReport 1994; 5: 2529–33.
6. Watt JA, Pike CJ, Walencewicz-Wasserman AJ, Cotman CW. Ultrastructural analysis of β-amyloid-induced apoptosis in cultured hippocampal neurons. Brain Res 1994; 661: 147–56.
7. LaFerla FM, Tinkle BT, Bieberich CJ, Haudenschild CC, Jay G. The Alzheimer's Aβ peptide induces neurodegeneration and apoptotic cell death in transgenic mice. Nature Genet 1995; 9: 21–30.
8. Kroemer G, Petit P, Zamzami N, Vayssiere J-L, Mignotte B. The biochemistry of programmed cell death. FASEB J 1995; 9: 1277–87.
9. Barinaga M. Death by dozens of cuts. Science 1998; 280: 32–4.
10. Kerr JF, Wyllie AH, Currie AR. Apoptosis: a basic biological phenomenon with wide-ranging implications in tissue kinetics. Br J Cancer 1972; 26: 239–57.

11. Majno G, Joris I. Apoptosis, oncosis and necrosis. An overview of cell death. Am J Pathol 1995; 146: 3–15.
12. Villa P, Kaufmann SH, Earnshaw WC. Caspases and caspase inhibitors. Trends Biochem Sci 1997; 22: 388–93.
13. Fernandes-Alnemri T, Litwack G, Alnemri ES. CPP32, a novel human apoptotic protein with homology to *Caenorhabditis elegans* cell death protein Ced-3 and mammalian interleukin-1 beta-converting enzyme. J Biol Chem 1994; 269: 30761–4.
14. Nicholson DW, Ali A, Thornberry NA, Vaillancourt JP, Ding CK, Gallant M, Gareau Y, Griffin PR, Labelle M, Lazebnik YA et al. Identification and inhibition of the ICE/CED-3 protease necessary for mammalian apoptosis. Nature 1995; 376: 37–43.
15. Vaux DL, Weissman IL, Kim SK. Prevention of programmed cell death in *Caenorhabditis elegans* by human bcl-2. Science 1992; 258: 1955–7.
16. Jacobson MD, Burne JF, King MP, Miyashita T, Reed JC, Raff MC. Bcl-2 blocks apoptosis in cells lacking mitochondrial DNA. Nature 1993; 361: 365–9.
17. Kaiser N, Edelman IS. Calcium dependence of glucocorticoid-induced lymphocytolysis. Proc Natl Acad Sci USA 1977; 74: 638–42.
18. Iseki R, Kudo Y, Iwata M. Early mobilization of Ca^{2+} is not required for glucocorticoid-induced apoptosis in thymocytes. J Immunol 1993; 151: 5198–207.
19. Beaver JP, Waring P. Lack of correlation between early intracellular calcium ion rises and the onset of apoptosis in thymocytes. Immunol Cell Biol 1994; 72: 489–99.
20. Kluck RM, McDougall CA, Harmon BV, Halliday JW. Calcium chelators induce apoptosis—evidence that raised intracellular ionised calcium is not essential for apoptosis. Biochim Biophys Acta 1994; 1223: 247–54.
21. Treves S, Trentini PL, Ascanelli M, Bucci G, Di Virgilio F. Apoptosis is dependent on intracellular zinc and independent of intracellular calcium in lymphocytes. Exp Cell Res 1994; 211: 339–43.
22. McConkey DJ, Orrenius S. The role of calcium in the regulation of apoptosis. J Leukoc Biol 1996; 59: 775–83.
23. Murrell RD, Tolkovsky AM. Role of voltage-gated Ca^{2+} channels and intracellular Ca^{2+} in rat sympathetic neuron survival and function promoted by high K^+ and cyclic AMP in the presence or absence of NGF. Eur J Neurosci 1993; 5: 1261–72.
24. Galli C, Meucci O, Scorziello A, Werge TM, Calissano P, Schettini G. Apoptosis in cerebellar granule cells is blocked by high KCl, forskolin, and IGF-1 through distinct mechanisms of action: the involvement of intracellular calcium and RNA synthesis. J Neurosci 1995; 15: 1172–9.
25. Beauvais F, Michel L, Dubertret L. Human eosinophils in culture undergo a striking and shrinkage during apoptosis. Role of K^+ channels. J Leukoc Biol 1995; 57: 851–5.
26. Ojcius DM, Zychlinsky A, Zheng LM, Young JD. Ionophore-induced apoptosis: role of DNA fragmentation and calcium fluxes. Exp Cell Res 1991; 197: 43–9.
27. Deckers CL, Lyons AB, Samuel K, Sanderson A, Maddy AH. Alternative pathways of apoptosis induced by methylprednisolone and valinomycin analyzed by flow cytometry. Exp Cell Res 1993; 208: 362–70.
28. Duke RC, Witter RZ, Nash PB, Young JD, Ojcius DM. Cytolysis mediated by ionophores and pore-forming agents: role of intracellular calcium in apoptosis. FASEB J 1994; 8: 237–46.
29. Yu SP, Farhangrazi ZS, Ying HS, Yeh C-H, Choi DW. β-Amyloid-induced enhancement of delayed rectifier K^+ current and attenuation of β-amyloid-induced neuronal death by tetraethylammonium. Soc Neurosci Abstr 1997; 23: 1629.

30. Yu SP, Farhangrazi ZS, Ying HS, Yeh C-H, Choi DW. Enhancement of outward potassium current may participate in β-amyloid peptide-induced cortical neuronal death. Neurobiol Dis 1998 (in press).
31. Yu SP, Yeh C-H, Sensi SL, Gwag BJ, Canzoniero LMT, Farhangrazi ZS, Ying HS, Tian M, Dugan LL, Choi DW. Mediation of neuronal apoptosis by enhancement of outward potassium current. Science 1997; 278: 114–17.
32. Gallo V, Kingsbury A, Balazs R, Jorgensen OS. The role of depolarization in the survival and differentiation of cerebellar granule cells in culture. J Neurosci 1987; 7: 2203–13.
33. Koike T, Martin DP, Johnson EM Jr. Role of Ca²⁺ channels in the ability of membrane depolarization to prevent neuronal death induced by trophic-factor deprivation: evidence that levels of internal Ca²⁺ determine nerve growth factor dependence of sympathetic ganglion cells. Proc Natl Acad Sci USA 1989; 86: 6421–5.
34. Franklin JL, Johnson EM Jr. Suppression of programmed neuronal death by sustained elevation of cytoplasmic calcium. Trends Neurosci 1992; 15: 501–8.
35. Johnson EM Jr, Koike T, Franklin J. A 'calcium set-point hypothesis' of neuronal dependence on neurotrophic factor. Exp Neurol 1992; 115: 163–6.
36. Jalonen TO, Charniga CJ, Wielt DB. β-Amyloid peptide-induced morphological changes coincide with increased K⁺ and Cl⁻ channel activity in rat cortical astrocytes. Brain Res 1997; 746: 85–97.
37. Furukawa K, Barger SW, Blalock EM, Mattson MP. Activation of K⁺ channels and suppression of neuronal activity by secreted β-amyloid-precursor protein. Nature 1996; 379: 74–8.
38. Simmons MA, Schneider CR. Amyloid β peptides act directly on single neurons. Neurosci Lett 1993; 150: 133–6.
39. Arispe N, Rojas E, Pollard HB. Alzheimer disease amyloid β protein forms calcium channels in bilayer membranes: blockade by tromethamine and aluminum. Proc Natl Acad Sci USA 1993; 90: 567–71.
40. Furukawa K, Abe Y, Akaike N. Amyloid beta protein-induced irreversible current in rat cortical neurones. NeuroReport 1994; 5: 2016–18.
41. Mirzabekov T, Lin MC, Yuan WL, Marshall PJ, Carman M, Tomaselli K, Lieberburg I, Kagan BL. Channel formation in planar lipid bilayers by a neurotoxic fragment of the beta-amyloid peptide. Biochem Biophys Res Commun 1994; 202: 1142–8.
42. Li WY, Czilli DL, Simmons LK. Neuronal membrane conductance activated by amyloid β peptide: importance of peptide conformation. Brain Res 1995; 682: 207–11.
43. Fraser SP, Suh Y-H, Djamgoz MB. Ionic effects of the Alzheimer's disease β-amyloid precursor protein and its metabolic fragments. Trends Neurosci 1997; 20: 67–72.
44. Sanchez DY, Blatz AL. Voltage-dependent block of fast chloride channels from rat cortical neurons by external tetraethylammonium ion. J Gen Physiol 1992; 100: 217–31.
45. Freeman LC, Kass RS. Expression of a minimal K⁺ channel protein in mammalian cells and immunolocalization in guinea pig heart. Circ Res 1993; 73: 968–73.
46. Holmes TC, Fadool DA, Ren R, Levitan IB. Association of Src tyrosine kinase with a human potassium channel mediated by SH3 domain. Science 1996; 274: 2089–91.
47. Yu SP, Kerchner GA. Endogenous voltage-gated potassium channels in human embryonic kidney (HEK 293) cells. J Neurosci Res 1998; 52: 612–17.
48. Keller JN, Germeyer A, Begley JG, Mattson MP. 17β-estradiol attenuates oxidative impairment of synaptic Na⁺/K⁺-ATPase activity, glucose transport, and

glutamate transport induced by amyloid β-peptide and iron. J Neurosci Res 1997; 50: 522–30.

49. Pike CJ, Balázs R, Cotman CW. Attenuation of β-amyloid neurotoxicity *in vitro* by potassium-induced depolarization. J Neurochem 1996; 67: 1774–7.

50. Colom LV, Diaz ME, Beers DR, Neely A, Xie WJ, Appel SH. Role of potassium channels in amyloid-induced cell death. J Neurochem 1998; 70: 1925–34.

51. Perregaux D, Gabel CA. Interleukin-1β maturation and release in response to ATP and nigericin. Evidence that potassium depletion mediated by these agents is a necessary and common feature of their activity. J Biol Chem 1994; 269: 15195–203.

52. Walev I, Reske K, Palmer M, Valeva A, Bhakdi S. Potassium-inhibited processing of IL-1β in human monocytes. EMBO J 1995; 14: 1607–14.

53. Hughes FM Jr, Bortner CD, Purdy GD, Cidlowski JA. Intracellular K^+ suppresses the activation of apoptosis in lymphocytes. J Biol Chem 1997; 272: 30567–76.

54. Yuan J, Shaham S, Ledoux S, Ellis HM, Horvitz HR. The *C. elegans* cell death gene ced-3 encodes a protein similar to mammalian interleukin-1β-converting enzyme. Cell 1993; 75: 641–52.

55. Bortner CD, Hughes FM Jr, Cidlowski JA. A primary role for K^+ and Na^+ efflux in the activation of apoptosis. J Biol Chem 1997; 272: 32436–42.

56. Bilney AJ, Murray AW. Pro- and anti-apoptotic effects of K^+ in HeLa cells. FEBS Lett 1998; 424: 221–4.

57. Dallaporta B, Hirsch T, Susin SA, Zamzami N, Larochette N, Brenner C, Marzo I, Kroemer G. Potassium leakage during the apoptotic degradation phase. J Immunol 1998; 160: 5605–15.

58. Wesseling H, Agoston S, Van Dam GB, Pasma J, DeWit DJ, Havinga H. Effects of 4-aminopyridine in elderly patients with Alzheimer's disease. N Engl J Med 1984; 310: 988–9.

59. Lavretsky EP, Jarvik LF. A group of potassium-channel blockers–acetylcholine releasers: new potentials for Alzheimer disease? A review. J Clin Psychopharmacol 1992; 12: 110–18.

60. Rose K, Goldberg MP, Choi DW. Cytotoxicity in murine neocortical cell culture. In: Tyson CA, Frazier JM (eds) Methods in Toxicology. San Diego, CA: Academic Press, 1993; 46–60.

61. Koh JY, Choi DW. Quantitative determination of glutamate mediated cortical neuronal injury in cell culture by lactate dehydrogenase efflux assay. J Neurosci Meth 1987; 20: 83–90.

Address for correspondence:

Shan Ping Yu,

Center for the Study of Nervous System Injury and Department of Neurology,

Box 8111, Washington University School of Medicine,

St. Louis, MO 63110, USA

Tel: 314 362 9460; fax: 314 362 9462; e-mail: yus@neuro.wustl.edu

41 Metal-catalyzed Redox Activity of Aβ—The Major Source of Amyloid-associated Oxidative Stress in Alzheimer's Disease

XUDONG HUANG, CRAIG S. ATWOOD,
LEE E. GOLDSTEIN, MARIANA A. HARTSHORN,
ALEISTER J. SAUNDERS, ROBERT D. MOIR,
RUDOLPH E. TANZI AND ASHLEY I. BUSH

INTRODUCTION

Oxygen radical involvement in human aging and human diseases was first proposed by Harman in 1956 [1]. An emerging body of data indicates that oxidative stress could play a role in the pathogenesis of Alzheimer's disease (AD), and that the neurotoxicity of Alzheimer Aβ peptides is mediated by reactive oxygen species (ROS). Apart from metabolic signs of oxidative stress in AD-affected neocortex, such as increased glucose-6-phosphate dehydrogenase activity [2] and increased heme oxygenase-1 levels [3], there are also numerous signs of oxygen radical-mediated chemical attack, such as increased protein and free carbonyls [4–6], lipid peroxidation adducts [7–8], peroxynitrite-mediated protein nitration [9–10] and mitochondrial and nuclear DNA oxidation adducts [11–12]. Recently, treatment of individuals with the antioxidant vitamin E has been reported to delay the onset of clinical AD [13].

A relationship seems likely to exist between the signs of oxidative stress and the characteristic Aβ collections [14–15] found in the cortical interstitium and cerebrovascular intima media in AD. Indeed, neurons cultured from subjects with Down's syndrome, a condition complicated by the invariable premature deposition of cerebral Aβ [16] and the over-expression of soluble Aβ1–42 in early life [17], exhibit lipid peroxidation and apoptotic cell death caused by increased generation of hydrogen peroxide [18]. Synthetic Aβ peptides have been shown to induce lipid peroxidation of synaptosomes [19], and to exert

Alzheimer's Disease and Related Disorders
Edited by K. Iqbal, D.F. Swaab, B. Winblad and H.M. Wisniewski
© 1999 John Wiley & Sons Ltd

neurotoxicity [20–21] or vascular endothelial toxicity through a mechanism that involves the generation of cellular superoxide/hydrogen peroxide (O_2^-/H_2O_2 and is abolished by the presence of SOD [22] or catalytic synthetic O_2^-/H_2O_2 scavengers [23]. Antioxidant vitamin E and the spin-trap compound PBN have been shown to protect against Aβ-mediated neurotoxicity *in vitro* [24–25].

Aβ, a 39–43 amino acid peptide, is produced [26–28] by constitutive cleavage of the amyloid protein precursor (APP) [29–30] as a mixture of polypeptides manifesting carboxyl-terminal heterogeneity. Aβ1–40 is the major soluble Aβ species in biological fluids [31] and is a minor soluble species, but is heavily enriched in interstitial plaque amyloid [15, 29, 32–34]. The discovery of pathogenic mutations of APP close to or within the Aβ domain [35–39] indicates that the metabolism of Aβ is involved with the pathophysiology of this predominantly sporadic disease. Familial AD-linked mutations of APP, Presenilin-1 and Presenilin-2 correlate with increased cortical amyloid burden and appear to induce an increase in the ratio of Aβ1–42 as part of their common pathogenic mechanism [40–41]. However, the mechanism by which Aβ1–42 specifically is more neurotoxic than Aβ1–40 and other Aβ peptides [42] is still unclear.

Aggregated or fibrillar forms of Aβ peptides are generally believed to account for observed Aβ neurotoxicity. One of the models proposed for Aβ neurotoxicity is based on the observation of Aβ-generated oxyradicals through a putative Aβ peptide fragmentation mechanism which is methionine-involved, O_2-dependent and metal-independent [19, 43]. Aβ25–35 peptide has been reported to exhibit H_2O_2-like reactivity towards aqueous Fe(II), nitroxide spin probes, and synaptosomal membrane proteins [44], and Aβ1–40 has also been reported to generate the hydroxyl radical by mechanisms that are unclear [45], but so far there has been no quantitative appraisal of the ROS-generating capacity of Aβ1–42 compared to Aβ1–40 and other Aβ variants.

Here we present a working model describing how interplay of Aβ, metals and O_2 can precipitate soluble Aβ, potentially lead to amyloid plaque formation, and engender oxidative stress associated with amyloid plaques.

ASSEMBLING Aβ DEPOSITS IN AD BY BIOMETALS

In vitro, Aβ is a metal-binding protein. It saturably binds zinc, manifesting histidine-mediated specific high affinity (K_D = 107 nM) and low affinity binding (K_D = 5.2 μM). The high-affinity zinc binding site was mapped to a stretch of contiguous residues between positions 6 and 28 of the Aβ sequence [46]. Concentrations of zinc ≥1 μM rapidly induce aggregation of human Aβ1–40 solutions [47], in reversible manner that is dependent upon the dimerization of the peptide in solution, its α-helical content and the concentration of NaCl

[48]. Rat/mouse Aβ1–40 (with substitutions of $R_5 \rightarrow G$, $Y_{10} \rightarrow F$, and $H_{13} \rightarrow R$) binds zinc less avidly (a single binding site, $K_A = 3.8$ μM) and, unlike the human peptide, is not precipitated by zinc at concentrations ≤ 25 μM. Since zinc is concentrated in the neocortex, we hypothesized that the differential solubility of the rat/mouse Aβ peptide in the presence of zinc may explain the scarcity with which these animals form cerebral Aβ deposits (49–50).

We have also observed interactions of Aβ with Cu(II), which stabilizes dimerization of Aβ1–40 on gel chromatography [46], and which induces Aβ aggregation under mildly acidic conditions [51]. Fe(II) has been observed to induce partial aggregation of Aβ [52].

In vivo, the levels of Cu and Fe and their binding proteins were discovered to be dysregulated in AD [53–58]. Histologic staining has revealed abnormal Zn accumulations in senile plaques, in the amyloid angiopathy surrounding diseased blood vessels, and in the somata of hippocampal neurons showing the characteristic neurofibrillary tangles of AD [59]. Moreover, a recent study indicates that concentrations of Cu, Fe and Zn are elevated in senile plaques compared to neuropil in AD [60]. In addition, specific Cu and Zn chelators resolubilize Aβ during homogenization of post-mortem AD-affected brain tissue [61]. Collectively, both *in vitro* and *in vivo* studies indicate that these biometals mediate the assembly of cerebral Aβ deposits in AD brain.

CHEMICAL BASIS OF AMYLOID-ASSOCIATED OXIDATIVE STRESS: METAL-CATALYZED Aβ REDOX CHEMISTRY

Evidence has implicated biometals, especially redox-active Fe and Cu, as playing roles other than being potent inducers of Aβ deposition in AD brain. Both Fe(II) and Cu(II) were found to induce SDS-resistant polymerization of Aβ peptide *in vitro* [62–63]. However, a direct interaction of Aβ in metal-dependent ROS generation has not been described, but seemed to us likely given the peptide's physiochemical interaction with transition metals, the presence of ferritin [64] and redox-reactive iron [65] in amyloid lesions, and the facilitation of Aβ1–40 neurotoxicity in cell culture by nanomolar concentrations of iron [66]. Thus, the interactions of Aβ with Fe and Cu may be of significance to lead to conditions that could catalyze ROS production which may partially account for observed oxidation insults in the AD-affected brain. This is because these amyloid-bound, redox-active metal ions in their reduced state may initiate the generation of ROS by transferring electrons to O_2. In fact, we have discovered the simultaneous production of H_2O_2 and reduced metal ions by Alzheimer Aβ itself, with the consequent generation of the hydroxyl radical. The amounts of reduced metal and ROS were both greatest when generated by Aβ1–42 > Aβ1–40 >> rat Aβ1–40, a chemical relationship that correlates with the relative neurotoxicity of these peptides [67]. This novel, O_2- and biometal-dependent pathway of ROS generation by Alzheimer $A\beta$ peptides is described in the following reactions:

$A\beta$ peptides reduce $M^{(n+1)+}$ (M = Fe or Cu) and radicalize.

$$2A\beta + M^{(n+1)+} \rightarrow A\beta + A\beta\cdot + M^{n+} \qquad \text{Reaction (1)}$$

Reduced Fe/Cu reacts with molecular oxygen to generate H_2O_2 through two electron reduction of O_2.

$$2M^{n+} + O_2 + 2H^+ \rightarrow 2M^{(n+1)+} + H_2O_2 \qquad \text{Reaction (2)}$$

The reaction of reduced metals with H_2O_2 generates the highly reactive hydroxyl radical by the Fenton or more generic Haber–Weiss reaction.

$$M^{n+} + H_2O_2 \rightarrow M^{(n+1)+} + OH\cdot + OH^- \qquad \text{Reaction (3)}$$

The radicalized $A\beta$ may undergo further chemical modification by *in situ* generated OH· and become polymerized and fragmented. This may initiate mature amyloid plaque formation and engender neurotoxicity. Since this scenario mainly occurs within amyloid deposits, we hypothesize that it is the chemical basis for amyloid-associated oxidative stress in AD.

CONCLUSION

In summary, we have presented a working model showing that interplay among $A\beta$, O_2 and redox-active metals that may be the genesis of amyloid-associated oxidative stress. If proved *in vivo*, this model will offer a unified explanation for the observed differential neurotoxicity of $A\beta$ peptide variants and validate antioxidant therapy in delaying the onset of clinical AD. Moreover, this interplay will potentially trigger a pathogenic vicious cycle in which amyloidogenic processing of APP would be further enhanced by oxidative stress, as speculated [68]. Furthermore, metal chelation therapy may hold therapeutic value in removing the oxidative stress associated with AD because of the catalytic role of those redox-active metals in generation of ROS.

ACKNOWLEDGEMENTS

This work is supported by funds from the Prana Corp., the NIH (R29AG12686), Alzheimer's Association, International Life Sciences Institute and the American Federation for Aging Research/Alliance for Aging Research (Beeson Award to A.I.B.). X. Huang is a National Research Service Awardee from the NIH (F32AG05782).

REFERENCES

1. Harman D. Aging: a theory based on free radical and radiation chemistry. J Gerontol 1956; 11: 298–300.
2. Martins RN et al. Increased cerebral glucose-6-phosphate dehydrogenase activity in Alzheimer's disease may reflect oxidative stress. J Neurochem 1986; 46: 1042–5.
3. Smith MA et al. Hemeoxygenase-1 is associated with the neurofibrillary pathology of Alzheimer's disease. Am J Pathol 1994; 145: 42–7.
4. Smith CD et al. Excess brain protein oxidation and enzyme dysfunction in normal aging and Alzheimer disease. Proc Natl Acad Sci USA 1991; 88: 10540–43.
5. Hensley K et al. Brain regional correspondence between Alzheimer's disease histopathology and biomarkers of protein oxidation. J Neurochem 1995; 65: 2146–56.
6. Smith MA et al. Oxidative damage in Alzheimer's disease. Nature 1996; 382: 120–21.
7. Palmer AM, Burns MA. Selective increase in lipid peroxidation in the inferior temporal cortex in Alzheimer's disease. Brain Res 1994; 645: 338–42.
8. Sayre LM et al. 4-Hydroxynonenal-derived advanced lipid peroxidation end products are increased in Alzheimer's disease. J Neurochem 1997; 68: 2092–7.
9. Good PF et al. Evidence for neuronal oxidative damage in Alzheimer's disease. Am J Pathol 1996; 149: 21–8.
10. Smith MA et al. Widespread peroxynitrite-mediated damage in Alzheimer's disease. J Neurosci 1997; 17: 2653–7.
11. Mecocci P et al. Oxidative damage to mitochondrial DNA shows marked age-dependent increases in human brain. Ann Neurol 1993; 34: 609–16.
12. Mecocci P et al. Oxidative damage to mitochondrial DNA is increased in Alzheimer's disease. Ann Neurol 1994; 36: 747–51.
13. Sano M et al. A controlled trial of selegiline, alpha-tocopherol, or both as treatment for Alzheimer's disease. N Engl J Med 1997; 336: 1216–22.
14. Glenner GG, Wong C. Alzheimer's disease: initial report of the purification and characterization of a novel cerebrovascular amyloid protein. Biochem Biophys Res Commun 1984; 120: 885–90.
15. Masters CL et al. Amyloid plaque core protein in Alzheimer disease and Down syndrome. Proc Natl Acad Sci USA 1985; 82: 4245–9.
16. Rumble B et al. Amyloid A4 protein and its precursor in Down's syndrome and Alzheimer's disease. N Engl J Med 1989; 320: 1446–52.
17. Teller JK et al. Presence of soluble amyloid β-peptide precedes amyloid plaque formation in Down's syndrome. Nature Med 1996; 2: 93–5.
18. Busciglio J, Yankner BA. Apoptosis and increased generation of reactive oxygen species in Down's syndrome neurons *in vitro*. Nature 1995; 378: 776–9.
19. Butterfield DA et al. β-amyloid peptide free radical fragments initiate synaptosomal lipoperoxidation in a sequence-specific fashion: implications to Alzheimer's disease. Biochem Biophys Res Commun 1994; 200: 710–15.
20. Behl C et al. Hydrogen peroxide mediates amyloid β protein toxicity. Cell 1994; 77: 817–27.
21. Mattson MP et al. Neurotrophic factors attenuate glutamate-induced accumulation of peroxides, elevation of intracellular Ca^{2+} concentration, and neurotoxicity and increase antioxidant enzyme activities in hippocampal neurons. J Neurochem 1995; 65: 1740–51.
22. Thomas T et al. β-amyloid-mediated vasoactivity and vascular endothelial damage. Nature 1996; 380: 168–71.

23. Bruce AJ et al. β-amyloid toxicity in organotypic hippocampal cultures: protection by EUK-8, a synthetic catalytic free radical scavenger. Proc Natl Acad Sci USA 1996; 93: 2312–16.

24. Goodman Y, Mattson MP. Secreted forms of β-amyloid precursor protein protect hippocampal neurons against amyloid β-peptide-induced oxidative injury. Exp Neurol 1994; 128: 1–12.

25. Harris ME et al. Direct evidence of oxidative injury produced by the Alzheimer's β-amyloid peptide (1–40) in cultured hippocampal neurons. Exp Neurol 1995; 131: 193–202.

26. Haass C et al. Amyloid β-peptide is produced by cultured cells during normal metabolism. Nature 1992; 359: 322–5.

27. Seubert P et al. Isolation and quantification of soluble Alzheimer β-peptide from biological fluids. Nature 1992; 359: 325–7.

28. Shoji M et al. Production of Alzheimer amyloid β protein by normal proteolytic processing. Science 1992; 258: 126–9.

29. Kang J et al. The precursor of Alzheimer's disease amyloid A4 protein resembles a cell-surface receptor. Nature 1987; 325: 733–6.

30. Tanzi RE et al. Amyloid β protein gene: cDNA, mRNA distribution, and genetic linkage near the Alzheimer locus. Science 1987; 235: 880–84.

31. Vigo-Pelfrey C et al. Characterization of β-amyloid peptide from human cerebrospinal fluid. J Neurochem 1993; 61: 1965–8.

32. Prelli F et al. Differences between vascular and plaque core amyloid in Alzheimer's disease. J Neurochem 1988; 51: 648–51.

33. Roher AE et al. Structural alterations in the peptide backbone of β-amyloid core protein may account for its deposition and stability in Alzheimer's disease. J Biol Chem 1993; 268: 3072–83.

34. Miller DL et al. Peptide composition of the cerebrovascular and senile plaque core amyloid deposits of Alzheimer's disease. Arch Biochem Biophys 1993; 301: 41–52.

35. Van Broeckhoven C et al. Amyloid β protein precursor gene and hereditary cerebral hemorrhage with amyloidosis (in Dutch). Science 1990; 248: 1120–22.

36. Levy E et al. Mutation of the Alzheimer's disease amyloid gene in hereditary cerebral hemorrhage, Dutch type. Science 1990; 248: 1124–6.

37. Goate A et al. Segregation of a missense mutation in the amyloid precursor protein gene with familial Alzheimer's disease. Nature 1991; 349: 704–6.

38. Murrell J et al. A mutation in the amyloid precursor protein associated with hereditary Alzheimer disease. Science 1991; 254: 97–9.

39. Mullan M et al. A pathogenic mutation for probable Alzheimer's disease in the N-terminus of β-amyloid. Nature Genet 1992; 1: 345–7.

40. Suzuki N et al. An increased percentage of long amyloid beta protein secreted by familial amyloid beta protein precursor (beta APP717) mutants. Science 1994; 264: 1336–40.

41. Citron M et al. Mutant presenilins of Alzheimer's disease increase production of 42-residue amyloid β-protein in both transfected cells and transgenic mice. Nature Med 1997; 3: 67–72.

42. Doré S et al. Insulin-like growth factor I protects and rescues hippocampal neurons against β-amyloid- and human amylin-induced toxicity. Proc Natl Acad Sci USA 1997; 94: 4772–7.

43. Hensley K et al. A model for β-amyloid aggregation and neurotoxicity based on free radical generation by the peptide: relevance to Alzheimer's disease. Proc Natl Acad Sci USA 1994; 91: 3270–74.

44. Butterfield DA et al. Aβ(25–35) peptide displays H_2O_2-like reactivity towards aqueous Fe^{2+}, nitroxide spin probes, and synaptosomal membrane proteins. Life Sci 1996; 58: 217–28.

45. Tomiyama T et al. Inhibition of amyloid β protein aggregation and neurotoxicity by rifampicin. J Biol Chem 1996; 271: 6839–44.

46. Bush AI et al. Modulation of Aβ adhesiveness and secretase site cleavage by zinc. J Biol Chem 1994; 269: 12152–8.

47. Bush AI et al. Rapid introduction of Alzheimer Aβ amyloid formation by zinc. Science 1994; 265: 1464–7.

48. Huang X et al. Zinc-induced Alzheimer's Aβ1–40 aggregation is mediated by conformational factors. J Biol Chem 1997; 272: 26464–70.

49. Johnstone EM, et al. Conservation of the sequence of the Alzheimer's disease amyloid peptide in dog, polar bear and five other mammals by cross-species polymerase chain reaction analysis. Mol Brain Res 1991; 10: 299–305.

50. Shivers BD et al. Alzheimer's disease amyloidogenic glycoprotein: expression pattern in rat brain suggests a role in cell contact. EMBO J 1988; 7: 1365–70.

51. Atwood CS et al. Dramatic aggregation of Alzheimer Aβ by Cu(II) is induced by conditions representing physiological acidosis. J Biol Chem 1998; 273: 12817–26.

52. Bush AI et al. Rapid introduction of Alzheimer Aβ amyloid formation by zinc (comments). Science 1995; 268: 1921.

53. Deibel MA et al. Copper, iron, and zinc imbalances in severely degenerated brain regions in Alzheimer's disease. J Neurol Sci 1996; 143: 137–42.

54. Good PF et al. Selective accumulation of aluminum and iron in the neurofibrillary tangles of Alzheimer's disease: a laser microprobe (LAMMA) study. Ann Neurol 1992; 31: 286–92.

55. Robinson SR et al. Most amyloid plaques contain ferritin-rich cells. Alzheimer's Res 1995; 1: 191–6.

56. Thompson CM et al. Regional brain trace-element studies in Alzheimer's disease. Neurotoxicology 1988; 9: 1–8.

57. Kennard ML et al. Serum levels of the iron binding protein p97 are elevated in Alzheimer's disease. Nature Med 1996; 2: 1230–35.

58. Connor JR et al. Ceruloplasmin levels in the human superior temporal gyrus in aging and Alzheimer's disease. Neurosci Lett 1993; 159: 88–90.

59. Suh SW et al. Histologic evidence implicating zinc in Alzheimer's disease (submitted).

60. Lovell MA et al. Copper, iron and zinc in Alzheimer's disease senile plaques. J Neurol Sci 1998; 158: 47–52.

61. Cherny RA et al. Solubilization of Alzheimer's disease cerebral Aβ amyloid deposits by metal chelators (submitted).

62. Dyrks T et al. Amyloidogenicity of βA4 and βA4-bearing amyloid protein precursor fragments by metal-catalyzed oxidation. J Biol Chem 1992; 267: 18210–17.

63. Atwood CS et al. (unpublished data).

64. Grundke-Iqbal I et al. Ferritin is a component of the neuritic (senile) plaque in Alzheimer dementia. Acta Neuropathol 1990; 81: 105–10.

65. Smith MA et al. Iron accumulation in Alzheimer disease is a source of redox-generated free radical. Proc Natl Acad Sci USA 1997; 94: 9866–8.

66. Schubert D, Chevion M. The role of iron in beta amyloid toxicity. Biochem Biophys Res Commun 1995; 216: 702–7.

67. Huang X et al. The Alzheimer's disease Aβ peptide directly generates hydrogen peroxide through metal ion reduction (submitted).

68. Pappolla MA et al. Evidence of oxidative stress and *in vivo* neurotoxicity of β-amyloid in a transgenic mouse model of Alzheimer's disease. J Neurochem (in press).

Address for correspondence:
Ashley I. Bush MD PhD and Xudong Huang PhD,
Laboratory for Oxidation Biology, Genetics and Aging Unit,
Massachusetts General Hospital—East,
Building 149, 13th Street, Charlestown, MA 02129, USA
Tel: (617)726 8244 or (617)724 9774; fax: (617)724-9610;
e-mail: bush@helix.mgh.harvard.edu; huangx@helix.mgh.harvard.edu

42 Cleavage of the Alzheimer's Disease Amyloid Precursor Protein During Apoptosis by Activated Caspases

A. WEIDEMANN, K. PALIGA, U. DÜRRWANG,
F.B.M. REINHARD, G. EVIN, C.L. MASTERS AND
K. BEYREUTHER

INTRODUCTION

The main pathological features of Alzheimer's disease (AD) are extracellular deposits of amyloid β protein (Aβ), intraneuronal cytoskeletal abnormalities and neuronal degeneration. The aberrant formation of polymer amyloid fibers composed of Aβ is considered to be one of the primary events for the neurodegeneration because Aβ shows cytotoxic effects and induces apoptosis in neuronal cultures [1]. Additionally, expression of APP carrying familial Alzheimer's disease (FAD) mutations has been reported to induce apoptosis in cells, suggesting a probable link between apoptotic pathways and neurodegeneration in AD [2, 3].

Recently, mutations causative for the majority of FAD cases have been identified in genes encoding presenilin-1 (PS1) and presenilin-2 (PS2) [4–6]. Although the exact function of the presenilins is not known, overexpression of PS2 in transfected cells resulted in an increased susceptibility to apoptosis, also suggesting the participation of presenilins in pathways of programmed cell death. The latter is even more pronounced in cells expressing mutant PS2-I which encodes one of the known PS2 missense mutations, changing Asn_{141} into Ile [7, 8]. This hypothesis is further supported by the finding that presenilins are cleaved by caspases, the central executioners of apoptosis [9–11]. Here we describe that APP also represents a target molecule for activated caspases and that APP is involved in apoptotic pathways.

Alzheimer's Disease and Related Disorders
Edited by K. Iqbal, D.F. Swaab, B. Winblad and H.M. Wisniewski
© 1999 John Wiley & Sons Ltd

MATERIALS AND METHODS

The point mutations in the cytoplasmic domain of APP695 (APP695$_{D/A}$ and APP695$_{del664}$) were introduced by PCR and cloned into pBluescript SK+ (Stratagene). The open reading frames of the resulting constructs were verified by sequencing followed by cloning into the expression vector pCEP4 (Invitrogen). APP695$_{D/A}$ encodes a point mutation in which Asp$_{664}$ was exchanged for Ala. In APP695$_{del664}$ a stop codon was introduced after Asp$_{664}$. COS-7 cells were maintained and transfected as described [12]. Stably expressing cell lines were generated by selection with hygromycine (250 μg/ml). Apoptosis was induced for 8 h by adding either staurosporine (2 μM in DMSO) or doxorubicine (100 μM in distilled water) in serum-free medium.

For immunoblotting, cells were harvested, resuspended in 8 M urea followed by brief sonication and boiling with SDS-sample buffer. For Western blotting, APP was separated on 7.5% Tris–glycine gels and immunodetected with mAb 22C11 [13].

RESULTS

In previous studies we demonstrated that APP forms non-covalent complexes with PS2 [12]. Subsequently, a direct interaction with APP was specified not only for PS2 but also for PS1[14–16], suggesting a direct effect of presenilins on APP metabolism and proteolysis.

When we further analyzed APP and N-terminal truncated derivatives thereof (i.e. SPA4CT) in cells co-expressing PS2, we observed proteolytic processing of APP within its cytoplasmic domain. This proteolytic conversion was even augmented in the presence of mutated PS2-I. Calculation of the molecular weight of the proteolytical fragment and inspection of the corresponding region encoded by the APP cytoplasmic domain revealed a consensus sequence for caspase-like proteases (group III caspases: [(IVL)ExD], [17]; Figure 1). These proteases are among the key enzymes that become activated in cells undergoing programmed cell death. An involvement of activated caspases in the proteolytic conversion of the APP C-terminus in cells, which overexpress PS2 and PS2-I, is in agreement with recent publications demonstrating that presenilins induce programmed cell death [7, 8]. Moreover, the observed increase in APP proteolysis in cells transfected with PS2-I is consistent with the observation that cells over-expressing mutant PS2-I are more prone to undergo apoptosis than cells expressing wild-type PS2 [7–9]. To validate that the proteolytic processing within the APP C-terminal domain can be attributed to apoptotic pathways and to confirm that the proteolysis is mediated by caspases, cells expressing full-length APP and N-terminal truncated fragments thereof were analyzed after induction of apoptosis with different chemical compounds, such as staurosporine or doxorubicine (Figure 2). As

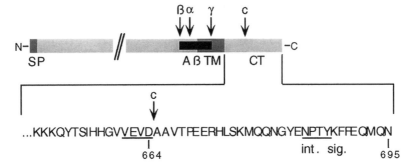

Figure 1. Schematic representation of APP and its carboxyterminal domain. The large extracellular domain of APP is followed by the Aβ sequence (Aβ), the transmembrane domain (TM) and the cytoplasmic domain (CT). SP, signal peptide. The positions of the proteolytic cleavage sites for α-, β- and γ-secretases are indicated. In its cytoplasmic domain, APP encodes an internalization signal (NPxY) and a consensus sequence for group III caspases (indicated as 'c') [(IVL)ExD]

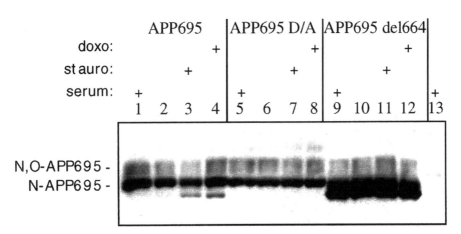

Figure 2. APP derivatives mutated at D_{664} are resistant to proteolytic conversion. Analysis of the corresponding APP derivatives. Cells were stably transfected with APP695 (lanes 1–4), APP695$_{D/A}$ (lanes 5–8) and APP695$_{del664}$ (lanes 9–12) and apoptosis was induced with either staurosporine (stauto; lanes 3, 7 and 11) or doxorubicine (doxo; lanes 4, 8 and 12). Total cellular homogenates were subjected to SDS–PAGE followed by imunoblotting with mAb22C11. In apoptotic cells, a C-terminal truncated species of APP695 is additionally detected at about 90 kDa (lanes 3 and 4), as compared with non-treated cells (lanes 1 and 2). Exchange of Asp$_{664}$ for Ala$_{664}$ completely abolishes APP cleavage in staurosporine or doxorubicine-treated cells (lanes 7 and 8). The N-glycosylated moiety of APP695$_{del664}$ (lanes 9–12) exhibits the same electrophoretic mobility as the caspase-derived fragments at about 90 kDa detected in lanes 3 and 4. The additional signals of about 95 kDa in APP695$_{del664}$-expressing cells represent posttranslationally higher glycosylated APP species

proposed for a participation of caspases, the proteolytic conversion of APP within its cytoplasmic domain is increased in apoptotic cells and inhibited by the addition of specific caspase inhibitors (not shown). Additionally, changing D_{664} into A_{664} at the cleavage site of the canonical sequence (Figure 1) completely abolished proteolytic conversion (Figure 2). Taken together, these novel results strongly suggest that APP represents a target for caspase-like proteases and that APP is involved in cell death pathways.

DISCUSSION

To date, evidence is accumulating that connects apoptotic pathways with neurodegeneration:

1. Apoptotic cell death has been reported to be a pathological feature of AD, as determined by histochemical studies [18, 19].
2. Expression of mutant APP carrying FAD mutations has been shown to induce apoptosis, indicating that apoptosis may therefore contribute to the neuronal loss in FAD [2, 3].
3. Over-expression of PS2 in neuronal and non-neuronal cells was found to enhance apoptosis, whereas transfection with a PS2 antisense construct rescued cells from apoptosis [7, 8, 20]. Inhibitory effects on apoptosis were also observed when a C-terminal portion of PS2 was expressed in cells [20, 21]. Additionally, the PS2 N_{141}–I FAD mutation was reported to confer enhanced basal activity for apoptosis [7, 22], similar to the L_{286}–V mutation in PS1 [23].
4. Both PS1 and PS2 have been shown to be targets for caspase-mediated proteolytic conversion [9–11]. The mutant PS2-I might be even converted to a higher extent as compared to the wild-type PS2 [9]. The corresponding PS fragments derived by caspase-mediated proteolysis were detected in all tissues and stages of animal development [10, 24], suggesting a role of PS processing in the cellular response to apoptotic signals.
5. Recently, Galli et al. demonstrated that cerebellar granule cells undergoing apoptosis show increased secretion of $\beta A4$ [25].

Taken together, all these data point to apoptotic pathways that participate in the observed neurodegeneration in Alzheimer's disease. As expected for a general mechanism for cellular death, apoptosis seems to be also closely linked with other neurodegenerative diseases, such as amyotrophic lateral sclerosis [26] or Huntington's disease [27].

REFERENCES

1. Loo D, Copani A, Pike C, Whittemore E, Walencewicz A, Cotman CW. Apoptosis is induced by β-amyloid in cultured central nervous neurons. Proc Natl Acad Sci USA 1993; 90: 7951–5.
2. Yamatsuji T, Matsui T, Okamoto T, Komatsuzaki K, Takeda S, Fukumoto H, Iwatsubo T, Suzuki N, Asamiodaka A, Ireland S, Kinane TB, Giambarella U, Nishimoto I. G-protein-mediated neuronal DNA fragmentation induced by familial Alzheimer's disease-associated mutants of APP. Science 1996; 272: 1349–52.
3. Zhao B, Chrest FJ, Horton WE, Sisodia SS, Kusiak JW. Expression of mutant amyloid precursor proteins induces apoptosis in PC12 cells. J Neurosci Res 1997; 47: 253–63.
4. Sherrington R, Rogaev EI, Liang Y, Rogaeva EA, Levesque G, Ikeda M, Chi H, Lin C, Li G, Holman K, Tsuda T, Mar L, Foncin JF, Bruni AC, Montesi MP, Sorbi S, Rainero I, Pinessi L, Nee L, Chumakov I, Pollen D, Brookes A, Sanseau P, Polinsky RJ, Wasco W, Da Silva HAR, Haines JL, Pericak-Vance MA, Tanzi RE, Roses AD, Fraser PE, Rommens JM, St George-Hyslop PH. Cloning of a gene bearing missense mutations in early-onset familial Alzheimer's disease. Nature 1995; 375: 754–60.
5. Levy-Lahad E, Wasco W, Pookaj P, Romano D, Oshima J, Pettingell P, Yu C, Jondro PD, Schmidt SD, Wang K, Crowley AC, Fu YH, Guenette SY, Galas D, Nemens E, Wijsman EM, Bird TD, Schellenberg GD, Tanzi RE. Candidate gene for the chromosome 1 familial Alzheimer's disease locus. Science 1995; 269: 973–7.
6. Rogaev EI, Sherrington R, Rogaeva EA, Levesque G, Ikeda M, Liang Y, Chi H, Lin C, Holman K, Tsuda T, Mar L, Sorbi S, Nacmias B, Placentini S, Amaducci L, Chumakov I, Cohen D, Lannfelt L, Fraser PE, Rommens JM, St George-Hyslop PH. Familial Alzheimer's disease in kindreds with missense mutations in a gene on chromosome 1 related to the Alzheimer's disease type 3 gene. Nature 1995; 376: 775–8.
7. Wolozin B, Iwasaki K, Vito P, Ganjei JK, Lacana E, Sunderland T, Zhao B, Kusiak JW, Wasco W, D'Adamio L. Participation of presenilin-2 in apoptosis: enhanced basal activity conferred by an Alzheimer mutation. Science 1996; 274: 1710–13.
8. Janicki S, Monteiro MJ. Increased apoptosis arising from increased expression of the Alzheimer's disease-associated presenilin-2 mutation (N141I). J Cell Biol 1997; 139: 485–95.
9. Kim TW, Pettingell WH, Jung YK, Kovacs DM, Tanzi RE. Alternative cleavage of Alzheimer-associated presenilins during apoptosis by a caspase-3 family protease. Science 1997; 277: 373–6.
10. Loetscher HR, Deuschle U, Brockhaus M, Reinhardt D, Nelboek P, Mous J, Gruenberg J, Haass C, Jacobsen H. Presenilins are processed by caspase-type proteases. J Biol Chem 1997; 272: 20655–9.
11. Grünberg J, Walter J, Loetscher H, Deuschle U, Jacobsen H, Haass C. Alzheimer's disease associated presenilin-1 holoprotein and its 18–20 kDa C-terminal fragment are death substrates for proteases of the caspase family. Biochemistry 1998; 37: 2263–70.
12. Weidemann A, Paliga K, Dürrwang U, Czech C, Evin G, Masters CL, Beyreuther K. Formation of stable complexes between two Alzheimer's disease gene products: presenilin-2 and β-amyloid precursor protein. Nature Med 1997; 3: 328–32.
13. Weidemann A, König G, Bunke D, Fischer P, Salbaum JM, Masters CL, Beyreuther K. Identification, biogenesis, and localization of precursors of Alzheimer's disease A4 amyloid protein. Cell 1989; 57: 115–26.
14. Xia W, Zhang J, Perez R, Koo EH, Selkoe DJ. Interaction between amyloid precursor protein and presenilins in mammalian cells: implications for the pathogenesis of Alzheimer disease. Proc Natl Acad Sci USA 1997; 94: 8208–13.

15. Wasco W, Tanzi RE, Moir RD, Crowley AC, Merriam DE, Romano DM, Jondro PD, Kellerman BA. Presenilin 2–APP interactions. In: Younkin SG, Tanzi RE, Christen Y (eds) Presenilins and Alzheimer's Disease. Heidelberg: Springer, 1998; 59–70.
16. Weidemann A, Paliga K, Dürrwang U, Reinhard F, Zhang D, Sandbrink R, Evin G, Masters CL, Beyreuther K. Interactions of the presenilins with APP. In: Hooper NM (ed) Methods in Molecular Medicine: Alzheimer's Disease, Methods and Protocols. Totowa, NJ: Humana, 1998 (in press).
17. Thornberry NA, Rano TA, Peterson EP, Rasper DM, Timkey T, Garcia Calvo M, Houtzager VM, Nordstrom PA, Roy S, Vaillancourt JP, Chapman KT, Nicholson DW. A combinatorial approach defines specificities of members of the caspase family and granzyme B. Functional relationships established for key mediators of apoptosis. J Biol Chem 1997; 272: 17907–11.
18. Cotman CW, Anderson AJ. A potential role for apoptosis in neurodegeneration and Alzheimer's disease. Mol Neurobiol 1995; 10: 19–45.
19. Lassmann H, Bancher C, Breitschopf H, Wegiel J, Bobinski M, Jellinger K, Wisniewski HM. Cell death in Alzheimer's disease evaluated by DNA fragmentation in situ. Acta Neuropathol 1995; 89: 35–41.
20. Vito P, Wolozin B, Ganjei JK, Iwasaki K, Lacana E, D'Adamio L. Opposing effect of ALG-3. J Biol Chem 1996; 271: 31025–8.
21. Vito P, Ghayur T, D'Adamio L. Generation of anti-apoptotic presenilin-2 polypeptides by alternative transcription, proteolysis, and caspase-3 cleavage. J Biol Chem 1997; 272: 28315–20.
22. Deng G, Pike CJ, Cotman CW. Alzheimer-associated presenilin-2 confers increased sensitivity to apoptosis in PC12 cells. FEBS Lett 1996; 397: 50–54.
23. Guo Q, Furukawa K, Sopher BL, Pham DG, Xie J, Robinson N, Martin GM, Mattson MP. Alzheimer's PS1 mutation perturbs calcium homeostasis and sensitizes PC12 cells to death induced by amyloid β-peptide. NeuroReport 1996; 8: 379–83.
24. Hartmann H, Busciglio J, Baumann KH, Staufenbiel M, Yankner BA. Developmental regulation of presenilin-1 processing in the brain suggests a role in neuronal differentiation. J Biol Chem 1997; 272: 14505–8.
25. Galli C, Piccini A, Ciotti MT, Castellani L, Calissano DZ, Tabaton M. Increased amyloidogenic secretion in cerebellar granule cells undergoing apoptosis. Proc Natl Acad Sci USA 1998; 95: 1247–52.
26. Friedlander RM, Brown RH, Gagliardini V, Wang J, Yuan J. Inhibition of ICE slows ALS in mice. Nature 1997; 388: 31.
27. Goldberg YP, Nicholson DW, Rasper DM, Kalchman MA, Koide HB, Graham RK, Bromm M, Kazemi-Esfarjani P, Thornberry NA, Vaillancourt JP, Hayden MR. Cleavage of huntingtin by apopain, a proapoptotic cysteine protease, is modulated by the polyglutamine tract. Nature Genet 1996; 13: 442–9.

Address for correspondence:
Andreas Weidemann,
Zentrum für Molekulare Biologie Heidelberg (ZMBH),
Universität Heidelberg,
Im Neuenheimer Feld 282, D-69120 Heidelberg, Germany
Tel: (49) 6221 546847; fax: (49) 6221 545891;
e-mail: weidemanna@sun0.urz.uni-heidelberg.de

43 X11 Modulation of β-Amyloid Precursor Protein Cellular Stabilization and Reduction of Amyloid β-Protein Secretion

EFRAT LEVY, MAGDALENA SASTRE AND
R. SCOTT TURNER

INTRODUCTION

β-amyloid precursor protein (β-APP) is a cell surface protein with a large extracellular amino-terminal domain, a single transmembrane segment, and a short cytoplasmic tail. Its location and structural features are characteristic of a receptor for signal transduction. Screening for potential proteins capable of interacting with the β-APP cytoplasmic domain led to the identification of proteins containing phosphotyrosine interaction/phosphotyrosine binding (PI/PTB) domains: Fe65, X11 and their homologues [1–5]. The X11 gene was originally isolated as a candidate gene for Friedreich ataxia, an autosomal recessive degenerative disorder that affects the cerebellum, spinal cord and peripheral nerves [6]. The X11 protein is a neuron-specific protein of unknown function that contains two postsynaptic density protein, disc-like, zo-1 (PDZ) domains at its carboxyl-terminus in addition to a PI/PTB domain [7].

Biochemical characterization of the interaction of X11 and Fe65 with β-APP indicated that the YENPTY motif located at the cytoplasmic carboxyl-terminus of β-APP is essential for its association with the PI/PTB domains [1, 2]. Alternative processing pathways of β-APP, by secretases with α-, β- and γ-cleavage activities, result in the release of amino-terminal soluble β-APP, sβ-APPα and sβ-APPβ, as well as amyloid-β protein (Aβ) and P3, into the extracellular compartment [8, 9]. Since it was demonstrated that the YENPTY sequence motif is involved in protein internalization and β-APP processing occurs in part following its internalization [10–12], association of PI/PTB domain containing proteins with the coated pit-mediated internalization signal of β-APP may affect the patterns of β-APP trafficking and generation of Aβ, as well as of sβ-APP and normal physiologic function.

Alzheimer's Disease and Related Disorders
Edited by K. Iqbal, D.F. Swaab, B. Winblad and H.M. Wisniewski
© 1999 John Wiley & Sons Ltd

RESULTS

We have previously analyzed the binding sites on β-APP for the X11 PI domain, using site-directed mutagenesis of the cytoplasmic domain of β-APP (Figure 1A). Deletion of the carboxyl-terminal 18 amino acids of β-APP (CD18) and two mutations within the YENPTY motif, Y682G and N684A, severely inhibit the binding of the PI/PTB domain of X11 to β-APP [2]. In order to study the effect of these mutations on β-APP processing, pulse-chase experiments were performed with mouse neuroblastoma N2a and human embryonic kidney 293 cell lines transiently transfected with the wild-type (β-APPwt) or mutated β-APP cDNAs. Immunoprecipitation of labeled cell lysate proteins with anti-Aβ$_{1-17}$ antibody (6E10) revealed that mutations within the X11 interactive domain of β-APP did not significantly affect the decrease of intracellular β-APP (Figure 1B). Immunoprecipitation of media proteins revealed that the secretion of sβ-APPα was increased in cells transfected with β-APP lacking the 18 carboxyl-terminal amino acids, including the YENPTY motif, when compared to cells transfected with wild-type cDNA. These results are compatible with previous reports of the effect of deletion of either the cytoplasmic domain or the YENPTY sequence of β-APP on its processing [11, 13]. Furthermore, mutation of the amino-terminal tyrosine (Y682G) or asparagine (N684A) within the YENPTY motif also cause increased secretion of sβ-APPα (Figure 1B).

Conversely, pulse-chase experiments were performed with cells transiently co-transfected with β-APPwt and either vector or X11 cDNAs. Immunoprecipitation of cell lysate proteins showed that co-transfection of β-APPwt and X11 delayed intracellular β-APP depletion (Figure 1B). While X11 caused intracellular β-APP stabilization in both cell lines, the effect was much more pronounced in 293 cells than in N2a cells. Immunoprecipitation of conditioned media proteins demonstrated decreased secretion of sβ-APPα (Figure 1B). These results suggest that β-APP binding to X11 delays β-APP turnover, resulting in retention of intracellular β-APP and decreased sβ-APP secretion.

The effect of X11 association with β-APP with the K595N/M596L double mutation found in a Swedish kindred with familial Alzheimer's disease, β-APPsw, was studied in 293 cells co-transfected with β-APPsw and either X11 or vector cDNAs. X11 effect on β-APPsw turnover and secretion was compared to its effect on the wild-type protein. Retention of intracellular

---

Figure 1 (opposite). (A) Residues within the carboxyl-terminal domain of β-APP that are involved in X11 binding. (B) Effect of X11 binding to the YENPTY motif of β-APP on secretion of sβ-APPα. 293 and N2a cells transiently transfected with wild-type or mutated β-APP or co-transfected with β-APPwt and X11 cDNAs were labeled with ^{35}S methionine/cysteine for 20 min and chased for different time periods. Cell lysates and media proteins immunoprecipitated with anti-Aβ$_{1-17}$ antibody (6E10) were

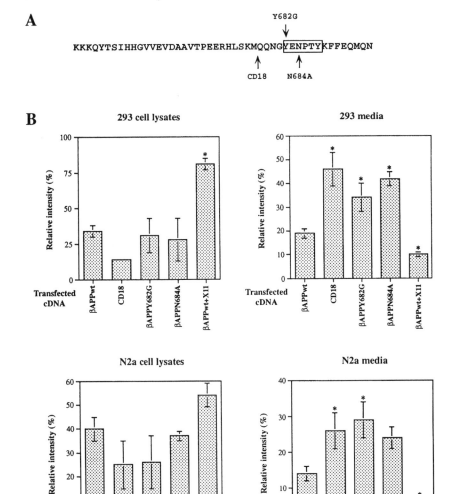

A

Y682G

KKKQYTSIHHGVVEVDAAVTPEERHLSKMQQNGYENPTYKFFEQMQN

CD18   N684A

B

293 cell lysates

293 media

N2a cell lysates

N2a media

separated by 8% SDS–PAGE and the gels were exposed to X-ray films. The protein bands were scanned using Adobe Photoshop software and quantitated using the NIH Image program. Relative intensity of the protein bands following chase for 4 h was calculated as a percentage of the intensity of the protein bands of cell lysates at the beginning of the chase (time zero). Means and standard deviations from five different experiments are presented. p Values < 0.05 for the comparison of the mutated β-APP or β-APPwt co-transfected with X11 with β-APPwt were considered to be statistically significant (*)

β-APP was observed in cells co-transfected with X11 and either β-APPwt or β-APPsw by immunoprecipitation of labeled cell lysates proteins with anti-$A\beta_{1-17}$ antibody (6E10) (Figure 2). Immunoprecipitation of conditioned media proteins revealed decreased secretion of sβ-APPα by cells co-transfected with either β-APPwt or β-APPsw and X11 compared to cells co-transfected with vector cDNA (Figure 2). These results indicate that the K595N/M596L double mutation does not affect X11 regulation of β-APP processing.

The effect of β-APP/X11 binding on Aβ secretion was studied by ELISA, as described previously [14]. The secretion of both $A\beta_{1-40}$ and $A\beta_{1-42}$ was lower in cells co-transfected with β-APPwt or β-APPsw and X11 as compared to cells co-transfected with vector cDNA (Figure 3). Furthermore, the secretion of both $A\beta_{1-40}$ and $A\beta_{1-42}$ was slightly lower in cells transfected with β-APPY682G, as compared to cells expressing β-APPwt cDNA (Figure 3).

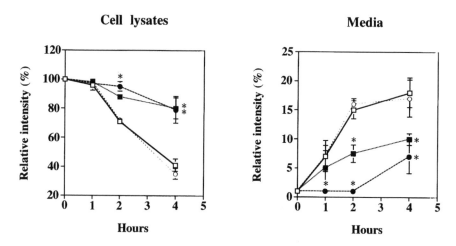

Figure 2. Effect of co-transfection of X11 and β-APPwt or β-APPsw on β-APP processing and secretion of sβ-APPα; 293 cells were labeled and analyzed as described in the legend to Figure 1B. Means and standard deviations from three different experiments are presented. Symbols represent co-transfection with: β-APPwt with vector (□); β-APPwt with X11 (■); β-APPsw with vector (○); and β-APPsw with X11 (●). p Values <0.05 for the comparison of β-APPsw co-transfected with X11 to the same β-APP cDNA co-transfected with vector alone were considered to be statistically significant (*)

DISCUSSION

These data demonstrate that X11 modulates β-APP processing via a direct protein–protein interaction, differentially affecting sβ-APP and Aβ secretion in neuronal and non-neuronal cells. While mutations in β-APP that impair interactions with X11 result in increased proteolysis by an α-secretase, co-

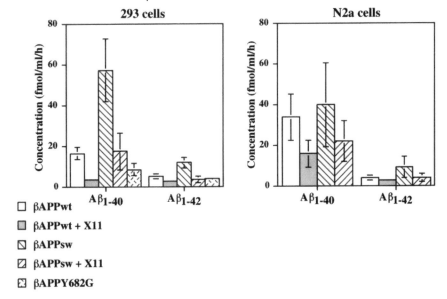

Figure 3. Reduced secretion of Aβ in cells over-expressing both X11 and β-APP. Cells were co-transfected with either β-APPwt or β-APPsw and vector or X11 cDNAs, or transfected with β-APPY682G and vector cDNAs. The conditioned media of 293 and N2a cells were collected 40 and 24 h after transfection, respectively. Three anti-Aβ antibodies were used for ELISA analysis of Aβ media proteins: anti-Aβ$_{1-10}$ antibody (BAN-50), anti-Aβ$_{x-40}$ antibody (BA-27) and anti-Aβ$_{x-42}$ antibody (BC-05). The concentrations of Aβ$_{1-40}$ and Aβ$_{1-42}$ are presented in fmol/ml/h as mean ± SE of six to seven different experiments

transfection of β-APP with X11 produces the opposite effect. Deletion of the carboxyl-terminal domain of β-APPwt inhibited very significantly the internalization of β-APP and inhibited the production of Aβ [15]. Our data demonstrate that an intact YENPTY motif is required for the production of some Aβ, since mutations within the YENPTY motif in β-APP leads to decreased Aβ secretion. Furthermore, over-expression of both X11 and β-APP results in prolongation of the half-life of cell-associated β-APP and decreased secretion of Aβ. A similar effect of X11–βAPP association was demonstrated in 293 [16], monkey kidney COS-1 and human glial U251 cell lines [17]. Since the YENPTY motif is implicated in internalization of β-APP via clathrin-mediated endocytosis [10–12], X11 may block clathrin-mediated endocytosis, possibly competitively interacting with the YENPTY motif of β-APP.

The double mutation K595N–M596L leads to over-production of Aβ [18]. As a consequence of early cleavage of β-APPsw by a β-secretase along the constitutive secretory pathway, the levels of full-length β-APPsw that arrive at the plasma membrane are considerably diminished [19–21]. We demonstrate that the double mutation does not affect X11 regulation of β-APP processing. Similar to β-APPwt, co-expression of β-APPsw with X11 decreases secretion of the soluble proteolytic peptides, sβ-APPα and Aβ. Thus, the specific inter-action of X11 with the YENPTY motif of β-APP may occur in multiple cellular locations, resulting in prolongation of the half-life of cellular β-APP, affecting both the secretory and endosomal pathways.

Since X11 has multiple protein interaction domains, other proteins may be complexed to the β-APP–X11 moiety, affecting β-APP processing or the nor-mal physiologic function of β-APP. Dimerization of the two PDZ motifs [22] may induce stabilization of the complex β-APP–X11–X11-dimerization-associate, blocking the accessibility of the secretase cleavage sites of β-APP, resulting in decreased secretion of both sβ-APP and Aβ. Alternatively, X11 may directly affect β-APP processing, preventing secretion of its soluble frag-ments and thereby leading to an accumulation of β-APP in the cell.

Cell-associated β-APP and secreted β-APP products have been implicated in cell growth, neuronal survival and viability, neurite outgrowth and neuro-protection [23]. Therefore, stabilization of the full-length protein within the cell surface as a result of β-APP/X11 coupling may be neuroprotective. Con-trary to the protective trophic activity of cell-associated β-APP as well as sβ-APP, many studies have shown that Aβ can be neurotoxic [24]. It was hypothesized that Aβ and sβ-APP are physiological ligands with reciprocal effects on neurons and alterations in the Aβ:sβ-APP ratio may have beneficial or deleterious effects on neuronal survival and growth [25]. Thus, stabiliza-tion of cellular β-APP and inhibition of the amyloidogenic processing pathway by stimulating the interaction of β-APP with an adaptor protein, such as X11 or another family member, may provide a novel approach for the phar-macological modulation of β-APP processing in Alzheimer's disease.

ACKNOWLEDGEMENTS

Supported by the National Institute on Aging, Grant No. AG13705.

REFERENCES

1. Fiore F, Zambrano N, Minopoli G, Donini V, Duilio A, Russo T. The regions of the Fe65 protein homologous to the phosphotyrosine interaction/phosphotyrosine binding domain of Shc bind the intracellular domain of the Alzheimer's amyloid precursor protein. J Biol Chem 1995; 270: 30853–6.
2. Borg JP, Ooi J, Levy E, Margolis B. The phosphotyrosine interaction domains of X11 and FE65 bind to distinct sites on the YENPTY motif of amyloid precursor protein. Mol Cell Biol 1996; 16: 6229–41.
3. Bressler SL, Gray MD, Sopher BL, Hu Q, Hearn MG, Pham DG, Dinulos MB, Fukuchi K, Sisodia SS, Miller MA, Disteche CM, Martin GM. cDNA cloning and chromosome mapping of the human Fe65 gene: interaction of the conserved cytoplasmic domains of the human β-amyloid precursor protein and its homo-logues with the mouse Fe65 protein. Hum Mol Genet 1996; 5: 1589–98.

4. Guenette SY, Chen J, Jondro PD, Tanzi RE. Association of a novel human FE65-like protein with the cytoplasmic domain of the β-amyloid precursor protein. Proc Natl Acad Sci USA 1996; 93: 10832–7.

5. McLoughlin DM, Miller CC. The intracellular cytoplasmic domain of the Alzheimer's disease amyloid precursor protein interacts with phosphotyrosine-binding domain proteins in the yeast two-hybrid system. FEBS Lett 1996; 397: 197–200.

6. Duclos F, Boschert U, Sirugo G, Mandel JL, Hen R, Koenig M. Gene in the region of the Friedreich ataxia locus encodes a putative transmembrane protein expressed in the nervous system. Proc Natl Acad Sci USA 1993; 90: 109–13.

7. Bork P, Margolis B. A phosphotyrosine interaction domain. Cell 1995; 80: 693–4.

8. Esch FS, Keim PS, Beattie EC, Blacher RW, Culwell AR, Oltersdorf T, McClure D, Ward PJ. Cleavage of amyloid β peptide during constitutive processing of its precursor. Science 1990; 248: 1122–4.

9. Sisodia SS, Koo EH, Beyreuther K, Unterbeck A, Price DL. Evidence that β-amyloid protein in Alzheimer's disease is not derived by normal processing. Science 1990; 248: 492–5.

10. Lai A, Sisodia SS, Trowbridge IS. Characterization of sorting signals in the β-amyloid precursor protein cytoplasmic domain. J Biol Chem 1995; 270: 3565–73.

11. Koo EH, Squazzo SL. Evidence that production and release of amyloid β-protein involves the endocytic pathway. J Biol Chem 1994; 269: 17386–9.

12. Chen WJ, Goldstein JL, Brown MS. NPXY, a sequence often found in cytoplasmic tails, is required for coated pit-mediated internalization of the low density lipoprotein receptor. J Biol Chem 1990; 265: 3116–23.

13. De Strooper B, Umans L, Van Leuven F, Van den Berghe H. Study of the synthesis and secretion of normal and artificial mutants of murine amyloid precursor protein (APP): cleavage of APP occurs in a late compartment of the default secretion pathway. J Cell Biol 1993; 121: 295–304.

14. Turner RS, Suzuki N, Chyung AS, Younkin SG, Lee VM-Y. Amyloids β40 and β42 are generated intracellularly in cultured human neurons and their secretion increases with maturation. J Biol Chem 1996; 271: 8966–70.

15. Essalmani R, Macq AF, Mercken L, Octave JN. Missense mutations associated with familial Alzheimer's disease in Sweden lead to the production of the amyloid peptide without internalization of its precursor. Biochem Biophys Res Commun 1996; 218: 89–96.

16. Borg JP, Yang Y, De Taddeo-Borg M, Margolis B, Turner RS. The X11α protein slows cellular amyloid precursor protein processing and reduces Aβ40 and Aβ42 secretion. J Biol Chem 1998; 273: 14761–6.

17. Sastre M, Turner RS, Levy E. X11 interaction with β-amyloid precursor protein modulates its cellular stabilization and reduces amyloid β-protein secretion. J Biol Chem 1998; 273: 22351–7.

18. Citron M, Oltersdorf T, Haass C, McConlogue L, Hung AY, Seubert P, Vigo-Pelfrey C, Lieberburg I, Selkoe DJ. Mutation of the β-amyloid precursor protein in familial Alzheimer's disease increases β protein production. Nature 1992; 360: 672–4.

19. Thinakaran G, Teplow DB, Siman R, Greenberg B, Sisodia SS. Metabolism of the 'Swedish' amyloid precursor protein variant in neuro2a (N2a) cells. Evidence that cleavage at the 'β-secretase' site occurs in the Golgi apparatus. J Biol Chem 1996; 271: 9390–97.

20. Schrader-Fischer G, Paganetti PA. Effect of alkalizing agents on the processing of the β-amyloid precursor protein. Brain Res 1996; 716: 91–100.

21. Perez RG, Squazzo SL, Koo EH. Enhanced release of amyloid β-protein from codon 670/671 'Swedish' mutant β-amyloid precursor protein occurs in both secretory and endocytic pathways. J Biol Chem 1996; 271: 9100–107.
22. Brenman JE, Chao DS, Gee SH, McGee AW, Craven SE, Santillano DR, Wu Z, Huang F, Xia H, Peters MF, Froehner SC, Bredt DS. Interaction of nitric oxide synthase with the postsynaptic density protein PSD-95 and α1-syntrophin mediated by PDZ domains. Cell 1996; 84: 757–67.
23. Mattson MP. Cellular actions of β-amyloid precursor protein and its soluble and fibrillogenic derivatives. Physiol Rev 1997; 77: 1081–132.
24. Yankner BA. Mechanisms of neuronal degeneration in Alzheimer's disease. Neuron 1996; 16: 921–32.
25. Larner AJ. Physiological and pathological interrelationships of amyloid β peptide and the amyloid precursor protein. Bioessays 1995; 17: 819–24.

Address for correspondence:
Efrat Levy,
Departments of Pharmacology and Pathology,
New York University Medical Center,
550 First Avenue, New York, NY 10016, USA

44 Amyloid β-Peptide-associated Free Radical Oxidative Stress and Alzheimer's Disease

D. ALLAN BUTTERFIELD

Amyloid β-peptide (Aβ) is the principal constituent in senile plaques (SP) in the Alzheimer's disease (AD) brain. A central role for Aβ in AD has been proposed [1], based on the following observations: certain genetic mutations in the amyloid precursor protein (APP), encoded on chromosome 21, lead to familial AD; essentially all Down's syndrome patients with chromosome 21 involvement eventually develop AD if they live sufficiently long; mutations in presenilin genes encoded on chromosomes 14 and 1, thought to be involved in APP processing and which lead to increased Aβ deposition, result in early-onset familial AD; and transgenic APP-over-expressing mice exhibit many, although not all, of the pathological characteristics of the AD brain, including Aβ deposition.

One of the most enigmatic aspects of AD research is the large number of reports of alterations in different enzymes, transport proteins, lipids, etc., in the AD brain. How can one disease have so many different alterations? This question led our group to consider the possibility that Aβ itself may be associated with free radical oxidative stress. If Aβ-associated free radical oxidative stress occurred, then neuronal membrane lipid peroxidation and protein oxidation would ensue, with subsequently altered function of membrane transport proteins and other moieties. In particular, if the Na^+/K^+-ATPase were inhibited by Aβ-associated free radicals or their byproducts, then the cell potential would be compromised. This would have the effect of opening voltage-gated Ca^{2+} channels, leading to large influx of intracellular Ca^{2+}. The latter could also cause the release of intracellularly-stored Ca^{2+}. If the Ca^{2+}-ATPase were also inhibited by the Aβ-associated free radicals or their byproducts, then the excess intracellular Ca^{2+} would not be removed from the neuron. Activation of Ca^{2+}-dependent degradative pathways, including proteases, endonucleases or apoptotic processes, would lead to neuronal death (Figure 1).

Alzheimer's Disease and Related Disorders
Edited by K. Iqbal, D.F. Swaab, B. Winblad and H.M. Wisniewski
© 1999 John Wiley & Sons Ltd

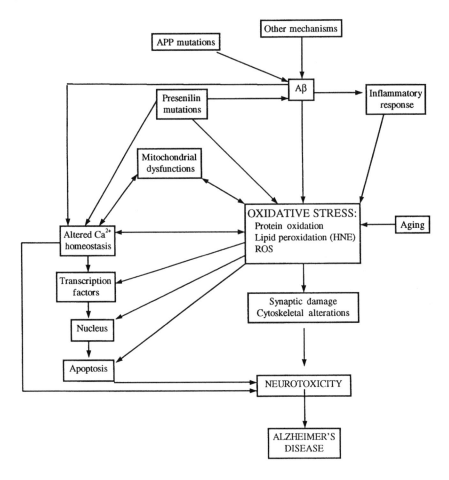

Figure 1. Amyloid β-peptide-associated oxidative stress model for neuronal death in Alzheimer's disease

The electron paramagnetic resonance (EPR) technique of spin trapping involves a non-paramagnetic nitrone, which, in the presence of a transient free radical, forms a stable, paramagnetic nitroxide that is detectable by EPR. Aβ(1–42), Aβ(1–40), or Aβ(25–35), when mixed with the spin trap, N-tert-butyl-α-phenylnitrone (PBN) in metal-chelating buffers, yields an EPR spectrum [2, 3], indicating that free radicals are associated with the peptide. The free radical formed is oxygen-dependent and, based on several different studies, may be peroxyl in nature (reviewed in [4, 5]). Should these processes occur in the AD brain, then alteration of many different enzymes, transport proteins, lipids, etc., in this disorder could be rationalized as discrete manifestations of the interactions of these moieties with Aβ-associated free radicals [4, 5] and the above-mentioned enigma might be better understood.

Recently, many laboratories have provided considerable evidence for oxidative stress in AD [6–9]. Among other alterations, AD brain regions rich in SP show evidence of protein oxidation, while the SP-poor cerebellum does not [6]. Lipid peroxidation also is observed in the AD brain [7]. Our group and many others have shown that Aβ, in ways inhibitable by free radical antioxidants, leads to lipid peroxidation [10–14] and protein oxidation [15–17] in various brain membrane systems; generates reactive oxygen species (ROS) [15, 16]; inhibits hippocampal neuronal and cortical synaptosomal membrane ion-motive ATPases, including Na^+/K^+-ATPase and Ca^{2+}-ATPase [18]; blocks glutamate uptake [16, 19, 20]; inhibits the activity of glutamine synthetase [2, 21, 22] (both the latter Aβ-induced alterations have the effect of increasing excitotoxic glutamate levels); causes intracellular Ca^{2+} levels to increase dramatically [15, 16, 23]; and leads to neurotoxicity in hippocampal neuronal or astrocytic cultures (reviewed in [5, 8]).

One way in which Aβ-associated free radical oxidative stress is manifested is by membrane lipid peroxidation [10–14]. Vitamin E protects against this peroxidation, expected for a free radical process [4, 5, 11]. The chief lipid peroxidation product, 4-hydroxy-2-*trans*-nonenal (4-HNE), rapidly modifies proteins through Michael addition of cysteine, lysine or histidine residues [24, 25]. Exposure of Aβ to cultured hippocampal neurons produces 4-HNE at a level of 5–10 μM [26]. This alkenal, like Aβ itself [18], inhibited ion-motive ATPases, led to increased intracellular Ca^{2+} and caused cell death in neuronal cultures and synaptosomes [26]. EPR studies, in conjunction with protein-specific spin labels, showed that 4-HNE, even at 1 μM, caused a significant alteration in the conformation of cortical synaptosomal membrane proteins [27], probably accounting for altered function of these membranes exposed to 4-HNE [28]. Glutathione, known to protect neurons from 4-HNE-induced toxicity [24, 26], prevented the conformational alterations in cortical synaptosomal membrane proteins by 4-HNE [27].

Aβ-associated free radical oxidative stress is prevented by various free radical antioxidants (reviewed in [4, 5]). Although there are undoubtedly other sources of oxidative stress in the AD brain, including, among others, activated microglia, transition metals and advanced glycation endproducts (reviewed in [8]), given the importance of Aβ in AD, free radical oxidative stress associated with this peptide most certainly plays an important role in neuronal death in the AD brain. In addition to direct oxidation of neuronal lipids and proteins or their modification by the lipid peroxidation product HNE, Aβ may also lead to neuronal death in AD by other mechanisms, e.g. induction of detrimental transcription factors leading to production of harmful proteins and apoptosis, inflammatory responses from microglia, or altered mitochondrial function. The common factor in all these processes is oxidative stress, and this suggests that brain-accessible free radical scavengers should be considered for potential therapeutic intervention/prophylaxis in AD. Initial reports using this strategy, consistent with our model for AD neuronal death (Figure 1), are encouraging [29].

In our laboratory, research continues on mechanistic investigations of Aβ-associated free radical oxidative stress. Methionine residue 35 appears to be involved since: Aβ(25–35) incubation leads to free radicals and formation of methionine sulfoxide; Aβ(25–35)-Met-SO, with the sulfoxide already synthesized in the peptide, yields no EPR signal, neither is this peptide toxic to the oxidatively-sensitive enyzme glutamine synthetase; substitution of methionine by norleucine in Aβ(25–35) (of similar length and hydrophobicity as Met, but with no sulfur), yields no EPR spectrum and is not toxic to GS; and Aβ(25–34), in which Met is absent, yields no EPR spectrum and is not toxic to GS. These negative results both point to the importance of Met-35 and suggest that metal-catalyzed processes are probably minimally involved, otherwise, one would have predicted similar reactions in Met-modified peptides, as in Aβ itself. Additional research on mechanisms of Aβ-associated free radicals, the membrane alterations that are induced by Aβ and its chief lipid peroxidation product 4-HNE, the relevance of Aβ-associated free radical oxidative stress to neurotoxicity in Alzheimer's brain, and potential pharmacological strategies to inhibit these processes [30], are in progress.

ACKNOWLEDGEMENTS

This work was supported in part by grants from NIH.

REFERENCES

1. Selkoe D. Alzheimer's disease: a central role of amyloid. J Neuropathol Exp Neurol 1994; 53: 438–47.
2. Hensley K, Carney J, Mattson M, Askenova M, Harris M, Wu JF, Floyd R, Butterfield DA. A new model for β-amyloid aggregation and neurotoxicity based on free radical-generating capacity of the peptide. Proc Natl Acad Sci USA 1994; 91: 3270–74.
3. Tomiyama T, Shaji A, Kataoka K, Suwa Y, Asano S, Kaneko H, Endo N. Inhibition of amyloid β-protein aggregation and neurotoxicity by rifampicin. Its possible function as a hydroxyl radical scavenger. J Biol Chem 1996; 271: 6839–44.
4. Butterfield DA, Hensley K, Hall N, Subramaniam R, Howard BJ, Cole P, Yatin S, LaFontaine M, Harris ME, Aksenova M, Aksenov M, Carney JM. In: Wasco W, Tanzi RE (eds) β-Amyloid-derived Free Radical Oxidation: A Fundamental Process in Alzheimer's Disease. New Jersey: Humana Press, 1996; 145–67.
5. Butterfield DA. β-amyloid-associated free radical oxidative stress and neurotoxicity: implications for Alzheimer's disease. Chem Res Toxicol 1997; 10: 495–506.
6. Hensley K, Hall N, Subramaniam R, Cole P, Harris M, Aksenov M, Aksenova M, Gabbita SP, Wu JF, Carney JM, Lovell M, Markesbery WR, Butterfield DA. Brain regional correspondence between Alzheimer's disease histopathology and biomarkers of protein oxidation. J Neurochem 1995; 65: 2146–56.
7. Markesbery WR, Lovell MA. 4-hydroxynonenal, a product of lipid peroxidation, is increased in the brain in Alzheimer's disease. Neurobiol Aging 1998; 19: 33–6.

8. Markesbery WR. Oxidative stress hypothesis in Alzheimer disease. Free Rad Biol Med 1997; 23: 134–47.

9. Behl C, Holsboer F. Oxidative stress in the pathogenesis of Alzheimer's disease and antioxidant neuroprotection. Fortschr Neurol Psychiatr 1998; 66: 113–21.

10. Butterfield DA, Hensley K, Harris M, Mattson M, Carney JM. β-Amyloid peptide free radical fragments initiate synaptosomal lipoperoxidation in a sequence-specific fashion: implications to Alzheimer's disease. Biochem Biophys Res Commun 1994; 200: 710–15.

11. Koppal T, Subramaniam R, Drake J, Prasad MR, Butterfield DA. Vitamin E protects against Alzheimer's amyloid peptide (25–35)-induced changes in neocortical synaptosomal membrane lipid structure and composition. Brain Res 1998; 786: 270–73.

12. Gridley KE, Green PS, Simpkins JW. Low concentrations of estradiol reduce β-amyloid (25–35)-induced toxicity, lipid peroxidation, and glucose utilization in human SK-N-SH neuroblastoma cells. Brain Res 1997; 778: 158–65.

13. Daniels WM, van Rensbury SJ, van Zyl JM, Taljaard JJ. Melatonin prevents β-amyloid-induced lipid peroxidation. J Pineal Res 1998; 24: 78–82.

14. Bruce-Keller AJ, Begley JG, Fu W, Butterfield DA, Bredesen DE, Hutchins JB, Hensley K, Mattson MP. Bcl-2 protects isolated plasma and mitochondrial membranes against lipid peroxidation induced by hydrogen peroxide and amyloid β-peptide. J Neurochem 1998; 70: 31–9.

15. Harris M, Hensley K, Butterfield DA, Leedle RA, Carney JM. Direct evidence of oxidative injury produced by the Alzheimer's amyloid β-peptide (1–40) in cultured hippocampal neurons. Exp Neurol 1995; 131: 193–202.

16. Harris ME, Wang Y, Pedigo NW, Hensley K, Butterfield DA, Carney JM. Aβ(25–35) inhibits Na$^+$-dependent glutamate uptake in rat hippocampal astrocyte cultures. J Neurochem 1996; 67: 277–86.

17. Subramaniam R, Koppal T, Green M, Yatin S, Jordan B, Drake J, Butterfield DA. The free radical antioxidant vitamin E protects cortical synaptosomal membranes from amyloid β-peptide (25–35) toxicity but not from hydroxynonenal toxicity: relevance to the free radical hypothesis of Alzheimer's disease. Neurochem Res 1998; 23: 1403–1410.

18. Mark RJ, Hensley K, Butterfield DA, Mattson MP. Amyloid β-peptide impairs ion-motive ATPase activities: evidence for a role in loss of neuronal Ca^{2+} homeostasis and cell death. J Neurosci 1995; 15: 6239–49.

19. Harris ME, Carney JM, Cole P, Hensley K, Howard BJ, Martin L, Bummer P, Wang Y, Pedigo N, Butterfield DA. β-amyloid peptide-derived, oxygen-dependent free radicals inhibit glutamate uptake in cultured astrocytes: implications to Alzheimer's disease. NeuroReport 1995; 6: 1875–9.

20. Keller JN, Pang Z, Gedded JW, Begley JG, Germeyer A, Waeg G, Mattson MP. Impairment of glucose and glutamate transport and induction of mitochondrial oxidative stress and dysfunction in synaptosomes by amyloid β-peptide: role of the lipid peroxidation product 4-hydroxynonenal. J Neurochem 199; 69: 273–84.

21. Aksenov MY, Aksenova MV, Harris ME, Hensley K, Butterfield DA, Carney JM. Enhancement of Aβ (1–40) neurotoxicity by glutamine synthetase. J Neurochem 1995; 65: 1899–1902.

22. Aksenov MY, Aksenova MV, Carney JM, Butterfield DA. Oxidative modification of glutamine synthetase by amyloid β-peptide. Free Radical Res 1997; 27: 267–81.

23. Mattson MP, Barger SW, Cheng B, Lieberburg L, Smith-Swintosky VL, Rydel RE. β-Amyloid precursor protein metabolites and loss of neuronal Ca^{2+} homeostasis in Alzheimer's disease. Trends Neurosci 1993; 16: 409–14.

24. Esterbauer H, Schaur RJ, Zollner H. Chemistry and biochemistry of 4-hydroxy-nonenal, malonaldehyde and related aldehydes. Free Radical Biol Med 1991; 11: 41–128.
25. Butterfield DA, Stadtman ER. Protein oxidation processes in aging brain. Adv Cell Aging Gerontol 1997; 2: 161–91.
26. Mark RJ, Lovell MA, Markesbery WR, Uchida K, Mattson MP. A role for 4-hydroxynonenal in disruption of ion homeostasis and neuronal death induced by amyloid β-peptide. J Neurochem 1997; 68: 255–64.
27. Subramaniam R, Roediger F, Jordan B, Mattson MP, Keller JN, Waeg G, Butterfield DA. The lipid peroxidation product, 4-hydroxy-2-*trans*-nonenal, alters the conformation of cortial synaptosomal membrane proteins. J Neurochem 1997; 69: 1161–9.
28. Mattson MP, Mark RJ, Furukawa K, Annadora JB. Disruption of brain cell ion homeostasis in Alzheimer's disease by oxy radicals, and signaling pathways that protect therefrom. Chem Res Toxicol 1997; 10: 507–17.
29. Sano M, Ernesto C, Thomas RG, Klauber MR, Schafer K, Grundman M, Woodbury P, Growdon J, Cotman CW, Pfeiffer E, Schneider LS, Thal LJ. A controlled trial of selegiline, α-tocopherol, or both as treatment for Alzheimer's disease. The Alzheimer's disease cooperative study. N Engl J Med 1997; 17: 1216–22.
30. Butterfield DA, Howard BJ, Yatin S, Allen KL, Carney JM. Free radical oxidation of brain proteins in accelerated senescence and its modulation by N-tert-butyl-α-phenylnitrone. Proc Natl Acad Sci USA 1997; 94: 674–8.

Address for correspondence:
D. Allan Butterfield PhD,
Department of Chemistry, Center for Membrane Sciences,
Sanders–Brown Center on Aging,
University of Kentucky, Lexington, KY 40506-0055, USA

45 Characterization of γ-Secretase Candidates from Human Brain Using a New Western Blot Assay

**G. EVIN, G. REED, J.E. TANNER, Q.-X. LI,
J.G. CULVENOR, S.J. FULLER, H. WADSWORTH,
D. ALLSOP, R.V. WARD, E.H. KARRAN, C.W. GRAY,
T. HARTMANN, S.F. LICHTENTHALER,
A. WEIDEMANN, K. BEYREUTHER AND C.L. MASTERS**

INTRODUCTION

βA4 (or Aβ), the principal component of Alzheimer's disease (AD) amyloid plaques [1, 2], is proteolytically derived from the amyloid precursor protein (APP) [3] by two sequential cleavages due to β- and γ-secretases. γ-Secretase cleavage, which releases the C-terminus of the peptide, generates two main species: βA4 1–40, which is fairly soluble and found in cerebrospinal fluid and cell culture media, and βA4 1–42/43, which has a tendency to aggregate and seeds amyloid deposition [4]. Missense mutations in the APP and presenilin genes which cause early-onset familial AD alter APP processing by elevating the ratio of long/short forms of βA4 [5]. This points to a possible abnormal processing of APP in AD, and in particular to γ-secretase cleavage. Thus, the identification of γ-secretase and the development of specific γ-secretase inhibitors are important goals of AD research and constitute a potential therapeutic approach.

Using a biotinylated probe derived from a peptide aldehyde inhibitor of βA4 secretion in cell culture, we have designed a novel assay involving SDS–polyacrylamide gel electrophoresis and Western blotting to characterize the proteases targeted by this class of inhibitor.

EXPERIMENTAL PROCEDURES

INHIBITORS AND BIOTINYLATED PROBES

Structures of the compounds studied are given in Figure 1. Compound A corresponds to the tripeptide aldehyde carbobenzoxy–leucyl–leucyl–leucinal

Alzheimer's Disease and Related Disorders
Edited by K. Iqbal, D.F. Swaab, B. Winblad and H.M. Wisniewski
© 1999 John Wiley & Sons Ltd

(Z–Leu–Leu–Leu–H). Compound B is the N-terminal biotin derivative of compound A, and compound C is the control biotin derivative of the inactive amide Z–Leu–Leu–Leu–NH$_2$. Because of its lack of cell penetrancy, compound B had little effect when tested for γ-secretase inhibition on cultured cells.

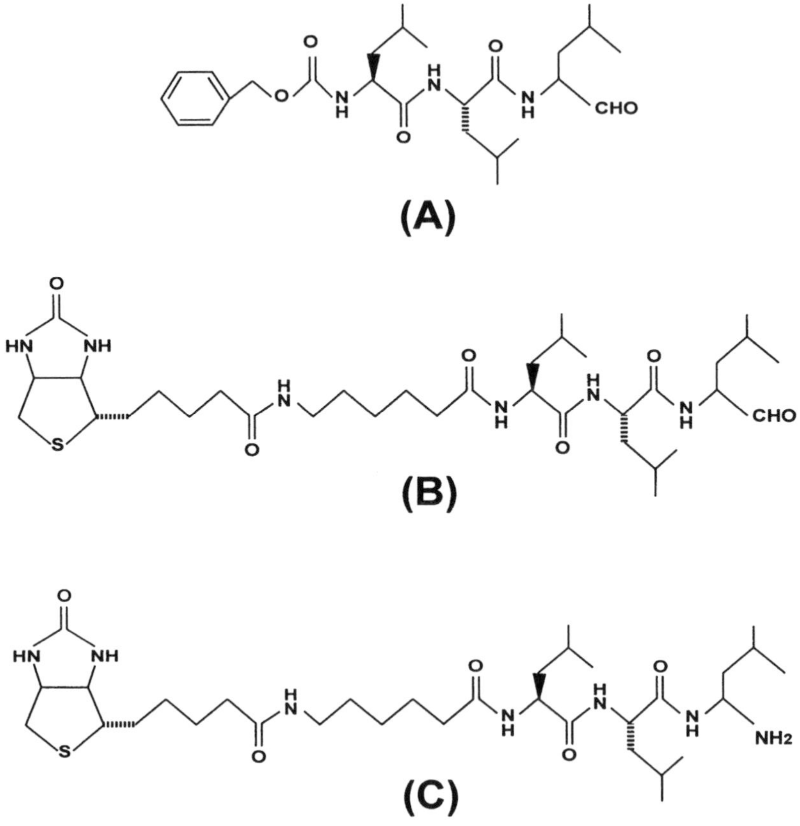

(A)

(B)

(C)

Figure 1. Structure of the peptide inhibitor derivatives (see text for details)

CELL CULTURE AND METABOLIC LABELLING

Human neuroblastoma SH-SY5Y cells were metabolically labelled, as described previously [6]. The inhibitor was added to the labelling medium as a DMSO solution (0.5% final volume). The control cell samples (without inhibitor) also contained 0.5% DMSO, a concentration which appeared to be non-toxic. After 3 h labelling, the medium was immunoprecipitated with mAb 1E8 (anti-βA4 18–22, which recognizes both βA4 and p3) [7]. The immunoprecipitates were resolved on 10–15% Tris–tricine gels, electroblotted onto 0.2 μM PVDF, and the blots were viewed by phosphorimaging, as reported previously [6]. sAPPα was quantitated by reprecipitating the medium with mAb WO2 (anti-βA4 1–16) [8], and sAPPβ by immunoprecipitation with mAb 1A9 (anti-APP$_{695}$ residues 591–596, which recognizes specifically APP-free Met$_{595}$) [9]. Measurement of ^{35}S-Met incorporation in the cell lysate gave an indication of the effect of the inhibitor on the cell metabolism. The cell morphology was also examined to assess inhibitor toxicity.

PREPARATION OF BRAIN HOMOGENATES AND SUBCELLULAR FRACTIONS

Homogenates from human brain cortex were prepared as described by Moir et al. [10]. Vesicles enriched in endosomal membranes were prepared according to Sabolic et al. [11], as follows: 5–10 g of cortex were homogenized in 0.3 M mannitol in 0.012 M Hepes, pH 7.4, centrifuged at 2500 × g for 15 min to remove nuclei and membrane debris, and then at 20 000 × g for 20 min. The supernatant was centrifuged at 100 000 × g for 1 h and the obtained pellet resuspended in homogenization buffer, sonicated and layered on top of an 18% Percoll solution. Centrifugation at 50 000 × g for 30 min yielded a dense pellet and a more diffuse one. Ultrastructure analysis by electron microscopy revealed that the dense pellet contained small membrane vesicles, with the morphology of endosomes.

INHIBITOR-LIGAND DETECTION ASSAY

Brain homogenates and fractions (5 μl) were incubated overnight at 37 °C with the biotinylated derivatives at 100 μM concentration, in a total volume of 30 μl of Tris–HCl (0.1 M, pH 7.5). For competition experiments, the samples were preincubated for 30 min at 37 °C with the appropriate inhibitors (Z–Leu–Leu–Leu–H, MDL 28170, calpeptin, antipain and pepstatin at 500 μM; iodoacetamide, E-64 and PMSF at 1 mM) before adding the biotinylated probe and proceeding as usual. The samples were boiled for 1 min, resolved by SDS–PAGE on 8–16% gradient gels, and electroblotted onto PVDF. The membrane was blocked with casein, incubated with Neutravidin–alkaline phosphatase conjugate, and developed with naphthol–Fast Red [12].

RESULTS AND DISCUSSION

INHIBITION OF γ-SECRETION BY Z–LEU–LEU–LEU–H

The human neuroblastoma cell line SH-SY5Y which has been shown to secrete amounts of βA4 readily detectable from the culture medium without transfection [6] was used for this study. Immunoprecipitation with βA4 antibodies [8] G2-10 (specific for βA4 1–40) and G2-11 (specific for βA4 1–42) characterized βA4 and p3 secreted species as the X-40 forms (Figure 2).

Z–Leu–Leu–Leu–H (compound A) was tested for its inhibition of βA4 secretion, at concentrations ranging from 5 to 100 μM (Figure 2). βA4 and p3 peptides were immunoprecipitated from the cell conditioned medium with mAb 1E8 [7]. At 100 μM concentration, complete inhibition of βA4 and p3 secretion was observed. The IC_{50} was estimated at 20 μM. The peptide toxicity was low as the cell morphology was unchanged during the 3 h incubation, and no significant alteration of protein metabolism occurred, as estimated from ^{35}S-Met incorporation. The amounts of sAPPα and sAPPβ secreted into the medium were not affected. These data indicate that Z–Leu–Leu–Leu–H inhibits γ-secretase, or the γ-secretase pathway. Small hydrophobic peptide aldehydes have been shown to inhibit βA4 secretion from transfected cells [7, 13–17] and we have reported previously that calpeptin (Z–Leu–Nle–H) and Z–Leu–Leu–Nle–H are efficient inhibitors, at 100 μM concentrations, when tested on transfected IMR-32 and SH-SY5Y cells [7], but compound A constitutes the most potent tripeptide aldehyde so far in our system. We noticed an increase in βA4 release at 5 μM and this result corroborates data reported by Yamazaki et al. [16] who used the same peptide aldehyde on transfected cells and obtained an increase of βA4 at concentrations in the low micromolar range.

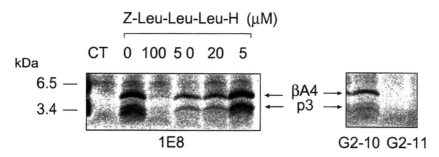

Figure 2. Effect of Z–Leu–Leu–Leu–H on the secretion of βA4 and p3 from untransfected SH-SY5Y cells

USE OF A BIOTINYLATED PROBE IN A WESTERN BLOT ASSAY FOR DETECTING POTENTIAL γ-SECRETASES

Small hydrophobic peptide aldehydes are known to inhibit calpains and the proteasome, which constitute possible γ-secretase candidates. To investigate the various proteases targeted by Z–Leu–Leu–Leu–H, an amino-terminal biotin derivative (compound B) was incubated with SH-SY5Y cell lysates and brain homogenates at 100 μM and the SDS-resistant complexes were analysed by Western blot developed with a Neutravidin conjugate. A series of bands was labelled with apparent molecular weights of 105, 85, 55 and 38 kDa (Figure 3A). The control compound C (biotin derivative of the inactive amide) showed only low and diffuse non-specific staining (Figure 3). The bands detected with compound B were present in both SH-SY5Y lysate and homogenates from human brain cortex, and a similar pattern was observed with AD and control samples.

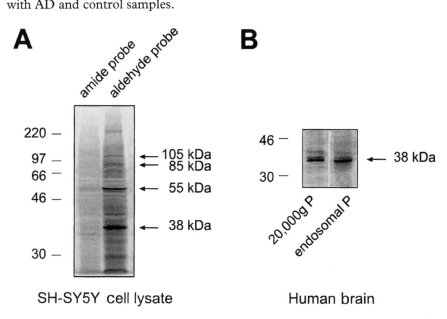

Figure 3. Analysis of SH-SY5Y lysate and of human brain fractions by Western blot assay after incubation with the biotinylated probes

PARTIAL PURIFICATION AND CHARACTERIZATION OF A 38 kDa SPECIES

The most prominent band, which corresponds to the 38 kDa species, was found associated with the membrane and present in membrane fractions of various densities, including a fraction enriched in endosome vesicles (Figure 3B). As the endosomes constitute a possible site for γ-secretase cleavage [18], we characterized further this 38 kDa protein and started its purification. Competition with various protease inhibitors showed that, as expected, the parent peptide, Z–Leu–Leu–Leu–H, and other small aldehydes, such as MDL 28170 [13] and calpeptin, could displace binding of the biotinylated probe. Among the cysteine protease inhibitors E-64, antipain, leupeptin and iodoacetamide, only E-64 competed with the biotinylated probe. The serine protease inhibitors TPCK and leupeptin had no effect, but PMSF was a competitor. Pepstatin also competed with the signal, indicating that the 38 kDa species exerts preference for hydrophobic aliphatic residues. It will be necessary to test pepstatin at concentrations in the nM range to conclude whether this 38 kDa species corresponds to an aspartyl protease. From its overall inhibition profile, it would correspond to a serine protease.

Purification of membrane extracts from human brains on Q-sepharose showed that the 38 kDa species binds at 250 mM NaCl concentration. Size-exclusion chromatography indicates that the purified species has a molecular weight much higher than that determined on SDS-reducing gels and thus may be part of a larger protein or complex. Larger-scale purification to obtain sequence data is in progress.

CONCLUSIONS

Using a biotinylated probe derived from a peptide inhibitor of βA4 and p3 release in cell culture, we have designed an assay to label protease candidates for γ-secretase and to monitor their purification. Used together with an assay for γ-secretase activity, this new Western blot assay may help with the characterization and isolation of γ-secretase from human brain.

REFERENCES

1. Glenner GG, Wong CW. Alzheimer's disease: initial report of the purification and characterization of a novel cerebrovascular amyloid protein. Biochem Biophys Res Commun 1984; 120: 885–90.
2. Masters CL, Simms G, Weinman NA, Multhaup G, McDonald B, Beyreuther K. Amyloid plaque core protein in Alzheimer disease and Down syndrome. Proc Natl Acad Sci USA 1985; 82: 4245–9.
3. Kang J, Lemaire H, Unterbeck A, Salbaum JM, Masters CL, Grzeschik K, Multhaup G, Beyreuther K, Müller-Hill B. The precursor of Alzheimer's disease amyloid A4 protein resembles a cell-surface receptor. Nature 1987; 325: 733–6.
4. Jarrett JT, Lansbury PT Jr. Seeding 'one-dimensional crystallization' of amyloid: a pathogenic mechanism in Alzheimer's disease and scrapie? Cell 1993; 73: 1055–8.
5. Scheuner D, Eckman C, Jensen M, Song X, Citron M, Suzuki N, Bird TD, Hardy J, Hutton M, Kukull W, Larson E, Levy-Lahad E, Viitanen M, Peskind E, Pookaj P, Schellenberg G, Tanzi R, Wasco W, Lannfelt L, Selkoe D, Younkin S. Secreted amyloid β-protein similar to that in the senile plaques of Alzheimer's disease is increased in vivo by the presenilin 1 and 2 and APP mutations linked to familial Alzheimer's disease. Nature Med 1996; 2: 864–70.
6. Fuller SJ, Storey E, Li Q-X, Smith AI, Beyreuther K, Masters CL. Intracellular production of βA4 amyloid of Alzheimer's disease: modulation by phosphoramidon and lack of coupling to the secretion of the amyloid precursor protein. Biochemistry 1995; 34: 8091–8.
7. Allsop D, Christie G, Gray C, Holmes S, Markwell R, Owen D, Smith L, Wadsworth H, Ward RG, Hartmann T, Lichtenthaler SF, Evin G, Fuller S, Tanner J, Masters CL, Beyreuther K, Roberts GW. Studies on inhibition of β-amyloid formation in APP751-transfected IMR-32 cells, and SPA4CT-transfected SHSY5Y cells. In: Iqbal K, Winblad B, Nishimura T, Takeda M, Wisniewski HM (eds) Alzheimer's Disease Biology, Diagnosis and Therapeutics. Chichester: Wiley, 1997; 716–27.

8. Ida N, Hartmann T, Pantel J, Schröder J, Zerfass R, Förstl H, Sandbrink R, Masters CL, Beyreuther K. Analysis of heterogenous βA4 peptides in human cerebrospinal fluid and blood by a newly developed sensitive Western blot assay. J Biol Chem 1996; 271: 22908–14.

9. Le Brocque D, Henry A, Cappai R, Li Q-X, Tanner JT, Galatis D, Gray C, Holmes S, Underwood JR, Beyreuther K, Masters CL, Evin G. Processing of the Alzheimer's Disease amyloid precursor protein in *Pichia pastoris:* immunocharacterization of α-, β- and γ-secretase products. Biochemistry 1998; 37: 14558–65.

10. Moir RD, Martins RN, Small DH, Bush AI, Milward EA, Multhaup G, Beyreuther K, Masters CL. Human brain βA4 amyloid protein precursor: purification and partial characterization. J Neurochem 1992; 59: 1490–98.

11. Sabolic I, Wuarin F, Shi L-B, Verkman AS, Ausiello D, Gluck S, Brown D. Apical endosomes isolated from kidney collecting duct principal cells lack subunits of the proton pumping ATPase. J Cell Biol 1992; 119: 111–22.

12. Evin G, Cappai R, Li Q-X, Culvenor JG, Small DH, Beyreuther K, Masters CL. Candidate γ-secretases in the generation of the carboxyl-terminus of the Alzheimer's disease βA4 amyloid: possible involvement of cathespin D. Biochemistry 1995; 34: 14185–92.

13. Higaki J, Quon D, Zhong Z, Cordell B. Inhibition of β-amyloid formation identifies proteolytic precursors and subcellular site of catabolism. Neuron 1995; 14: 651–9.

14. Citron M, Diehl TS, Gordon G, Biere AL, Seubert P, Selkoe DJ. Evidence that the 42- and 40-amino acid forms of amyloid β protein are generated from the β-amyloid precursor protein by different protease activities. Proc Natl Acad Sci USA 1996; 93: 13170–75.

15. Klafki HW, Abramowski D, Swoboda R, Paganetti PA, Staufenbiel M. The carboxyl termini of β-amyloid peptides 1–40 and 1–42 are generated by distinct γ-secretase activities. J Biol Chem 1996; 271: 28655–9.

16. Yamazaki T, Haass C, Saido TC, Omura S, Ihara Y. Specific increase in amyloid β-protein 42 secretion ratio by calpain inhibitors. Biochemistry 1997; 3: 8377–83.

17. Hartmann T, Bieger SC, Brühl B, Tienari PJ, Ida N, Allsop D, Roberts GW, Masters CL, Dotti CG, Unsicker K, Beyreuther K. Distinct sites of intracellular production for Alzheimer's disease Aβ-40/42 amyloid peptides. Nature Med 1997; 3: 1016–20.

18. Koo EH, Squazzo SL. Evidence that production and release of amyloid β-protein involves the endocytic pathway. J Biol Chem 1994; 269: 17386–9.

Address for correspondence:
Geneviève Evin PhD,
Department of Pathology, University of Melbourne,
Parkville, Victoria 3052, Australia

46 Vasoactivity of Soluble Aβ Peptides—*In Vitro* and *In Vivo*

M. MULLAN, D. PARIS, Z. SUO, T. TOWN, A. PLACZEK, T. PARKER, A. KUNDTZ, J. HUMPHREY AND F. CRAWFORD

Aβ VASOACTIVITY IS RELATED TO CONFORMATIONAL TRANSITION STATE OF Aβ

We have shown previously that Aβ peptides are vasoactive on isolated rings of rat aorta, particularly enhancing the effects of known vasoconstrictors, [1]. We have also shown that the vasoactivity of Aβ occurs with preparations of peptides that do not particularly favor β sheet formation (freshly solubilized, nanomolar concentrations of less amyloidogenic peptides ($A\beta_{1-40}$)) [2]. These conditions do not generally favor cytotoxicity and we have previously proposed that mechanisms other than those active in standard Aβ cytotoxicity assays are operating in Aβ vasoactivity. We now show that vasoactivity of Aβ peptides, individually or in combination, is related to the percentage of β sheet content, suggesting that transitional forms of peptides (between random coil and β sheet conformation) are most able to enhance endothelin-1 (ET-1)-induced vasoactivity (Figure 1). The percentage of β-sheet content of each peptide and combinations of peptides was estimated by analysis of CD spectra using the Lincomb algorithm and plotted against the percentage of vasoconstriction produced by 1 μM of Aβ peptide at a 3 nM dose of ET-1. $A\beta_{1-40}$ is more vasoactive than $A\beta_{1-42}$ and the HCHWA-D mutant ($A\beta(22Q)_{1-40}$) displays almost no vasoactive effect. When mixtures of freshly solubilized peptides are added, but molarity is maintained, we see significant increases in vasoactivity. These increases in vasoactivity correlate with less β-sheet conformation than that exhibited by either native $A\beta_{1-42}$ or $A\beta(22Q)_{1-40}$ [3].

These findings are significant as they show that Aβ can be biologically active without adopting extensive β-sheet formation. It is also of interest that the mutant Aβ associated with the most prominent cerebrovascular damage can have the most biological activity in this system when mixed with wild-type Aβ. In life, carriers of the HCHWA-D mutant are heterozygous for the mutant allele and therefore express the forms of the protein mixed here.

Alzheimer's Disease and Related Disorders
Edited by K. Iqbal, D.F. Swaab, B. Winblad and H.M. Wisniewski
© 1999 John Wiley & Sons Ltd

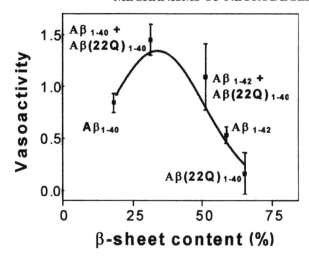

Figure 1. Relationship between vasoactivity and conformation of Aβ peptides. Vaso-activity of Aβ peptides. Aortic rings were constricted by addition of various doses of endothelin (ET-1). Following equilibration, 1 μm of peptide or peptide combinations were added as indicated and the constriction repeated with the same ET-1 doses. The percentage increase over baseline in the pre-treatment contraction was subtracted from the percentage increase over baseline in the post-treatment contraction, the mean difference for each treatment at each dose was calculated, and adjusted values (calculated against control constrictions showing zero increase over baseline) were plotted as shown. Reproduced from reference [3], © 1998, FEBS Lett 436; 445–8, with permission from Elsevier Science

Aβ ENHANCEMENT OF ENDOTHELIN VASOACTIVITY IS MEDIATED BY A PRO-INFLAMMATORY PATHWAY

Since ET-1 vasoconstriction is enhanced by Aβ, and ET-1 together with NO is largely responsible for regulating vasotonus in the cerebrovasculature, we investigated the effect of $A\beta_{1-40}$ on the known signal transduction pathways of both ET-1 and NO.

Stimulation of ET-1 is known to result in vasoconstriction via stimulation of the PLC/PLD DAG/IP3 pathways which raise intracellular calcium levels, and activate PKC and other kinases resulting in vasoconstriction. NO stimulates soluble guanylyl cyclase to produce cGMP, the level of which is also controlled by cGMP-phosphodiesterase (cGMP-PDE) which reduces calcium levels and causes vasorelaxation. We eliminated PKC as important in the transduction of the Aβ vasoactivity signal as we find only additive (as opposed to statistically interactive) effects with stimulators and inhibitors of PKC (data not shown). However, when we investigated the possible contribution of the PLA2 pathway to the vasoactive properties of Aβ, we find evidence that this is the pathway which mediates most of the Aβ vasoactivity. We evaluated the effect of two peptides in conjunction with ET-1 and $A\beta_{1-40}$, melittin and mastoparan, both of which are potent and specific stimulators of PLA2. We find that melittin (Figure 2) and mastoparan alone enhance the vasoconstriction induced by ET-1, mimicking the vasoactive effect of Aβ. In addition, statistical interaction among $A\beta_{1-40}$, melittin and ET-1, and among $A\beta_{1-40}$, mastoparan and ET-1, was observed, suggesting that $A\beta_{1-40}$ vasoactivity is mediated through the PLA2 pathway. Moreover, by directly adding secretory PLA2 (sPLA2) in our vessel bath system, we are able to enhance the vasoconstriction induced by ET-1, again mimicking Aβ vasoactivity (data not shown). A statistical interaction was also noted among $A\beta_{1-40}$, PLA2 and ET-1, further substantiating the hypothesis that $A\beta_{1-40}$ vasoactivity is mediated through the PLA2 pathway.

We then investigated the effects of a specific inhibitor of sPLA2 (oleyloxy-ethylphosphocholine) on the vasoactivity mediated by $A\beta_{1-40}$ and $A\beta_{1-42}$. Oleyloxyethylphosphocholine completely blocks the enhancement of vasoactivity induced by either $A\beta_{1-40}$ or $A\beta_{1-42}$, again suggesting that Aβ is able to stimulate secretory PLA2 (Figure 3).

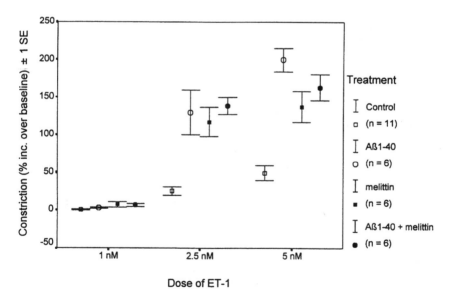

Figure 2. Interaction among melittin, Aβ, and ET-1 on vasoconstriction. Aortic rings were treated with 1 μM freshly solubilized $A\beta_{1-40}$, 1 μM melittin, or melittin + Aβ, or were untreated, 5 min prior to the addition of a dose range of ET-1. Results are expressed as a mean ± 1 S.E. of the percentage vasoconstriction increase over baseline. ANOVA showed significant main effects of ET-1 dose ($p < 0.001$), Aβ ($p < 0.001$) and melittin ($p < 0.001$), as well as significant interactive terms between ET-1 dose and either Aβ ($p < 0.001$) or melittin ($p < 0.05$). Furthermore, there was a significant interactive term among ET-1 dose, Aβ and melittin ($p < 0.01$)

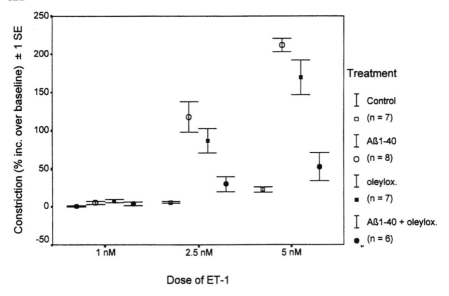

Figure 3. Interaction among oleyloxyethylphosphocholine (oleylox; inhibitor of secretory PLA2), Aβ, and ET-1 on vasoconstriction. Aortic rings were treated with 1 μM freshly solubilized Aβ$_{1-40}$, 1μM oleylox or oleylox + Aβ, or were untreated, 5 min prior to the addition of a dose range of ET-1. There were significant main effects by ANOVA of ET-1 dose ($p < 0.001$) and Aβ ($p < 0.01$) but not of oleylox ($p > 0.05$). There was also a significant interactive term among ET-1 dose, Aβ and oleylox ($p < 0.001$)

We went on to investigate the contribution of arachidonic acid (AA) metabolism in Aβ$_{1-40}$ vasoactivity. Arachidonic acid can be metabolized essentially through two distinct pathways involving the cyclo-oxygenases (COX) and lipoxygenases (LOX). The COX pathway gives rise to prostaglandins and thromboxanes, while the LOX pathway results in the production of leukotrienes and lipoxins. We show that aspirin, an irreversible COX inhibitor (at doses ranging from 1 mM to 40 mM) is not able to reverse the vasoconstrictive properties of Aβ$_{1-40}$, suggesting that COXs do not mediate Aβ$_{1-40}$ vasoactivity (Figure 4). By using a specific and potent inhibitor of 5-lipoxygenase, MK-886, we were able to completely inhibit the vasoactive properties of Aβ$_{1-40}$ (Figure 5) or Aβ$_{1-42}$. Taken together, our data demonstrate that the vasoactive properties of Aβ peptides are mediated through the stimulation of the PLA2-AA-5-LOX pro-inflammatory pathway [4].

Aβ AND THE NO/cGMP PATHWAY

We showed that the relaxation induced by sodium nitroprusside (SNP) is reduced in rat aortae pre-treated with Aβ, suggesting that Aβ is able to

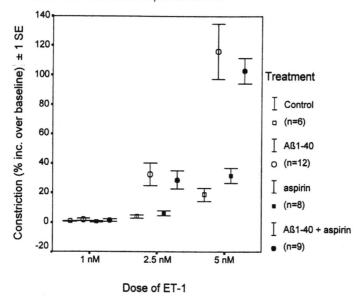

Figure 4. Effect of aspirin on Aβ enhancement of ET-1-induced vasoconstriction. Aortic rings were treated with 1 μM freshly solubilized Aβ$_{1-40}$, 40 mM aspirin or aspirin + Aβ, or were untreated, 5 min prior to the addition of a dose range of ET-1. ANOVA showed significant main effects of ET-1 dose ($p < 0.001$) and Aβ ($p < 0.001$) but not aspirin ($p > 0.05$). There was also a significant interactive term between ET-1 dose and Aβ ($p < 0.001$) but not among ET-1, Aβ and aspirin ($p > 0.05$)

interfere with the nitric oxide/cGMP pathway. These data led us to further investigate the role of soluble guanylyl cyclase in the vasoactivity mediated by Aβ. Most of the previous studies that have examined the role of soluble guanylyl cyclase in vessels have used methylene blue and LY-83583, compounds that generate superoxide anions and are not specific for inhibition of soluble guanylyl cyclase. We used a novel and highly selective inhibitor of soluble guanylyl cyclase, 1H-[1,2,4]oxadiazolo[4,3,-a]quinoxalin-1-one (ODQ). We showed that the vasoconstriction induced by ET-1 is synergistically enhanced after Aβ or ODQ treatment, but is only statistically additive with Aβ and ODQ co-treatment, suggesting that Aβ is not able to modulate the activity of soluble guanylyl cyclase or the production of NO. In order to block the hydrolysis of cGMP, we inhibited cGMP-PDE by using dipyridamole. We observed no significant difference in dipyridamole-induced relaxation between Aβ-treated and control vessels, showing that dipyridamole blocks the opposition to relaxation normally induced by Aβ. We also showed that dipyridamole is able to block Aβ enhancement of ET-1-induced constriction in an interactive manner (data not shown here), and that, in Aβ-treated aortae, cGMP levels are reduced (data not shown here). Taken together, these data show that Aβ is not able to modulate the synthesis of cGMP via the

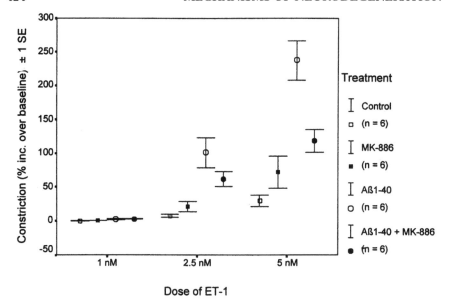

Figure 5. Effect of MK-886 on Aβ enhancement of ET-1-induced vasoconstriction. Aortic rings were treated with 1 μM freshly solubilized Aβ$_{1-40}$, 1 μM MK-886, or MK-886 + Aβ, or were untreated, 5 min prior to the addition of a dose range of ET-1. ANOVA showed significant main effects of ET-1 dose (p < 0.001), Aβ (p < 0.001), and MK-886 (p < 0.05). There was also a significant interaction among ET-1, Aβ and MK-886 (p = 0.001)

NO-activated soluble guanylyl cyclase, but is able to impair the level of cGMP by activating cGMP-PDE, leading to an enhancement of the vasotension in response to ET-1 [5].

IN VIVO EVIDENCE THAT Aβ CAN INDUCE CEREBROVASCULAR CONSTRICTION

Male Sprague–Dawley rats (7–8 months old) were cannulated at the right common carotid artery, positioned at the aortic arch for arterial blood pressure (BP) measurements and (following stabilization of blood pressure), intra-arterial infusions with either 40 nmol/kg human Aβ$_{1-40}$ (AB), rat Aβ$_{1-40}$ (rAB), rat amylin (rAmylin), or vehicle control (0.5 ml 0.9% NaCl). Animals were also cannulated at the left femoral artery for withdrawal of a reference blood sample. Four minutes after infusion, fluorescent microspheres (1 ml of a solution of 1×10^5 15 μm diameter spheres/ml, Molecular Probes) were infused at the carotid cannula at a rate of 1 ml/min, while simultaneously withdrawing reference blood from the femoral artery at the same rate. After 10 min animals were sacrificed by decapitation and the target tissues (kidney, heart and cerebral cortex) were removed. The tissues were separated, weighed, homogenized and then digested along with the reference blood samples to release the fluorescent dye for fluorometric quantification.

Figure 6 shows a specific reduction in cerebrovascular blood flow as calculated by this method. Given that there was no change in blood pressure during these experiments, it is concluded that the reduction in flow is due to increased resistance of the microcerebrovasculature—suggesting vasoconstriction of these vessels after Aβ treatment [6].

This effect was specific for the brain, as neither heart nor kidney showed decreased blood flow by this method (Figure 7).

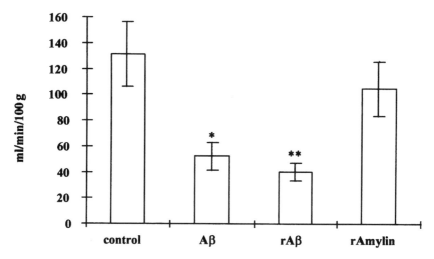

Figure 6. Effects of infusion of human Aβ, rat Aβ and rat amylin on microcerebrovascular flow. Cerebrovascular flow was calculated from fluorescent measurement of microsphere retention in the cortex as described in rats infused with the above treatments. Infusion with either rat or human Aβ produced a significant reduction in cerebral blood flow, as indicated. *p < 0.05; **p = 0.01 compared with control. Reproduced from reference [6], © 1998, Neurosci Lett 257(2): 77–80, with permission from Elsevier Science

CONCLUSIONS

We have previously demonstrated that soluble Aβ peptides display vasoactive properties, and have suggested that this could contribute to the AD process by damaging vascular endothelial cells and reducing cerebral blood flow [1]. The most vasoactive Aβ peptides have mixtures of random coil and β-sheet structure. The finding that peptides containing low or high levels of β-pleated conformation are less vasoactive than those containing intermediate amounts leads us to propose the existence of a transitional form of Aβ between random

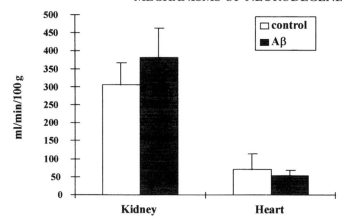

Figure 7. Absence of effects of Aβ on microvascular flow in heart and kidney of animals infused in Figure 6. By contrast with the cerebrovascular effects, infusion with Aβ had no effect on blood flow through peripheral organs, as shown above. Reproduced from reference [6], © 1998, Neurosci Lett 257(2): 77–80, with permission from Elsevier Science

coil and β-pleat structure that is the vasoactive species. This is the first time that Aβ conformational intermediates have been suggested and a biological activity associated with them [3].

Phospholipase A2 (PLA2), a key enzyme involved in inflammatory processes, initiates the arachidonic acid cascade leading to the generation of multiple eicosanoid products. Our data demonstrate that $A\beta_{1-40}$ and $A\beta_{1-42}$ mediate vasoactivity by activating PLA2. The arachidonic acid product of PLA2 is metabolized through two distinct pathways: the cyclo-oxygenase and lipoxygenase pathways. Our findings suggest that Aβ vasoactivity is mediated through the latter pathway but that the prostaglandin synthetic pathway is also likely to be activated and may have important consequences in other cell types [4].

Through examination of the possible clinical relevance of Aβ vasoactivity, we find that *in vivo* infusion of low doses of freshly solubilized $A\beta_{1-40}$ results in a specific reduction of cerebral blood flow in rats [6]. High circulating levels of soluble Aβ thus have a direct and specific constrictive effect on cerebral vessels *in vivo*, which may contribute to the cerebral hypoperfusion observed early in the AD process.

REFERENCES

1. Thomas T, Thomas G, McLendon C, Sutton T, Mullan M. β-amyloid-mediated vasoactivity and vascular endothelial damage. Nature 1996; 380: 168–71.
2. Crawford F, Suo Z, Fang C, Mullan M. Characterization of the *in vitro* vasoactivity of Aβ peptides. Exp Neurol 1998; 150: 159–68.

3. Crawford F, Soto C, Suo Z, Fang C, Parker T, Sawar A, Frangione B, Mullan M. Alzheimer's β-amyloid vasoactivity: identification of a novel β-amyloid conformational intermediate. FEBS Lett 1998; 436: 445–8.
4. Paris D, Town T, Parker T, Tan J, Humphrey J, Mullan M. Alzheimer's disease β-amyloid peptides mediate vasoactivity through a pro-inflammatory pathway: the phospholipase A2/arachidonic acid/5-lipoxygenase cascade (submitted).
5. Paris D, Town T, Parker T, Tan J, Humphrey J, Crawford F, Mullan M. Inhibition of Alzheimer's β-amyloid induced vasoactivity and pro-inflammatory response in microglia by a cGMP-dependent mechanism. Exp Neurol (in press).
6. Suo Z, Humphrey J, Kundtz A, Sethi F, Placzek A, Crawford F, Mullan M. Soluble Alzheimer's β-amyloid constricts the cerebral vasculature *in vivo*. Neurosci Lett 1998; 257(2): 77–80.

Address for correspondence:
Mike Mullan,
Roskamp Institute, University of South Florida,
3515 E. Fletcher Avenue,
Tampa, FL 33613, USA

.

47 Neuro-inflammatory Mechanisms in Alzheimer's Disease

PATRICK L. McGEER, KOJI YASOJIMA AND
EDITH McGEER

INTRODUCTION

In this chapter we will describe briefly the general parameters of neuro-inflammation, the role this phenomenon plays in the pathogenesis of Alzheimer's disease (AD), and the therapeutic possibilities that have been revealed by studying its nature.

Inflammation is commonly considered to be caused by hyperemia induced by blood-borne elements. Inflammation in the brain, it has been argued, cannot exist in the absence of obvious monocytic or other cellular and serum infiltration into brain tissue. But intensive studies of the pathology of AD have taught us that the brain generates its own inflammatory and innate immune response, and that neurons, as well as glia, are active participants [1]. Work on the heart suggests that other tissues of the body also have their own inflammatory and innate immune response systems [2]. While the responses are intended to deal with injury and infection, they can also be autodestructive. It follows that interference with the process should have significant therapeutic benefit.

More than a century ago, Metchnikoff injected starfish larvae, which have no circulatory system, with rose thorns. He found that the thorns became surrounded by local cells, which he named phagocytes. He concluded that such cells, which were indicative of a local response, were fundamental to defense of the organism. His idea of exclusive defense by phagocytes was supplemented by the experiments of his student Jules Bourdet. Bourdet showed that lysis of bacteria could be achieved by sensitized serum in the absence of any cells. Paul Ehrlich supplied the name 'complement'. Killing by the twin methods of phagocytosis and complement are the most potent of the body's defenses. The discovery that phagocytes exist in the brain was made by del Rio Hortega. Hortega developed a silver carbonate modification of the

Alzheimer's Disease and Related Disorders
Edited by K. Iqbal, D.F. Swaab, B. Winblad and H.M. Wisniewski
© 1999 John Wiley & Sons Ltd

Golgi stain and, in 1919, described microglia as part of the 'el terco elemento' that had so confused Ramon y Cajal; oligodendroglia were the other part. Hortega recognized that microglia were of mesodermal origin, entering the brain in late embryonic life. When he irritated the brain with a stab wound, these cells became phagocytic, just as did Metchnikoff's cells when starfish were wounded with rose thorns.

A concept linking the ideas of Metchnikoff, Hortega and others was put forward by van Furth in 1963. He proposed the monocyte phagocytic system, which is comprised of cells of the monocyte line, which enter tissues to become the resident phagocytes. Microglia were the representatives in the brain. Long after the time of Hortega and van Furth, and even into the present decade, the idea that microglia belonged to the monocytic line and were resident brain phagocytes was denied (see [1] for references). Data confirming the concepts of Hortega and van Furth have now come from a number of laboratories, especially those studying AD. These data establish that reactive microglia migrate to the consolidated plaques and extracellular tangles of AD, that they are indeed phagocytic, and that they are of monocytic origin. They further establish that the lesions of AD are decorated with active components of the classical complement pathway, including the autodestructive membrane attack complex. Interaction between the two main systems of defense, phagocytosis and complement activation, is provided by immunohistochemical data showing that reactive microglia express prodigious levels of complement receptors. What is new, and formerly not suspected, is that the complement system is produced and activated within the brain, and that the activation is independent of antibodies. The complement system of the brain is independent of the liver or serum.

IMMUNOHISTOCHEMICAL EVIDENCE FOR NEUROINFLAMMATION IN AD

Many studies in our laboratory and others indicate that a chronic inflammation appears to exist in the AD brain, as evidenced by the appearance of activated microglia and at least 40 proteins associated with immune reactions (reviewed in [1]). These include proteins of the classical complement cascade, complement inhibitors, acute phase reactants, inflammatory cytokines, proteases and protease inhibitors. Such activated microglia and immune system proteins either do not appear or appear at very low levels in normal adult brain.

The microglia are clearly members of the monocyte phagocytic system and express many surface receptors characteristic of leukocytes generally, and monocytes specifically. They include complement receptors, immunoglobulin receptors, major histocompatibility class I and class II glycoproteins, leucocyte common antigens, plasmin activator inhibitor, and receptors for vitronectin, intracellular adhesion molecules and colony stimulating factor, all of which are upregulated in the reactive microglia of AD tissue (reviewed in [1]). Microglia, like all professional phagocytes, possess a system which can generate prodigious quantities of superoxide anions from oxygen molecules. Hydroxyl radicals, singlet oxygen species and hydrogen peroxide are downstream products. The system is one of the main methods by which phagocytes kill invading organisms and tumor cells. The purpose, of course, is phagocytosis, and some might argue that the activated microglia in AD are there only to clean up the debris. But the oxidative stress may not distinguish friend from foe, so the possibility must be kept in mind that microglia, acting through this mechanism alone, may contribute substantially to autotoxic tissue damage. That this may well be true is supported by evidence from studies on mixed neuronal/microglial cultures, indicating that activated microglia secrete products toxic to neurons [3, 4, 5].

Proteins of the classical complement cascade (Table 1) are of particular importance. This cascade produces not only proteins which mark structures for opsonization but also anaphylotoxins, which spur on the immune system and, if the pathway is fully activated, the membrane attack complex (the MAC, C5b-9). Opsonizing components of the complement cascade may mistakenly mark host tissue for opsonization, thus leading to damage, but it is the MAC which is designed for killing cells. The most compelling immunohistochemical evidence for autodestruction of neurons and their processes is the presence of the MAC on dystrophic neurites in senile plaques. Such dystrophic neurites appear in classical senile plaques but not diffuse amyloid deposits. The MAC inserts into the membranes of intact cells, causing lysis and death of the cell. The MAC is intended to destroy foreign cells and viruses, but host cells are at significant risk of bystander lysis.

Table 1. Components of the classical complement pathway

Native protein		Active fragments	Function
C1	$\rightarrow$	C1q	Activation
C2			
C4	$\rightarrow$	C2a4b3b	Opsonization
C3		C3a, C4a, C5a	Anaphylotoxic stimulants
C5			
C6			
C7	$\rightarrow$	C5b-(C9)n	Membrane attack complex
C8			
C9			

SOURCE OF COMPLEMENT PROTEINS

Complement has traditionally been thought of as a blood-borne system activated by antigen–antibody complexes. However, *in situ* hybridization studies and immunohistochemical studies have shown that both the mRNAs for all the complement proteins and the proteins themselves are located prominently in neurons, especially in the cortical pyramidal neurons, which are severely affected in AD [6, 7]. Whether complement-producing neurons are particularly vulnerable to immune system attack remains to be explored.

Recent work in our laboratory quantifying the mRNAs for all the complement proteins in a number of regions of AD and normal brains has revealed a dramatic upregulation in those regions of the AD brain which are particularly affected by the pathology. This is illustrated in Figure 1, which shows data obtained on the mRNAs for C1q and C9. These examples are selected because C1q is required for the initiation of the cascade and C9 is necessary for formation of an active membrane attack complex. What these data show, and others like them for the complement components in between, is that there is a spectacular increase in complement message, consistent with its involvement in driving the pathology.

ACTIVATORS OF THE COMPLEMENT SYSTEM

The presence of activated complement in AD tissue inspired a search for immunoglobulin antibodies that might be responsible for activating the complement. But these could not be found. Moreover, in experimental models of brain injury, activation of the complement pathway and appearance of reactive microglia occur much too rapidly to allow for the production of autoantibodies [8, 9]. It is now clear that the complement cascade can be activated in the absence of antibodies. Several of the proteins occurring in association with the lesions in AD have been found to activate the complement cascade *in vitro*. These include β-amyloid protein, amyloid P, Hageman factor and C-reactive protein [1].

AUTOTOXIC HYPOTHESIS

It is well known from seminal studies by the Braaks [10, 11] that neurofibrillary tangles, diffuse amyloid deposits, and even some consolidated deposits occur in people at an age well below that of typical onset of clinical AD. These lesions are not the result of normal aging because they do not universally occur. A better interpretation is that they represent a benign, preclinical phase of AD that can go on for years. However, if one examines objective measures, such as serial PET scans of glucose metabolism [12] or serial CT scans of the width of the medial temporal lobe [13], AD cases show precipitous declines. Similar sharp declines have been noted in cognitive tests [13, 14]. Indeed, all of these parameters show a similar percentage loss (Figure 2). What all of this says is that AD goes through a benign phase which may last several years, but this is converted into a malignant phase. In the malignant phase, brain

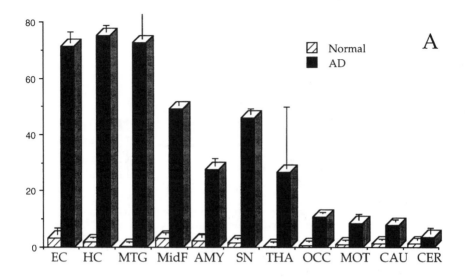

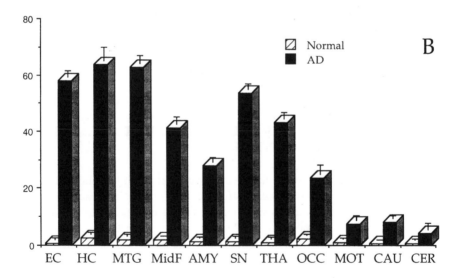

Figure 1. Levels of the mRNA for C1q (A) and C9 (B) in various brain regions of AD and neurologically normal controls. EC, entorhinal cortex; HC, hippocampus; MTG, midtemporal gyrus; MidF, mid-frontal gyrus; AMY, amygdala; SN, substantia nigra; THA, thalamus; OCC, occipital cortex; MOT, motor cortex; CAU, caudate; CER, cerebellum (unpublished data)

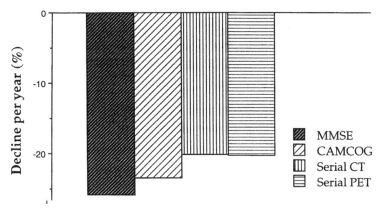

Figure 2. Percentage change per year in various indexes reported in AD. MMSE studies from reference [14], CAMCOG measurements and serial CT scans on the thickness of the medial temporal lobe from reference [13], and serial PET studies measuring glucose metabolism in the medial temporal lobe from reference [12]

substance is lost in vulnerable regions, brain metabolism drops in those same brain regions, and mental decline occurs, all in parallel time fashion. We suggest that the conversion from a benign to a malignant phase in AD disease is caused by the inflammatory burden exceeding the defensive threshold of neurons and their processes. In other words, the inflammation takes over the pathology, just as it does in other human diseases such as arthritis. If this hypothesis is true, then much can be achieved in a therapeutic way by the use of anti-inflammatory agents.

EVIDENCE FOR A THERAPEUTIC EFFECT OF ANTI-INFLAMMATORY AGENTS IN AD

There are now some 20 studies showing that people who take anti-inflammatory drugs, or who suffer from conditions where such drugs are routinely administered, have a significantly reduced prevalence of AD compared with the general population. These studies come from nine different countries. They involve many thousands of patients. They represent a variety of epidemiological approaches. Figure 3 shows a meta-analysis of 17 of these studies in which they have been grouped according to methodology [15]. The reduction in risk was highly significant in groups on anti-inflammatory medication, and it suggests that the use of such agents might reduce the prevalence by at least half. In one of these epidemiological studies [16], carried out by Stewart and colleagues as part of the Baltimore longitudinal study on aging, it was possible to group the patients according to how long they had been taking non-steroidal anti-inflammatory drugs (NSAIDs). For those who had been on

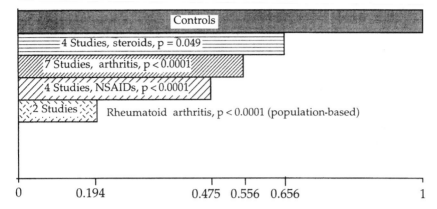

Figure 3. Results of a meta-analysis of homogeneous studies on arthritis or use of anti-inflammatory drugs as a risk factor for Alzheimer's disease. The calculated odds ratio and p value are shown for each group. All groups involved case-controlled studies except where population based is specified. This graph includes data from reference [16], as well as the 17 studies reported in our published meta-analysis [15]

NSAIDs for less than 2 years, the odds ratio was 0.65, but for those who had been on NSAIDs for more than 2 years, the odds ratio was reduced to 0.40, again indicating that 60% of the people expected to come down with AD were spared.

The epidemiological studies test prevention but not necessarily treatment. There has been one small, double-blind, placebo-controlled clinical trial led by Joe Rogers [17]. In this 6 month trial, indomethacin patients held their own, while placebo patients deteriorated at the expected rate.

CONCLUSIONS

AD lesions have high concentrations of inflammatory proteins associated with them. These proteins are produced in the brain, many of them by neurons. Conversion of AD from a benign to a malignant state correlates with the activation of inflammatory processes. Epidemiological studies indicate that populations using anti-inflammatory drugs have a reduced prevalence of AD. The NSAID indomethacin seems to be capable of holding AD in check. Hence, effective anti-inflammatory therapy may both prevent and significantly retard progression of AD. The best data we have to date are for NSAIDs, but these agents strike at the outer edges and not the central core of inflammatory processes. More effective anti-inflammatory agents may be able to hold incipient AD indefinitely in the benign phase. That would be a worthy goal. The complement system appears to be a most important target for studies aimed at developing more effective anti-inflammatory agents.

ACKNOWLEDGEMENTS

Supported by grants from the Alzheimer Society of British Columbia and the Jack Brown and Family AD Research Fund, as well as donations from individual British Columbians.

REFERENCES

1. McGeer PL, McGeer EG. The inflammatory response system of brain: implications for therapy of Alzheimer and other neurodegenerative diseases. Brain Res Rev 1995; 21: 195–218.
2. Yasojima K, Kilgore KS, Washington RA, Lucchesi BR, McGeer PL. Complement gene expression by rabbit heart: upregulation by ischemia and reperfusion. Circ Res 1998; 82: 1224–30.
3. McMillian MK, Vainio PJ, Tuominen RK. Role of protein kinase C in microglia-induced neurotoxicity in mesencephalic cultures. J Neuropath Exp Neurol 1997; 56: 301–7.
4. Giulian D, Haverkamp LJ, Yu JH, Karshin W, Tom D, Li J, Kirkpatrick J, Kuo LM, Roher AE. Specific domains of beta-amyloid from Alzheimer plaque elicit neuron killing in human microglia. J Neurosci 1996; 16: 6021–37.
5. Roher AE, Chaney M, Kuo YM, Webster SD, Stine WB, Haverkamp LJ, Woods AS, Cotter RJ, Tuohy JM, Krafft GA, Bonnell BS, Emmerling MR. Morphology and toxicity of Aβ-(1–42) dimer derived from neuritic and vascular amyloid deposits of Alzheimer's disease. J Biol Chem 1996; 271: 20631–5.
6. Shen Y, Li R, McGeer EG, McGeer PL. Neuronal expression of mRNAs for complement proteins of the classical pathway in Alzheimer brain. Brain Res 1997; 769: 391–5.
7. Terai K, Walker DG, McGeer EG, McGeer PL. Neurons express proteins of the classical complement pathway in Alzheimer disease. Brain Res 1997; 769: 385–90.
8. Akiyama H, Tooyama I, Kondo H, Ikeda K, Kimura H, McGeer EG, McGeer PL. Early response of brain resident microglia to kainic acid-induced hippocampal lesions. Brain Res 1994; 635: 257–68.
9. Pasinetti GM, Johnson SA, Rozovsky I, Lampert-Etchells M, Morgan DG, Gordon MN, Morgan TE, Willoughby D, Finch CE. Complement C1qB and C4 mRNAs responses to lesioning in rat brain. Exp Neurol 1992; 118: 117–25.
10. Braak H, Braak E, Bohl J, Reintjes R. Age, neurofibrillary changes, Aβ-amyloid and the onset of Alzheimer's disease. Neurosci Lett 1996; 210: 87–90.
11. Braak H, Braak E. Frequency of stages of Alzheimer-related lesions in different age categories. Neurobiol Aging 1997; 18: 351–7.
12. McGeer EG, Peppard RP, McGeer PL, Tuokko H, Crockett D, Parks R, Akiyama H, Calne DB, Beattie BL, Harrop R. [18]Fluorodeoxyglucose positron emission tomography studies in presumed Alzheimer cases, including 13 serial scans. Can J Neurol Sci 1990; 17: 1–11.
13. Jobst KA, Smith AD, Szatmari M, Esiri MM, Jaskowski A, Hindley N, McDonald B, Molyneux AJ. Rapidly progressing atrophy of medial temporal lobe in Alzheimer's disease. Lancet 1994; 343: 829–30.
14. Mortimer JA, Ebbutt B, Jun SP, Finch MD. Predictors of cognitive and functional progression in patients with probable Alzheimer's disease. Neurology 1992; 42: 1689–96.

15. McGeer PL, Schulzer M, McGeer EG. Arthritis and antiinflammatory agents as possible protective factors for Alzheimer's disease: a review of 17 epidemiological studies. Neurology 1996; 47: 425–32.
16. Stewart WF, Kawas C, Corrada M, Metter EJ. Risk of Alzheimer's disease and duration of NSAID use. Neurology 1997; 48: 626–32.
17. Rogers J, Kirby LC, Hempelman SR, Berry DL, McGeer PL, Kaszniak AW, Zalinski J, Cofield M, Mansukhani L, Willson P, Kogan F. Clinical trial of indomethacin in Alzheimer's disease. Neurology 1993; 43: 1609–11.

Address for correspondence:
    Dr Patrick L. McGeer,
    Kinsmen Laboratory of Neurological Research,
    University of British Columbia, 2255 Wesbrook Mall,
    Vancouver, BC V6T 1Z3, Canada
    Tel: 604 822 7377; fax: 604 822 7086;
    e-mail: mcgeerpl@interchange.ubc.ca

48 β-Amyloid-induced Inflammatory Molecular Cascades in Vascular Cells

ZHIMING SUO, JUN TAN, FIONA CRAWFORD, ANDON PLACZEK, CHUNHONG FANG, AMY KUNDTZ, GEORGE SU, PATRICK POMPL AND MIKE MULLAN

INTRODUCTION

A large body of evidence suggests that inflammation is involved in the Alzheimer's disease (AD) process. Increased β-amyloid (Aβ) production, one of the pathological features of AD, is believed to play a central role in the pathogenesis of this disorder. Studies attempting to understand the mechanisms by which Aβ may drive AD pathogenesis have revealed multiple aspects of the properties of Aβ, one of which is its ability to stimulate inflammation [1]. The upregulated expression of cell adhesion molecules, increased cytokine production and activation of the complement system and microglial cells in the brain parenchyma of AD patients are closely associated with Aβ deposits [1–4]. *In vitro* experiments have demonstrated the capacity of Aβ to activate these inflammatory processes in glial cells [3, 5, 6]. These data suggest that the increase in Aβ may be partially responsible for the initiation of the inflammatory processes in the brain parenchyma of AD.

More than 83% of AD patients display cerebral amyloid angiopathy (CAA) [7]. In these cases, extensive cerebral vascular degeneration is closely associated with Aβ deposition [8]. A recent immunopathological observation revealed that infiltration of macrophages, and both CD4+ and CD8+ T-cells occur with Aβ deposits in cerebral vessels in CAA [9]. This leads us to propose that increased Aβ production in AD may not only initiate inflammatory processes in the brain parenchyma but may also trigger an inflammatory response in cerebral vessels.

We have recently found that Aβ induces expression of cell adhesion molecules (CAMs) in cultured human vascular endothelial (EC) and smooth muscle (SM) cells. Cytokines, such as interleukin-1β (IL-1β) and interferon-γ

Alzheimer's Disease and Related Disorders
Edited by K. Iqbal, D.F. Swaab, B. Winblad and H.M. Wisniewski
© 1999 John Wiley & Sons Ltd

(IFN-γ), and interaction of CD40 and CD40 ligand (CD40L), further increase the Aβ-induced expression of adhesion molecules in these same cells. Since upregulation of CAMs in EC is responsible for activation and extravasation of circulating leukocytes and monocytes in typical inflammatory processes, these findings implicate the capacity of Aβ to initiate an inflammatory process in vascular walls. Because aggregated Aβ is not easily degraded [1], once these inflammatory processes in vascular walls are initiated, they may be prolonged by the continuous presence of the antigen and result in inflammatory damage to the surrounding vascular or brain parenchymal cells.

CD40–CD40L interactions and cytokine secretion are important regulatory events in inflammatory processes which determine the efficiency and consequences of the inflammatory reaction. To further characterize the Aβ-induced inflammatory responses in vascular cells, we evaluated the capacity of Aβ to stimulate cytokine secretion (IL-1β and IFN-γ) and upregulate expression of CD40 and IFN-γ receptor (IFN-γR), in addition to investigating the interactions between the Aβ-induced inflammatory molecules.

RESULTS

CELL TOXICITY AND PROLIFERATION INDUCED BY Aβ

For all ELISAs and CELISAs, no significant proliferation was observed in either EC or SM cells resulting from Aβ treatment. Also, Aβ did not induce significant cell death in SM cells. However, a significant amount of cell death was observed in EC treated with either 10 or 20 μM of Aβ_{1-42} or Aβ_{25-35}, measured by MTS assay (data not shown). Corrections to the assays were not employed since this effect would only serve to increase the significance of the results reported.

Aβ PEPTIDES INDUCE SECRETION OF IL-1β AND IFN-γ FROM EC

EC were treated with increasing concentrations of either Aβ_{1-40} or Aβ_{1-42} for 24 h. The resulting cell culture media were assayed for IL-1β or IFN-γ using ELISA (see Figure 1). Aβ_{1-42} increased the secretion of IL-1β and IFN-γ in a dose-dependent manner ($p < 0.001$ by ANOVA). The lowest effective concentration was determined to be 100 nM for IFN-γ ($p < 0.01$) and 1 μM for IL-1β ($p < 0.01$). In contrast, Aβ_{1-40} does not show a dose-dependent effect on the induction of secretion of either cytokine in the tested concentrations. However, the largest dose of Aβ_{1-40} (20 μM) does induce a significant production of IFN-γ vs. control ($p < 0.05$) and has no effect on IL-1β secretion. These data suggest that Aβ_{1-42} is capable of activating EC and increasing the secretion of cytokines. Furthermore, the activation of EC is more sensitive to Aβ_{1-42} than Aβ_{1-40}.

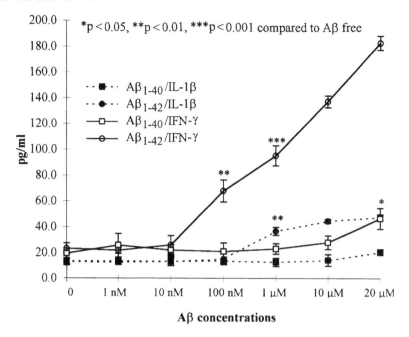

Figure 1. Aβ peptides dose-dependently induce cytokine release from EC. One-way ANOVA and *post hoc* comparison of means revealed the significant differences at the levels indicated above. Reproduced from reference [11], © 1998, Brain Res 807: 110–17, with permission from Elsevier Science

Aβ PEPTIDES UPREGULATE THE EXPRESSION OF IFN-γR

As shown in Figure 2A, there is no expression of IFN-γR in normal EC, and neither $Aβ_{1-40}$ nor $Aβ_{25-35}$ is able to induce such expression. However, 10 μM of $Aβ_{1-42}$ dramatically increases IFN-γR expression ($p < 0.001$) in EC. By contrast, untreated SM cells express IFN-γR, and neither $Aβ_{1-42}$ nor $Aβ_{25-35}$ modulate the IFN-γR expression. Only $Aβ_{1-40}$ induces a significant effect on IFN-γR ($p < 0.05$) in SM cells. These results suggest that Aβ not only increases the cytokine secretion but also upregulates receptor expression, and that $Aβ_{1-42}$ preferentially activates endothelial cells rather than smooth muscle cells, while $Aβ_{1-40}$ has the opposite effect. Further confirmation of this effect was provided with Western blotting (Figure 2B).

Aβ PEPTIDES INDUCE THE EXPRESSION OF CD40 IN A DOSE-DEPENDENT MANNER

To characterize the inducibility of CD40 by Aβ, we examined the dose effect of both $Aβ_{1-40}$ and $Aβ_{1-42}$ on CD40 expression in EC (Figure 3). The results show that $Aβ_{1-42}$ and $Aβ_{1-40}$ dose-dependently increase CD40 expression in

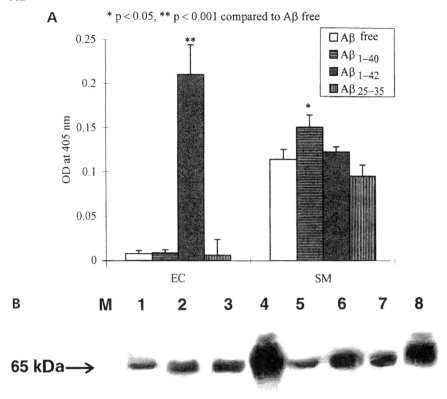

Figure 2. (A) Aβ peptides upregulate the expression of IFN-γR in EC and SM cells. One-way ANOVA and *post hoc* comparison of means revealed the differences indicated above. (B) Western blot of IFN-γ expression in EC. M = protein ladder; lane 1, vehicle; lane 2, IFN-γ; lane 3, $Aβ_{1-40}$; lane 4, $Aβ_{1-42}$; lane 5, mAb (3/23); lane 6, IFN-γ + mAb (3/23); lane 7, $Aβ_{1-40}$ + mAb (3/23); lane 8, $Aβ_{1-42}$ + mAb (3/23). Reproduced from reference [11], © 1998, Brain Res 807: 110–17, with permission from Elsevier Science

EC. The lowest effective concentrations were 100 nM of $Aβ_{1-42}$ ($p < 0.01$) and 10 μM of $Aβ_{1-40}$ ($p < 0.01$), respectively. These data show that concentrations of $Aβ_{1-42}$ in the nanomolar range can still induce a significant increase in CD40 expression in EC; and that the differential effects of Aβ types are consistent with those of the previous observations. The Aβ-induced CD40 expression has also been confirmed by Western blotting (Figure 3B) and RT–PCR (Figure 3C).

Figure 3. (opposite) (A) Aβ peptides dose-dependently induce CD40 expression in EC. Two-way ANOVA showed that both factors and the interactive term (dose, Aβ type, and dose *Aβ type) were all significant ($p < 0.001$). The significance of post hoc comparison of mean treatment response vs. Aβ-free is shown above. (B) Western blotting for expression of CD40 induced by Aβ peptides in EC and SM. M = protein

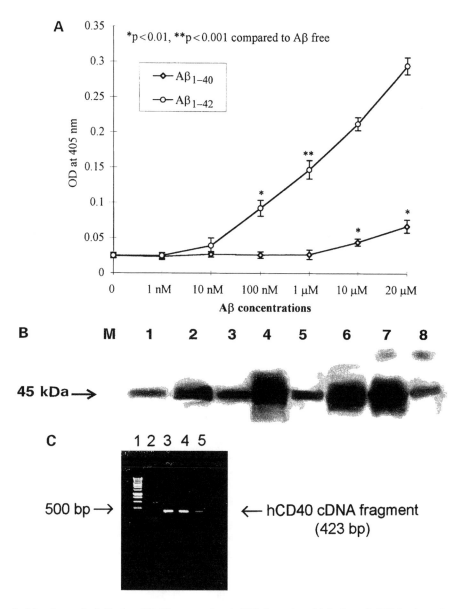

ladder; lanes 1–4 display CD40 expression in EC (lane 1, vehicle; lane 2, IFN-γ; lane 3, Aβ$_{1-40}$; lane 4, Aβ$_{1-42}$); lanes 5–8 show CD40 expression in SM cells (lane 5, vehicle; lane 6, IFN-γ; lane 7, Aβ$_{1-40}$; lane 8, Aβ$_{1-42}$). (C) RT–PCR for CD40 mRNA level changes induced by Aβ peptides in EC. Lane 1, 1 kb DNA ladder; lane 2, cDNA prepared from control peptide-treated EC; lane 3, cDNA prepared from EC treated with Aβ$_{1-40}$; lane 4, cDNA prepared from EC treated with Aβ$_{1-42}$; lane 5, cDNA prepared from IFN-γ-treated EC. Reproduced from reference [11], © 1998, Brain Res 807: 110–17 with permission from Elsevier Science

IL-1β AND IFN-γ INCREASE THE EXPRESSION OF CD40 AND IFN-γR

The results in Figure 4 show the effects of cytokines on the expression of CD40 and IFN-γR. Both IL-1β and IFN-γ significantly (p < 0.001) upregulate the expression of CD40 and IFN-γR in both EC and SM cells. This suggests that the Aβ-induced increase of cytokines in the culture media may further increase Aβ upregulation of expression of CD40 and IFN-γR. This conclusion is confirmed by the data shown in Figure 5; the mAbs against either IL-1β or IFN-γ significantly reduce the $Aβ_{1-42}$ upregulated expression of CD40 (p < 0.001) and IFN-γR (p < 0.01) in EC.

ACTIVATION OF CD40 SIGNALING FURTHER INCREASES THE Aβ-INDUCED EFFECTS

As shown in Figures 6–8, the ligation of CD40 further increases the Aβ-induced IFN-γ secretion and IFN-γR expression. For Aβ-induced IFN-γR expression in EC, only $Aβ_{1-42}$ displays a significant effect (p < 0.001) and a significant interaction with the mAb (p < 0.001). Western blotting for Aβ-induced IFN-γR expression after treatment with mAb (3/23) confirms the enhancement of this effect by ligation of CD40 (Figure 2B). These results

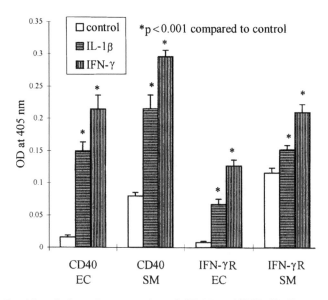

Figure 4. Cytokines induce the expression of CD40 and IFN-γR. One-way ANOVA and *post hoc* comparison of means revealed the differences indicated above. Reproduced from reference [11], © 1998, Brain Res 807: 110–17, with permission from Elsevier Science

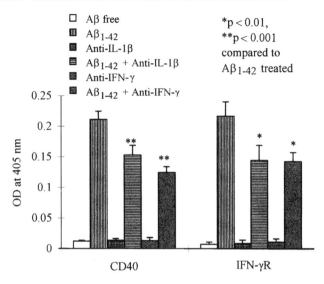

Figure 5. The effects of mAbs against IL-1β or IFN-γ on the expression of CD40 and IFN-γR induced by $A\beta_{1-42}$ in EC. Two-way ANOVA and *post hoc* comparison of means showed the significant effects of the mAb treatments at the indicated levels. In addition, a significant interaction between both mAb types and $A\beta_{1-42}$ (interactive term, $p < 0.001$ for CD40 expression, $p < 0.01$ for IFN-γR expression) was observed. Reproduced from reference [11], © 1998, Brain Res 807: 110–17, with permission from Elsevier Science

suggest that the activation of CD40 signaling amplifies the Aβ-induced effects via a common signal transduction pathway. Figure 8 shows that ligation of CD40 by mAb (3/23) further increases IFN-γR expression in SM cells in an additive way for $A\beta_{1-42}$ and $A\beta_{25-35}$, and in a synergistic way for $A\beta_{1-40}$ (interactive term, $p < 0.001$ by ANOVA).

DISCUSSION

In the current study, we report that Aβ directly induces both CD40 expression and the secretion of IL-1β and IFN-γ from EC in a dose-dependent manner. An increased expression of IFN-γR in either endothelial or smooth muscle cells can also be directly induced by specific types of Aβ. These data suggest that, although cytokines such as IL-1β and IFN-γ may be mainly produced by recruited circulating T-cells and macrophages, Aβ can activate vascular cells and stimulate the production of functional cytokines. Moreover, using either recombinant human cytokines or mAbs against the cytokines, we show that both IL-1β and IFN-γ can upregulate the expression of both CD40 and IFN-γR. These data are consistent with previous reports that different

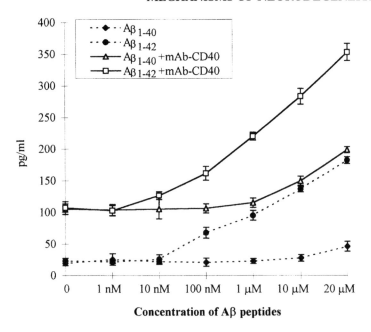

Figure 6. The effect of interaction of CD40–CD40L on Aβ-induced IFN-γ secretion from EC. Separate two-way ANOVAs revealed significant main effects of Aβ dose (p < 0.001), Aβ type (p < 0.001) and mAb (3/23) treatment (p < 0.001). Additionally, a significant effect (p < 0.01) was evident for the Aβ dose and type interaction. Reproduced from reference [11], © 1998, Brain Res 807: 110–17, with permission from Elsevier Science

cytokines can synergistically modulate the expression of multiple genes, including their own and those of their receptors [10]. These results imply that Aβ-induced cytokine production can amplify the Aβ effects by auto-regulation or a further increase in CD40 expression. This study shows that the activation of CD40 signaling further increases production of all the tested molecules. Also, infiltration of T-cells/macrophages into the vasculature, which may be mediated by the increased expression of adhesion molecules observed in our previous studies (unpublished data), would result in a further increase in cytokine production.

We have shown that Aβ dose-dependently increases expression of CD40 and cytokine secretion in EC. The effective concentration of Aβ which induces both cytokine secretion and CD40 expression starts in the nanomolar range, a much lower concentration than that required to induce direct cytotoxicity (10–100 μM). It is also evident that for a given cell type, the induction of an inflammatory cascade is dependent upon the type of Aβ peptide. Both physiologically produced Aβ peptides (Aβ$_{1-40}$ and Aβ$_{1-42}$) are able to induce inflammatory responses, with Aβ$_{1-42}$ inducing much stronger effects in endothelial cells than in smooth muscle cells. By contrast, Aβ$_{1-40}$ is a

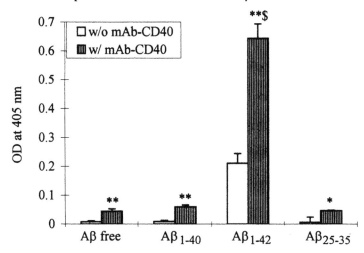

*p < 0.01, **p < 0.001 compared to w/o mAb-CD40

$p < 0.001 interaction between Aβ and mAb-CD40

Figure 7. The effect of interaction of CD40–CD40L on Aβ-induced IFN-γR expression in EC. Significant differences between means were identified by one-way ANOVA and *post hoc* comparisons, while the interactive term showed here is significant by two-way ANOVA (p < 0.001). Reproduced from reference [11], © 1998, Brain Res 807: 110–17, with permission from Elsevier Science

more potent stimulator of smooth muscle cells than endothelial cells. These results imply that *in vivo*, $Aβ_{1-42}$ may mainly activate the vascular endothelial cells, which may contribute to disruption of the blood–brain barrier in CAA and AD. Furthermore, the presence of $Aβ_{1-40}$, which is the predominant vascular isoform of Aβ in CAA and AD, may contribute to the development of inflammatory processes in the smooth muscle layer and result in smooth muscle degeneration in these diseases.

Collectively, these results imply that Aβ can function as an immunogen to activate vascular cells and is responsible for an auto-amplified inflammatory molecular cascade, specifically mediated by interactions among adhesion molecules, CD40–CD40L and cytokines. If the Aβ-induced inflammatory cascade can be validated in cerebral vascular tissues *in vivo*, it may demonstrate its role in cerebral vascular degeneration in CAA and AD. Moreover, blockage of the CD40–CD40L interaction, or neutralization of the effects of IL-1β and IFN-γ, are then implicated as therapeutic targets for CAA and AD.

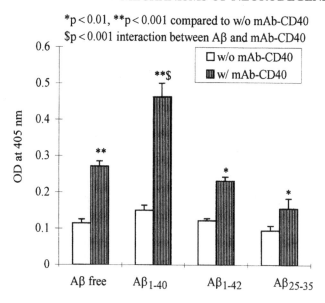

Figure 8. The effect of interaction of CD40–CD40L on Aβ-induced IFN-γR expression in SM. One-way ANOVA and *post hoc* comparison of means identified the significant differences noted above. The interactive term was significant by two-way ANOVA ($p. < 0.001$). Reproduced from reference [11], © 1998, Brain Res 807: 110–17, with permission from Elsevier Science

ACKNOWLEDGEMENTS

We would like to thank Mr and Mrs Robert Roskamp for their generous support.

REFERENCES

1. McGeer PL, McGeer EG. The inflammatory response system of brain: implications for therapy of Alzheimer and other neurodegenerative diseases. Brain Res Rev 1995; 21: 195–218.
2. Altstiel LD, Sperber K. Cytokines in Alzheimer's disease. Prog Neuropsychopharmacol Biol Psychiat 1991; 15: 481–95.
3. Eikelenbloom P, Veerhuis R. The role of complement and activated microglia in the pathogenesis of Alzheimer's disease. Neurobiol Aging 1996; 17: 673–80.
4. Singh VK. Studies of neuroimmune markers in Alzheimer's disease. Mol Neurobiol 1994; 9: 73–81.
5. Aisen PS. Inflammation and Alzheimer disease. Mol Chem Neuropathol 1996; 28: 83–8.
6. Kalaria RN et al. Molecular aspects of inflammatory and immune responses in Alzheimer's disease. Neurobiol Aging 1996; 17: 687–93.

7. Snowdon DA, Greiner LH, Mortimer JA, Riley KP, Greiner PA, Markesbery WR. Brain infarction and the clinical expression of Alzheimer disease. The Nun Study. JAMA 1997; 277: 813–17.
8. Cohen DL, Hedera P, Premkumar DR, Friedland RP, Kalaria RN. Amyloid-β protein angiopathies masquerading as Alzheimer's disease? Ann NY Acad Sci 1997; 826: 390–95.
9. Yamada M et al. Immune reactions associated with cerebral amyloid angiopathy. Stroke 1996; 27: 1155–62.
10. Raitano AB, Korc M. Tumor necrosis factor upregulates γ-IFN binding in a human carcinoma cell line. J Biol Chem 1990; 265: 10466–72.
11. Suo Z, Tan J, Placzek A, Crawford F, Fang C, Mullan M. Alzheimer's β-amyloid peptides induce inflammatory cascade in human vascular cells: the roles of eytokines and CD40. Brain Res 1998; 807: 110–17.

Address for correspondence:
   Zhiming Suo,
   Roskamp Institute,
   University of South Florida,
   3515 E. Fletcher Ave.,
   Tampa, FL 33613, USA

49 Enhanced Expression of Microglial NADPH-oxidase (p22-phox) in Alzheimer's Disease

FREEK L. VAN MUISWINKEL,
CORLINE J.A. DE GROOT,
J.M. ROZEMULLER-KWAKKEL AND
PIET EIKELENBOOM

From neuropathological, biochemical and clinical studies, the picture emerges that the progression of Alzheimer's disease (AD) is closely associated with both inflammation and oxidative stress in the diseased brain [1]. Although numerous factors might be implicated, such as inherited- and/or age-dependent deficits in cellular energy metabolism, iron homeostasis and/or a general decrease in the activity of anti-oxidant defense systems, it is tempting to speculate that activated microglial cells contribute to the oxidative challenge observed in the AD brain. Recently, this concept has gained strong impetus from the results of *in vitro* studies which showed that amyloid-β (Aβ), i.e. the major constituent of the senile plaques that are found in the AD brain, is capable of priming and/or triggering the respiratory burst of cultured rat microglia and human phagocytes [2]. Thus, in mononuclear phagocytes the NADPH-oxidase-catalyzed reduction of molecular oxygen and consequent release of the superoxide free radical is enhanced upon exposure to Aβ. In respect to pathological mechanisms, the pivotal role of microglia-derived reactive oxygen species (ROS) is illustrated by the fact that ROS not only exert direct neurotoxic effects but may also influence neuronal integrity indirectly, e.g. via the redox-sensitive (NF-κB-mediated) transcription of pro-inflammatory and/or anti-apoptotic genes in surrounding astrocytes and neurons. Reportedly, the superoxide generating NADPH-oxidase is a multicomponent complex consisting of a membrane-associated flavocytochrome b558, which by itself comprises a low molecular weight α- (p22-phox) and a high molecular weight β-subunit (gp91phox), and at least four cytosolic proteins termed p40-phox, p47-phox, P67-phox and Rac. In resting phagocytes, the

Alzheimer's Disease and Related Disorders
Edited by K. Iqbal, D.F. Swaab, B. Winblad and H.M. Wisniewski
© 1999 John Wiley & Sons Ltd

cytochrome b558 is thought to be located in the membranes of intracellular organelles which, upon activation of the cells, will fuse with the plasma membrane, resulting in the expression of gp-91phox and p22-phox in the cell membrane. At the same time, upon phosphorylation by tyrosine kinases, the cytosolic subunits will translocate to the membrane to assemble with the cytochrome b558, hence forming an active superoxide generating NADPH-oxidase complex. Interestingly, in cultured human phagocytes the Aβ-induced respiratory burst has been linked to changes in tyrosine kinase-dependent intracellular signal transduction and/or alterations in the expression of distinct NADPH-oxidase subunits [3, 4]. To investigate whether (Aβ-induced) activation of microglial respiratory burst might also occur in the AD brain, we studied the cellular expression of NADPH-oxidase in post-mortem AD brain tissue, using antibodies raised against the NADPH-oxidase subunits of human neutrophils, including p22-phox. Therefore, brain tissue obtained at autopsy from patients suffering from AD (Braak VI), Down's syndrome (Braak VI) and non-demented control subjects were studied. In brief, cryostat sections of snap-frozen cortical brain tissue were mounted onto poly-L-lysine-coated glass slides, air-dried and fixed in acetone prior to overnight incubation with MoAb 449; 1:200 diluted in phosphate-buffered saline (pH 7.4) containing 1% bovine serum albumin. Thereafter, sections were washed, incubated with bio-tinylated rabbit anti-mouse secondary antibodies (Dako, Denmark), followed by incubation with avidin–biotin–peroxidase complexes (ABC, Vector Laboratories). Subsequently, peroxidase activity was visualized using 3,3-diaminobenzidine tetrahydrochloride dihydrate and H_2O_2 as chromogen substrate. Finally, sections were counterstained with hematoxylin and Congo red, dehydrated and cover-slipped. The results obtained with the MoAb 449, a mouse monoclonal directed against p22-phox ([5]; courtesy of Dr A.J. Verhoeven), are shown in Figure 1. As shown in panel 1A, negative staining was observed when sections were incubated with PBS only, i.e. without the primary antibody. Although some p22-phox-immunoreactive microglial cells were found in the neuropil of non-demented controls, p22-phox staining was mainly seen in the mononuclear granulocytes located in the lumen of blood vessels (Figure 1B, C). Interestingly, as illustrated in Figure 1D–G, in AD brains the number as well as the staining intensity of these p22-phox expressing parenchymal microglial cells was dramatically enhanced. Moreover, in contrast to controls, in AD and Down's syndrome tissue microglial cells generally showed a reactive morphology with abbreviated short cellular processes and enlarged cell somata. In addition, as illustrated in Figure 1D, E, dense clusters of intensely stained microglial cells were found to be associated with neuritic plaques. Finally, as shown in Figure 1F, G, p22-phox immunoreactivity was found in so-called perivascular microglial cells surrounding (congophilic) cerebral blood vessels.

Reportedly, in human phagocytes the cellular content of p22-phox and enhanced immunoreactivity for MoAb 449 have been shown to correlate well

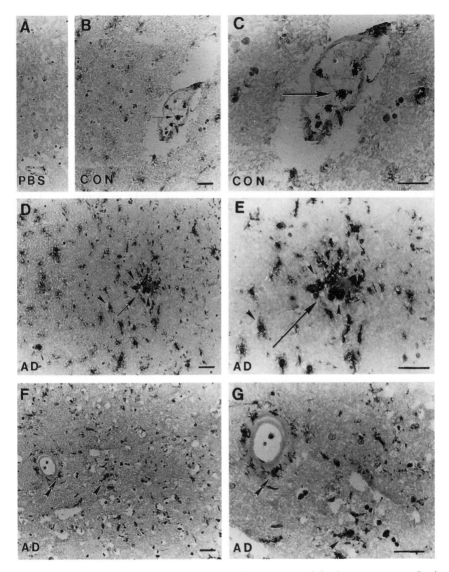

Figure 1. Photomicrographs show p22-phox immunoreactivity in post-mortem brain tissue obtained at autopsy from control (B, C) and Alzheimer's disease patients (A, D–G). As indicated by the arrow, in the control brain immunoreactivity is mainly seen in granulocytes located in the lumen of blood vessels, while p22-phox-immunoreactive cells in the neuropil are scanty (B, C). In panels D and E, the arrow and arrowheads indicate the presence of a congophylic neuritic plaque and plaque-associated microglia cells, respectively. In panels F and G, double arrowheads indicate p22-phox immunoreactivity in perivascular microglial cells in an AD brain. Bars = 40 μm

with the respiratory burst activity of these cells [5, 6]. Hence, provided that the levels of gp91phox and p47-phox/p67-phox/Rac are sufficient to support full NADPH-oxidase activity, our neuropathological data suggest that microglial cells in the AD brain exhibit profound respiratory burst activity. Since markers of oxidative damage are apparently lacking around Aβ plaques—which might be explained by the fact that senile plaques and plaque-associated factors are thought to have considerable scavenging capacity—a pro-oxidative role of plaque-associated microglial cells has been argued. It was noteworthy, therefore, that in the present study, p22-phox immunoreactivity was also observed in parenchymal and perivascular microglial cells randomly distributed throughout the cortical and hippocampal area and was not restricted to the plaque-associated microglial cells only. Hence, it is postulated that at least the parenchymal and perivascular cells are likely to contribute to the oxidative challenge in the AD brain. Given the widespread distribution of these cells, the question arises as to whether fibrillar Aβ in the neuritic plaque and/or plaque-associated factors are to be considered as the only naturally occurring trigger for the microglial respiratory burst. Rather, on the basis of our own studies and those of others, showing *inter alia* the ability of non-fibrillar Aβ to activate microglial superoxide production, it is tempting to speculate that microglia activation in the AD brain is the result of pathogenic mechanisms driven by diffusible factors, e.g. pro-inflammatory cytokines and/or soluble non-fibrillar Aβ oligomers [7].

ACKNOWLEDGEMENTS

The authors thank The Netherlands Brain Bank of The Netherlands Brain Institute for Brain Research, Amsterdam, for providing the tissue, Dr W. Kamphorst for the neuropathological evaluation of the tissue used, Ing. E.L. Montagne for excellent technical assistance, and Dr A.J. Verhoeven of the Central Laboratory of The Netherlands Red Cross Blood Transfusion Service (CLB, Amsterdam, The Netherlands) for kindly providing the antibodies raised against the NADPH-oxidase subunits. This study was supported by Grant No. 903-41-141 from the Dutch Organization of Scientific Research (NWO).

REFERENCES

1. Van Muiswinkel FL, Eikelenboom P. Inflammation and oxidative stress in Alzheimer's disease. In: Cacabelos R, Winblad B, Eikelenboom P (eds) Neurogerontology and Neurogeriatrics, vol 2: Inflammation and Neuroimmunotrophic Activity in Alzheimer's Disease. Barcelona, Philadelphia: Prous Science, 1998; 43–55.

2. Van Muiswinkel FL, Veerhuis R, Eikelenboom P. Amyloid-β protein primes cultured rat microglia cells for an enhanced phorbol 12-myristate 13-acetate-induced respiratory burst. J Neurochem 1996; 66: 2468–76.
3. McDonald DR, Bamberger ME, Combs CK, Landreth G. β-amyloid fibrils activate parallel mitogen-activated protein kinase pathways in microglia and THP1 monocytes. J Neurosci 1998; 18: 4451–60.
4. Meda L, Bonaiuto C, Baron P, Otvos L, Rossi F, Cassatella MA. Priming of monocyte respiratory burst by β-amyloid fragment Aβ(25–35). Neurosci Lett 1996; 219: 91–4.
5. Verhoeven AJ, Bolscher BGJM, Meerhof LJ, van Zwieten R, Keijer J, Weening RS, Roos D. Characterization of two monoclonal antibodies against cytochrome b558 of human neutrophils. Blood 1989; 73: 1686–94.
6. Yagisawa M, Yuo A, Yonemaru M, Imajoh-Ohmi S, Kanegaski S, Yazaki Y, Takaku F. Superoxide release and NADPH oxidase components in mature human phagocytes: correlation between functional capacity and amount of functional proteins. Biochem Biophys Res Comm 1996; 228: 510–16.
7. Lambert MP, Barlow AK, Chromy BA, Edwards C, Freed R, Liosatos M, Morgan TE, Rozovsky I, Trommer B, Viola KL, Wals P, Zhang C, Finch CE, Krafft GA, Klein WL. Diffusable, non-fibrillar ligands derived from Aβ1–42 are potent central nervous system neurotoxins. Proc Natl Acad Sci USA 1998; 95: 6448–53.

Address for correspondence:
    F.L. van Muiswinkel,
    Graduate School Neurosciences Amsterdam,
    Faculty of Medicine, Department of Psychiatry, Vrije Universiteit,
    Van der Boechorststraat 7, 1081 BT Amsterdam, The Netherlands
    e-mail: FLV.Muiswinkel.Pharm@med.vu.nl

50 The Amyloid-β1–42-induced Respiratory Burst of Primary Human Macrophages Is Enhanced in the Presence of Amyloid-β25–35

HESSEL A. SMITS, FREEK L. VAN MUISWINKEL,
N. MACHIEL DE VOS, JAN VERHOEF AND
HANS S.L.M. NOTTET

INTRODUCTION

Previously, we and others have shown that amyloid-β (Aβ), which is the full-length homolog to the Aβ actually deposited in the Alzheimer's disease brain, is capable of priming and/or triggering the respiratory burst of cultured rat microglial cells [1]. Using primary cultures of human monocyte-derived macrophages as a model of human microglial cells, we recently discovered that the amino-terminus of Aβ is critical for the cellular binding and consequent activation of the phagocytic respiratory burst (Van Muiswinkel et al., unpublished observations). Furthermore, in line with previous studies of Giulian and colleagues [2, 3], we found that Aβ1–16 behaves like a pharmacological antagonist. Thus, using flow cytometry with Aβ1–42–FITC and lucigenin-enhanced chemiluminescence, it was found that Aβ1–16, which has been described as containing a cell attachment domain [2, 3], inhibited both the cellular binding and the Aβ1–42-induced release of superoxide in human macrophages. In the present study, we have used the same experimental model to investigate the effects of Aβ25–35 on the Aβ1–42-induced oxidative burst.

MATERIALS AND METHODS

AMYLOID-β PEPTIDES

The synthetic Aβ peptides Aβ1–42 and Aβ25–35 (Bachem AG, Switzerland), prepared as stock solutions in sterile water at a concentration of

Alzheimer's Disease and Related Disorders
Edited by K. Iqbal, D.F. Swaab, B. Winblad and H.M. Wisniewski
© 1999 John Wiley & Sons Ltd

500 μM, were stored at −20 °C. FITC-labeled Aβ1–42 was prepared by incubating Aβ1–42 at a concentration of 10 mg/ml with 0.1 mg/ml FITC in PBS (pH = 7.4) for 1 h at 22 °C. Subsequently, using a 1 kDa Spectra/Por dialyzation membrane, Aβ1–42–FITC was dialyzed overnight against PBS to remove unbound FITC, diluted to a concentration of 220 μM and stored at −20 °C.

HUMAN MONOCYTE-DERIVED MACROPHAGES

Monocytes were derived from peripheral blood mononuclear cells by Ficoll–Paque (Pharmacia Biotech, Sweden) density gradients and purified by centrifugal elutriation as described previously [4]. Cells were seeded at a concentration of 2×10^6 cells/ml in Teflon Erlenmeyer flasks (Nalgene, USA) and grown as suspension at 37 °C in a humidified atmosphere of 5% CO_2/95% air. Culture medium was composed of Iscove's modified Dulbecco's medium (Gibco Life Technologies, The Netherlands) supplemented with 10% heat-inactivated human AB serum, 2 mM L-glutamine, 19 mM sodium bicarbonate, 10 μg/ml gentamicin and 10 μg/ml ciprofloxacin. After 7 days, monocyte-derived macrophages (MDMs) were harvested from the flasks, washed with Hanks' balanced salt solution (HBSS) and used for the experiments.

SUPEROXIDE PRODUCTION

Superoxide production was measured as lucigenin-enhanced chemiluminescence [4]. Briefly, cells were transferred to polystyrene vials (2×10^5/vial), placed into a luminometer (Packard Instruments, Belgium) and incubated for 30 min at 37 °C in HBSS containing 250 nM bis-N-methylacridinum (Lucigenin; Sigma Chemical Co., The Netherlands) to assess the spontaneous release of superoxide. Subsequently, Aβ peptides were added and chemiluminescence (expressed as millivolts, mV) was monitored for 30–60 min.

FLOW CYTOMETRY

For Aβ1–42–FITC binding studies, 2×10^5 cells were incubated at 37 °C with HBSS containing 2.5 μM Aβ1–42–FITC, either alone or in combination with 50 μM Aβ25–35. After 30 min, the cells were washed with HBSS and fixed for 15 min with PBS containing 2% paraformaldehyde. Thereafter, flow cytometry analysis was performed by analyzing 10 000 cells per experimental condition on an FACScan flow cytometer (Becton Dickinson and Co., USA) equipped with a computer-assisted data analysis system.

RESULTS

EFFECT OF Aβ25–35 ON THE Aβ1–42-INDUCED SUPEROXIDE ANION RELEASE

To investigate the effect of Aβ25–35 on the Aβ1–42 induced superoxide production, MDMs were incubated with Aβ1–42, either alone or in combination with various amounts of Aβ25–35. Results are shown in Figure 1. While the spontaneous burst amounted to 6.9 ± 1.3 mV, it was found that the respiratory burst was enhanced to 18.8 ± 0.4 mV by 10 µM Aβ1–42. Moreover, while Aβ25–35 did not trigger the respiratory burst by itself, Aβ25–35 dramatically enhanced the Aβ1–42 release of superoxide anion, i.e. in the presence of 200 µM Aβ25–35 the Aβ1–42-induced release amounted to 67.8 ± 2.1 mV.

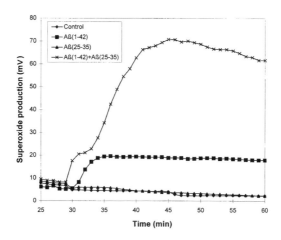

Figure 1. Effect of Aβ25–35 on the Aβ1–42 induced superoxide anion release from human monocyte-derived macrophages. Superoxide release was measured in MDMs, incubated with either HBSS (control), 10 µM Aβ1–42, 200 µM Aβ25–35 or a combination thereof

EFFECT OF Aβ25–35 ON THE CELLULAR BINDING OF Aβ1–42–FITC

To characterize the nature of the aforementioned effects of Aβ25–35 on the Aβ1–42-stimulated superoxide release, we next investigated the effect of Aβ25–35 on the cellular binding of Aβ1–42 to human macrophages. Therefore, MDMs were incubated with Aβ1–42–FITC, either alone or in combination with Aβ25–35. As shown in Figure 2, it was found that 2.5 µM Aβ1–42–FITC readily binds to MDMs. Control experiments performed at 4 °C or in the presence of 10 µg/ml cytochalasine B revealed that under our conditions Aβ1–42–FITC accumulates predominantly at the cell surface. Interestingly, whereas preincubation of cells with Aβ25–35 did not have any effect, the cellular binding was markedly enhanced when 2.5 µM Aβ1–42–FITC was added together with 50 µM Aβ25–35. This phenomenon was even more pronounced when Aβ1–42–FITC and Aβ25–35 were first incubated for 30 min prior to adding the peptides to the cells (Figure 2).

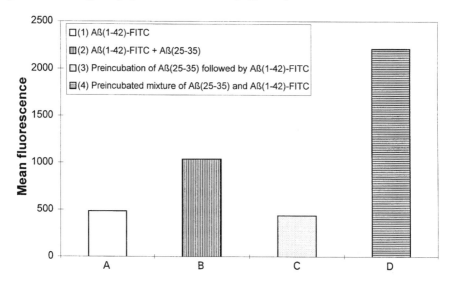

Figure 2. Effect of Aβ25–35 on the binding of Aβ1–42–FITC to human monocyte-derived macrophages. Cells were incubated for 30 min with either 2.5 µM Aβ1–42–FITC (A); or Aβ1–42–FITC together with 50 µM Aβ25–35 (B); or preincubated with Aβ25–35 followed by Aβ1–42–FITC (C); or preincubation with a mixture of Aβ25–35 and Aβ1–42–FITC (D)

DISCUSSION

In summary, the results of the current study demonstrate that the cellular binding of Aβ1–42 and consequent activation of the respiratory burst of MDMs is enhanced in the presence of Aβ25–35. Intriguingly, this effect was only observed when Aβ1–42 and Aβ25–35 were first preincubated in the absence of cells or when both peptides were added as a mixture. Although the nature of this effect is, as yet, largely enigmatic, various cellular mechanisms might be implicated. For example, Aβ25–35 is known to induce changes in intracellular calcium homeostasis and/or to trigger tyrosine kinase-dependent intracellular signal-transduction pathways [5, 6], phenomena which are both thought to be implicated in the activation and/or regulation of the respiratory burst [6, 7]. Thus, in such a way Aβ25–35 might be able to prime MDMs for an enhanced Aβ1–42-induced respiratory burst. Alternatively, the effects of Aβ25–35 might be due to its direct influence on the biophysical properties and/or the assembly state of Aβ1–42. Particularly since preincubation of cells with Aβ25–35 prior to the addition of Aβ1–42 did not have any effect, in our opinion the latter explanation seems the more plausible. Hence, notwithstanding the fact that Aβ25–35 fragment, as such, does not exist in the AD brain, the results obtained in our study might be relevant in that they provide new insight into the structural features required for Aβ–microglia interactions and consequent microglia-driven pathogenetic mechanisms.

ACKNOWLEDGEMENTS

This work was supported by Grant No. 903-51-104 from the Dutch Organization for Scientific Research (NWO) to H.S.L.M.N.

REFERENCES

1. Van Muiswinkel FL, Veerhuis R, Eikelenboom P. Amyloid β protein (Aβ) primes cultured rat microglial cells for an enhanced phorbol-myristate-acetate induced respiratory burst activity. J Neurochem 1996; 66: 2468–76.
2. Giulian D, Haverkamp LJ, Yu JH, Karshin W, Tom D, Li J, Kirkpatrick J, Kuo Y-M, Roher AE. Specific domains of β-amyloid from Alzheimer plaque elicit neuron killing in human microglia. J Neurosci 1996; 16: 6021–37.
3. Giulian D. Immune responses and dementia. Ann NY Acad Sci 1997; 835: 91–110.
4. Nottet HSLM, de Graaf L, de Vos NM, Bakker L, van Strijp JAG, Visser MR, Verhoef J. Phagocytic function of monocyte-derived macrophages is not affected by human immunodeficiency virus type 1 infection. J Infect Dis 1993; 168: 84–91.
5. Korotzer AR, Whittemore ER, Cotman CW. Differential regulation by β-amyloid peptides of intracellular free Ca^{2+} concentration in cultured rat microglia. Eur J Pharm 1995; 288: 125–30.
6. McDonald DR, Bamberger ME, Combs CK, Landreth GE. β-Amyloid fibrils activate parallel mitogen-activated protein kinase pathways in microglia and THP1 monocytes. J Neurosci 1998; 18(12): 4451–60.
7. Colton CA, Jia M, Li MS, Gilbert DL. K^+ modulation of microglial superoxide production: involvement of voltage-gated Ca^{2+} channels. Am J Physiol Cell Physiol 1994; 266: C1650–55.

Address for correspondence:
  Hessel A. Smits,
  Eijkman-Winkler Institute,
  Section of Neuroimmunology, Utrecht University,
  Heidelberglaan 100, 3584 CX, Utrecht, The Netherlands

51 Amyloid-β Induces Chemokine Secretion and Monocyte Migration across the Blood–Brain Barrier

MILAN FIALA, LING ZHANG, XIAOHU GAN,
OMRI BERGER, MICHAEL C. GRAVES,
BARBARA SHERRY AND DENNIS TAUB

INTRODUCTION

A large number of inflammatory components have been identified in Alzheimer's disease (AD) lesions, among them the activated complement proteins (from C1q to C5b–C9 membrane attack complex), acute phase reactants, cytokines and chemokines [1, 2]. The principal cell mediating this response appears to be activated microglia [3, 4, 5]. The potential contribution of circulating monocytes/macrophages to the inflammatory process of AD has not, however, previously been considered. We present here experiments demonstrating the responses of blood-derived monocytes to stimulation by amyloid-β (Aβ).

The brain parenchyma is separated from the circulation by a selective and efficient blood–brain barrier (BBB). However, circulating monocytes could traverse the BBB if attracted by powerful chemotactic stimuli, as occurs in some experimental inflammatory states of the brain [6, 7] or following intraparenchymal injections of chemokines [8]. A disturbed BBB in AD is also supported by gross anatomical and functional alterations of the cerebral microvessels [9, 10], by the occasional absence of endothelial cells [11] and the presence of amyloid deposits, often associated with microvessels [12]. These observations lend support to the possibility of monocytes transmigrating into the vicinity of Aβ deposits and transformation into microglia-like cells surrounding the amyloid plaque cores. Transformation of peripheral monocytes into microglia-like cells has been demonstrated *in vitro* on monolayers of astrocytes [13], and recently *in vivo* during autoimmune inflammation of the axotomized rat facial nucleus [7].

Alzheimer's Disease and Related Disorders
Edited by K. Iqbal, D.F. Swaab, B. Winblad and H.M. Wisniewski
© 1999 John Wiley & Sons Ltd

In the present investigation, we have used a model of the human BBB which displays physiological regulation of molecular permeability and permits monocyte transmigration [14, 15]. We used this paradigm to explore the possibility of transmigration of peripheral monocytes facilitated by inflammatory cytokines and chemokines, and we also studied the ability of Aβ to induce the secretion of these molecules in the model.

MATERIALS AND METHODS

CHEMICALS

Synthetic Aβ1–42 peptide was from California Peptide Research Inc., Napa, CA. The Aβ was dissolved as 1.0 mM stock in concentrated dimethylsulfoxide. The solution was negative for endotoxin (less than 10 pg/ml) by the Limulus Lysate Test (Sigma, St Louis, MO). The stock solution was diluted in RPMI 1640 medium (Irvine Scientific, Santa Ana, CA) with 10% fetal calf serum (Hyclone, Logan, UT) as indicated. The tissue culture media, either alone or with DMSO at 1%, were used as control media.

DIFFERENTIATION OF MONOCYTES INTO MACROPHAGES

Human blood monocytes were obtained from the peripheral blood of healthy donors by a modification of the Recalde procedure [16]. In 1 ml of RPMI medium with 10% autologous serum, 1×10^6 monocytes were incubated for 8 days alone or in the presence of Aβ1–42 at indicated concentrations or control medium. The adherent cell density was estimated using the 3-(4,5-dimethylthiazol-2-yl)-2,5-diphenyl tetrazolium bromide (MTT) assay.

CULTURES OF PERIPHERAL MONOCYTES

Monocytes (1×10^6) were cultured in 1 ml in 24-well plates, in the presence of various concentrations of Aβ1–42. After 48 h incubation, the medium was harvested for cytokine assays. RPMI media containing 10% autologous serum with or without DMSO at 1% or 0.1% were used as controls.

ELISA ASSAYS OF CYTOKINES AND CHEMOKINES

TNF-α, IL-6, IL-10 and IL-12 levels in the culture media were determined by a sandwich ELISA, as previously described [17]. Interleukin-1β (IL-1β), human monocyte chemoattractant protein-1 (MCP-1) and interleukin-8 (IL-8) levels were determined using Quantikine ELISA kits (R&D Systems, Minneapolis, MN) following the manufacturer's instructions. Human macrophage inflammatory protein-1α (MIP-1α) was determined by a sandwich ELISA, as described previously with some modifications [18].

BLOOD–BRAIN BARRIER MODEL

The endothelial cell–astrocyte BBB model was constructed using human brain microvascular endothelial cells (BMVEC) in 24-well tissue culture plate inserts with a Cyclopore R polyethylene terephthalate membrane bottom. The surfaces of the membrane were coated with rat tail collagen type I and with human fibronectin (Collaborative Biomedical Products), as previously described [15].

TRANSMIGRATION OF MONOCYTES

To assess monocyte/macrophage migration through the BBB model, 160 μg of Aβ1–42 in 35 μl of medium were placed in the bottom of the lower chamber of six wells and air-dried. Another six wells without Aβ were used as null controls. To three of the Aβ-containing wells and three of the null control wells, 2×10^4 monocytes in 1 ml DME-S medium were added. After 16 h of incubation, 5×10^5 monocytes in DME-S medium were added to each of the 12 upper chambers. Following a period of 24 h incubation, the number of monocytes present in each of the chambers was determined using a hemocytometer chamber.

RESULTS

Aβ1–42 ELICITS THE DIFFERENTIATION OF MONOCYTES INTO MACROPHAGES

Human peripheral blood monocytes were cultured in the presence of Aβ1–42 and evaluated by the MTT method with respect to differentiation into macrophages. Monocytes exposed to various doses of AA ranging from 1.5 to 12.5 μg/ml differentiated into adherent macrophages with maximum effect at 3–6 μg/ml, whereas higher doses were increasingly toxic, and this effect was also time-dependent.

Aβ1–42 INDUCES SECRETION OF CYTOKINES BY CULTURED MONOCYTES

Human monocytes were cultured in presence of increasing concentrations of Aβ to induce secretion of cytokines. At 0.25 μg/ml, Aβ had no effect on cytokine secretion. However, significant secretion of cytokines was noticed at 2.5 μg/ml, with the largest response at 25 μg/ml (Table 1). At this concentration the secretion of TNF-α by 1×10^6 monocytes amounted to 1400 pg/ml, three times more than that stimulated by the control media containing DMSO. At the same concentration of Aβ (25 μg/ml), the secretions of IL-6 and IL-12 were also increased, equivalent to about seven and 20 times, respectively, more than those observed in control values. Aβ1–42 had no significant effect on the secretion of IL-10 up to 25 μg/ml. Aβ1–42 increased monocyte secretion of IL-1β 2.5-fold.

Table 1. Effects of amyloid-β on cytokine secretion by peripheral monocytes[1]

Cytokine	Amyloid-β concentration (μg/ml)	Cytokine concentration (pg/ml)[2]	DMSO Control (%)[3]
TNF-α	0.25	501.2 + 23.7	100.58
	2.5	789.3 + 51.6	158.40
	25	1401.8 + 22.1	281.32
IL-12	0.25	12 + 0.51	141.18
	2.5	6.8 + 0.46	832.01
	25	10.6 + 0.82	1247.06
IL-6	0.25	17.9 + 3.4	91.33
	2.5	108.8 + 6.2	555.10
	25	147.7 + 9.3	753.57
IL-10	0.25	211.3 + 15.6	76.50
	2.5	323.5 + 13.2	117.13
	25	319.4 + 14.8	115.64

[1] Monocytes (5×10^5) were cultivated in RPMI medium with 10% autologous serum in the presence of control DMSO (not shown) and indicated concentrations of Aβ. Media were harvested after 48 h.
[2] Cytokine concentrations in the media were determined by cytokine ELISA assay.
[3] (Cytokine concentration in presence of Aβ/cytokine concentration in presence of control DMSO) × 100.

During the course of this investigation we noticed individual donor fluctuations in the amount of cytokine secretion when the monocytes were stimulated with Aβ1–42. Therefore, we investigated these variations in seven individual donors, whose monocytes were treated by 2.5 μM Aβ1–42, and expressed the degree of cytokine secretion as the percentage of secretion with Aβ/DMSO in the medium. With respect to TNF-α, monocyte cultures from four out of seven individuals showed a significant elevation of this cytokine, but cultures of two individuals showed an inhibition. IL-6 and IL-12 demonstrated a substantial increase in six and four donors, respectively. Interestingly, three individual cultures showed significant depression of IL-12 secretion (data not shown).

Aβ1–42 INDUCES SECRETION OF CC AND CXC CHEMOKINES BY CULTURED MONOCYTES

As with cytokine induction, in comparison to DMSO control, Aβ induced secretion of the CXC chemokine IL-8 and the CC chemokines MIP-1α and MCP-1, in a dose-responsive fashion in the range 0.5–50 μg/ml (Table 2). As with the cytokines, there was a striking heterogeneity between donors (data not shown).

Aβ1–42 WITH MONOCYTES STIMULATE MONOCYTE TRANSMIGRATION ACROSS THE BBB MODEL

The BBB model was then used to test whether Aβ can attract the cells across a monolayer of human endothelial cells, derived from cerebral microvessels, and

Table 2. Effects of amyloid-β on chemokine secretion by peripheral monocytes[1]

Chemokine family	Chemokine	Amyloid-β concentration (μg/ml)	Chemokine concentration (pg/ml)[2]	DMSO Control (%)[3]
C-X-C	IL-8	0.5	113.7 + 19.04	227.40
		5	657.7 + 415.9	1315.40
		50	3247 + 1905	6494.00
C-C	MIP-1α	0.5	703.3 + 308.1	1406.60
		5	2603 + 1747	5206.00
		50	8868 + 1794	17736.00
	MCP-1	0.5	340.3 + 172.2	680.60
		5	410.7 + 183.1	821.40
		50	893 + 176.4	1786.00

[1] Monocytes (5×10^5) were cultivated in RPMI medium with 10% autologous serum in the presence of control DMSO (not shown) and indicated concentrations of Aβ. Media were harvested after 48 h.

[2] Chemokine concentrations in the media were determined by chemokine ELISA assay.

[3] (Chemokine concentration in presence of Aβ/chemokine concentration in presence of control DMSO) × 100.

human astrocytes, separating the vascular side (upper chamber) from the brain parenchymal side (lower chamber). In a control experiment, 5×10^5 human monocytes were placed in the upper chamber and only medium in the lower chamber (Table 3). After 24 h 0.83% of the input monocytes were found in the lower chamber. When small numbers of monocytes were introduced into the lower chamber prior to the experiment, the migration of monocytes from the upper to the lower chamber increased 2.3-fold. Addition of Aβ1–42 at the bottom of the lower chamber resulted in a 10-fold increase in the transmigration of monocytes. The transmigration of monocytes was increased 30.7-fold when the lower chamber contained both Aβ1–42 and 20 000 monocytes.

Table 3. Effects of amyloid-β on monocyte migration across the blood–brain barrier model

Lower chamber content[1]	Monocyte migration to the lower chamber (%)[2]
Medium	0.83 ± 0.62
Monocytes	1.87 ± 0.12
Aβ1–42	8.63 ± 2.23
Monocytes + Aβ1–42	25.47 ± 3.56

[1] The BBB models were prepared for migration by placing control medium, a dot of Aβ (160 μg), monocytes (2×10^4), or both Aβ and monocytes in the lower chamber.

[2] Monocytes (5×10^5) were added into the upper chamber, and 24 h later cell counts in each chamber were determined using a hemocytometer chamber.

DISCUSSION

A subtle and chronic inflammatory reaction induced by reactive glial cells is one of the major pathological events in the AD brain. The hypothesis that amyloid deposits cause neuronal loss in AD by a mechanism involving activated microglia and pro-inflammatory molecules has gained support from several different experimental approaches [1, 2]. One of the key questions is the source of the microglia which are active in causing AD. We have begun to explore a process whereby circulating monocytes are continually recruited into the brain from the circulation and transform into microglia during the course of AD. We have shown that blood-derived monocytes can differentiate into adherent macrophages in the presence of Aβ. We have shown that monocytes from the peripheral blood of normal donors have the property of secreting the pro-inflammatory cytokines that are implicated in the pathogenesis of AD. We have also shown that Aβ induces monocytes to secrete chemokines. Chemokines are cytokines which can induce the chemotaxis of more inflammatory cells. Lastly, the recruitment of monocytes into the brain would require that the cells pass the blood–brain barrier. We have used a model of the BBB, constructed with human cellular components and having many of the characteristics of the intact barrier. In this model, the findings suggest that Aβ can stimulate a small number of monocytes on the brain side of the barrier to secrete chemokines. The presence of chemokines results in opening of the barrier and recruitment of additional monocytes across the barrier. All of these steps thus represent hypothetical targets for blocking ongoing recruitment of monocytes and possibly stopping the pathology of AD from progressing. One of our salient findings is the wide heterogeneity of chemokine and cytokine responses to Aβ by monocytes from different donors. A future research question is to determine whether this is a characteristic of the individual donor that may thus represent a risk factor for the future development of AD.

One might postulate that common insults that can compromise the BBB even transiently, such as head trauma, small hemorrhagic and ischemic lesions common in older people, or even aging itself, might initiate AD in susceptible individuals by seeding a few monocytes from the circulation into the brain parenchyma. These cells may provoke recruitment of more cells by a mechanism such as that outlined above, involving chemokines.

In conclusion, numerous studies have shown that Aβ can invoke the secretion of pro-inflammatory factors by monocytic cells. In AD, increased chemokine and cytokine concentrations in brain parenchyma may attract circulating monocytes/macrophages to migrate across the BBB. The recruitment of peripheral monocytic cells into the cerebral cortex could further intensify the already existing inflammatory reaction but may be limited to individuals whose peripheral monocytes are hyper-reactive to Aβ. Identification of such individuals among AD patients and in the general population may shed light on the role played by the inflammatory reaction in AD.

ABSTRACT

Background: Inflammation is an important mechanism in the pathogenesis of Alzheimer's disease. Activated microglia in the AD brain are the likely source of many pro-inflammatory cytokines. These cytokines may permit the passage of peripheral monocytes into the brain parenchyma, where monocytes could transform into macrophages, and thereby contribute to the pathogenesis of AD.

Materials and Methods: Monocytes, from human donors, were exposed to Aβ1–42, and then tested for differentiation into macrophages and for ability to secrete cytokines and chemokines. In an *in vitro* model of the blood–brain barrier, we determined the ability of monocytes/macrophages to transmigrate when challenged by Aβ1–42 on the brain side of the blood–brain barrier model.

Results: Aβ1–42 induced peripheral monocytes to secrete the cytokines TNF-α, IL-1β, and IL-12 in a dose-related fashion. Aβ1–42 also induced the CC chemokines MCP-1, MIP-1α and MIP-1β and the CXC chemokine IL-8. In the blood–brain barrier model, Aβ1–42 together with monocytes in the brain-side chamber resulted in monocyte transmigration from the blood-side to the brain-side of the blood–brain barrier. In addition, Aβ1–42 stimulated differentiation of monocytes into adherent macrophages in a dose-related fashion. The magnitude of these effects of Aβ1–42 varied dramatically between different monocyte donors.

Conclusion: Monocytes could be recruited from circulation into the brain by a mechanism involving chemokines. There they may differentiate into macrophages and microglia, and may add to the inflammatory process of Alzheimer's disease.

REFERENCES

1. McGeer PL, McGeer EG. The inflammatory response system of the brain: implications for therapy of Alzheimer and other neurodegenerative diseases. Brain Res Rev 1995; 21: 195–218.
2. Rogers J, O'Barr S. Inflammatory mediators in Alzheimer's disease. In Wasco W, Tanzi RE (eds) Molecular Mechanisms of Dementia. Totowa, NJ: Humana Press, 1997; 177–98.
3. Haga S, Akai K, Ishii T. Demonstration of microglial cells in and around senile (neuritic) plaques in the Alzheimer brain. Acta Neuropathol 1989; 77: 569–75.
4. Mackenzie IRA, Hao CH, Munoz DG. Role of microglia in senile plaque formation. Neurobiol Aging 1995; 16: 797–804.
5. Perlmutter LS, Scott SA, Barron E, Chui HC. MHC class II-positive microglia in human brain: association with Alzheimer lesions. J Neurosci Res 1992; 33: 549–58.
6. Butter C, Baker D, O'Neill JK, Turk JL. Mononuclear cell trafficking and plasma protein extravasation into the CNS during chronic relapsing experimental allergic encephalomyelitis in Biozzi AB/H mice. J Neurol Sci 1991; 104: 9–12.

7. Fluegell A, Kreutzberg GW, Graeber MB. Transformation of bone marrow-derived macrophages into ramified microglia during autoimmune inflammation of the axotomized rat facial nucleus. Fifth International Congress of Neuroimmunology, Montreal, Canada, 1998.

8. Bell MD, Taub DD, Perry VH. Overriding the brain's intrinsic resistance to leukocyte recruitment with intraparenchymal injections of recombinant chemokines. Neuroscience 1996; 74: 283–92.

9. Buee L, Hof PR, Delacourte A. Brain microvascular changes in Alzheimer's disease and other dementias. Ann NY Acad Sci 1997; 826: 7–24.

10. Kalaria RN, Harik SI. Reduced glucose transporter at the blood–brain barrier in cerebral cortex in Alzheimer's disease. J Neurochem 1989; 53: 1083–8.

11. Kalaria RN. Cerebral vessels in ageing and Alzheimer's disease. Pharmacol Ther 1996; 72: 193–214.

12. Roher AE, Lowenson JD, Clarke S, Woods AS, Cotter RJ, Gowing E, Ball MJ. β-Amyloid-(1–42) is a major component of cerebrovascular amyloid deposits: implications for the pathology of Alzheimer disease. Proc Natl Acad Sci USA 1993; 90: 10836–40.

13. Sievers J, Parwaresch R, Wottge H-U. Blood monocytes and spleen macrophages differentiate into microglia-like cells on monolayers of astrocytes: morphology. Glia 1994; 12: 245–58.

14. Persidsky Y, Stins M, Way D, Witte MH, Weinand M, Kim K-S, Bock P, Gendelman HE, Fiala M. A model for monocyte migration through the blood–brain barrier during HIV-1 encephalitis. J Immunol 1997; 158: 3499–510.

15. Fiala M, Looney DJ, Stins M, Way D, Zhang L, Gan X, Chiappelli F, Shapshak P, Weinand M, Graves M, Witte M, Kim K-S. TNF-α opens a paracellular route for HIV-1 invasion across the blood–brain barrier. Molec Med 1997; 3: 553–64.

16. Fogelman AM, Elahi F, Sykes K, Van Lenten BJ, Territo MC, Berliner JA. Modification of the Recalde method for the isolation of human monocytes. J Lipid Res 1988; 29: 1243–7.

17. Gan X-H, Robin JP, Huerta JMM, Braquet P, Bonavida B. Inhibition of TNF-α and IL-1β secretion but not IL-6 from activated human peripheral blood monocytes by a new synthetic demethylpodophyllotoxin derivative. Clin Immunol 1994; 14: 280–88.

18. Schmidtmayerova N, Nottet HSLM, Nuovo G, Raabe T, Flanagan CR, Dubrovsky L, Gendelman HE, Cerami A, Bukrinsky M, Sherry B. HIV-1 infection alters chemokine β peptide expression in human monocytes: implications for recruitment of leukocytes into brain and lymph nodes. Proc Natl Acad Sci USA 93: 700–704.

Address for correspondence:
  Milan Fiala,
  Department of Medicine,
  UCLA School of Medicine,
  Los Angeles, CA, USA

52 Lipoprotein Oxidation and Alzheimer's Disease

SVEN SCHIPPLING, ANATOL KONTUSH, SÖNKE ARLT,
DIANA DAHER, CARSTEN BUHMANN,
HANS JÖRG STÜRENBURG, ULRIKE MANN,
TOMAS MÜLLER-THOMSEN AND ULRIKE BEISIEGEL

INTRODUCTION

The central nervous system (CNS) is especially vulnerable to oxidative stress as a result of the brain's high oxygen consumption rate, its high lipid content, and the relative paucity of antioxidants [1]. Strong evidence exists for increased oxidative damage in the Alzheimer's disease (AD) brain [2]. However, the exact mechanisms responsible for this effect remain unclear.

Amyloid β (Aβ) has been implicated as a key oxidant involved in the pathogenesis of AD [3]. It is a major component of AD plaques and can spontaneously generate free radicals [4]. Aβ is found in biological fluids such as cerebrospinal fluid (CSF), where it is complexed to lipoproteins [5]. Lipoproteins in the density range of plasma high-density lipoproteins (HDL) have been found in CSF [6, 7]. They contain polyunsaturated fatty acids, a major substrate for lipid peroxidation, and lipophilic antioxidants, e.g. tocopherols. Plasma lipoproteins are known to be highly susceptible to oxidation [8], a mechanism playing a crucial role in the pathogenesis of atherosclerosis.

Here we raise the question of whether lipoprotein oxidation is also involved in the pathogenesis of AD. To assess this hypothesis, we analyzed plasma and CSF samples from 29 AD patients and 29 non-demented subjects for their lipid content, levels of lipophilic and hydrophilic antioxidants and their oxidizability *in vitro*.

METHODS

SUBJECTS

AD patients were recruited in the psychiatric clinic of the Hamburg University Hospital and diagnosed according to the NINCDS–ADRDA and DSM-IV

Alzheimer's Disease and Related Disorders
Edited by K. Iqbal, D.F. Swaab, B. Winblad and H.M. Wisniewski
© 1999 John Wiley & Sons Ltd

criteria. Subjects without degenerative disorders or cognitive impairment who attended the local neurological clinic and underwent lumbar puncture for diagnostic purposes were recruited as controls. Informed consent was obtained from all subjects. The study was approved by the ethical committee of Hamburg.

SAMPLE COLLECTION

CSF (1 ml) and EDTA blood (10 ml) were sampled at the same visit and immediately placed on ice. Blood was centrifuged at 4 °C to obtain plasma. CSF and plasma were frozen under argon at −80 °C for no longer than 3 months and thawed directly before analysis.

CSF AND PLASMA OXIDATION KINETICS

CSF was diluted 10-fold with phosphate-buffered saline (PBS), containing 0.6 M NaCl, pH 7.4, and treated with Chelex 100 ion-exchange resin to remove transition metal ions. The samples were oxidized at 37 °C for 50 h, either in the absence (auto-oxidation) or in the presence of the exogenous oxidant 2,2'-azobis-(2-amidinopropane) hydrochloride (AAPH) at 100 µM. Plasma was diluted 150-fold with PBS and incubated at 37 °C for 20 h in the absence of exogenous oxidants (auto-oxidation) or in the presence of AAPH (330 µM) and soybean lipoxygenase (25 U/ml) [9]. Oxidation was monitored as a change in the sample absorbance at 234 nm. This parameter is known to reflect the level of lipid hydroperoxides, oxidation products of the lipid component of lipoproteins having conjugated diene structure [10]. The absorbance was measured at 5 min intervals.

ANTIOXIDANTS

α-Tocopherol, α- and β-carotene, ubiquinol-10 and ubiquinone-10 were measured in plasma and α-tocopherol and β-carotene were measured in CSF as major lipophilic antioxidants, using reversed-phase HPLC with electrochemical detection [11]. Ascorbate, a major hydrophilic antioxidant in CSF, was measured by ion-pairing HPLC with UV detection at 267 nm [12]. Plasma ascorbate was measured photometrically [12].

STATISTICAL ANALYSIS

Between-group differences in continuous variables were analyzed by Student's t-test for independent groups. Differences in dichotomous variables were analyzed by Fisher's exact test. All results are expressed as mean ± SD.

RESULTS

CHARACTERIZATION OF PATIENTS

AD patients had significantly higher mean age than control subjects (71.7 ± 10.1 vs. 55.1 ± 18.8 years, $p < 0.01$). To evaluate the possible influence of age on our data we formed two subgroups, excluding all individuals younger than 60 years; 26 subjects remained in the AD subgroup (11 males and 15 females; mean age 73.9 ± 7.6) and 14 in the control subgroup (eight males and six females; mean age 70.3 ± 8.3). All data were analyzed in parallel for the whole study population and the age-matched subgroups. Between-group comparison revealed a significantly higher number of current smokers amongst the controls (9 vs. 2, $p < 0.05$). No other parameter related to oxidative stress, such as coronary heart disease, hypertension, diabetes and plasma lipids or sex, showed a significant difference (data not shown). As expected, the apoE $\varepsilon 4$ allele frequency was significantly higher in the AD patients (0.36 vs. 0.07, $p < 0.01$). The AD patients reached a mean Mini-Mental Status Examination score of 18.8 ± 5.1 points. The age of AD onset was 68.1 ± 10.3 and the mean time since diagnosis of the disease was 3.6 ± 2.9 years.

LIPOPROTEIN OXIDATION IN CSF

A typical time-course of the absorbance at 234 nm exhibited three consecutive phases: the lag phase, during which the oxidation rate was close to zero; the propagation phase, presenting a fast accumulation of lipid peroxides; and the plateau phase, with an oxidation rate close to zero again [13]. The absorbance of oxidizing CSF paralleled the time-course of phosphatidylcholine hydroperoxides measured by HPLC with UV detection and correlated with the consumption of antioxidants in the sample.

When the oxidation kinetics of CSF from AD patients were compared to those of the control group, the oxidizability of AD CSF was found to be significantly higher. The duration of the oxidation lag phase was significantly shorter in the AD collective (Figure 1), whereas the mean oxidation rate during the initial phase was significantly higher (data not shown). The differences between the two groups concerning lag phase duration and initial oxidation rate were similarly pronounced when AAPH, a chemical initiator of oxidation, was used to induce CSF oxidation (data not shown). The age of the patients showed no influence on the sample's oxidizability (Figure 1), so that the difference remained similarly significant in the age-matched subgroups.

The amount of hydrophilic as well as lipophilic antioxidants in the CSF of patients and controls was in accordance with the results of the oxidation kinetic measurements (Table 1). Ascorbate, the major antioxidant in CSF, was significantly lower in both the whole and the age-matched AD groups, compared to the corresponding control groups. α-Tocopherol was decreased in

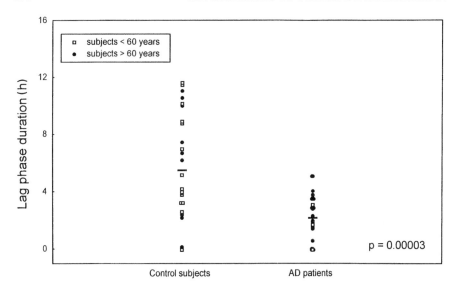

Figure 1. Auto-oxidation lag phase of CSF obtained from AD patients and control subjects. CSF was diluted 10-fold with PBS and incubated at 37 °C in the absence of exogenous oxidants. Bars correspond with the mean values calculated for each group. Each filled circle corresponds to one subject older and each open square to a subject younger than 60 years old. Significance of the difference between the groups is shown as a p value

AD CSF but the decrease did not reach statistical significance, whereas the difference in β-carotene values was negligible. There was no significant difference in the CSF samples of AD patients and the control groups as far as total protein, CSF:plasma albumin ratio and cholesterol level were concerned (Table 1).

Table 1. CSF and plasma parameters of AD patients and control subjects

	AD patients (n = 29)		Control subjects (n = 29)	
CSF				
Total protein (mg/l)	439	± 131	438	± 167
CSF/plasma albumin ratio	6.7	± 3.1	6.9	± 3.8
Cholesterol (mg/l)	6.8	± 2.5	7.5	± 2.6
Ascorbate (µM)	166.7	± 40.9**	193.4	± 27.7
α-Tocopherol (nM)	45.5	± 34.6	56.7	± 28.4
β-Carotene (nM)	2.1	± 0.9	1.9	± 1.4
Plasma				
Ascorbate (µM)	35.0	± 18.6*	48.8	± 18.5
α-Tocopherol (µM)	22.3	± 10.8	24.6	± 7.7
α-Carotene (µM)	0.06 ±	0.07***	0.18 ±	0.06
β-Carotene (µM)	0.54 ±	0.51	0.56 ±	0.34

[a] Percentage of total fatty acids; *** p < 0.001, ** p < 0.01, * p < 0.05 vs. control group.

LIPOPROTEIN OXIDATION IN PLASMA

Under the oxidizing conditions employed, plasma oxidation kinetics were monotonic, in accordance with previously reported data [9]. When the mean oxidation rates were compared, AD plasma samples presented with a highly significant increase compared to the samples of controls. This was the case for all three oxidizing conditions: auto-oxidation, oxidation by lipoxygenase and AAPH (Figure 2). As in CSF, plasma oxidation rates did not differ between the corresponding whole and age-matched groups (data not shown).

The levels of antioxidants were in accordance with the results of the oxidation kinetics (Table 1). In the whole AD group the hydrophilic antioxidant ascorbate was significantly lower than in controls. The only lipophilic antioxidant that revealed a significant difference between the AD and control group was α-carotene, which was lower in the patients (Table 1). There was no difference in the levels of α-tocopherol, β-carotene (Table 1), ubiquinol-10 and ubiquinone-10 (data not shown). These results were consistent with the age-matched analysis of the same parameters and the lipid-normalized values expressed as pmol/mg total cholesterol and triglycerides (data not shown). When plasma lipids of AD patients and controls were compared, neither triglycerides nor total cholesterol showed any difference (data not shown).

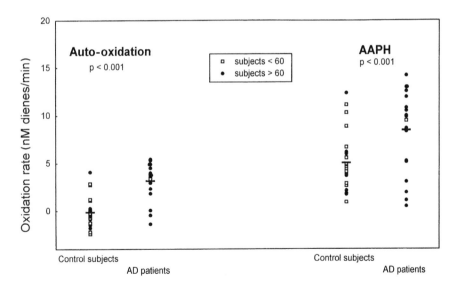

Figure 2. Initial oxidation rate of plasma obtained from AD patients and control subjects. Plasma was diluted 150-fold with PBS and incubated at 37 °C in the absence of exogenous oxidants (auto-oxidation) and in the presence of AAPH (330 μM). Bars correspond with the mean values calculated for each group. Each filled circle and open square corresponds with one subject older and younger than 60 years of age, respectively. Significance of the difference between the groups is shown as a p value

DISCUSSION

Oxidation has been proposed as an important factor in the pathogenesis of AD [2] and Aβ is considered to be a key oxidant [3]. Aβ is found in biological fluids complexed to lipoproteins [5]. On the basis of these findings, we investigated the potential role of lipoprotein oxidation in the pathology of AD. Our study revealed a highly significant increase in the *in vitro* lipoprotein oxidizability in AD compared to controls for both CSF and plasma samples. In addition, a significant decrease in antioxidant levels in both biological fluids could be demonstrated.

These data strongly support the concept of oxidation as an important factor in the pathogenesis of AD. They also suggest that lipoprotein oxidation may be important for the development of AD. Oxidation of plasma lipoproteins is known to be an important factor in development of atherosclerosis [8]. Lipoproteins in CSF have, however, not yet been fully characterized and no data on oxidation of CSF lipoproteins are as yet available. We found an accelerated formation of conjugated dienes in CSF of AD patients during *in vitro* oxidation. Conjugated dienes are lipid hydroperoxides, intermediate oxidation products of unsaturated fatty acids [10]. Most of the CSF fatty acids as well as the lipophilic antioxidants, α-tocopherol and β-carotene, are associated with lipoproteins. The finding that antioxidants were decreased among the AD patients strongly suggests that lipoprotein oxidation is a feature of AD pathology *in vivo*.

These data are also supported by findings of increased amounts of pro-oxidants, such as transition metal ions, in the brains of AD patients [14]. Aβ, another potential pro-oxidant in AD, can generate free radicals [4], and tissue samples of the frontal pole region from the AD brain, showing a heavy burden of senile plaques, can produce free radicals *in vitro* [15]. This suggests that the process of oxidation is secondary to the formation of plaques and Aβ, thus promoting the course of the disease rather than being causal. This is similar to other degenerative diseases, such as atherosclerosis, where oxidation seems to be secondary to high plasma lipid levels and immune responses.

Methodologically, it should be emphasized that the concept of *in vitro* measurement of oxidation to evaluate the *in vivo* situation is technically difficult and its biological relevance must be considered. We have developed a method to measure lipoprotein oxidation in diluted plasma using photometrical registration of the formation of conjugated dienes [9] and adapted it for lipoprotein oxidation in CSF. To verify this method, which determines oxidation products, levels of antioxidants were measured in the same samples. The good agreement between the pro- and antioxidant parameters verified the validity of our approach.

AD, being a multifunctional disease, is neither genetically fully elucidated nor do we know all factors influencing its pathogenesis. With the presented data on the oxidation status of CSF of AD patients, we are adding one meaningful process, oxidation of CSF lipoproteins, to understanding the mechanism of this disease.

REFERENCES

1. Coyle JT, Puttfarcken P. Oxidative stress, glutamate, and neurodegenerative disorders. Science 1993; 262: 689–95.
2. Markesbery WR. Oxidative stress hypothesis in Alzheimer's disease. Free Radic Biol Med 1997; 23: 134–47.
3. Davis JB. Oxidative mechanisms in beta-amyloid cytotoxicity. Neurodegeneration 1996; 5: 441–4.
4. Hensley K, Carney JM, Mattson MP, Aksenova M, Harris M, Wu JF et al. A model for beta-amyloid aggregation and neurotoxicity based on free radical generation by the peptide: relevance to Alzheimer disease. Proc Natl Acad Sci USA 1994; 91: 3270–74.
5. Koudinov AR, Koudinova NV, Kumar A, Beavis RC, Ghiso J. Biochemical characterization of Alzheimer's soluble amyloid beta protein in human cerebrospinal fluid: association with high density lipoproteins. Biochem Biophys Res Commun 1996; 223: 592–7.
6. Pitas RE, Boyles JK, Lee SH, Hui D, Weisgraber KH. Lipoproteins and their receptors in the central nervous system. J Biol Chem 1987; 262: 14352–60.
7. Borghini I, Barja F, Pometta D, James RW. Characterization of subpopulations of lipoprotein particles isolated from human cerebrospinal fluid. Biochim Biophys Acta 1995; 1255: 192–200.
8. Heinecke JW. Mechanisms of oxidative damage of low density lipoprotein in human atherosclerosis. Curr Opin Lipidol 1997; 8: 268–74.
9. Kontush A, Beisiegel U. Measurement of oxidizability of blood plasma. Methods Enzymol 1998 (in press).
10. Esterbauer H, Striegl G, Puhl H, Rotheneder M. Continuous monitoring of *in vitro* oxidation of human low density lipoprotein. Free Radic Res Commun 1989; 6: 67–75.
11. Kontush A, Meyer S, Finckh B, Kohlschütter A, Beisiegel U. Alpha-tocopherol as a reductant for Cu(II) in human lipoproteins. J Biol Chem 1996; 271: 11106–12.
12. Karten B, Beisiegel U, Gercken G, Kontush A. Mechanisms of lipid peroxidation in human blood plasma: a kinetic approach. Chem Phys Lipids 1997; 88: 83–96.
13. Schippling S, Kontush A, Arlt S, Daher D, Buhmann C, Stürenburg HJ, Mann U, Müller-Thomsen T, Beisiegel U. Lipoprotein oxidation and Alzheimer's disease. Nature Med 1998 (submitted).
14. Dedman DJ, Treffry A, Candy JM, Taylor GA, Morris CM, Bloxham CA et al. Iron and aluminium in relation to brain ferritin in normal individuals and Alzheimer's disease and chronic renal dialysis patients. Biochem J 1992; 287: 509–14.
15. Zhou Y, Richardson JS, Mombourquette MJ, Weil JA. Free radical formation in autopsy samples of Alzheimer and control cortex. Neurosci Lett 1995; 195: 89–92.

Address for correspondence:
Professor Ulrike Beisiegel,
Medical Clinic, University Hospital Eppendorf,
Martinistrasse 52, 20246 Hamburg, Germany
Tel: +49 40 47173917; fax: +49 40 47174592;
e-mail: beisiegel@uke.uni-hamburg.de

53 Ectopic Expression of Cell Cycle Components Predicts Neuronal Death in Alzheimer's Disease

K. HERRUP, J. BUSSER AND D.S. GELDMACHER

The occurrence of neuronal cell death during the progress of Alzheimer's disease (AD) has several characteristics that remain to be adequately explained. One of these traits is the characteristic regional variation of the cell loss; a second is the precise biological/biochemical mechanism that mediates the death. This chapter examines the hypothesis that the unscheduled initiation of a cell division cycle in a mature, normally postmitotic neuron leads to an abortive re-activation of a variety of cell cycle components and ultimately the demise of the nerve cell.

CELL DIVISION

Cell division is among the most basic of biological processes. All life forms, from blue-green algae to human hepatocytes, ultimately depend for their survival on the ability of one cell to create two. But while unicellular creatures such as bacteria, protozoa and yeasts are free to divide whenever the nutrient source is adequate, multicellular organisms must tightly regulate the division of their constituent cells if they are to maintain their correct size and shape. Indeed, since life itself depends on the existence of a vigorous cell division process, it is nearly axiomatic that complex organisms must have an equally robust series of mechanisms to hold the cell cycle in check. Nowhere is this need for cellular restraint more crucial than in the adult central nervous system.

The mitotic cell cycle has four recognized phases: G1, S, G2 and M (for recent reviews, see [1, 2]) (Figure 1). The proteins that regulate this process are diverse in both form and function, and a full recapitulation of the protein components is beyond the scope of this chapter. Several salient proteins were utilized in our study, however, and they interface in a known way with the cell

Alzheimer's Disease and Related Disorders
Edited by K. Iqbal, D.F. Swaab, B. Winblad and H.M. Wisniewski
© 1999 John Wiley & Sons Ltd

cycle. When a cell is ready to commit to cell division and leave the G1 phase, the levels of cyclin D increase. Cyclin D is a regulatory subunit of the cell cycle-dependent kinases, cdk4 and cdk6. The cell then enters S phase, where its DNA is replicated. During this period, the levels of proliferating cell nuclear antigen (PCNA—a subunit of the DNA polymerase holoenzyme) are increased. Following S phase, cyclin B (a regulatory subunit of cdk2) increases. Mitosis (M phase) follows shortly thereafter.

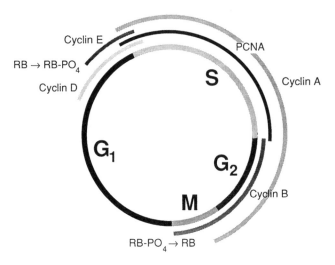

Figure 1. The phases of the cell cycle, with the expression pattern of a few relevant regulators and enzymes illustrated

CELL DEATH

The death of a nerve cell in most advanced vertebrates is a paradox of development and a scourge of old age. In the CNS, nearly all neurons are mitotically generated during embryogenesis. Once neurogenesis is completed, if a neuron is lost for any reason it cannot be replaced. Despite this, the developmental process of many nervous structures normally includes the loss of 50% or more of the originally generated nerve cells [3, 4]. This seemingly wasteful process has been postulated to serve as a means of sculpting a precise numerical balance among neurons and their target populations [5]. During development, target-related cell death, although paradoxical, seems to perform a function that has the potential to enhance the performance of the organism. The same cannot be said for nerve cell deaths that occur later in life. There is little evidence for statistically significant loss of neurons as part of the normal aging process. The extensive cell losses that occur in Alzheimer's disease, therefore, are abnormal and most likely lie at the root of the observed behavioral changes. As with other neurodegenerative disorders, Alzheimer's disease is marked by cell loss that is highly regional in its severity.

AN EMERGING SYNTHESIS

Until recently, the concepts of cell division and cell death seemed not only separate, but polar opposite concepts. Yet during the past few years a substantial body of evidence has accumulated suggesting that the two processes, far from being separate, are intimately related and use many of the same mechanisms for their execution. Some of the first hints of this came from the analyses of transgenic mice, in which researchers attempted to create immortalized cell lines of specific neuronal cell types. Curiously, driving oncogenes such as T-antigen with cell type-specific promoters led to cell death rather than cell division [6, 7]. Careful study of one such case [8] revealed that when T-antigen expression is driven by a cerebellar Purkinje cell specific promoter, (a) expression of the gene can be detected in dying Purkinje cell nuclei; (b) the dying Purkinje cells can be labeled by BrdU before their demise; and (c) the ability of T-antigen to perform this function depended on its ability to bind the tumor suppressor gene, RB. This is significant, since engineered mutations in the mouse Rb-1 gene lead to massive amounts of nerve cell death and prenatal embryo lethality [9–11].

These observations led to the speculation that once a neuroblast made the commitment to stop dividing and begin differentiation, any event that forced it back into the cell cycle would result in its death [11]. Additional evidence for the linkage between the cell cycle and cell death came from tissue culture studies of both PC12 cells and primary cultures of sympathetic neurons. When deprived of NGF, cell cultures of newborn rat superior cervical ganglia undergo a stereotyped cell death. Freeman et al. [12] used quantitative PCR techniques to search for those mRNAs that were increased as the cells began to die. Unexpectedly, one of these genes was cyclin D. At the same time our laboratory was developing *in vivo* evidence in the mouse that target-related cell death in two neurological mutant models was accompanied by the re-expression in the dying cells of several cell cycle markers, including DNA synthesis [13]. Subsequent to this, a series of studies in sympathetic neurons and PC12 cells showed that several drugs that block the cell cycle at a G1/S checkpoint are efficient at preventing the death of both PC12 cells and sympathetic neurons following NGF withdrawal, while agents that block in S, G2 or M phase are ineffective [14–17]. Further evidence in support of the strong linkage between cell cycle and cell death emerged though the increasing association of traditional cell cycle genes with apoptotic cell death [18–20]. The p53 protein, for example, appears to monitor the integrity of the genome as a cell enters division. If DNA damage is too great, it steers the cell into an apoptotic pathway rather than let it divide [21].

All of the above evidence is derived either from trophic factor-treated cell lines or developing neuronal populations. More recently, it appears as if the linkage between apoptosis and the cell cycle is equally relevant to neuro-degenerative diseases of aging. The cdc2 kinase (cdk1) and its associated cyclin B1 have been found to be elevated in the hippocampus of the AD brain [22, 23]. Further, the cdc2/cyclin B complex isolated from these brains has been shown to effectively phosphorylate tau [22]. This is significant, since hyperphosphorylated tau is a major constituent of the neurofibrillary tangles that are a hallmark of AD brain pathology. Cyclin B and cdc2 are both markers for the G2 phase of the cell cycle. Additional evidence for the involvement of cell cycle components in hippocampal cell loss has been developed in several other laboratories [24–26].

Overall, the data from both developing and aging systems establish a strong link between cell death and ectopic cell cycle components. This linkage leads to the following three principles: (a) driving the cell cycle in postmitotic neurons leads to cell death; (b) blocking the cell cycle after trophic factor withdrawal prevents cell death; (c) neuronal cell death in many different situations is correlated with the ectopic appearance of cell cycle components.

CELL CYCLE AND NEURONAL SURVIVAL IN ALZHEIMER'S DISEASE

The persistent correlation of ectopic cell cycle events and neuronal degeneration led us to question whether this same principle applied to nerve cell deaths that occur as part of the aging process. The virtual absence of CNS tumors of neuronal origin is consistent with the hypothesis that the cell cycle–cell death relationship is maintained for the life of the organism. To test its applicability later in life, we turned to autopsy material obtained from individuals who had died with AD. In neuropathological examinations, it is well known that the most common abnormalities are an unusually high density of senile plaques and neurofibrillary tangles, predominantly in hippocampus and entorhinal cortex, with lower densities elsewhere [27, 28]. In addition to the plaques and tangles, there is evidence of significant neuronal cell death, also with distinct regional variability. In some regions, such as the hippocampus, cell loss occurs in conjunction with high densities of plaques and tangles. In other regions, neuronal death is found while the density of plaques and tangles is low. Examples of this latter situation are the basal forebrain [29] and discrete nuclei of the brainstem, such as the dorsal raphe and locus coeruleus [30, 31].

We investigated the brains of 12 neuropathologically verified cases of AD and eight age-matched disease-free controls for the presence of cell cycle proteins. Using immunocytochemical techniques, we found evidence of ectopic expression of cell cycle proteins only in the brains of individuals who have died with AD [32]. Six regions were examined: hippocampus, subiculum, locus coeruleus, dorsal raphe, inferotemporal cortex and cerebellum. In clinically affected individuals, neurons in the first four of these locations are depleted, and in each of these areas we find significant numbers of cells that are immunopositive for one or more of the four cell cycle proteins we studied: cyclin D, cdk4, PCNA and cyclin B1 (Table 1). By contrast, neurons in the same brain sites in non-demented, age-matched control brains showed little to no evidence of immunoreactivity; neither was staining found in the regions of the AD brain where no exceptional cell death was identified. These findings argue for an association between these cell cycle-related proteins and the death of neurons in AD. This conclusion is further strengthened by our observations in the larger neurons of Ammon's horn and the subiculum, where antibodies against hyperphosphorylated tau are found co-localized with the cell cycle components.

We find that the percentages of cyclin D-positive cells are much smaller than the percentages of PCNA- or cyclin B1-positive cells. In agreement with Vincent et al. [22], we do not find mitotic figures. The relationship between the state of these four proteins and a typical cell cycle is unclear. Normally, cyclin D is elevated late in G1 phase; cdk4 levels rise during G1 but remain high; PCNA is present only during S-phase and early G2; and cyclin B1 is elevated only in G2 phase. Superficially, therefore, the cells we have observed in the AD brain would appear to have begun a 'cycle' in which they finish G1, only to become blocked in the later stages. It is very important to consider, however, that the term 'cycle' is a misleading one here, since in a well-regulated cell cycle PCNA levels should go down as cyclin B1 levels rise. Further, the localization of the PCNA and cyclin B1 proteins should be predominantly nuclear, while in our material they can be either nuclear or, more commonly, cytoplasmic. For PCNA this may result in part from the use of formaldehyde fixation [33] but overall it would appear that while the AD neurons can begin a cascade of gene expression that includes various cell cycle components, the tight coordination that characterizes a normal cycle is soon lost.

Table 1. Percentage of immunopositive cells (Normal/AD)

	Cyclin D	PCNA	Cyclin B	cdk4
Hippocampus	0/0.6	0.5/9.0	0.1/8.8	0.1/3.9
Locus coeruleus	0/0.3	0.2/8.3	1.2/4.0	0/10.5
Dorsal raphe	0/0.4	0/11	0.8/11	0/8.9

CONCLUSIONS

The emerging view that reactivation of the cell cycle in a normally postmitotic cell, such as a neuron, is a lethal decision that leads to cell death has many implications for both the biology of neurodegeneration and the development of new therapeutic approaches to AD. It would seem to be a productive approach to begin to consider anti-mitotic compounds as potential agents to arrest the cell loss in AD. These agents would be fundamentally different from those most commonly used in cancer therapy, where the goal is to stop cell cycling by killing any cell that tries to divide. In AD, our hypothesis predicts that this approach would only make a bad situation worse. Rather, compounds need to be developed that prevent the initiation of the cycle. The cell cycle–cell death linkage also suggests a parallel strategy of research aimed at identifying the source of the 'pressure' that coerces a normally postmitotic neuron to attempt to divide. Relief from this pressure may also serve as an alternative therapeutic approach to Alzheimer's disease and possibly many other neurodegenerative conditions.

ACKNOWLEDGEMENTS

This work was supported by funding from the National Institutes of Health (NS20591, A608012).

REFERENCES

1. Weinberg R. The retinoblastoma protein and cell cycle control. Cell 1995; 81: 323–30.
2. Dirks P, Rutka J. Current concepts in neuro-oncology: the cell cycle—a review. Neurosurgery 1997; 40: 1000–1013.
3. Oppenheim R. Cell death during development of the nervous system. Ann Rev Neurosci 1991; 14: 453–501.
4. Williams R, Herrup K. The control of neuron number. Ann Rev Neurosci 1988; 11: 423–53.
5. Herrup K, Sunter K. Numerical matching during cerebellar development: quantitative analysis of granule cell death in staggerer mouse chimeras. J Neurosci 1987; 7: 829–36.
6. al-Ubaidi MR, Hollyfield JG, Overbeek PA, Baehr W. Photoreceptor degeneration induced by the expression of simian virus 40 large tumor antigen in the retina of transgenic mice. Proc Natl Acad Sci USA 1992; 89: 1194–8.
7. Feddersen RM, Ehlenfeldt R, Yunis WS, Clark HB, Orr HT. Disrupted cerebellar cortical development and progressive degeneration of Purkinje cells in SV40 T antigen transgenic mice. Neuron 1992; 9: 955–66.
8. Feddersen R, Clark H, Yunis W, Orr H. In vivo viability of postmitotic Purkinje neurons required pRb family member function. Mol Cell Neurosci 1995; 6: 153–67.
9. Clarke A et al. Requirement for a functional Rb-1 gene in murine development. Nature 1992; 359: 328–30.
10. Jacks T, Fazeli A, Schmitt E, Bronson R, Goodell M, Weinberg R. Effects of an Rb mutation in the mouse. Nature 1992; 359: 295–300.
11. Lee EY et al. Mice deficient for Rb are non-viable and show defects in neurogenesis and haematopoiesis. Nature 359: 288–94.

12. Freeman R, Estus S, Johnson E. Analysis of cell cycle-related gene expression in postmitotic neurons: selective induction of cyclin D1 during programmed cell death. Neuron 1994; 12: 343–55.

13. Herrup K, Busser JC. The induction of multiple cell cycle events precedes target-related neuronal death. Development 1995; 121: 2385–95.

14. Farinelli S, Greene L. Cell cycle blockers mimosine, ciclopirox, and deferoxamine prevent the death of PC12 cells and postmitotic sympathetic neurons after removal of trophic support. J Neurosci 1996; 16: 1150–62.

15. Park D, Farinelli S, Greene L. Inhibitors of cyclin-dependent kinases promote survival of post-mitotic neuronally differentiated PC12 cells and sympathetic neurons. J Biol Chem 1996; 271: 8161–9.

16. Park D, Levine B, Ferrari G, Greene L. Cyclin dependent kinase inhibitors and dominant negative cyclin dependent kinase 4 and 6 promote survival of NGF-deprived sympathetic neurons. J Neurosci 17: 8975–83.

17. Park D, Morris E, Greene L, Geller H. G1/S cell cycle blockers and inhibitors of cyclin-dependent kinases suppress camptothecin-induced neuronal apoptosis. J Neurosci 1997; 17: 1256–70.

18. Meikrantz W, Schlegel R. Apoptosis and the cell cycle. J Cell Biochem 1995; 58: 160–74.

19. Ross M. Cell division and the nervous system: regulating the cycle from neural differentiation to death. Trends Neurosci 1996; 19: 62–8.

20. Heintz N. Cell death and the cell cycle: a relationship between transformation and neurodegeneration? Trends Biochem Sci 1993; 18: 157–9.

21. Morgan S, Kastan M. p53 and ATM: cell cycle, cell death, and cancer. Adv Cancer Res 1997; 71: 1–25.

22. Vincent I, Jicha G, Rosado M, Dickson D. Aberrant expression of mitotic cdc2/cyclin B1 kinase in degenerating neurons of Alzheimer's disease brain. J Neurosci 1997; 17: 3588–98.

23. Vincent I, Rosado M, Davies P. Mitotic mechanisms in Alzheimer's disease? J Cell Biol 1996; 132: 413–25.

24. McShea A, Harris P, Webster K, Wahl A, Smith M. Abnormal expression of the cell cycle regulators p16 and cdk4 in Alzheimer's disease. Am J Pathol 1997; 150: 1933–9.

25. Nagy Z, Esiri M, Cato A, Smith A. Cell cycle markers in the hippocampus in Alzheimer's disease. Acta Neuropathol (Berl) 1997; 94: 6–15.

26. Nagy Z, Esiri M, Smith A. Expression of cell division markers in the hippocampus in Alzheimer's disease and other neurodegenerative conditions. Acta Neuropathol 1997; 93: 294–300.

27. Alzheimer A. Über eine eigenartige Erkangkung der Hirnrinde. Allgemaine Zeitschr Psychiat Psych Gerichtl Med 1907; 64: 146–8.

28. Blessed G, Tomlinson B, Roth M. The association between quantitative measures of dementia and of senile dementia in the cerebral gray matter of elderly subjects. Br Psychiat 1968; 114: 797–811.

29. Whitehouse P, Price D, Struble R, Clark A, Coyle J, DeLong M. Alzheimer's disease and senile dementia: loss of neurons in the basal forebrain. Science 1982; 215: 1237–9.

30. Zweig R et al. The neuropathology of aminergic nuclei in Alzheimer's disease. Ann Neurol 1988; 24: 233–42.

31. Bondareff W, Mountjoy C, Roth M. Loss of neurons of origin of the adrenergic projection to cerebral cortex (nucleus locus coeruleus) in senile dementia. Neurology 1982; 32: 164–8.

32. Busser J, Geldmacher DS, Herrup K. Ectopic cell cycle proteins predict the sites of neuronal cell death in Alzheimer's disease brain. J Neurosci 1998; 18: 2801–7.
33. Bravo R, Frank R, Bludnell P, MacDonald-Bravo H. Cyclin/PCNA is the auxiliary protein of DNA polymerase δ. Nature 1987; 326: 515–17.

Address for correspondence:
   K. Herrup,
   University Alzheimer Center,
   Department of Neurology, Case Western Reserve University,
   10900 Euclid Avenue, Cleveland, OH 44106, USA

54 Neuronal Activity and Genetic Background in Alzheimer's Disease

A. SALEHI, E.J.G. DUBELAAR, T.A. ISHUNINA AND D.F. SWAAB

INTRODUCTION

Alzheimer's disease (AD) is the most common cause of dementia in the elderly. This disorder is characterized by progressive memory loss and other cognitive impairments and by neuropathological lesions, i.e. neuritic plaques (NPs), neurofibrillary tangles (NFTs) and neuropil threads [1]. A series of observations have indicated that, in addition to plaques and tangles, decreased neuronal activity is an essential characteristic of AD and that high or enhanced neuronal activity may protect against the degenerative changes of AD. The brain of AD patients shows a lower total amount of protein, total cytoplasmic RNA, mRNA and glucose metabolism (see [2]). The changes in regional cerebral glucose metabolism, as measured by positron emission tomography (PET), are correlated with Mini-Mental State Examination (MMSE) score in AD patients [3]. The suggestion that reduced neuronal activity in AD brains may by itself be a crucial hallmark for AD [4, 5] raised questions on the nature of the relationship between AD pathology and neuronal activity. As a measure of neuronal metabolic activity, we used the size of the Golgi apparatus (GA), since it has been established that all newly synthesized proteins destined for fast axonal transport are processed through the GA [6] and that a decreased size of the neuronal GA reflects an impairment of protein processing. In a series of studies we established that plaques, tangles and decreased neuronal activity, as determined by the size of the GA, occur independently from each other in various brain areas of AD patients [5, 7–9].

Epidemiological and molecular genetic studies have revealed that the genetic variation in apolipoprotein E (ApoE) is an important risk factor for AD [10]. The inheritance of one or two ApoE ε4 alleles increases the risk of AD and decreases the age of onset of this disease, while ApoE ε2 appears to reduce the risk of AD and to increase the age of onset.

Alzheimer's Disease and Related Disorders
Edited by K. Iqbal, D.F. Swaab, B. Winblad and H.M. Wisniewski
© 1999 John Wiley & Sons Ltd

The lack of relationship between neuronal activity and AD hallmarks (plaques and tangles) prompted us to study the relationship between the number of ApoE ε4 alleles and neuronal metabolism.

MATERIALS AND METHODS

TISSUE COLLECTION

Brains from 30 non-demented controls ranging in age from 29 to 94 years (58.4 ± 3; mean ± SEM) and 41 AD patients ranging in age from 40 to 98 years (72.8 ± 2) were obtained at autopsy. AD was diagnosed clinically based on NINCDS–ADRDA criteria and the diagnosis 'probable AD' was established by excluding other causes of dementia [11]. No significant differences were found in age (p = 0.296), brain weight (p = 0.249), post-mortem delay (p = 0.507), fixation time (p = 0.872), GDS ([12]; p = 0.652) or duration of the disease (p = 0.451) among the three groups of AD patients with either one or two or without any ApoE ε4 alleles.

IMMUNOCYTOCHEMISTRY AND MORPHOMETRY

A polyclonal antibody was raised against immunoaffinity-purified MG-160, a sialoglycoprotein of the medial cisternae of the rat neuronal GA [13] in the nucleus basalis of Meynert (NBM), which is neuropathologically severely affected in AD and also shows severely decreased neuronal activity [5]. Since the NBM is a very extensive cell system, the measurements were performed in a standardized part of the NBM, i.e. the medial subdivision of Ch4a [14], using an IBAS image analysis system (Kontron KAT-based system; [5]). ApoE genotyping was performed on frozen tissue from the cerebellum of the AD patients [15].

RESULTS

The immunocytochemical visualization of the GA in the NBM neurons revealed a cytoplasmic staining with a perinuclear distribution in both neurons and glia. Qualitative microscopic analysis showed that the area occupied by the GA in the cytoplasm of NBM neurons in control subjects was clearly larger than that of AD patients. Furthermore, the GA size of AD patients with ApoE genotype ε3/3 was generally larger than that of AD patients with ApoE genotype ε3/4 or ε4/4. The mean area of the GA in control subjects (127.8 ± 10.4 μm²; mean GA size ± SEM) was significantly larger (p < 0.001) than that of AD patients (63.7 ± 4.3 μm²). As far as the AD group was concerned, the Kruskal–Wallis test showed significant differences (p = 0.002) in GA size and mean profile area among the three groups of patients with different ApoE genotypes.

AD patients with ApoE genotype ε3/3 had a mean GA size of 85.1 ± 5.2 μm², while AD patients with ApoE genotype ε3/4 had a mean GA size of 51.9 ± 5.9 μm² [16]. The patients with ApoE genotype ε4/4 had a mean GA size of 48.8 ± 8.1 μm². The mean GA size of AD patients with ApoE genotype ε3/4 or ε4/4 was significantly (p < 0.001) lower than the mean GA size of AD patients with ApoE genotype ApoE ε3/3. The size of the GA of AD patients with ApoE genotype ε4/4 was not different (p = 0.760) from that of AD patients with ApoE genotype ε3/4. The cell profile area of AD patients with ApoE genotype ε3/4 (254.1 ± 17.0 μm²) or 4/4 (187.3 ± 23.0 μm²) was significantly lower (p < 0.001) than that of AD patients with ApoE genotype ε3/3 (346.1 ± 12.1 μm²).

DISCUSSION

Mutations in different genes located in chromosomes 21, 14 and 1 are invariably associated with AD [17, 18]. In contrast, the ApoE ε4 variant associated with AD can also be found in quite elderly, cognitively normal individuals, indicating that ApoE ε4 should be considered a risk factor for AD. Polymorphism in specific regions of the ApoE gene might be of importance for the occurrence of AD [19]. The mechanism of involvement of ApoE in AD is not known. It has been hypothesized that ApoE affects the deposition of amyloid or interacts with the microtubule associated protein tau. In addition, a role of ApoE in neuronal repair and degeneration has been suggested [20–23], and it was proposed that ApoE ε4 might be less able to support neuronal survival during neurodegeneration than ApoE ε2 or ε3. The prevalence of ApoE indeed correlates with β-amyloid accumulation [10, 24] and neurofibrillary tangle formation [24, 25]. However, in a recent study, we did not find any clear relationship between the number of ApoE ε4 alleles and the occurrence of early cytoskeletal alterations [26]. Moreover, the role of ApoE in the cascade of cholesterol and phospholipid transport and re-uptake and the involvement of these mechanisms in repair in brain aging and AD [20–23] should be taken into consideration. Because the transport of cholesterol and other lipoproteins plays a central role in synaptogenesis, it is possible that AD patients differing in their ApoE phenotype also differ in their capacities of synaptogenesis. Recent *in vitro* data have shown that in the presence of a lipid source, ApoE ε3 enhances and ApoE ε4 inhibits neurite outgrowth in neuronal cell cultures [27]. As far as amyloid is concerned, an enhanced dose-dependent burden of β-amyloid has been observed in ApoE ε4 carriers [10, 24, 25]. Furthermore, it has been shown that inhibition of energy metabolism can influence APP processing, leading to decreased secretion of non-amyloidogenic fragments of APP [28]. One may suggest, therefore, that ApoE ε4 alleles increase the burden of amyloid by inhibition of energy metabolism. On the other hand, we found no clear relationship between GA size and the distance of neurons from NPs [29], pleading against such a local inhibitory effect of amyloid on neuronal metabolism.

Our study shows that one of the possible mechanisms by which ApoE ε4 participates in the pathogenesis of AD is through regulation of metabolic activity of neurons. Interestingly, it has been shown that a decrease in cerebral glucose metabolism may precede cognitive impairment. Cognitively normal subjects homozygous for ApoE ε4 alleles already appear to have reduced glucose metabolism in the same regions of the brain as the ones affected in AD patients [30].

We could not find any significant difference in the GA size between AD patients with ApoE genotype ε4/4 and those with ε3/4. This indicates that the relationship between the size of the GA and the number of ApoE ε4 alleles is not dose-dependent and that there may be a threshold effect in the NBM, as was found for the cholinergic deficit in the NBM [21]. It may well be that the GA itself is a direct target of ApoE ε4 alleles. In support of this possibility, Verde et al. [28] showed that ATP depletion blocks the export of proteins from the endoplasmic reticulum to the intermediate compartment of the Golgi complex, which may lead to GA shrinkage.

One of the most consistent neurochemical abnormalities in AD brains is a cholinergic deficit, as evidenced by a loss of ChAT and AChE in the neocortex and hippocampus, and a degeneration of cholinergic neurons in the NBM [5, 28]. Recent studies have indicated that AD patients carrying an ApoE ε4 allele have a more severe cholinergic deficit in several areas of the brain. All these data support the notion that ApoE plays a crucial role in the metabolic activity of the cholinergic neurons of the NBM. Our data suggest that ApoE ε4 may be a risk factor for the development of AD by reducing neuronal metabolism. It may be presumed that a lower protein synthetic ability of the NBM neurons in AD predisposes them to neurodegeneration [4].

Recently we found that there is a clear relationship between the expression of low affinity neurotrophin receptors, i.e. P75, and the size of the GA in the hypothalamic supraoptic nucleus (Ishunina et al., in preparation). This increased size of the GA may indicate enhanced response of neurons to neurotrophins. This suggests that an enhanced supply of neurotrophins goes together with enhanced metabolic rate of neurons, which is in line with data of Arendt et al. [31] showing a clear negative relationship between the number of ApoE ε4 alleles and the expression of p75 receptors in the nucleus basalis of AD patients. Furthermore, this possibility is in accordance with our own data showing a dramatic reduction in the expression of both tyrosine kinase trk receptors [32] and the GA size [5] in the NBM of Alzheimer patients.

The proposal that ApoE type influences the metabolic activity of neurons may have clinical implications, since it supports the idea that in cholinergic treatment of AD patients the ApoE genotype should be taken into account. The differential responses to drugs with cholinergic-enhancing effects, such as tacrine, by AD individuals with different ApoE types could be explained by our data. Poirier [21] indeed showed that patients without ε4 alleles responded significantly better to a 30-week period of tacrine treatment than AD patients carrying the ApoE ε alleles.

ACKNOWLEDGEMENTS

This work was supported by a grant from Internationale Stichting Alzheimer Onderzoek (ISAO; A.S.).

REFERENCES

1. Trojanowski JQ, Schmidt ML, Shin RW et al. PHFt (A68): from pathological marker to potential mediator of neuronal dysfunction and degeneration in Alzheimer's disease. Clin Neurosci 1993; 1: 184–91.
2. Swaab DF, Lucassen PJ, Salehi A et al. Reduced neuronal activity and reactivation in Alzheimer's disease. In: van Leeuwen FW, Salehi A, Giger RJ, Holtmaat AJGD, Verhaagen J (eds) Neuronal Degeneration and Regeneration: From Basic Mechanisms to Prospects for Therapy. Progress in Brain Research, Vol. 117. Amsterdam: Elsevier; 343–77.
3. Mielke R, Herholz K, Grond M et al. Clinical deterioration in probable Alzheimer's disease correlates with progressive metabolic impairment of association areas. Dementia 1994; 5: 36–41.
4. Swaab DF. Brain aging and Alzheimer's disease, 'wear and tear' versus 'use it or lose it'. Neurobiol Aging 1991; 12: 317–24.
5. Salehi A, Lucassen PJ, Pool CW et al. Decreased neuronal activity in the nucleus basalis of Alzheimer's disease as suggested by the size of the Golgi. Neuroscience 1994; 59: 871–80.
6. Hammerschlag R, Stone GC, Bolen FA et al. Evidence that all newly synthesized proteins destined for fast axonal transport pass through the Golgi apparatus. J Cell Biol 1982; 93: 568–75.
7. Salehi A, Van de Nes JAP, Hofman MA et al. Early cytoskeletal changes as shown by Alz-50 are not accompanied by decrease neuronal activity. Brain Res 1995; 678: 29–39.
8. Salehi A, Heyn S, Gonatas NK, Swaab DF. Decreased protein synthetic activity of the hypothalamic tuberomamillary nucleus in Alzheimer's disease, as suggested by smaller Golgi aparatus. Neurosci Lett 1995; 193: 29–32.
9. Salehi A, Ravid R, Gonatas NK, Swaab DF. Decreased activity of hippocampal neurons in Alzheimer's disease is not related to the presence of neurofibrillary tangles. J Neuropathol Exp Neurol 1995; 54: 704–9.
10. Corder EH, Saunders AM, Strittmatter WJ et al. Gene dose of apolipoprotein E type 4 allele and the risk of Alzheimer's disease in late-onset families. Science 1993; 261: 921–3.
11. McKhann G, Drachman D, Folstein M et al. Clinical diagnosis of Alzheimer's disease: report of NINCDS–ADRDA work group under the auspices of Department of Health and Human Service Task Force on Alzheimer's disease. Neurology 1984; 34: 939–44.
12. Reisberg B, Ferris SH, Leon De MJ et al. The Global Deterioration Scale for assessment of primary degenerative dementia. Am J Psychiat 1982; 139: 1136–9.
13. Croul S, Mezitis SGE, Stieber A et al. Immunocytochemical visualization of the Golgi apparatus in several species, including human, and tissues with an antiserum against MG-160, a sialoglycoprotein of rat Golgi apparatus. J Histochem Cytochem 1990; 38: 957–63.
14. Mesulam MM, Mufson EJ, Levey AI, Wainer BH. Atlas of cholinergic neurons in the forebrain and upper brainstem of the macaque based on monoclonal choline acetyltransferase immunohistochemistry and acetylcholinesterase histochemistry. Neuroscience 1984; 12: 669–86.
15. Crook R, Hardy J, Duff KJ. Single-day apolipoprotein E genotyping. J Neurosci Methods 1994; 53: 125–7.

16. Salehi A, Dubelaar EJG, Mulder M, Swaab DF. Aggravated decrease in the activity of nucleus basalis neurons in Alzheimer's disease is ApoE type dependent. Proc Natl Acad Sci USA 1998; 95: 11445–9.
17. Sherrington R, Rogaev EI, Liang Y et al. Cloning of a gene bearing missense mutations in early-onset familial Alzheimer's disease. Nature 1995; 375: 754–60.
18. Rogaev EI, Sherrington R, Rogaev EA et al. Familial Alzheimer's disease in kindreds with missense mutations in a gene in chromosome 1 related to the Alzheimer's disease type 3 gene. Nature 1995; 376: 775–8.
19. Bullido MJ, Artiga MJ, Recuero M et al. A polymorphism in the regulatory region of APOE associated with risk for Alzheimer's dementia. Nature Genet 1998; 18: 69–71.
20. Beffert U, Danik M, Krzywkowski P et al. The neurobiology of apolipoproteins and their receptors in the CNS and Alzheimer's disease. Brain Res Rev 1998; 27: 119–41.
21. Poirier J, Delisle M-C, Quirion R et al. Apolipoprotein E4 allele as a predictor of cholinergic deficits and treatment outcome in Alzheimer's disease. Proc Natl Acad Sci USA 1995; 92: 12260–64.
22. Poirier J, Davignon J, Bouthillier D, Kogan S, Bertrand P, Gauthier S. Apolipoprotein E polymorphism and Alzheimer's disease. Lancet 1993; 342: 697–9.
23. Masliah E, Mallory M, Alford M et al. Neurodegeneration in the central nervous system of apoE-deficient mice. Exp Neurol 1995; 136: 107–22.
24. Strittmatter WJ, Weisgraber KH, Huang DY et al. Binding of human apolipoprotein E to synthetic amyloid-β isoform-specific effects and implications for late-onset disease. Proc Natl Acad Sci USA 1993; 90: 8098–102.
25. Nagy Z, Esiri MM, Jobst KA et al. Influence of the apolipoprotein E genotype on amyloid deposition and neurofibrillary tangle formation in Alzheimer's disease. Neuroscience 1995; 69: 757–61.
26. Salehi A, Gonzalez-Martinez V, Swaab DF. A sex difference and no effect of ApoE type on the amount of cytoskeletal alterations in the nucleus basalis of Meynert in Alzheimer's disease. Neurobiol Aging (in press).
27. Lovestone S, Anderton BH, Hartley C et al. The intracellular fate of apolipoprotein E is tau dependent and ApoE allele-specific. NeuroReport 1996; 7: 1005–8.
28. Verde C, Pascale MC, Martire G et al. Effect of ATP depletion and DTT on the transport of membranes from endoplasmatic reticulum and the intermediate compartment to the Golgi complex. Eur J Cell Biol 1995; 67: 267–74.
29. Salehi A, Pool CW, Mulder M et al. Activity of hippocampal CA1 neurons in Alzheimer's disease is not affected by the presence of adjacent neuritic plaques. J Alz Dis (in press).
30. Reiman EM, Caselli RJ, Yun LS et al. Preclinical evidence of Alzheimer's disease in persons homozygous for the ε4 alleles for apolipoprotein E. N Engl J Med 1996; 334: 252–8.
31. Arendt T, Schindler C, Brückner MK et al. Plastic neuronal remodeling is impaired in patients with Alzheimer's disease carrying apolipoprotein e4 alele. J Neuroscience 1997; 17: 516–29.
32. Salehi A, Verhaagen J, Dijkhuizen PJ, Swaab DF. Co-localization of high-affinity neurotrophin receptors in nucleus basalis of Meynert neurons and their differential reduction in Alzheimer's disease. Neuroscience 1996; 75: 373–87.

Address for correspondence:
A. Salehi,
Netherlands Institute for Brain Research,
Meibergdreef 33, 1105 AZ Amsterdam, The Netherlands
Tel: 031 20 5665503; fax: 031 20 6961006;
e-mail: A.Salehi@nih.knaw.nl

55 L-Deprenyl Protects Vascular Endothelium from Amyloid-β Toxicity and Stimulates Production of Nitric Oxide

TOM THOMAS, CHRIS McLENDON AND
GEORGE THOMAS

INTRODUCTION

Selegiline (L-deprenyl, Eldepryl) is an irreversible inhibitor of mitochondrial monoamine oxidase type-B (MAO-B) and has been used clinically in combination with levo-dopa (L-dopa) to treat Parkinson's disease [1]. MAO inhibitors (e.g. iproniazid) were among the first psychotropic agents to be discovered as antidepressants and introduced into clinical practice [1]. It has been reported that selegiline alone can significantly delay the onset of disability associated with early untreated PD [2]. The drug has also been shown to improve the clinical condition of Alzheimer's disease (AD) patients [3] and depression [4]. A plethora of evidence suggests that the clinical efficacy of selegiline may be due to novel and hereto unrecognized properties that are unrelated to the inhibition of MAO-B activity. Much of the current interest in MAO-B inhibitors is based on the possibility that these compounds possess neuroprotective effects and may retard the progression of neurodegenerative diseases. AD is a heterogeneous and complex disorder but Aβ toxicity mediated by free radical generation, altered calcium homeostasis and inflammatory changes is believed to contribute to the disease process. Parkinson's disease (PD) is characterized by progressive destruction of dopaminergic neurons, possibly mediated by the generation of free radicals. There is considerable overlap between AD and PD in terms of age of occurrence, presence of dementia, role of free radical-mediated oxidative stress and Aβ deposits in the brain.

We recently demonstrated [5–7] that vascular damage induced by Aβ may be an early event in the pathology of AD and this free radical-mediated damage was prevented by antioxidants. Since selegiline has been shown to

Alzheimer's Disease and Related Disorders
Edited by K. Iqbal, D.F. Swaab, B. Winblad and H.M. Wisniewski
© 1999 John Wiley & Sons Ltd

have a protective effect against the progression of AD and PD, we investigated the action of this compound on vasoactivity and Aβ-induced vascular damage.

METHODS

Nitric oxide was quantified by measuring accumulation of nitrites using the Griess assay for nitrites, as previously described [8]. Brain tissue from various regions or segments of isolated middle cerebral artery were incubated (30 min at 37 °C) in 2.5 ml of oxygenated Krebs buffer solution in the presence or absence of test compounds.

Thoracic rat aorta and/or bovine middle cerebral arteries with intact endothelium were maintained in a perfusion bath containing oxygenated Krebs bicarbonate buffer at 37 °C, as previously described [5–7]. The vessels were preconstricted submaximally, as previously described, and relaxed with increasing doses of ACH, 5-HT or L-deprenyl ($0.1–400 \times 10^{-6}$ M). These contraction/relaxations were repeated following incubation with various antagonists, or enzyme inhibitors. To assess the *in vivo* effects of selegiline, adult male Sprague–Dawley rats weighing 200–250 g (n = 4 per group) were injected intraperitoneally (IP) with 10 mg/kg body weight of freshly prepared L-deprenyl in saline. Control animals were injected with saline alone. After 1 h the animals were sacrificed and the aorta were isolated and sectioned as described above. Points marked by (*) in the figures are significantly different from respective control values, as determined by one-way analysis of variance (ANOVA) ($p < 0.05$).

RESULTS

STIMULATION OF NO PRODUCTION BY SELEGILINE

Selegiline produced a significant increase in NO production, whereas the endogenous NOS stimulant, L-glutamate, had only a minimal effect in rat brain (Figure 1A). In bovine cerebellum both 10 and 100 µM selegiline produced significantly more NO than 1 mM glutamate. D-deprenyl, which is the biologically less active isomer, had considerably less activity. Selegiline stimulated NO production in all the brain regions examined as well as a midcerebral artery (Figure 1B).

To investigate the *in vivo* vascular effect of selegiline, aortas from selegiline- or saline-injected rats were dissected 1 h following injection. The enhanced sensitivity of the selegiline-treated aorta to the vasodilator acetylcholine is illustrated in Figure 2A. The aorta from the treated animal retained the effect of the drug even after extensive washing of the tissue. This would indicate that the effects of the drug on the vasculature persists for a significant period of time.

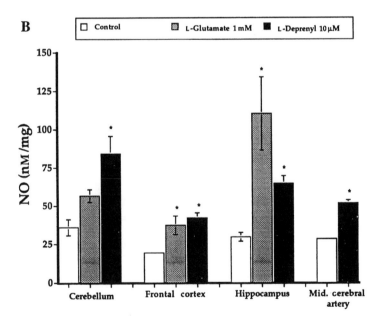

Figure 1. Stimulation of NO production induced by deprenyl. (A) In whole rat brain L-deprenyl (10 μM) produced considerable amounts of NO at concentrations 100-fold lower than that of L-glutamate (1 mM). In bovine cerebellum L-deprenyl produced NO in a dose-dependent manner. L-deprenyl generated considerably more NO than the clinically inactive isomer D-deprenyl or the endogenous activator L-glutamate. (B) Comparison of NO production by L-glutamate (1 mM) or L-deprenyl (10 μM) in various brain regions and middle cerebral arteries showed that L-deprenyl produced significantly more NO than L-glutamate. ★ See text for explanation

A

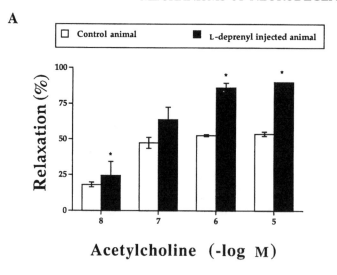

Acetylcholine (-log M)

B

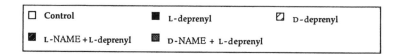

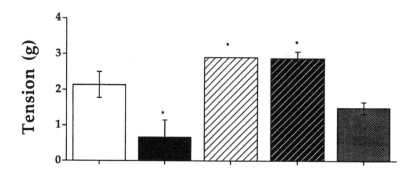

Figure 2. (A) *In vivo* vascular effect of L-deprenyl. Enhanced response to acetyl-choline in the L-deprenyl injected rat aorta is evident from the increased response to low concentrations of ACH. (B) Effect of L-deprenyl on PE-induced vasoconstriction of peripheral arteries. L-deprenyl significantly reduced vasoconstriction, while the bio-logically inactive isomer D-deprenyl had a detectable stimulatory effect on the contraction. L-deprenyl significantly diminished PE-induced vasoconstriction. Pretreatment with NOS inhibitor L-NAME nearly abolished the L-deprenyl effect. The inactive isomer D-NAME was considerably less effective in blocking the L-deprenyl effect. * See text for explanation

Comparison of the activities of the biologically active L-deprenyl and the less active isomer D-deprenyl clearly demonstrates the superior ability of L-deprenyl in antagonizing the PE-induced contraction (Figure 2B). Pretreatment of the intact aortic rings with the nitric oxide synthase inhibitor L-NAME abolished the inhibitory action of selegiline.

Figure 3A demonstrates the dose-dependent vasodilation of cerebral arteries with L-deprenyl. Lower doses (≤25 μM) produced rapid and transient vasodilatory responses in vessels with intact endothelium. Higher doses (≥50 μM) produced slower, more sustained relaxations.

Figure 3B demonstrates the ability of L-deprenyl to attenuate vascular damage produced by the Alzheimer's protein β-amyloid. Preincubation with $A\beta_{1-40}$ produced a significant increase in vasoconstriction induced by 5-HT in bovine middle cerebral artery. Pretreating the vessels with L-deprenyl 10 min prior to the addition of $A\beta_{1-40}$ completely abolished this increase in vasoconstriction.

DISCUSSION

Selegiline (L-deprenyl) is one of the few compounds that are capable of delaying functional deterioration in neurodegenerative diseases [2, 3]. The renewed interest in selegiline is based on the possibility that it could be a prototype drug for agents with neuroprotective and life-extending properties [9]. Dysfunction of the normal endothelial mechanisms has been found in aging and cardiovascular diseases. The blood–brain barrier is composed of endothelial cells and, by protecting the endothelium, selegiline would ensure the viability of the blood–brain barrier. Reduced cerebral blood flow implicating a vascular component in the pathology of AD and PD has been previously reported [10]. Cerebral deposits of Aβ are hallmarks of AD and to a lesser extent PD [11, 12]. Recent reports [5–7] of a rapid and direct action of the AD peptide Aβ on endothelium could account for many of the vascular abnormalities observed in the brains of patients with AD. The Aβ-induced vascular damage could be an early event relative to the development of neurodegenerative diseases. The prevention of Aβ toxicity to endothelial cells by selegiline represents another mechanism whereby the drug may play a cytoprotective role.

Studies of AD patients have shown a consistent relationship between neuronal and vascular pathology. A number of vascular diseases often precede or accompany the onset of AD, including hypertension, atherosclerosis, coronary artery disease, vasospasm, stroke and cerebral ischemia [13].

The role of oxidative stress in degenerative diseases may account for the cumulative damage associated with the delayed onset and progressive nature of these disorders. Free radical generation by Aβ could contribute to an imbalance between the production of nitric oxide and oxygen radicals and precipitate an oxidative stress [14]. The rapid stimulation of NO production in

A

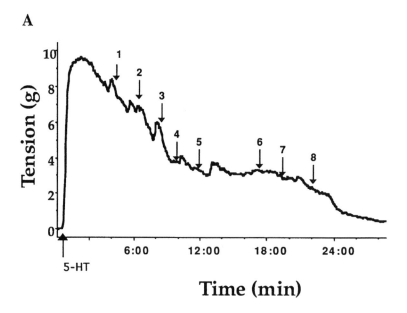

B

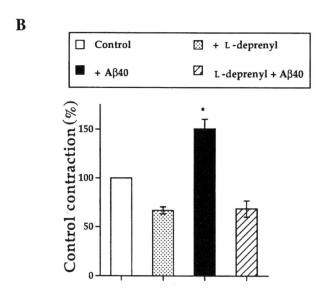

Figure 3. Cerebrovascular effects of L-deprenyl. (A) In bovine middle cerebral arteries with intact endothelium, low doses (≤10 μM) of L-deprenyl were capable of eliciting a rapid vasodilatory response, while high doses relaxed the vessel nearly to basal levels. (B) L-deprenyl is capable of antagonizing the Aβ-induced enhancement of contraction in bovine cerebral vessels. * See text for explanation

brain tissue and blood vessel by selegiline indicates the activation of the constitutive form of NO synthase, which could potentially alleviate the oxidative stress and prevent degenerative changes. The facilitation of LTP and synaptic plasticity by NO might be a factor in the neuroprotective ability of selegiline. The stimulation of NO production by selegiline might enhance motor functions in PD. Selegiline readily crosses the blood–brain barrier, has minimal adverse effects in the elderly and can be administered orally or transdermally [15]. The novel actions of L-deprenyl reported here—stimulation of NO production, vasodilation and protection of vascular endothelium from Aβ toxicity—might contribute to the clinical efficacy of the drug. Prophylactic use of low doses of L-deprenyl may accord protection against vascular diseases, stroke and neurodegenerative disorders associated with aging.

REFERENCES

1. Youdim MBH, Finberg JPM. Monoamine oxidase inhibitor antidepressants. In: Grahme-Smith DH, Hippius A, Winoker H. Psychopharmacology. Amsterdam: Excerpta Medica, 1985; 37–62.
2. The Parkinson Study Group. Effects of tocopherol and deprenyl on the progression of disability in early Parkinson's disease. N Engl J Med 1993; 328: 176–83.
3. Sano M, Ernesto C, Thomas RG, Klauber MR, Schafer K, Grundman M, Woodbury P, Growden J, Cotman CW, Pfieffer E, Schneider LS, Thal LJ. A controlled trial of selegiline, alpha tocopherol, or both as treatment for Alzheimer's disease. N Engl J Med 1997; 336: 1216–22.
4. Gerlach M, Reiderer P, Youdim MBH. The molecular pharmacology of L-deprenyl. Eur J Pharmacol 1992; 226: 97–108.
5. Thomas T, Thomas G, McLendon C et al. β-Amyloid-mediated vasoactivity and endothelial dysfunction. Nature 1996; 380: 168–71.
6. Thomas T, Sutton ET, McLendon C, Thomas G. Cerebrovascular endothelial dysfunction mediated by β-amyloid. NeuroReport 1997; 8: 1387–91.
7. Thomas T, Sutton ET, Bryant M, Rhodin J. *In vivo* leukocyte activation and inflammatory response induced by β-Amyloid. J Submicrosc Cytol Pathol 1997; 29: 293–304.
8. Cook JA, Kim SY, Teague D, Krishna MC, Pacelli R, Mitchell JB, Vodovots Y, Nims RW, Christodoulou D, Miles AM, Grisham MB, Wink D. Convenient colorimetric and fluorometric assays for S-nitrosothiols. Anal Biochem 1996; 238: 150–58.
9. Birkmayer WJ, Knoll P, Riederer P. Increased life expectancy resulting from addition of L-deprenyl to madopar treatment in Parkinson's disease: a long term study. J Neur Transm 1985; 64: 113–27.
10. Oishi MN, Mochizuki Y, Hara M, Du CM, Takasu T. Effects of intravenous L-dopa on P300 and regional cerebral flow in parkinsonism. Intern J Neurosci 1996; 85: 147–54.
11. Guiroy DC, Mellini M, Miyazaki M, Hilbich C, Safar J, Garruto RM, Yanagihara R, Beyreuther K, Gajdusek DC. Neurofibrillary tangles of Guamanian amyotrophic lateral sclerosis, parkinsonism-dementia and neurologically normal Guamanians contain a 4–4.5 kilodalton protein which is immunoreactive to anti-amyloid β/A4-protein antibodies. Acta Neuropathol 1993; 86: 265–74.

12. Kalaria RN. Cerebral vessels in aging and Alzheimer's disease. Pharmacol Ther 1996; 72: 193–214.
13. Hofman A, Ott A, Breteler MM, Bots ML, Slooter AJ, van Harskamp F, van Duijn CN, Van Broeckhoven C, Grobbee DE. Atherosclerosis, apolipoprotein E, and prevalence of dementia and Alzheimer's disease in the Rotterdam Study. Lancet 1997; 349: 151–4.
14. Stamler JS. Alzheimer's disease: a radical vascular connection. Nature 1996; 380: 108–11.
15. Barret JS, Hochadel TJ, Morales RJ, Rohatagi S, DeWilt KE, Watson SK, DiSanto AR. Pharmacokinetics and safety of a selegiline transdermal system relative to single-dose oral administration in the elderly. Am J Therapeut 1996; 3: 688–98.

Address for correspondence:

Tom Thomas MD PhD,
Woodlands Medical and Research Center,
3150 Tampa Road,
Oldsmar, Florida 34677, USA
Tel: (727) 786 5587; fax: (727) 785 3254;
e-mail: tthomas1@tampabay.rr.com

56 A Family with Late-onset Alzheimer's Disease Carrying a Val91Met Mutation of the Apolipoprotein A-II Gene Suggests Altered Plasma Lipid Metabolism in Alzheimer's Disease

KOUZIN KAMINO, ELLEN WIJSMAN, LEO ANDERSON,
ELLEN NEMENS, HIDEHISA YAMAGATA,
SHIGEO OHTA, THOMAS D. BIRD AND
GERARD D. SCHELLENBERG

INTRODUCTION

Apolipoprotein E (APOE)-ε4 allele modifies the risk for familial and sporadic late-onset Alzheimer's disease (AD) in a gene–dose-dependent manner [1, 2]. The APOE-ε4 allele is associated with high plasma LDL cholesterol level [3], and the APOE-ε4 allele could also induce elevated LDL cholesterol levels in the brain, possibly leading to elevation of oxidized LDL cholesterol that could cause both necrotic and apoptotic neuronal death [4]. On the other hand, plasma high-density lipoprotein (HDL) cholesterol, apolipoprotein (apo) A-I and A-II levels in late-onset AD are decreased [5, 6]. Since the interaction between LDL and HDL cholesterol could affect the delivery of oxidized lipoproteins from neurons into the cerebral blood circulation, the APO A-II locus, shown to link to the plasma apo A-II level and to affect the plasma HDL-cholesterol level [7, 8], could modify the risk for AD. To examine the genetic relationship between late-onset AD and the APO A-II gene, we performed a screening for sequence alterations of the APO-AII gene in Caucasian familial cases with late-onset AD, and also examined the relationship between a polymorphism within an Alu sequence 3' to the APO-AII gene [9] and sporadic cases with AD.

Alzheimer's Disease and Related Disorders
Edited by K. Iqbal, D.F. Swaab, B. Winblad and H.M. Wisniewski
© 1999 John Wiley & Sons Ltd

SUBJECTS AND METHODS

Sixty-seven unrelated Caucasian familial cases with late-onset AD reported previously [10, 11] were screened for sequence alterations of the APO A-II gene. One hundred and fourteen patients with sporadic AD and 184 non-demented age-matched control subjects in the Caucasian population, and 107 sporadic patients with probable late-onset AD and 218 age-matched control subjects in the Japanese population were investigated in the association study of an APO A-II polymorphism. Patients with probable late-onset AD were diagnosed according to the criteria of the National Institute of Neurological and Communicative Disorders and the Stroke–Alzheimer's Disease and Related Disorders Association (NINCDS–ADRDA) [12].

Direct sequencing of four exons of the APO A-II gene was performed, based on the sequence information reported previously [13]. Briefly, the whole genomic region of the APO A-II gene was amplified using LA-Taq kit (TAKARA, Kyoto), and applied to direct sequencing with primers for each exon, using the Dye-terminator Sequencing Kit and the ABI Sequencer (Applied Biosystems).

A Val-to-Met mutation at codon 91 of the APO A-II gene (Val91Met) was screened for by PCR-RFLP, in 15 µl reaction volume with 10 ng DNA, 7.5 pmol of each primer, AK8: CCTTTTCCTTCCTCTTCTCCTCCCTTAC and AK27: TGCTCTGACCTCCCACCACCACC, 200 mM each dNTP, 2.5 mM $MgCl_2$, 0.375 unit of Taq polymerase, by thermal cycling of 30 cycles of 94 °C for 30 s and 63 °C for 1 min; after digestion with Nla III, the PCR product was subjected to 3% agarose electrophoresis, where the Val allele shows 385 bp and the Met mutant allele shows 169 and 216 bp. For DNA extracted from paraffin-embedded slices, short PCR product (73 bp) was amplified in a 10 µl reaction volume composed of 1 pmol of ^{32}P-end-labeled and 4 pM of unlabeled primer AK28B: AGAAGGCTGGAACGGAAC-TGGT, 5 pM of primer AK29: CACTGGGTGGCAGGCTGTGT, 20 mM each dNTP, 1.5 mM $Mgcl_2$, and 0.25 unit of Taq polymerase with the reaction buffer (Promega), by thermal cycling of 35 cycles of 94 °C for 30 s and 60 °C for 1 min, and after digestion with Nla III, subjected in denaturing polyacrylamide gel electrophoresis and autoradiography.

The genotype of a Msp I polymorphism within an Alu sequence 3' to the APO A-II gene was determined [9], where the rare M1 allele encoding T at nucleotide (nt) 2769 according to the base numbering by Knott et al. [13] loses the Msp I site, which the common M2 allele encoding C harbors. P value less than 0.05 by χ^2 statistics was considered significant.

RESULTS

Among 67 unrelated cases with late-onset AD, one case (the BOB family) disclosed a base change of guanine to adenine at nt2157 according to the base numbering by Knott et al. (1985), resulting in amino acid substitution at codon 91 of Val to Met (Val91Met). This Val91Met mutation creates a novel Nla III site. Among four affected in the BOB family, the Val91Met mutation was found in three patients, but not in one patient with age at onset of 87 years. This mutation was not found in unaffected siblings except for one subject who died aged 67 without dementia, according to the genotyping of his/her descendants (Figure 1). None of sporadic patients with AD and control subjects harbored this mutation in either the Caucasian or the Japanese population.

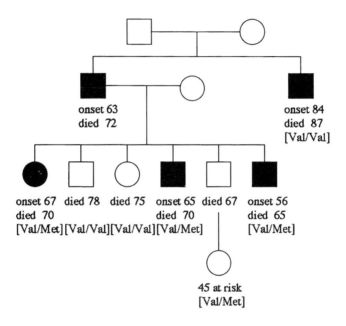

Figure 1. Genotyping of a family carrying the Val91Met mutation

The Msp I polymorphism within an Alu sequence 3' to the APO A-II gene was genotyped and examined the association with AD. In the Japanese subjects, the frequency of the rare M1 allele was slightly higher in the patient group than in the control group (0.313 vs. 0.288; p = 0.50), and the frequency of subjects with M1/M1 genotype was also higher in the patient group (0.140 vs. 0.084; p = 0.11) (Table 1). In the Caucasian group, the frequency of subjects with the M1/M1 genotype was lower than in the Japanese group, and the same trend was found (M1 allele frequency, 0.158 vs. 0.122; M1/M1 genotype frequency, 0.018 vs. 0.005). However, these differences were not statistically significant.

Table 1. Genotype frequency of the Msp I polymorphism within an Alu sequence 3' to the APO A-II gene

Genotype	M1/M1	M1/M2	M2/M2	Total
Japanese				
Late-onset AD	15 (0.140)	37 (0.346)	55 (0.514)	107
Control	20 (0.084)	97 (0.408)	121 (0.320)	218
Caucasion				
AD	2 (0.018)	32 (0.280)	80 (0.702)	114
Control	1 (0.005)	43 (0.234)	140 (0.761)	184

Allele frequencies of the M1 allele (patient vs. control) were 0.313 vs. 0.288 in Japanese and 0.158 vs. 0.122 in Caucasian. The differences of the M1/M1 genotype frequency between patient and control groups were not significant, though the same trend was found in both populations (p = 0.11 for Japanese, p = 0.30 for Caucasian, respectively).

DISCUSSION

We identified a novel Val91Met mutation of the APO A-II gene in patients with familial late-onset AD, and genomic analysis of patients' families indicated incomplete penetrance of the effect of this mutation for development of late-onset AD.

Apo A-II is synthesized mainly in the liver and partly in the small intestine and transported in the blood circulation, in contrast to apoE, which is synthesized in a wide range of tissues. Human apo A-II exists in plasma HDL mainly as disulfide-linked homodimers (17.4 kDa) [14] and heterodimers with apoD (38 kDa) and apoE (43 kDa) [15, 16]. Apo A-II, B and C-II are not detectable in the brain, while apo A-I, A-IV, D, E and J are present [17]. It was shown that mice deficient for apo E developed lipid deposition in the brain on a high-fat/high-cholesterol diet [18], and that rabbits fed with 2% cholesterol diet showed accumulation of intracellular β-amyloid [19]. Although lipid transport mediated by the blood–brain barrier remains undetermined, given that apoE and apoD work as molecular chaperons to scavenge the oxidative product in the brain, apo A-II could deliver the oxidized product through the blood vessels and participate in scavenging the oxidized products. It was speculated that plasma lipid contents could affect lipid metabolism and β-amyloid production in the brain. On the other hand, altered lipid metabolism could be causative for the neuronal membrane alteration [20, 21] and impaired cerebral microcirculation [22] noted in AD.

The Msp I polymorphism examined here has been proposed to associate with plasma lipid levels and coronary artery disease [9, 23], but this association remains controversial. We found a trend of an association between the APO A-II gene and sporadic late-onset AD, but this association was not statistically significant. However, variability of plasma apo A-II levels in monozygotic twin pairs was significantly restricted in subjects with the M2/M2 genotype, suggesting the existence of a 'variability gene' close to the APO A-II locus, which could modify the response of plasma apo A-II levels to dietary changes [24]. This hypothesis might be examined by linkage analysis of familial late-onset AD.

REFERENCES

1. Corder EH, Saunders AM et al. Gene dose of apolipoprotein E type 4 allele and the risk of Alzheimer's disease in late onset families. Science 1993; 261: 921–3.
2. Farrer LA, Cupples LA et al. Effects of age, sex, and ethnicity on the association between apolipoprotein E genotype and Alzheimer's disease. JAMA 1997; 278: 1349–56.
3. Sing CF, Davignon J. Role of the apolipoprotein E polymorphism in determining normal plasma lipid and lipoprotein variation. Am J Hum Genet 1985; 37: 268–85.
4. Escargueil-Blanc I, Salvayre R, Negre-Salvayre A. Necrosis and apoptosis induced by oxidized low density lipoproteins occur through two calcium-dependent pathways in lymphoblastoid cells. FAESB J 1994; 8: 1075–80.
5. Kuriyama M, Takahashi K et al. Low levels of serum apolipoprotein AI and AII in senile dementia. Jpn J Psychiat Neurol 1994; 48: 589–93.
6. Kawano M, Kawakami M et al. Marked decrease of plasma apolipoprotein AI and AII in Japanese patients with late-onset non-familial Alzheimer's disease. Clin Chim Acta 1995; 239: 209–11.
7. Bu X, Warden CH et al. Linkage analysis of the genetic determinants of high density lipoprotein concentrations and composition: evidence for involvement of the apolipoprotein A-II and cholesteryl ester transfer protein loci. Hum Genet 1994; 93: 639–48.
8. Warden CH, Daluiski A et al. Evidence for linkage of the apolipoprotein A-II locus to plasma apolipoprotein A-II and free fatty acid levels in mice and humans. Proc Natl Acad Sci USA 1993; 90: 10886–90.
9. Scott J, Knott TJ et al. High-density lipoprotein composition is altered by a common DNA polymorphism adjacent to apolipoprotein AII gene in man. Lancet 1985; 1: 771–3.
10. Kamino K, Orr HT et al. Linkage and mutational analysis of familial Alzheimer disease kindreds for the APP gene region. Am J Hum Genet 1992; 51: 998–1014.
11. Yu C-E, Payami H et al. The apolipoprotein E/CI/CII gene cluster and late-onset Alzheimer disease. Am J Hum Genet 1994; 54: 631–42.
12. McKhann G, Drachman D et al. Clinical diagnosis of Alzheimer's disease. Neurology 1984; 34: 939–44.
13. Knott TJ, Wallis SC et al. The human apolipoprotein AII gene: structural organization and sites of expression. Nucleic Acids Res 1985; 13: 6387–98.
14. Brewer HB, Lux SE et al. Amino acid sequence of human apoLp-GlnII (apo A-II), an apolipoprotein isolated from the high density lipoprotein complex. Proc Natl Acad Sci USA 1972; 69: 1304–8.
15. Blance-Vaca F, Via DP et al. Characterization of disulfide-linked heterodimers containing apolipoprotein D in human plasma lipoproteins. J Lipid Res 1992; 33: 1785–96.
16. Weisgraber KH, Mahley RW. Apolipoprotein (E–A-II) complex of human plasma lipoproteins. I. Characterization of this mixed disulfide and its identification in a high density lipoprotein subfraction. J Biol Chem 1978; 253: 6281–8.

17. Harr SD, Uint L et al. Brain expression of apolipoproteins E, J, and A-I in Alzheimer's Disease. J Neurochem 1996; 66: 2429–35.
18. Walker LC, Parker CA et al. Cerebral lipid deposition in aged apolipoprotein-E-deficient mice. Am J Pathol 1997; 151: 1371–7.
19. Sparks DL, Scheff SW et al. Induction of Alzheimer-like β-amyloid immunoreactivity in the brains of rabbits with dietary cholesterol. Exp Neurol 1994; 126: 88–94.
20. Mason RP, Shoemaker WI et al. Evidence for changes in the Alzheimer's disease brain cortical membrane structure mediated by cholesterol. Neurobiol Aging 1992; 13: 413–19.
21. Roth GS, Joseph JA, Mason RP. Membrane alterations as cause of impaired signal transduction in Alzheimer's disease and aging. Trends Neurosci 1995; 18: 203–6.
22. de la Torre JC. Cerebromicrovascular pathology in Alzheimer's disease compared to normal aging. Gerontology 1997; 43: 26–43.
23. Civeira F, Genest J et al. The Msp I restriction fragment length polymorphism 3' to the apolipoprotein A-II gene: relationships with lipids, apolipoproteins, and premature coronary artery disease. Atherosclerosis 1992; 92: 165–76.
24. Thorn JA, Stocks J et al. Variability of plasma apolipoprotein (apo) A-II levels associated with an apo A-II gene polymorphism in monozygotic twin pairs. Biochem Biophys Acta 1993; 1180: 299–303.

Address for correspondence:
    Kouzin Kamino,
    Department of Biochemistry and Cell Biology,
    Institute of Gerontology, Nippon Medical School,
    1-396 Kosugi-cho, Nakahara-ku, Kawasaki 211-8533, Japan
    e-mail: kamino@nms.ac.jp

VI Related Neurodegenerative Conditions

57 Cracking An Enigma: The Puzzle of Unusual Dementias

P.L. LANTOS

INTRODUCTION

It is customary to use the term 'unusual dementias' synonymously with 'non-Alzheimer dementia'. Accepting this definition of unusual dementias, there is a large group of clinicopathological entities belonging to this complex, increasingly interesting and challenging area of neurodegeneration. However, this review does not cover prion diseases, Pick's disease, Huntington's disease, argyrophilic grain dementia, tangle-only dementia and frontal lobe degeneration of non-Alzheimer type. Instead the focus will be on dementia with Lewy bodies, progressive supranuclear palsy, corticobasal degeneration, motor neuron disease-associated dementia and frontotemporal dementia and parkinsonism associated with chromosome 17.

There has been spectacular progress in the understanding of unusual dementias. These developments fall into three major areas: definition of clinicopathological entities, investigations into cellular and molecular mechanisms and genetic discoveries. The clinicopathological entities reviewed here all have the common feature of subcortical pathology playing the major role in bringing about neurodegeneration. These diseases have previously been considered to be predominantly subcortical, but now the widespread involvement of the cerebral cortex has been realized. It is also timely to review here important neuropathological developments: these include the characterization of the extensive cortical involvement, the glial changes and the cytoskeletal abnormalities. Although the approach is from a neuropathological aspect, these disorders will be described in the context of clinical symptomatology and basic neuroscience. Thus, the review will lead from clinical features through gross lesions and cellular pathology to molecular pathology and genetic alterations.

Alzheimer's Disease and Related Disorders
Edited by K. Iqbal, D.F. Swaab, B. Winblad and H.M. Wisniewski
© 1999 John Wiley & Sons Ltd

DEMENTIA WITH LEWY BODIES

The association of dementia with Parkinson's disease has long been established and only its frequency has been disputed. It was the observation of cortical Lewy bodies which transformed the view of the pathogenesis of dementia in Parkinson's disease. Although Okazaki et al. [1] described 'intra-cytoplasmic ganglionic inclusions' as early as 1961, it was Kosaka and his colleagues [2] who drew attention to the widespread occurrence of these intranuclear inclusions in the cerebral cortex and focused attention on the existence of a spectrum of Lewy body diseases in 1980. In a study of 55 cases of Parkinson's disease, three groups could be distinguished according to the frequency and distribution of Lewy bodies and Alzheimer-type changes [3]. Consequently, these groups later were termed 'diffuse', 'transitional' and 'brainstem' types of Lewy body disease and only this last was equated with classical idiopathic Parkinson's disease [4]. Subsequently, various terms, including 'Lewy body variant of Alzheimer's disease' [5], 'senile dementia of the Lewy body type' [6] and 'Lewy body dementia' [7], were used to describe the same condition. A consensus meeting in Newcastle upon Tyne, UK, defined the clinical as well as the neuropathological criteria and suggested the now-accepted term of 'dementia with Lewy bodies' [8].

The incidence of dementia with Lewy bodies (DLB) varies in different series. In California, 5% of 260 consecutive autopsy cases had DLB [9]; a finding similar to that in Nottingham, UK, where this figure is 7% of 216 referred brains but 27% of clinically diagnosed dementias [10]. In New York, 13% of 216 consecutive brains referred with the diagnosis of neurodegenerative disorders showed DLB [11]. The clinical features of DLB fall into three major groups: progressive dementia, visual hallucinations and parkinsonism. Progressive dementia is the central clinical feature characterized by fluctuating cognition with variations in attention and alertness. The visual hallucinations are recurrent, complex and detailed. The parkinsonian features include flexed posture, shuffling gait, rigidity and hyperkynesia.

Macroscopically the brain usually shows atrophy; this may be diffuse or may be more severe in the frontotemporal or frontal regions. The pigmented nuclei of the brainstem, particularly the substantia nigra and the locus coeruleus, show pallor. The histological abnormalities include Lewy bodies, neuronal loss, abnormal neurites, astrocytosis and vacuolation of the cortex. The histological hallmark lesion of the disease is the Lewy body. These are spherical, intraneuronal cytoplasmic inclusions which stain uniformly pink with haematoxylin and eosin. Three subtypes can be distinguished: the brainstem, the cortical and the intra-neuritic. The brainstem Lewy bodies show the classical configuration of spherical inclusions surrounded by a clear halo. This latter is not obvious in cortical Lewy bodies, which are more difficult to discern. According to the distribution and densities of Lewy bodies, the Newcastle consensus criteria distinguish three subtypes of DLB: neocortical, transitional and limbic. This distribution is based on a semiquantitative assessment with scoring the density of Lewy bodies in various prescribed cortical areas [8]. Lewy bodies are ubiquitous structures; in addition to the pigmented nuclei of the brainstem and cerebral cortex, they may occur in the basal ganglia, hypothalamus, autonomic nervous system and spinal cord. Electron microscopy reveals a complex inclusion composed of filamentous, granular and vesicular structures. They immunostain positively with antibodies to cytoskeletal proteins, including neurofilaments, tubulin, MAP 1 and 2, ubiquitin, chromogranin A, synaptophysin and α-synuclein. Until recently the method of choice for the demonstration of Lewy bodies has been ubiquitin staining, but since the discovery of the involvement of the synuclein gene in Parkinson's disease, α-synuclein proves to be a reliable and consistent method [12]. In addition to Lewy bodies, there are abnormal neurites which stain positively with ubiquitin and α-synuclein which are most often seen in the CA2 and CA3 region of the hippocampus. The severe neuronal loss in the cortex, usually in the temporal lobe, results in vacuolation of the cortex, with accompanying astrocytosis best demonstrated by GFAP immunostaining.

The neurochemical abnormalities of DLB involves loss of dopaminergic neurons in the substantia nigra, resulting in reduced dopamine in the caudate nucleus. In addition, there is abnormality of the cholinergic system with degeneration of cholinergic neurons in the nucleus basalis of Meynert, which leads to a decrease of cortical choline acetyltransferase. There is reduced nicotinic receptor binding and increased muscarinic receptor binding (for review, see [13]). The severity of dementia appears to be related to the density of Lewy bodies. In addition, there may be Alzheimer-type pathology, including the formation of senile plaques with the deposition of βA4. However, neurofibrillary tangles, although they may occur, are not a prominent feature. The concurrence of DLB and AD may present considerable diagnostic problems. The first case of familial AD with a point mutation in the APP gene at codon 717, resulting in valine-to-isoleucine substitution, showed not only severe AD but also brainstem and cortical Lewy bodies. Subsequently, two further members of the same family also developed both AD and DLB [14].

Two genes have been identified which are thought to predispose to Lewy body formation. The first was the cytochrome P450 gene CYP2D6B, which appears to be a relatively weak risk factor [15]. More importantly, a mutation link to chromosome 4q21–q23 [16] is associated with autosomal dominant Parkinson's disease. Subsequently, an alanine-to-threonine amino acid substitution at position 53 (Ala53Thre) has been identified in *SNCA*, the gene encoding α-synuclein [17]. Most recently Ala30Pro mutation in the gene encoding α-synuclein in Parkinson's disease has been reported [18]. The association of apolipoprotein E ε4 gene type with DLB may reflect a secondary factor [13].

PROGRESSIVE SUPRANUCLEAR PALSY

Progressive supranuclear palsy (PSP) was defined as a clinical and neuro-pathological entity in 1964 by Steele, Richardson and Olszewski, whose names later served to be eponymous alternatives for the designation of the disease. They reported nine cases of progressive brain disease characterized by supranuclear ophthalmoplegia, pseudobulbar palsy, dysarthria and dystonic rigidity of the neck and upper trunk [19]. The incidence of the disease is difficult to assess. Approximately 4% of parkinsonian patients have PSP [20] or four cases per 10^6 population per year [21]. A minimum estimate of prevalence in New Jersey is 1.39 per 10^6 [22].

The average age of onset is 59 years with a variation between 12 and 80 years. There is a slight male preponderance, the ratio of male:female is 60:40%. The duration of the disease is on average 5.7 years, ranging from 1 year to 23 years (for review, see [23]). The clinical features include parkinsonism, vertical supranuclear palsy, cognitive decline, dysarthria and dysphasia. The parkinsonian symptomatology consists of bradykinesia, rigidity, gait disorders, masked facies, neck dystonia and falls; but there is no tremor and the patient does not respond to levodopa.

Macroscopically the brains show variation: they may be normal or atrophied. The atrophy may include the globus pallidus, the thalamus, and occasionally the brainstem and the cerebellum. The 3rd and 4th ventricles may be enlarged. Usually there is pallor of the substantia nigra and the locus coeruleus. Cortical atrophy may be present, but it is difficult to assess. The histology of PSP includes the presence of neurofibrillary tangles, neuropil threads, glial inclusions, neuronal loss and astrocytosis. Neurofibrillary tangles are the predominant histological hallmarks of PSP. Depending on the type of neurons in which they occur, two configurations can be distinguished: globose tangles, usually in the brainstem, and flame-shaped or triangular tangles in the pyramidal cells of the cerebral cortex. More irregular, round or cone-shaped neurofibrillary tangles are also seen in smaller neurons. Neurofibrillary tangles are present in the substantia nigra, the globus pallidus, the subthalamic nucleus, the nucleus basalis of Meynert, the pretectal region, the tegmentum of the midbrain and pons, including the periaqueductal grey matter, the locus coeruleus, the raphe nuclei and in the nuclei of various cranial nerves. They occur less frequently in the red nucleus, corpus striatum, thalamus and inferior olives. More recently attention has focused on neurofibrillary tangles in the cortex (for review, see [24]).

Neurofibrillary tangles can be demonstrated by silver impregnation techniques, including modified Bielshowsky and the Gallyas techniques. They immunostain with antibodies to tau, but their reaction for ubiquitin and neurofilament proteins are more variable. Neuropil threads, which are also observed in PSP, show similar tinctorial and antigenic properties. Electron microscopy reveals the neurofibrillary tangle to be composed of straight filaments of 12–15 nm, which in turn are composed of six or more protofilaments of 2–5 nm. They also contain twisted or paired filaments and intermediate forms between the straight and the twisted filaments (for reviews, see [23, 24]).

There is neuronal loss in various nuclei of the brainstem, diencephalon and cerebellum. The severity of nerve cell loss appears to be related to neurofibrillary tangle formation: areas with the most severe neuronal depletion show the largest number of tangles. In the cerebellum the dentate nucleus, in addition to neuronal loss and neurofibrillary tangles, may develop grumose degeneration—perineuronal eosinophilic granular structures which, in silver impregnation, appear as argyrophilic rings or knobs. Electron microscopy reveals that they consist of clusters of axon terminals and preterminal axons. Neuronal loss in various areas of the brain is accompanied by astrocytosis. In addition to this stereotypic response of astrocytes there is, more significantly, glial pathology. Many astrocytes show inclusions, the so-called astrocytic tangles, and tuft-shaped or thorn-shaped astrocytes have also been observed. These are always tau-positive and electron microscopy reveals bundles of straight filaments. In addition, oligodendroglial cells may also contain inclusions referred to as 'coiled bodies'. These are not to be confused with the glial cytoplasmic inclusions of multiple system atrophy (for review, see [25]).

The chief biochemical abnormality of PSP is tau pathology. All the inclusions, including neurofibrillary tangles, neuropil threads and glial inclusions, contain abnormal tau. This tau, however, is different from the biochemical lesion of AD and is composed of a doublet of 64 and 69 kDa, whilst the third major band of 55 kDa tau to be seen in Alzheimer's disease is not present in PSP. The neurochemical pathology of PSP involves chiefly the dopaminergic and the cholinergic systems and these abnormalities have been recently reviewed [24].

PSP is a sporadic disease. However, familial cases indicating autosomal dominant inheritance have been reported [26, 27]. Recently a dinucleotide repeat polymorphism in a tau intron has been identified: a homozygous tau AO allele was found in 95.5% of PSP cases compared to 50% in controls and in AD. The putative mutation may be a tau coding mutation or it may determine tau expression or splicing pattern [28]. PSP has a considerable neuropathological and clinical heterogeneity which makes the diagnosis sometimes difficult [29]. Criteria for the neuropathological diagnosis of PSP, as a result of a series of consensus meetings, have been published [30]. The diagnosis is based on a semiquantitative assessment of the distribution of neurofibrillary tangles. The criteria also take account of the presence of neuropil threads and tau-positive astrocytes. Based on neuropathological criteria, three types of PSP can be distinguished: typical, atypical and combined. Typical cases show pathological features as originally described, while atypical cases are variants of the histological changes characteristic of PSP: either the severity or the distribution of abnormalities, or both of these, deviate from the typical pattern. In combined cases, in addition to PSP there is another disease process; this may be another neurodegenerative disorder, for example AD or vascular disease [23].

CORTICOBASAL DEGENERATION

Originally the clinical and pathological features of corticobasal degeneration (CBD) were reported in three patients by Rebeiz et al. in 1968 [31], who termed the disease 'corticodentatonigral degeneration with neuronal achromasia'. Clinically the cases resembled progressive supranuclear palsy, while some of the pathological features were similar to those of Pick's disease. Further cases have been reported and corticobasal degeneration has been recently reviewed [32, 33]. Synonymous terms include corticobasal ganglionic degeneration and corticonigral degeneration with neuronal achromasia. The prevalence and incidence of CBD are not known, but it is a relatively rare disease. One large clinical series showed a mean age of 60.9 years, ranging from 40 to 76 years [34]. Both sexes appear to be equally affected, without obvious familial cases. The disease duration varies from 5 to 10 years. A re-evaluation of 40 consecutive cases of non-Alzheimer, non-Lewy body dementia in Toronto, collected between 1981 and 1996, revealed nine cases (22%) with features of corticobasal degeneration. In this particular series, CBD appeared to be the second commonest form of non-Alzheimer's, non-Lewy body dementia after frontotemporal dementia, being more frequent than classical Pick's disease [33]. Clinical features include asymmetrical motor impairment, the 'alien limb' phenomenon, pyramidal deficits, cortical sensory disturbance, supranuclear gaze palsy and cognitive dysfunction.

Macroscopically the brain usually shows atrophy of the frontal, temporal and parietal lobes. The distribution of atrophy may vary. In the classical form, the peri-Rolandic areas are most affected, in cases with severe dementia frontal atrophy is predominant and in patients with aphasia there is a striking atrophy of the temporal lobes. There may be changes in the caudate nucleus, the amygdala and the hippocampus. The substantia nigra is often pale.

Histology reveals swollen achromatic neurons, the so-called corticobasal inclusions, and neuronal loss accompanied by astrocytosis. In addition to the increase in astrocytes, there is a striking glial, particularly astrocytic, pathology. Abnormal neurons are large, swollen and achromatic: the round nucleus is often eccentric. The cytoplasm may show vacuolation. These cells are obvious on haematoxylin-and-eosin-stained sections and silver impregnation. They can be demonstrated by immunohistochemistry: the best immunocytochemical marker is αB-crystallin, but they are also positive with antibodies to phosphorylated neurofilament epitopes, as well as to tau. Immunostaining with antibodies to ubiquitin is more variable and more controversial. The swollen neurons occur mainly in the layers V and VI of the cortex and to some extent in layer III. They may be also found in the deep grey matter, including the substantia nigra, the thalamus, the corpus striatum, the sub-thalamus, the globus pallidus and nucleus basalis of Meynert, amongst others. Electron microscopy of swollen neurons shows that the cytoplasm contains loose bundles of straight or curved filaments approximately 10–14 nm in diameter, interspersed with various cell organelles including mitochondria, lysosomes and vesicular structures. Tubular structures with a diameter exceeding 20 nm, similar to microtubules, were also seen in these neurons.

Of the deep grey matter, the substantia nigra is most severely affected. There is neuronal loss with ample extraneuronal pigment in the neuropil and in the macrophages, swollen neurons and intraneuronal cytoplasmic inclusions termed 'corticobasal inclusions' [35]. These are argyrophilic and tau-positive, but ubiquitin-negative. They have a faintly fibrillary basophilic structure and are similar to globose tangles. In addition to the substantia nigra they are to be found in other areas of the deep grey matter. Ultrastructurally the corticobasal inclusions are composed of straight tubules with a diameter of 20 nm.

There is neuronal loss and astrocytosis in the affected areas of the cortex and in the deep grey matter. In the cortex, particularly in the superficial layers, there are tau-positive inclusions in the small neurons and neuropil threads. Another striking feature of CBD is the presence of widespread and severe astroglial pathology. This glial pathology includes the so-called 'astrocytic plaques', 'abnormal astrocytes' and 'oligodendroglial coiled bodies'. The white matter also shows a variety of abnormal tau-positive profiles. The most typical glial lesion is the astrocytic plaques: they are amyloid-negative cortical plaques composed of collections of dilated distal processes of tau-positive astrocytes. They are also argyrophilic by Gallyas silver impregnation [35, 36].

CBD is best characterized by its extensive and varied tau pathology. Hyper-phosphorylated tau is the major component of all these inclusions which on immunoblot shows a doublet of 64 and 69 kDa, thus being different from the triplet of Alzheimer's disease. Despite the superficial similarity of abnormal tau in CBD and PSP, the tau isoforms are different in these two diseases: in CBD it is without exon 3 and in PSP it is with exon 3.

Views concerning the nosological entity of corticobasal degeneration has been divided but now seems to be accepted as a clinicopathological entity. Its differential diagnosis from Alzheimer's disease and Parkinson's disease, at least on a neuropathological basis, does not present serious differential diagnostic problems. However, the separation from PSP and Pick's disease may be more difficult. Although there are clearly features overlapping between PSP, CBD and Pick's disease [36, 37], the differential diagnosis is now becoming clearer on the basis of molecular pathology. It has been possible more recently to distinguish between the abnormal tau inclusion in corticobasal degeneration and Pick's disease, which previously represented the most difficult diagnostic problem. Another diagnostic problem is the neuropathological and clinical heterogeneity of CBD, as demonstrated in a review of 11 cases. All showed the typical features of swollen neurons, tau-positive neuronal and glial inclusions, neuropil threads and grains, as well as nigral degeneration. However, six out of 11 showed overlapping neuropathological features of one or more disorders, including Alzheimer's disease, PSP, Parkinson's disease and hippocampal sclerosis [38].

MOTOR NEURON DISEASE DEMENTIA

The association between motor neuron disease (MND) and dementia was originally recognized as part of the dementia–parkinsonism complex of Guam [39, 40]. Since then, cases have been reported both from Western countries and from Japan. The occurrence of dementia with motor neuron disease raises two important questions. First, what is the underlying neuropathological substrate of the patient's mental impairment? Second, how do these changes found correlate with other neurodegenerative disorders in general and with frontal lobe dementia of non-Alzheimer-type in particular?

Motor neuron disease associated dementia has a world-wide distribution. It is predominantly sporadic, but apparently some 15–20% of the cases are familial. The age group most frequently affected includes those in their 50s and 60s and there is a preponderance of male to female, the ratio being 2:1. The clinical features fall into two major categories. First, there is dementia of frontotemporal type, with a progressive decline in personal and social conduct, repetitive stereotypic and ritualistic behaviour and reduced language; however, navigational ability and day-to-day memory are relatively well preserved. As the disease progresses, the memory impairment becomes more striking. The second group of clinical features include neurological signs typical of motor neuron disease, both pyramidal (amyotrophy, weakness, fasciculation) and extrapyramidal (tremor, bradykinesia and rigidity). Usually dementia is the initial clinical presentation with the neurological signs appearing later. Often the clinical symptomatology of MND is not obvious.

Macroscopically there is cerebral atrophy affecting mainly the anterior frontal, temporal and parietal lobes. The lateral ventricles are enlarged, while the corpus callosum is thin. The substantia nigra may appear paler than usual. Histology shows neuronal loss, vacuolar degeneration, astrocytosis and intraneuronal inclusions in the cortex. The neuronal loss can be profound in the affected areas, leaving severe status spongiosus in layers II and III of the cortex. There may be striking astrocytosis, the distribution of which may be laminar or occasionally involving the entire thickness of the cortex. The intraneuronal inclusions occur in the superficial small cortical neurons, together with neuropil threads. These are ubiquitin-positive but tau-negative. However, neuronal inclusions are most abundant in the dentate gyrus of the hippocampal formation. The substantia nigra is severely affected, with neuronal loss and astrocytosis. In addition, there are the typical lesions of motor neuron disease which involve both the brainstem nuclei and the spinal cord.

More recently a variety of motor neuron disease-associated dementia was described and the term 'motor neuron disease inclusion dementia' was suggested [41]. This is characterized by the clinical features of dementia but without the clinical features of motor neuron disease. Histologically, the intraneuronal inclusions are the same as in motor neuron disease-associated dementia and there are also ubiquitin-positive dystrophic neurites, white matter pallor with astrocytosis and severe neuronal loss and astrocytosis in the cortex, basal ganglia and substantia nigra. The inclusions are ubiquitin-positive and composed of abnormal filaments of 10–15 nm in diameter [42].

The underlying neuropathological lesions responsible for dementia in these cases appear to be the extensive neuronal loss with cortical vacuolation and neuronal inclusions, both in the hippocampus and in the affected areas of the cortex. In addition, there is a sub-cortical involvement. The relationship with other predominantly frontotemporal dementias is more complex and these issues have been recently addressed in several reviews [43–45].

FRONTOTEMPORAL DEMENTIA AND PARKINSONISMS LINKED TO CHROMOSOME 17

Many cases of frontotemporal dementia with non-specific neuropathology, often referred to as neurodegeneration without distinctive histology, are familial. Dementia in one of these families was linked to chromosome 17 [46]. This initial discovery resulted in a consensus conference on frontotemporal dementia and parkinsonism linked to chromosome 17 (FTDP-17). The participants, after assessing 25 previously identified families, have agreed that eight families have disease definitely linked to the critical region of chromosome 17 because of LOD score greater than 3 and they further classified five families having disease that is probably linked because of LOD score between 1 and 3.

The symptomatology varies within the same kindred and between kindreds, but some of the features appear to be common to all. The disease usually starts insidiously with behavioural or motor manifestations typically in the fifth decade, but occasionally in the third, fourth and sixth decades. The duration of the disease is variable, on average about 10 years ranging from 3 to 30 years. The course is slowly progressive. Presenting symptoms may include dementia, parkinsonism, non-fluent aphasia, personality changes or obvious psychosis. The principal clinical features fall into three categories of behavioural, cognitive and motor disturbances. The clinical features are clearly distinct from those of Alzheimer's disease in which memory and cognitive decline predominate. The motor abnormalities usually consist of parkinsonian extrapyramidal disorders with rigidity, bradykinesia and postural instability but without resting tremor. Neuroimaging on CT and MRI shows focal, usually frontal, atrophy. Functional neuroimaging reveals frontotemporal hypometabolism.

Macroscopically there is frontotemporal atrophy, some atrophy of the basal ganglia and the substantia nigra, and the lateral ventricles are enlarged. The overall histology shows neuronal loss, with superficial vacuolation and astrocytosis of the affected cortex. In addition there is astrocytosis in the white matter. The caudate nucleus, the putamen, the amygdala, the hypothalamus and the substantia nigra also show neuronal loss and astrocytosis. In addition there may be neuronal and glial inclusions, as well as large swollen cells. The argentophilic and tau-positive neuronal inclusions are to be found in the neocortex, the basal ganglia, the hypothalamus, the brainstem and the spinal cord. Glial inclusions occur chiefly in oligodendrocytes, but some astrocytes are also affected. Electron microscopy reveals the neuronal inclusions to be reminiscent of paired helical filaments, whereas in oligodendrocytes there are tightly packed filaments. Based on the presence of tau-positive inclusions and of ballooned neurons, four groups can be distinguished: tau- and ballooned neuron-positive, tau-positive, ballooned neuron-positive and ballooned neuron-negative [47].

Thus, it appears that in some FTDP-17 cases tau pathology plays a prominent role. There are tau-positive neuronal and glial, chiefly oligodendroglial, inclusions and the tau appears to be in the form of twisted filaments. These are, however, different from the paired helical filaments of Alzheimer's disease; their diameter varies between 6 and 22 nm at their narrowest and widest, with a periodicity of 140–300 nm. They immunostain with both phosphorylation-independent and -dependent tau antibodies. The biochemistry shows a minor 72 kDa band as well as two major bands of 64 and 68 kDa. These contain hyperphosphorylated four-repeat tau isoforms of 383 and 412 amino acids [48, 49].

Three recent reports of molecular genetic investigations implicate tau mutations in FTDP-17. The first shows a point mutation of valine to methionine in the coding region of tau in a family with FTDP-17 [50]. The second paper reports on glycine-to-alanine transition in an intron of tau in another family [51]. The third describes a mixture of exon and intron tau mutations in 10 different families [52]. None of these tau mutations were present in any of the controls. A large number of the mutations are seen to be at the exon 10 splice site. This mutation could result in more frequent alternative splicing at exon 10 and a higher proportion of tau-protein molecules that have four rather than three binding domain repeats. In some of the FTDP-17 families, the neurofibrillary tangles consist of tau with four repeats, suggesting that a larger amount of protein with four repeats could be the cause of the disease.

FRONTOTEMPORAL DEMENTIAS

This is a clinical term and the underlying pathology may include Pick's disease, corticobasal degeneration, motor neuron disease-associated dementia, frontal lobe degeneration of non-Alzheimer-type, FTDP-17 and Alzheimer's disease. Although the differential diagnosis in some cases can be difficult, with immunocytochemistry and molecular genetics there are clear differences between these disorders. For the neuropathologists the presence or absence of neuronal and glial inclusions, and their distribution and antigenicity, provide the most useful diagnostic landmarks. Pick's disease is characterized by the typical tau- and ubiquitin-positive Pick inclusions in the affected areas of the cortex, deep grey matter and the dentate gyrus of the hippocampal formation. They are usually, but not always, accompanied by the presence of swollen achromatic Pick cells. The distribution of lesions in corticobasal degeneration is different; moreover, Pick inclusions do not occur, although swollen cells are the hallmark lesions. Another prominent feature of CBD is the widespread presence of glial inclusions, particularly astrocytic plaques. Monoclonal antibodies to tau-protein can now distinguish between the cellular abnormalities of Pick's disease and corticobasal degeneration. In motor neuron disease-associated dementia, the inclusions in the neurons are ubiquitin-positive but tau-negative. In addition there are abnormal ubiquitin-positive neurites in the cortex. The frontal lobe degeneration of non-Alzheimer-type does not show obvious neuronal or glial inclusions, but only non-specific changes of neuronal loss, vacuolation of the cortex and astrocytosis. FTDP-17 shows tau-positive neuronal and glial inclusions in some, but not in all the cases. The genetic abnormality provides the diagnostic hallmark to distinguish these latter cases from the non-specific changes of frontal lobe dementia of non-Alzheimer-type. Thus, the combination of immunocytochemistry, molecular pathology and genetics will secure a more sound diagnosis of these occasionally overlapping clinicopathological disorders.

FUTURE DEVELOPMENTS

The results of the last few years are encouraging to plan further strategies to a more scientific approach to unusual dementias. Although considerable achievements, the definition of clinicopathological entities and the investigation of phenotypic heterogeneity remain an important and basic goal. The characterization of the molecular pathology and biochemistry of cytoskeletal abnormalities is likely to provide further vital pathogenetic clues. Studies of the role and nature of glial lesions have expanded the pathological spectrum and concentrated our attention on a previously neglected component of the central nervous system. There is now little doubt that glial cells may play an important role in pathogenesis. Analyses of selective neuronal vulnerability in neurodegenerative disorders have hardly commenced in earnest and research in this area should be a future priority. The search for genetic abnormalities will continue, particularly in the light of recent discoveries of mutations in the tau gene, which may give an additional insight into the pathogenesis of

Alzheimer's disease. Finally, identification of the molecular pathology underlying the mechanisms of neurodegeneration remains a most important goal. Our knowledge of clinical symptomatology, cellular and molecular pathology, biochemistry and genetics should be synthesized in order to gain a full understanding of these diseases.

REFERENCES

1. Okazaki H, Lipkin LE, Aronson SM. Diffuse intracytoplasmic ganglionic inclusions (Lewy type) associated with progressive dementia and quadriparesis in flexion. J Neuropathol Exp Neurol 1961; 20: 237–44.
2. Kosaka K, Marsushita M, Oyanagi S. A clinicopathological study of 'Lewy body disease'. Psychiat Neurol Japan 1980; 82: 292–311.
3. Yoshimura N. Cortical changes in the parkinsonian brain: a contribution to the delineation of 'diffuse Lewy body disease'. J Neurol 1983; 229: 17–23.
4. Kosaka K, Yoshimura M, Ikeda K, Budka H. Diffuse type of Lewy body disease: progressive dementia with abundant cortical Lewy bodies and senile changes of varying degree—a new disease? Clin Neuropathol 1984; 3: 185–92.
5. Hansen LA, Salmon D, Galasko D et al. The Lewy body variant of Alzheimer's disease: a clinical pathological entity. Neurology 1990; 40: 1–8.
6. Perry RH, Irving D, Blessed G, Fairburn A, Perry EK. Senile dementia of Lewy body type. A clinically and neuropathologically distinct form of Lewy body dementia in the elderly. J Neuro Sci 1990; 95: 119–39.
7. Gibb WRG, Esiri MM, Lees AJ. Clinical and pathological features of diffuse cortical Lewy body disease (Lewy body dementia). Brain 1987; 110: 1131–53.
8. McKeith IG, Galasko D, Kosaka K et al. Consensus guidelines for the clinical and pathological diagnosis of dementia with Lewy bodies (DLB): report of the Consortium of DLB International Workshop. Neurology 1996; 47: 1113–24.
9. Forno LS, Langston JW. The amygdala parahippocampal region: a predilection site of Lewy bodies. J Neuropathol Exp Neurol 1988; 47: 354.
10. Byrne EJ, Lennox G, Lowe J, Godwin-Austin RB. Diffuse Lewy body disease: clinical features in 15 cases. J Neurol Neurosurg Psychiat 1989; 52: 709–17.
11. Dickson DW, Crystal H, Mattiace LA et al. Diffuse Lewy body disease: light and electron microscopic immunocytochemistry of senile plaques. Acta Neuropathol (Berl) 1989; 78: 572–84.
12. Spillantini MG, Crowther RA, Jakes R et al. α-Synuclein in filamentous inclusions of Lewy bodies from Parkinson's disease and dementia with Lewy bodies. Proc Natl Acad Sci USA 1998; 95: 6469–73.
13. Lennox GG, Lowe JS. In: Markesbery WR (ed) Neuropathology of Dementing Disorders. London: Arnold, 1998; 181–90.
14. Lantos PL, Luthert PJ, Hanger D et al. Familial Alzheimer's disease with the amyloid precursor protein position 717 mutation and sporadic Alzheimer's disease have the same cytoskeletal pathology. Neurosci Lett 1992; 137: 221–4.
15. Rempfer R, Crook R, Houlden H et al. Parkinson's disease, but not Alzheimer's disease, Lewy body variant associated with mutant alleles at cytochrome P450 gene. Lancet 1994; 344: 815.
16. Polymeropoulos MH, Hoggins JJ, Golbe LI et al. Mapping of a gene for Parkinson's disease to chromosome 4q21–q23. Science 1996; 274: 1197–9.
17. Polymeropoulos MH, Lavedan C, Leroy E et al. Mutation in the α-synuclein gene identified in families with Parkinson's disease. Science 1997; 276: 2045–7.

18. Krüger R, Kuhn W, Müller T et al. Ala30Pro mutation in the gene encoding α-synuclein in Parkinson's disease. Nature Genet 1998; 18: 106–8.

19. Steele JC, Richardson JC, Olszewski T. Progressive supranuclear palsy. Arch Neurol 1964; 10: 333–59.

20. Jackson JA, Jankovic J, Ford J. Progressive supranuclear palsy: clinical features and response to treatment in 16 patients. Ann Neurol 1983; 13: 273–8.

21. Mastaglia FL, Grainger K, Kee F et al. Progressive supranuclear palsy (the Steele–Richardson–Olszewski syndrome): clinical and electrophysiological observations in eleven cases. Proc Aust Assoc Neurol 1973; 10: 35–44.

22. Golbe LI, Davis PH, Schoenberg BS et al. Prevalence and natural history of progressive supranuclear palsy. Neurology 1998; 38: 1031–4.

23. Lantos PL. The neuropathology of progressive supranuclear palsy. J Neural Transm 1994; 42: 127–52.

24. Hauw J-J, Verny M, Ruberg M, Duyckaerts C. In: Markesbery WR (ed) Neuropathology of Dementing Disorders. London: Arnold, 1998; 193–212.

25. Lantos PL. Cellular and molecular pathology of multiple system atrophy: a review and recent developments. Brain Pathol 1997; 7: 1293–7.

26. Brown J, Lantos P, Stratton M et al. Familial progressive supranuclear palsy. J Neurol Neurosurg Psychiatry 1993; 56: 473–6.

27. de Yébenes JG, Sarasa JL, Daniel SE et al. Familial progressive supranuclear palsy. Description of a pedigree and review of the literature. Brain 1995; 118: 1095–103.

28. Conrad C, Andreadis A, Trojanowski JQ et al. Genetic evidence for the involvement of τ in progressive supranuclear palsy. Ann Neurol 1997; 4: 277–81.

29. Gearing M, Olson DA, Watts RL et al. Progressive supranuclear palsy: neuropathological and clinical heterogeneity. Neurology 1994; 44: 1015–24.

30. Hauw J-J, Daniel SE, Dickson D et al. Preliminary NINDS neuropathologic criteria for Steel–Richardson–Olszewski syndrome (progressive supranuclear palsy). Neurology 1994; 44: 2015–19.

31. Rebeiz JJ, Kolodny EH, Richardson EP Jr. Corticodentatonigral degeneration with neuronal achromasia. Arch Neurol 1968; 18: 20–33.

32. Revesz T, Daniel SE. In: Markesbery WR (ed) Neuropathology of Dementing Disorders. London: Arnold, 1998; 257–65.

33. Bergeron C, Davis A, Lang AE. Corticobasal ganglionic degeneration and progressive supranuclear palsy presenting with cognitive decline. Brain Pathol 1998; 8: 355–65.

34. Rinne JO, Lee MS, Thompson PD et al. Corticobasal degeneration. A clinical study of 35 cases. Brain 1994; 117: 1183–96.

35. Gibb WRG, Luthert PJ, Marsden CD. Corticobasal degeneration. Brain 1989; 112: 1171–92.

36. Feany MB, Dickson DW. Widespread cytoskeletal pathology characterizes corticobasal degeneration. Am J Pathol 1995; 146: 1388–96.

37. Feany MB, Mattiace LA, Dickson DW. Neuropathologic overlap of progressive supranuclear palsy, Pick's disease and corticobasal degeneration. J Neuropathol Exp Neurol 1996; 55: 53–67.

38. Schneider JA, Watts RL, Gearing M et al. Corticobasal degeneration: neuropathologic and clinical heterogeneity. Neurology 1997; 48: 959–69.

39. Hirano A, Kurland LT, Krooth RS et al. Parkinsonism–dementia complex, an endemic disease on the island of Guam. Brain 1961; 84: 642–61.

40. Hirano A, Malamud N, Kurland LT. Parkinsonism–dementia complex, an endemic disease on the island of Guam. II. Pathological features. Brain 1961; 84: 662–79.

41. Jackson M, Lennox G, Lowe J. Motor neurone disease-inclusion dementia. Neurodegeneration 1996; 5: 339–50.
42. Kinoshita A, Tomimoto H, Suenaga T et al. Ubiquitin-related cytoskeletal abnormality in frontotemporal dementia: immunohistochemical and immunoelectron microscope studies. Acta Neuropathol (Berl) 1997; 94: 67–72.
43. Ince PG, Lowe J, Shaw PJ. Amyotrophic lateral sclerosis: current issues in classification, pathogenesis and molecular pathology. Neuropathol Appl Neurobiol 1998; 24: 104–17.
44. Brun A, Gustafson L. In: Markesbery WR (ed) Neuropathology of Dementing Disorders. London: Arnold, 1998; 158–66.
45. Mann DA. Dementia of frontal type and dementias with subcortical gliosis. Brain Pathol 1998; 8: 325–38.
46. Wilhelmsen KC, Lynch T, Pavlou E et al. Localization of disinhibition–dementia–parkinsonism–amyotrophy complex to 17q21–22. Am J Hum Genet 1994; 55: 1159–65.
47. Foster NL, Wilhelmsen K, Anders AF et al. Frontotemporal dementia and parkinsonism linked to chromosome 17: a consensus conference. Ann Neurol 1997; 41: 706–15.
48. Spillantini MG, Goedert M, Crowther RA et al. Familial multiple system tauopathy with presenile dementia: a disease with abundant neuronal and glial tau filaments. Proc Natl Acad Sci USA 1997; 94: 4113–18.
49. Spillantini MG, Bird TD, Ghetti B. Frontotemporal dementia and parkinsonism linked to chromosome 17: a new group of tauopathies. Brain Pathol 1998; 8: 387–402.
50. Poorkaj P, Bird TD, Wijsman E et al. Tau is a candidate gene for chromosome 17 frontotemporal dementia. Ann Neurol 1998; 43: 815–25.
51. Spillantini MG, Murrell JR, Goedert M et al. Mutation in the tau gene in familial multiple system tauopathy with presenile dementia. Proc Natl Acad Sci USA 1998; 95: 7737–41.
52. Hutton M, Lendon CL, Rizzu P et al. Association of missense and 5'-splice-site mutations in *tau* with the inherited dementia FTDP-17. Nature 1998; 393: 702–5.

Address for correspondence:
Professor P.L. Lantos,
Department of Neuropathology,
Institute of Psychiatry, King's College London University,
De Crespigny Park, Denmark Hill,
London SE5 8AF, UK

58 The Interaction Between Vascular Disorders and Alzheimer's Disease

INGMAR SKOOG

ASSOCIATIONS BETWEEN ALZHEIMER'S DISEASE AND VASCULAR DISORDERS

Alzheimer's disease (AD) is a primary degenerative dementia and is not considered to be of vascular origin. However, several recent lines of evidence suggest that there may be an association between vascular disorders and AD (Table 1). Since Alois Alzheimer's first case it has been recognized that AD is associated with changes in the cerebral microvessels. These changes include cerebral amyloid angiopathy [1], degeneration of the endothelium [2] and vascular basement membrane alterations [3]. Since the 1980s, ischemic white matter lesions, associated with lipohyalinosis and narrowing of the lumen of the small perforating arteries and arterioles which nourish the deep white matter, have been described in both clinical and autopsied cases of AD [4, 5]. The main hypothesis is that long-standing hypertension causes the lipohyalinosis and thickening of the vessel walls [6]. De la Monte [7], in a study of non-demented individuals with extensive neuropathology of AD, suggested that the white matter degeneration precedes the cortical atrophy in AD.

Table 1. Vascular risk factors in Alzheimer's disease

Hypertension
ApoE ε4 allele
Generalized atherosclerosis
Coronary heart disease
Changes in cardiac innervation
Atrial fibrillation
Diabetes mellitus
Ischemic white matter lesions
Changes in cerebral microvessels

Alzheimer's Disease and Related Disorders
Edited by K. Iqbal, D.F. Swaab, B. Winblad and H.M. Wisniewski
© 1999 John Wiley & Sons Ltd

Since 1993 numerous studies have reported an increased frequency of the apoE ε4 allele in individuals with AD [8, 9]. The frequency of this allele is also increased in middle-aged individuals with coronary heart disease [10] and atherosclerosis [11]. In 1993, Sparks et al. [12] reported an increased amount of neurofibrillary tangles and senile plaques in the brains of non-demented individuals with hypertension and a year later it was reported from an epidemiological study that both systolic and diastolic blood pressure was increased 10–15 years before the onset of AD [13]. AD has also been associated with coronary heart disease [14], generalized atherosclerosis [15], atrial fibrillation [16], diabetes mellitus [17] and changes in the cardiac innervation [18].

POSSIBLE MECHANISMS FOR THE ASSOCIATION BETWEEN ALZHEIMER'S DISEASE AND VASCULAR FACTORS (TABLE 2)

DIAGNOSTIC ERRORS

It is often difficult to differentiate between AD and vascular dementia [19], and different criteria may result in substantial differences in the proportion of demented individuals diagnosed as having vascular dementia or AD [20, 21]. The findings of an association between AD and vascular factors may thus reflect an over-diagnosis of AD in individuals with vascular dementia [20].

Cerebrovascular diseases may also increase the possibility that individuals with Alzheimer lesions in their brains will express a dementia syndrome [22].

Table 2. Possible mechanisms for the association between Alzheimer's disease and vascular factors

---

Over-diagnosis of Alzheimer's disease in cases of vascular dementia
Cerebrovascular disease affects the clinical expression of Alzheimer's disease
Shared pathogenesis
Vascular disease causes or stimulates Alzheimer's disease
Alzheimer's disease causes or stimulates vascular diseases

SHARED PATHOGENESIS

The association between AD and vascular factors may also reflect shared pathogenic pathways (Table 3).

Apolipoprotein E

Apolipoprotein E (ApoE) may play a role both in vascular disorders and in Alzheimer's disease. ApoE is a constituent of several plasma lipoproteins. It is

Table 3. Shared pathogenetic pathways between AD
and vascular disorder

Apolipoprotein ε4
Oxidative stress
Disturbance in the renin–angiotensin system
Apoptosis
Psychological stress

essential in the transport and redistribution of lipids [23] and may also be involved in the injury–repair response in the artery wall, and thus in the progression and regression of atherosclerotic lesions [23]. Apolipoprotein E4 is associated with elevated levels of plasma cholesterol and low-density lipoprotein (LDL). Elevation in plasma cholesterol is linked to atherosclerosis. LDL is the main carrier of cholesterol in the blood and is considered to be the most atherogenic of the plasma lipoproteins [24]. It is also the lipoprotein that is most closely associated with coronary artery disease [25]. It has been suggested that part of the effect of the apoE ε4 allele on the risk for AD may be mediated through high serum cholesterol levels [26].

ApoE is also present in the brain. After injury, ApoE scavenges cholesterol and other membrane lipids from the degenerating axons and myelin sheaths. At the time of sprouting and remyelination, neuronal growth cones take up and re-use the lipids in membrane and myelin synthesis [23, 27]. This membrane lipid re-utilization may be of importance as a repair mechanism for neuronal degeneration. An increased re-utilization of ApoE-lipid complexes may explain our recent finding that ApoE in CSF is decreased in both Alzheimer's disease and vascular dementia [28]. However, low levels of ApoE may also result in a diminished repair function in the brain, increasing the risk of neuronal damage. In addition, other mechanisms are possible [29]. An interaction between generalized atherosclerosis [15], as well as ischemic white matter lesions [30], and the apoE ε4 genotype in the etiology of Alzheimer's disease has recently been reported.

Oxidative Stress

Oxidative stress with the formation of free radicals has been suggested to be involved in the etiology of both vascular disorders and Alzheimer's disease [31]. It has now been shown that β-amyloid induces oxidative stress in both neurons [32, 33] and endothelial cells [34]. One mediating factor may be the receptor for advanced glycation end products (RAGE) [33]. This receptor, which is found on the surface of neurons, microglia and vascular endothelium, is activated by β-amyloid [33]. This activation results in the generation of damaging reactive oxygen species. RAGE is also important in vascular disease, and its activation may damage the integrity of the endothelial lining [35].

The Renin–Angiotensin System

The renin–angiotensin system (RAS) is an example of a system that may be involved in the pathogenesis of both vascular disorders and Alzheimer's disease. This system has been ascribed a role in both peripheral and central blood pressure regulation via the effector peptide angiotensin II. This peptide is generated via an enzymatic cascade initiated by renin [36]. Renin cleaves angiotensinogen to angiotensin I. The angiotensin I-converting enzyme (ACE) converts the largely inactive decapeptide angiotensin I to the active octapeptide angiotensin II. This enzyme also inactivates bradykinin. Angiotensin II has several blood pressure increasing effects, such as direct vasoconstriction, stimulation of aldosterone secretion, sodium retention and activation of the sympathetic nervous system [36]. Angiotensin II also promotes hyperplasia and hypertrophy in vascular smooth muscle cells, independent of its effect on blood pressure [37].

The RAS also exists within the brain, where it may have a role in the regulation of behavioral and physiological responses, such as tonic control over blood pressure and the autoregulation of cerebral blood flow [38]. In experimental models of cognitive function, elevated levels of angiotensin II impair learning, especially acquisition and recall of newly learned material, and other memory functions [38]. The results are, however, contradictory and it may be that at very high levels, angiotensin II may facilitate learning [38]. Angiotensin II receptor antagonists improve cognitive function in mice [39]. Similar effects are reported for ACE inhibitors [38]. An increased activity of the ACE in the brains of victims of Alzheimer's disease has been reported [40, 41].

Apoptosis

The differentiated cells of multicellular organisms seem to share the ability to induce their own death by the activation of an internally encoded suicide program [42]. When activated, this suicide program initiates a characteristic form of cell death called apoptosis, which is characterized by specific changes in the cytoplasm of cells with fragmentation of chromatin, while cell membranes remain preserved. Apoptosis may be triggered by a number of stimuli, including free radicals, glutamate, dopamine, glucocorticoids, ischemia and the β-amyloid peptide [42]. Hamet et al. [43] reported an increased apoptosis in organs of spontaneously hypertensive mice, including heart, kidney and brain (cortex, striatum, hippocampus and thalamus), underlying the importance of cell death dysregulation in hypertension.

Psychological Stress

Traumatic events during early life have in humans been associated with hypertension [44] and with an increased incidence of Alzheimer's disease [45], and in rats with impairments associated with the hippocampus [46], which is impaired early in Alzheimer's disease. In rats, stress may lead to increased glucocorticoid levels, associated with early aging and damage to the hippocampus [47]. It is noteworthy that stressors that increase ACTH secretion also appear to influence the renin–angiotensin system, with increased levels of plasma renin and angiotensin II [38].

VASCULAR DISEASES CAUSE OR STIMULATE AD

Vascular diseases may also cause or stimulate AD. Both hypertension [48] and Alzheimer's disease [49] have been associated with increased vascular permeability with protein extravasation in brain parenchyma. The association between hypertension and AD may thus be mediated through a blood–brain barrier (BBB) dysfunction, suggested to be involved in the etiology and pathogenesis of Alzheimer's disease [50]. The cerebrospinal fluid (CSF):serum albumin ratio is a method of assessing the BBB function in living subjects. We recently reported from a population-based study on 85 year-olds that individuals with Alzheimer's disease had a higher CSF:serum albumin ratio than non-demented individuals, and that there were indications of a disturbed BBB function even before onset of the disease [51]. A relative BBB dysfunction may increase the possibility that substances from serum penetrate the BBB and reach the brain, where they may interact with neurons [49, 50], perhaps starting a cascade with amyloid accumulation and Alzheimer encephalopathy.

ALZHEIMER'S DISEASE CAUSES OR STIMULATES VASCULAR DISEASES

Alzheimer's disease may also lead to lesions in the cerebral microvasculature. Thomas et al. [34] reported that the interaction of β-amyloid with endothelial cells of the rat aorta produced excess of superoxide radicals, which caused endothelial damage. Olichney et al. [52] reported that there was a strong interaction effect between severity of cerebral amyloid angiopathy, i.e. amyloid infiltration of the media and adventitia, and hypertension for the development of cerebral infarctions in patients with Alzheimer's disease.

CONCLUSION

It seems clear that there is a connection between Alzheimer's disease and vascular factors. The exact mechanism behind this association is not clear. One reason may be over-diagnosis of Alzheimer's disease in cases of vascular dementia, or that cerebrovascular disease affects the clinical expression of Alzheimer's disease. However, as shown in this review, other possible reasons for the association have to be considered, such as that vascular factors may stimulate the Alzheimer's disease process, that similar mechanisms may be involved in the pathogenesis of both vascular disorders and Alzheimer's disease, and that Alzheimer's disease may stimulate vascular disorders.

ACKNOWLEDGEMENT

This work was supported by a working grant from the Swedish Medical Research Council Project No. 11337.

REFERENCES

1. Vinters HV. Cerebral amyloid angiopathy: a critical review. Stroke 1987; 18: 311–24.
2. Kalaria RN, Hedera P. β-amyloid vasoactivity in Alzheimer's disease [letter]. Lancet 1996; 347: 1492–3.
3. Perlmutter LS, Chui HC. Microangiopathy, the vascular basement membrane and Alzheimer's disease: a review. Brain Res Bull 1990; 24: 677–86.
4. Brun A, Englund E. A white matter disorder in dementia of the Alzheimer type: a pathoanatomical study. Ann Neurol 1986; 19: 253–62.
5. Skoog I, Palmertz B, Andreasson L-A. The prevalence of white matter lesions on computed tomography of the brain in demented and non-demented 85 year-olds. J Geriatr Psychiatry Neurol 1994; 7: 169–75.
6. Skoog I. The relationship between blood pressure and dementia: a review. Biomed Pharmacother 1997; 51: 367–75.
7. De la Monte SM. Quantitation of cerebral atrophy in preclinical and end-stage Alzheimer's disease. Ann Neurol 1989; 25: 450–59.
8. Poirier J, Davignon J, Bouthillier D, Kogan S, Bertrand P, Gauthier S. Apolipoprotein E polymorphism and Alzheimer's disease. Lancet 1993; 342: 697–9.
9. Saunders AM, Strittmatter WJ, Schmechel D, St George-Hyslop PH, Pericak-Vance MA, Joo SH, Rosi BL, Gusella JF, Crapper-MacLachlan DR, Alberts MJ, Hulette C, Crain B, Goldgaber D, Roses AD. Association of apolipoprotein E allele ε4 with late-onset familial and sporadic Alzheimer's disease. Neurology 1993; 43: 1467–72.
10. Wilson PWF, Myers RH, Larson MG, Ordovas JM, Wolf PA, Schaefer EJ. Apolipoprotein E alleles, dyslipidemia, and coronary heart disease: the Framingham offspring study. JAMA 1994; 272: 1666–71.
11. Davignon J, Gregg RE, Sing CF. Apolipoprotein E polymorphism and atherosclerosis. Arteriosclerosis 1988; 8: 1–21.
12. Sparks DL, Scheff SW, Liu H, Landers TM, Coyne CM, Hunsaker III JC. Increased incidence of neurofibrillary tangles (NFT) in non-demented individuals with hypertension. J Neurol Sci 1995; 131: 162–9.
13. Skoog I, Lernfelt B, Landahl S, Palmertz B, Andreasson L-A, Nilsson L, Persson G, Odén A, Svanborg A. A 15-year longitudinal study on blood pressure and dementia. Lancet 1996; 347: 1141–5.
14. Sparks DL, Hunsaker III JC, Scheff SW, Kryscio RJ, Henson JL, Markesbery WR. Cortical senile plaques in coronary artery disease, aging and Alzheimer's disease. Neurobiol Aging 1990; 11: 601–7.
15. Hofman A, Ott A, Breteler MMB, Bots ML, Slooter AJC, van Harksamp F, van Duijn CN, Van Broeckhoven C, Grobbee DE. Atherosclerosis, apolipoprotein E, and the prevalence of dementia and Alzheimer's disease in the Rotterdam Study. Lancet 1997; 349: 151–4.

16. Ott A, Breteler MMB, de Bruyne MC, van Harskamp F, Grobbee DE, Hofman A. Atrial fibrillation and dementia in a population-based study. The Rotterdam Study. Stroke 1997; 28: 316–21.
17. Leibson CL, Rocca WA, Hanson VA, Cha R, Kokmen E, O'Brien PC, Palumbo PJ. Risk of dementia among persons with diabetes mellitus: a population-based cohort study. Am J Epidemiol 1997; 145: 301–8.
18. Aharon-Peretz J, Harel T, Revach M, Ben-Haim SA. Increased sympathetic and decreased parasympathetic cardiac innervation in patient's with Alzheimer's disease. Arch Neurol 1992; 49: 919–22.
19. Skoog I. Risk factors for vascular dementia. A review. Dementia 1994; 5: 137–44.
20. Skoog I, Nilsson L, Palmertz B, Andreasson L-A, Svanborg A. A population-based study of dementia in 85 year-olds. N Engl J Med 1993; 328: 153–8.
21. Wetterling T, Kanitz R-D, Borgis K-J. Comparison of different diagnostic criteria for vascular dementia (ADDTC, DSM-IV, ICD-10, NINDS-AIREN). Stroke 1996; 27: 30–36.
22. Snowdon DA, Greiner LH, Mortimer JA, Riley KP, Greiner PA, Markesbery WR. Brain infarction and the clinical expression of Alzheimer disease. The Nun Study. JAMA 1997; 277: 813–17.
23. Mahley RW. Apolipoprotein E: cholesterol transport protein with expanding role in cell biology. Science 1988; 240: 622–30.
24. Davignon J, Bouthillier D, Nestruck AC, Sing CF. Apolipoprotein E polymorphism and atherosclerosis: insight from a study in octagenerians. Trans Am Clin Climeritol Ass 1987; 99: 100–10.
25. Campbell JH, Campbell GR. Pathogenesis of atheroma. In: Swales JD (ed) Textbook of Hypertension. Oxford: Blackwell Scientific Publications, 1994.
26. Notkola I-L, Sulkava R, Pekkanen J, Erkinjuntti T, Ehnholm C, Kivinen P, Tuomilehto J, Nissinen A. Serum total cholesterol, apolipoprotein E ε4 allele, and Alzheimer's disease. Neuroepidemiology 1998; 17: 14–20.
27. Poirier J, Baccichet A, Dea D, Gauthier S. Cholesterol synthesis and lipoprotein reuptake during synaptic remodelling in hippocampus in adult rat. Neuroscience 1993; 55: 81–90.
28. Skoog I, Hesse C, Fredman P, Andreasson L-A, Palmertz B, Blennow K. Apolipoprotein E in cerebrospinal fluid in 85 year-olds. Relation to dementia, apolipoprotein E polymorphism, cerebral atrophy, and white-matter lesions. Arch Neurol 1997; 54: 267–72.
29. Mahley RW. Heparan sulfate proteoglycan/low density lipoprotein receptor-related protein pathway involved in type III hyperlipoproteinemia and Alzheimer's disease. Israel J Med Sci 1996; 32: 414–29.
30. Skoog I, Hesse C, Aevarsson O, Landahl S, Wahlström J, Fredman P, Blennow K. A population study of ApoE genotype at the age of 85: relation to dementia, cerebrovascular disease and mortality. J Neurol Neurosur Psychiatr 1998; 64: 37–43.
31. Lethem R, Orrell M. Antioxidants and dementia. Lancet 1997; 349: 1189–90.
32. El Khoury J, Hickman SE, Thomas CA, Cao L, Silverstein SC, Loike JD. Scavenger receptor-mediated adhesion of microglia to β-amyloid fibrils. Nature 1996; 382: 716–19.
33. Yan SD, Chen X, Fu J, Chen M, Zhu H, Roher A, Slattery T, Zhao L, Nagashima M, Morser J, Migheli A, Nawroth P, Stern D, Schmidt AM. RAGE and amyloid-β peptide neurotoxicity in Alzheimer's disease. Nature 1996; 382: 685–91.
34. Thomas T, Thomas G, McLendon C, Sutton T, Mullan M. β-amyloid-mediated vasoactivity and vascular endothelial damage. Nature 1996; 380: 168–71.
35. Finkel E. Pinning the suspect to the crime in Alzheimer's. Lancet 1996; 348: 1506.
36. Bader M, Paul M, Fernandez-Alfonso M, Kaling M, Ganten D. Molecular biology and biochemistry of the renin–angiotensin system. In: Swales JD (ed) Textbook of Hypertension. Oxford: Blackwell Scientific Publications, 1994.

37. Stuijker Boudier HAJ. Vascular growth and hypertension. In: Swales JD (ed) Textbook of Hypertension. Oxford: Blackwell Scientific Publications, 1994.
38. Wright JW, Harding JW. Brain angiotensin receptor subtypes in the control of physiological and behavioral responses. Neurosci Biobehav Rev 1994; 18: 21–53.
39. Barnes NM, Costall B, Kelly ME, Murphy DA, Naylor RJ. Cognitive enhancing actions of PD 123177 detected in a mouse habituation paradigm. NeuroReport 1991; 2: 351–3.
40. Arregui A, Perry E, Rossor M, Tomlinson BE. Angiotensin converting enzyme in Alzheimer's disease: increased activity in caudate nucleus and cortical areas. J Neurochem 1982; 82: 1490–92.
41. Barnes NM, Cheng CH, Costall B, Naylor RJ, Williams TJ, Wischik CM. Angiotensin converting enzyme density is increased in temporal cortex from patients with Alzheimer's disease. Eur J Pharmacol 1991; 20: 289–92.
42. Thompson CB. Apoptosis in the pathogenesis and treatment of disease. Science 1995; 267: 1456–62.
43. Hamet P, Richard L, Dam T-V, Teiger E, Orlov SN, Gaboury L, Gossard F, Tremblay J. Apoptosis in target organs of hypertension. Hypertension 1995; 26: 642–8.
44. Ekeberg O, Kjeldsen SE, Eide I, Leren P. Childhood traumas and psychosocial characteristics of 50 year-old men with essential hypertension. J Psychosom Res 1990; 34: 643–9.
45. Persson G, Skoog I. A prospective population study of psychosocial risk factors for late-onset dementia. Int J Geriatric Psychiatry 1996; 11: 15–22.
46. Meaney MJ, Aitken DH, van Berkel C, Bhatnagar S, Sapolsky RM. Effect of neonatal handling on age-related impairments associated with the hippocampus. Science 1988; 239: 766–8.
47. Sapolsky R, Armanini M, Packan D, Tombaugh G. Stress and glucocorticoids in aging. Endocrinol Metabol Clin N Am 1987; 16: 965–80.
48. Johansson BB. Cerebral vascular bed in hypertension and consequences for the brain. Hypertension 1984; 6 (suppl 3): 81–6.
49. Wisniewski HM, Kozlowski PB. Evidence for blood–brain barrier changes in senile dementia of the Alzheimer type (SDAT). Ann NY Acad Sci 1982; 396: 119–31.
50. Hardy J, Mann D, Wester P, Winblad B. An integrative hypothesis concerning the pathogenesis and progression of Alzheimer's disease. Neurobiol Aging 1986; 7: 489–502.
51. Skoog I, Wallin A, Fredman P, Hesse C, Aevarsson O, Karlsson I, Gottfries CG, Blennow K. A population-study on blood–brain barrier function in 85 year-olds. Relation to Alzheimer's disease and vascular dementia. Neurology 1998; 50: 966–71.
52. Olichney JM, Hansen LA, Hofstetter CR, Grundman M, Katzman R, Thal LJ. Cerebral infarction in Alzheimer's disease is associated with severe amyloid angiopathy and hypertension. Arch Neurol 1995; 52: 702–8.

Address for correspondence:
Ingmar Skoog, MD, PhD,
Department of Psychiatry, Sahlgrenska University Hospital,
S-413 45 Göteborg, Sweden
Tel: +46 31 342 12 89; fax: +46 31 82 81 63;
e-mail: Ingmar.Skoog@psychiat.gu.se

59 Prevalence and Neuropathological Diagnostic Criteria in Argyrophilic Grain Disease

E. BRAAK AND H. BRAAK

Argyrophilic grain disease (AGD) is a progressive degenerative disorder of the human brain which becomes increasingly prevalent with advancing age [1]. The pathological process underlying this disease is associated with the formation of abnormal tau protein in a few select neuronal types and in a subpopulation of oligodendroglial cells. The presence of small spindle-shaped argyrophilic grains in the cellular processes of nerve cells is essential for the neuropathological diagnosis of AGD [1–19]. Argyrophilic grains are not found to occur regularly in non-demented individuals of advanced age and cannot be regarded, therefore, as typical age-changes of the human brain.

An initial turning point in the development of the disease is hyperphosphorylation of the microtubule-associated tau protein. A hydrophilic material emerges which, at the outset, is non-argyrophilic in nature [20]. Immunoreactions for demonstration of the abnormally phosphorylated tau protein (antibody: AT8) display the altered neurons and glial cells with all of their cellular processes. In a second facultative step, abnormal material aggregates and then adopts a pronounced argyrophilia, recognizable when using conventional silver stains or the Gallyas silver iodide method [21]. Only a fraction of the emerging abnormal material in AGD eventually consists of argyrophilic fibers which constitute, none the less, the central feature, the argyrophilic grains. Owing to the characteristic grains, the disorder can be easily differentiated from other tauopathies, such as Alzheimer's disease (Figure 1), Pick's disease, progressive supranuclear palsy or corticobasal degeneration [1, 9].

The anteromedial portion of the temporal lobe bears the brunt of the lesions (Figure 1). Grains generally can be found in abundance in the pyramidal layers of the first Ammon's horn sector, the entorhinal layer pre-β (Figure 1), layer III of the adjoining temporal, insular and orbitofrontal neocortex, the

Alzheimer's Disease and Related Disorders
Edited by K. Iqbal, D.F. Swaab, B. Winblad and H.M. Wisniewski
© 1999 John Wiley & Sons Ltd

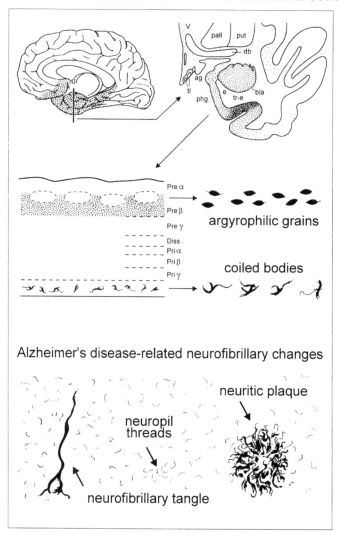

Figure 1. *Upper row:* summary diagram showing the distribution pattern of the lesions associated with AGD. The brunt of the pathology is borne by the nuclear complex of the amygdala, portions of the temporal allocortex, and adjoining territories of the basal temporal, insular and orbitofrontal neocortex: ag, ambient gyrus; bla, basolateral nuclei of the amygdala; db, diagonal band; e, entorhinal region; pall, pallidum; phg, parahippocampal gyrus; put, putamen; tl, lateral tuberal nucleus; tr-e, transentorhinal region. *Central row:* lamination pattern of the entorhinal cortex and distribution of the key lesions (argyrophilic grains in neuronal processes and coiled bodies in oligodendroglial cells) throughout the entorhinal cortex: Diss, lamina dissecans; Pre-α-γ, layers of the external principal stratum; Pri-α-γ, layers of the internal principal stratum. *Lower row:* characteristic intraneuronal lesions developing in the course of Alzheimer's disease. The size, shape and distribution pattern of these lesions are easily differentiated from cytoskeletal alterations associated with AGD

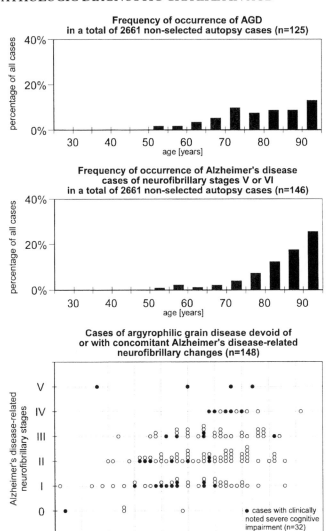

Figure 2. Frequency in the occurrence of AGD in different age categories (upper diagram) as compared with the prevalence of fully developed Alzheimer's disease at neurofibrillary stages V and VI (central diagram). Both diagrams are derived from evaluation of a total of 2661 non-selected autopsy cases. Note that AGD is a relatively frequently occurring disorder and shows a marked increase in prevalence with advancing age. Lower diagram: age distribution of AGD cases with and without concomitant Alzheimer's disease-related neurofibrillary changes. Most AGD cases exhibit co-occurrence of mild Alzheimer's disease-associated lesions corresponding to stages I–III. Note that AGD cases with more advanced Alzheimer's stages gradually become more prevalent with greater age. Reproduced from reference [1], by permission of Springer-Verlag, Vienna

subcortical nuclear complex of the amygdala, and the hypothalamic lateral tuberal nucleus [1–3].

The material evaluated for this study includes 125 cases of AGD found in 2661 non-selected brains obtained at autopsy (5%). The fact that the same material contains 146 cases of fully developed Alzheimer's disease at neurofibrillary stages V or VI (6%) supports the view that AGD is not a rare disorder. Figure 2 permits comparison between the prevalence of AGD cases in different age categories with that of fully developed Alzheimer's disease. Note the increasing prevalence of AGD cases with greater age. Frequently, the lesions of AGD coexist with those found in Alzheimer's disease or in other tauopathies [22, 23]. Most often encountered are cases of AGD in combination with mild Alzheimer's disease-associated neurofibrillary changes corresponding to stages I–III (Figure 2). Note that AGD cases with more advanced stages of Alzheimer's disease become more prevalent with increasing age.

In the material presently available to us, a progressive mental deterioration is documented clinically in 22% of the cases [1]. It is to be expected that correct neuropathological diagnosis of AGD will reduce considerably the number of enigmatic and unexplained cases of adult-onset dementia. AGD merits attention because of its frequent occurrence and its potential to cause severe brain dysfunction.

ACKNOWLEDGEMENTS

This work was supported by the Deutsche Forschungsgemeinschaft and the Bundesministerium für Bildung, Wissenschaft, Forschung und Technologie, the Alzheimer Research Center Frankfurt (AFZF) and Degussa, Hanau. The skilful assistance of Ms Szasz (drawings) is gratefully acknowledged.

REFERENCES

1. Braak H, Braak E. Argyrophilic grain disease: frequency of occurrence in different age categories and neuropathological diagnostic criteria. J Neural Transm 1998; 105: 801–19.
2. Braak H, Braak E. Argyrophilic grains: characteristic pathology of cerebral cortex in cases of adult onset dementia without Alzheimer changes. Neurosci Lett 1987; 76: 124–7.
3. Braak H, Braak E. Cortical and subcortical argyrophilic grains characterize a disease associated with adult onset dementia. Neuropathol Appl Neurobiol 1989; 15: 13–26.
4. Cras P, Perry G. Dementia with argyrophilic grains. Ann Neurol 1991; 30: 853–4.

5. Davis DG, Ross GW, Petrovitch H, White LR, Hardman JM, Nelson JS, Thiessen P, Wang HZ, Patel E, Markesbery WR. Quantitation of argyrophilic grains in hippocampal CA-1 of aged Japanese-American men. J Neuropathol Exp Neurobiol 1997; 56 (abstr): 587.

6. De Vos RAI, Jansen ENH, Wesseling P, Braak H. Parkinson's disease and dementia with argyrophilic grains. Neuropathol Appl Neurobiol 1996; 22 (suppl) (abstr): 74–5.

7. Ikeda K, Akiyama H, Kondo H, Haga C. A study of dementia with argyrophilic grains. Possible cytoskeletal abnormality in dendrospinal portion of neurons and oligodendroglia. Acta Neuropathol 1995; 89: 409–14.

8. Itagaki S, McGeer PL, Akiyama H, Beattie BL, Walker DG, Moore GRW, McGeer EG. A case of adult-onset dementia with argyrophilic grains. Ann Neurol 1989; 26: 685–9.

9. Jellinger KA. Dementia with grains (argyrophilic grain disease). Brain Pathol 1998; 8: 377–86.

10. Martinez-Lage P, Munoz DG. Prevalence and disease association of argyrophilic grains of Braak. J Neuropathol Exp Neurol 1997; 56: 157–64.

11. Masliah E, Hansen LA, Quijada S, DeTeresa R, Alford M, Kauss J, Terry R. Late-onset dementia with argyrophilic grains and subcortical tangles or atypical progressive supranuclear palsy? Ann Neurol 1991; 29: 389–96.

12. Tolnay M, Probst A. Ballooned neurons expressing αB-crystallin as a constant feature of the amygdala in argyrophilic grain disease. Neurosci Lett 1998; 246: 165–8.

13. Tolnay M, Spillantini MG, Goedert M, Ulrich J, Langui D, Probst A. Argyrophilic grain disease: widespread hyperphosphorylation of tau protein in limbic neurons. Acta Neuropathol 1997; 93: 477–84.

14. Tolnay M, Schwietert M, Monsch AU, Staehelin HB, Langui D, Probst A. Argyrophilic grain disease: distribution of grains in patients with and without dementia. Acta Neuropathol 1997; 94: 353–8.

15. Tolnay M, Ipsen S, Mistl C, Probst A. Argyrophilic grain disease: occurrence of grains inside dendritic branches of neurons containing hyperphosphorylated tau protein. Brain Pathol 1997; 7: 1176 (abstr).

16. Tolnay M, Mistl C, Ipsen S, Probst A. Argyrophilic grains of Braak: occurrence in dendrites of neurons containing hyperphosphorylated tau protein. Neuropathol Appl Neurobiol 1998; 24: 53–9.

17. Ulrich J. Demenz infolge der Hirnkrankheit mit argyrophilen Körnchen. Neurol Psychiat 1989; 3: 500–502.

18. Yamada T, McGeer PL. Oligodendroglial microtubular masses: an abnormality observed in some human neurodegenerative diseases. Neurosci Lett 1990; 120: 163–6.

19. Yamada T, McGeer PL, McGeer EG. Some immunohistochemical features of argyrophilic grain dementia with normal cortical choline acetyltransferase levels but extensive subcortical pathology and markedly reduced dopamine. J Geriat Psychiat Neurol 1992; 5: 3–13.

20. Braak E, Braak H, Mandelkow E-M. A sequence of cytoskeleton changes related to the formation of neurofibrillary tangles and neuropil threads. Acta Neuropathol 1994; 87: 554–67.

21. Gallyas F. Silver staining of Alzheimer's neurofibrillary changes by means of physical development. Acta Morphol Acad Sci Hung 1971; 19: 1–8.

22. Braak H, Braak E. Neuropathological stageing of Alzheimer-related changes. Acta Neuropathol 1991; 82: 239–59.

23. Braak H, Braak E. Frequency of stages of Alzheimer-related lesions in different age categories. Neurobiol Aging 1997; 18: 351–7.

Address for correspondence:
    E. Braak,
    Department of Anatomy, J.W. Goethe University,
    Theodor Stern Kai 7, D-60590 Frankfurt, Germany
    Tel: +49 69 6301 6914; fax: +49 69 6301 6425;
    e-mail: Braak@em.uni-frankfurt.de

60 Argyrophilic Grain Disease: A Neurodegenerative Disorder Distinct from Alzheimer's Disease

MARKUS TOLNAY AND ALPHONSE PROBST

INTRODUCTION

Argyrophilic grain disease (AGD) constitutes one cause of late-onset dementia in which the main morphological finding consists of abundant argyrophilic neuropil grains (ArGs) [1, 2]. ArGs are densely distributed through various parts of the limbic area, including the CA1 sector of the hippocampus, layer II (pre-α-layer) and III (pre-β-layer) of the entorhinal and transentorhinal cortices, the amygdala and the hypothalamic lateral tuberal nuclei. ArGs are associated with oligodendroglial inclusions (coiled bodies) in the subcortical white matter [1, 2, 3]. Ultrastructurally, ArGs mainly consist of aggregates of 9–18 nm filaments [2, 4, 5] and of bundles of 25 nm diameter smooth tubules [3, 6]. The microtubule-associated protein tau encountered in ArGs and coiled bodies has been shown to share a number of abnormally phosphorylated sites with tau of neurofibrillary tangles (NFT) and neuropil threads (NTh) in Alzheimer's disease (AD) [5], whereas, so far, paired helical filaments (PHFs) have not been reported in AGD. We previously reported that up to 80% of pyramidal cells in sector CA1 showed diffuse staining in their somata and dendrites when using the phosphorylation-dependent anti-tau antibody, AT8. We have shown that a subset of ArGs are formed within dendrites of neurons containing hyperphosphorylated tau [5, 7], which corroborates the idea of Ikeda and co-workers [3] that the origin of ArGs is within dendrites and dendritic spines of neurons, rather than within axons.

Although AGD constitutes a morphologically well-defined disease entity, its nosological status is still unclear because most of the reported AGD cases have associated AD-type changes. These changes mainly consist of NFT [5, 8], in a distribution that rarely exceeds Braak stages I–III [9], which generally are not associated with a cognitive decline.

Alzheimer's Disease and Related Disorders
Edited by K. Iqbal, D.F. Swaab, B. Winblad and H.M. Wisniewski
© 1999 John Wiley & Sons Ltd

In a previous study of 301 consecutive autopsies of patients older than 65, we found 28 (9.3%) cases with ArGs as the main histopathological finding. A late-onset dementia was retrospectively documented in only half of these patients [5] but surprisingly changes of the AD-type were not found to be more severe in demented patients than in subjects without cognitive decline. Similar results have been reported by Martinez-Lage and Munoz [10], who found 11 AGD cases among 300 non-selected autopsies (4%). However, only two out of the 11 AGD cases had presented dementia. These results indicate that ArGs *per se* are not necesssarily associated with a cognitive decline. Furthermore, intellectual impairment observed in some patients with ArGs is obviously not explained by the presence or the severity of associated morphological changes.

As the presence or absence of a cognitive decline in subjects with ArGs could be accounted for by the distribution and the density of ArGs, we decided to investigate the relationship between these parameters and the intellectual status of 35 subjects with ArGs [11]. Moreover, as the ε4 allele of the apolipoprotein E gene (ApoE) is a strong susceptibility factor for AD (for review, see [12]) we analyzed the ApoE genotypes in subjects with ArGs [13] to investigate whether AgD is distinct from AD not only morphologically but also genetically.

MATERIALS AND METHODS

Brains from 35 subjects with ArGs as the main histopathological findings were investigated. The detailed clinicopathological background of these cases has been described elsewhere [11]. Nineteen patients (8 females, 11 males; mean age 84.9 ± 17.5 years) were retrospectively diagnosed as demented and 16 patients (6 females, 10 males; mean age 17.6 years) as cognitively normal, according to the Diagnostic and Statistical Manual of Mental Disorders, 4th edn (DSM-IV) [14]. The anterior and posterior hippocampal regions were investigated on both sides, including the head, body and tail of the cornu ammonis, the dentate gyrus, the subiculum, the entorhinal/transentorhinal cortex, parts of the gyrus fusiformis near the rhinal sulcus and the parahippocampal gyrus with adjacent temporobasal neocortex. Further regions from various parts of the brain were examined as well. Paraffin-embedded histological sections stained with hematoxylin and eosin, Holmes Luxol, periodic acid–methenamin silver stain and the Gallyas silver technique [15] were used for diagnostic assessment and the ArG distribution study.

DNA was extracted from paraffin-embedded tissue blocks of liver, kidney or cerebellum as described [16]. ApoE genotypes were determined by a polymerase chain reaction (PCR) assay using primer pair Wbp ½ or a PCR assay which allowed analysis of DNA isolated from paraffin-embedded brain tissue [17]. Yates's corrected Chi-square test was used to compare the demented and non-demented groups and the differences in the distribution of ApoE ε2, ε3 and ε4 alleles.

RESULTS

DISTRIBUTION OF ArGS IN DEMENTED AND NON-DEMENTED PATIENTS

ArGs were found in the limbic area of all cases, irrespective of the presence or absence of dementia. However, there were important differences in the density and in the distribution of ArGs between demented and non-demented patients. The overall amount of ArGs in structures of the limbic area (e.g. sector CA1, entorhinal/transentorhinal and parahippocampal cortices) was significantly higher in demented than in non-demented patients (p < 0.0002). In contrast to the rostral half of the CA1 sector, a significant difference was found in its caudal half. Whereas all demented patients showed ArGs (84.2% in both sides), the caudal part of CA1 was affected in only 9 (56.3%) of the non-demented patients (p < 0.01). Moreover, semiquantitative assessment of grain density revealed that the densities of grains in the caudal cornu ammonis was higher in demented than in non-demented patients.

Demented patients showed more severe and more frequent involvement of the entorhinal/transentorhinal region than the non-demented (p < 0.05). This cortical region was affected in all demented patients but in only 75% of the non-demented. In the more caudal parahippocampal cortex, as in the caudal half of sector CA1, ArGs were found more frequently and in a higher density in demented than in cognitively normal patients (78.9% and 37.5%, respectively; p < 0.05).

In summary, AGD cases with dementia showed more abundant ArGs and a more widespread rostrocaudal extension of ArGs in the limbic area than cases without dementia.

ASSOCIATED NEUROPATHOLOGICAL FINDINGS

Mild to moderate changes of the AD type were found in all AGD cases. The distribution of NFT corresponded to early Braak stages I–III. Senile plaques (SP) shown by methenamin silver stain and/or Aβ-immunohistochemistry were found in 25 out of our 35 cases. Vascular lesions (e.g. old cerebral infarcts, not larger than 3 cm in diameter, or deep lacunar infarcts) were found in 18 cases. Braak stages, the presence or absence of SP or vascular lesions did not significantly differ in patients with dementia and those without dementia. Two cases with clinically known Parkinson's disease (one demented and one non-demented case) showed loss of pigmented cells and Lewy body inclusions in the substantia nigra. Ballooned cells were found in the amygdala of all AGD cases, as previously described [18].

ApoE GENOTYPE

PCR analysis revealed the following ApoE genotypes for the AGD cases: 24 patients (68.6%) ε3/3; six patients (17.1%) ε2/3; four patients (11.4%) ε3/4; and one patient (2.9%) ε2/4. The ApoE ε2, ε3 and ε4 allele frequencies were 0.10, 0.83 and 0.07, respectively. The ApoE ε4 allele frequency in AGD patients significantly differed from the ε4 allele frequencies reported in AD patients (0.24–0.38), but not from age-matched control subjects (0.09–0.13; for details see Table 1) [19–23]. ApoE allele frequencies did not differ significantly between AGD patients with or without SP, or between demented and non-demented AGD patients.

Table 1. ApoE allele frequencies in AGD, controls and AD

	ApoE ε2	ApoE ε3	ApoE ε4	p vs. AGD
AGD (n = 70)	0.10	0.83	0.07	
Controls (n = 108)[a]	0.037	0.852	0.111	n.s.
Controls (n = 5008)[b]	0.077	0.789	0.134	n.s.
Controls (octogenarian) (n = 472)[c]	0.09	0.82	0.09	n.s.
Braak I–III (n = 206)[d]	0.09	0.083	0.08	n.s.
AD (n = 54)[a]	0.00	0.65	0.35	< 0.0005
AD (n = 2896)[b]	0.044	0.588	0.380	< 0.0001
AD (octogenarian) (n = 72)[e]	0.01	0.75	0.24	< 0.005

[a] Controls (mean age: 71.2 ± 9.5 years) and AD (mean age: 77.9 ± 8.1 years). Data from [19].
[b] Controls and AD, pooled data from [20].
[c] Octogenarian controls (mean age: 84.7 ± 4.2 years). Data from [21].
[d] AD (Braak stages I–III). Data from [22].
[e] Octogenerian AD (mean age: 83.5 ± 7.3 years). Data from [23].
n = Number of alleles; n.s. = not significant.

DISCUSSION

A significantly more widespread rostrocaudal extension of ArGs change was found in the limbic area in subjects with documented cognitive decline than in non-demented subjects [11]. Whereas no differences in distribution and density of ArGs were found in the rostral part of CA1, the caudal half of CA1 was significantly more often affected in demented AGD cases. Moreover, ArGs were significantly more widespread in the entorhinal/transentorhinal region and the parahippocampal cortex of demented patients. The finding that none of our AGD cases showed an exclusive involvement of the posterior hippocampal region without an involvement of the anterior part suggests that the earliest changes in AGD occur in the rostral aspects of the hippocampus, e.g. sector CA1. Thus, the progression of pathological changes in AGD significantly differs from the progression of neurofibrillary changes in AD, where the initial lesions are observed in the entorhinal cortex, followed by sector CA1 of the hippocampus and eventually by the neocortex.

We previously reported that in AGD up to 80% of pyramidal cells of sector CA1 show hyperphosphorylation of tau protein in their soma and dendrites [5, 7], thus looking very similar to the 'stage 0 tangles' of Bancher et al. [24] and the 'group 1 neurons' of Braak et al. [25]. However, whereas in AD hyperphosphorylation of tau is believed to precede PHFs assembly [24, 25], this association seems to be less stringent in cortical areas where ArGs develop, since NFT only rarely develop in nerve cell perikarya despite large numbers of neurons containing hyperphosphorylated tau [5]. We found that at least a subset of ArGs are formed within dendritic branches of neurons containing hyperphosphorylated tau protein in AGD [7]. An additional important feature of AGD consisted in a progressive shrinkage and loss of dendritic branches bearing ArGs [7]. One possible explanation for the dementia observed in some subjects with AGD is that there is a more severe and widespread loss of postsynaptic structures, including synaptic contacts, throughout the hippocampus–entorhinal/parahippocampal complex, and probably the amygdaloid nuclei.

A roughly three-fold increase in the frequency of the ApoE ε4 allele has been reported in late-onset AD [12]. However, in AGD we found a very low ApoE ε4 allele frequency (0.07) [13], which significantly differed from the ε4 allele frequencies reported in AD patients (0.24–0.38), but not from age-matched control subjects (0.08–0.13) [13–19]. Recently, Braak's group reported quite similar results, although they found a higher incidence of the ApoE ε2 allele in their AGD cases than in age-matched control patients [26]. However, both studies suggest that the ApoE ε4 allele does not constitute a risk factor for the development of AGD [13, 26].

In conclusion, our findings suggest that AGD is, indeed, a distinct disease entity separate from AD by both morphological and genetic criteria.

ACKNOWLEDGEMENTS

The help of Rupert Egensperger (Neuropathology, Hannover, Germany) and Andreas Monsch (Geriatric University Clinic, Basel, Switzerland) is gratefully acknowledged. M.T. is supported by grants from the Swiss National Science Foundation, the Royal Society of London and the L & Th La Roche Foundation.

REFERENCES

1. Braak H, Braak E. Argyrophilic grains: characteristic pathology of cerebral cortex in cases of adult onset dementia. Neurosci Lett 1987; 76: 124–7.
2. Braak H, Braak E. Cortical and subcortical argyrophilic grains characterize a disease associated with adult onset dementia. Neuropathol Appl Neurobiol 1989; 15: 13–26.

3. Ikeda K, Akiyama H, Kondo H, Haga C. A study of dementia with argyrophilic grains. Possible cytoskeletal abnormality in dendrospinal portion of neurons and oligodendroglia. Acta Neuropathol 1995; 89: 409–14.

4. Itagaki S, McGeer PL, Akiyama H, Beattie BL, Walker DG, Moore GRW, McGeer EG. A case of adult-onset dementia with argyrophilic grains. Ann Neurol 1989; 26: 685–9.

5. Tolnay M, Spillantini MG, Goedert M, Ulrich J, Langui D, Probst A. Argyrophilic grain disease: widespread hyperphosphorylation of tau protein in limbic neurons. Acta Neuropathol 1997; 93: 477–83.

6. Masliah E, Hansen LA, Quijata S, DeTeresa R, Alford M, Kauss J, Terry R. Late onset dementia with argyrophilic grains and subcortical tangles or atypical progressive supranuclear palsy? Ann Neurol 1991; 29: 389–96.

7. Tolnay M, Mistl C, Ipsen S, Probst A. Argyrophilic grains of Braak: occurrence in dendrites of neurons containing hyperphosphorylated tau protein. Neuropathol Appl Neurobiol 1998; 24: 53–9.

8. Braak H, Braak E. Argyrophilic grain disease: frequency of occurrence in different age categories and neuropathological diagnostic criteria. J Neural Transm 1998; 105: 801–19.

9. Braak H, Braak E. Neuropathological staging of Alzheimer-related changes. Acta Neuropathol 1991; 82: 239–59.

10. Martinez-Lage P, Munoz DG. Prevalence and disease association of argyrophilic grains of Braak. J Neuropathol Exp Neurol 1997; 56: 157–64.

11. Tolnay M, Schwietert M, Monsch AU, Staehelin HB, Langui D, Probst A. Argyrophilic grain disease: distribution of grains in patients with and without dementia. Acta Neuropathol 1997; 94: 353–8.

12. Strittmatter WJ, Roses AD. Apolipoprotein E and Alzheimer's disease. Ann Rev Neurosci 1996; 19: 53–77.

13. Tolnay M, Probst A, Monsch AU, Staehelin HB, Egensperger R. Apolipoprotein E allele frequencies in argyrophilic grain disease. Acta Neuropathol 1998; 96: 225–27.

14. American Psychiatric Association. Diagnostic and Statistical Manual of Mental Disorders, 4th edn. Washington, DC: American Psychiatric Association, 1991.

15. Gallyas F. Silver staining of Alzheimer's neurofibrillary changes by means of physical development. Acta Morphol Acad Sci Hung 1971; 19: 1–8.

16. Koesel S, Graeber MB. Use of neuropathological tissue for molecular genetic studies: parameters affecting DNA extraction and polymerase chain reaction. Acta Neuropathol 1994; 88: 19–25.

17. Egensperger R, Koesel S, Schnabel R, Mehraein P, Graeber MB. Apolipoprotein E genotype and neuropathological phenotype in two members of a German family with chromosome 14-linked early-onset Alzheimer's disease. Acta Neuropathol 1995; 90: 257–65.

18. Tolnay M, Probst A. Ballooned neurons expressing αB-crystallin as a constant feature of the amygdala in argyrophilic grain disease. Neurosci Lett 1998; 246: 165–8.

19. Egensperger R, Bancher C, Koesel S, Jellinger K, Mehraein P, Graeber MB. The apolipoprotein E ε4 allele in Parkinson's disease with Alzheimer lesions. Biochem Biophys Res Commun 1996; 244: 484–6.

20. Harrington CR, Louwagie J, Rossau R, Vanmechelen E, Perry EK, Xuereb JH, Roth M, Wischik CM. Influence of apolipoprotein E genotype on senile dementia of the Alzheimer and Lewy body types. Significance for etiological theories of Alzheimer's disease. Am J Pathol 1994; 145: 1472–84.

21. Davignon J, Gregg RE, Sing CF. Apolipoprotein E polymorphism and athero-sclerosis. Arteriosclerosis 1988; 8: 1–21.
22. Ohm TG, Kirca M, Bohl J, Scharnagl H, Gross W, Marz W. Apolipoprotein E polymorphism influences not only cerebral senile plaque load but also Alzheimer-type neurofibrillary tangle formation. Neuroscience 1995; 69: 757–67.
23. Brousseau T, Legrain S, Berr C, Gourlet V, Vidal O, Amouyel P. Confirmation of the ε4 allele of the apolipoprotein E gene as a risk factor for late-onset Alzheimer's disease. Neurology 1994; 44: 342–4.
24. Bancher C, Brunner C, Lassmann H, Budka H, Jellinger K, Wiche G, Seitelberger F, Grundke-Iqbal K, Wisniewski HM. Accumulation of abnormally phosphory-lated tau precedes the formation of neurofibrillary tangles in Alzheimer's disease. Brain Res 1989; 477: 90–99.
25. Braak E, Braak H, Mandelkow E-M. A sequence of cytoskeleton changes related to the formation of neurofibrillary tangles and neuropil threads. Acta Neuropathol 1994; 87: 554–67.
26. Ghebremedhin E, Schultz C, Botez G, Rueb U, Sassin I, Braak E, Braak H. Argyrophilic grain disease is associated with apolipoprotein E ε2 allele. Acta Neuropathol 1998; 96: 222–4.

Address for correspondence:
Markus Tolnay MD,
Institute of Pathology, Division of Neuropathology,
Schoenbeinstrasse 40, CH-4003 Basel, Switzerland
Tel: +41 61 265 2896; fax: +41 61 265 3194; e-mail: mtolnay@uhbs.ch

61 On the Possible Lifetime of a Tangled Neuron in the Parkinsonism–Dementia Complex of Guam

C. SCHWAB, J.C. STEELE, M. SCHULZER AND
P.L. McGEER

INTRODUCTION

Neurofibrillary pathology in the form of neurofibrillary tangles (NFTs), dystrophic neurites (DNs) and neuropil threads occurs in several neurodegenerative diseases. Such pathology is considerably more severe in the parkinsonism–dementia complex of Guam (PDC) than in Alzheimer's disease (AD) or any of the other neurodegenerative disorders where tangles appear. NFTs contain paired helical filaments (PHFs), consisting of abnormally phosphorylated tau [1–4]. The abnormal tau in PDC is indistinguishable from that in AD by immunohistochemistry and Western blotting [5, 6]. Intracellular NFTs (iNFTs) develop in neurons, particularly pyramidal neurons of the allocortex and isocortex. Eventually these neurons die, leaving behind extracellular NFTs (eNFTs) or ghost tangles [7, 8]. The hierarchical appearance of NFTs is similar in PDC and AD, except that in PDC they extend more extensively into subcortical structures, thus accounting for the appearance of a parkinsonian syndrome. Also, neocortical tangles in PDC are most prominent in layers II and III, while in AD they are most prominent in layers III and V [9].

In PDC, as in AD, the appearance of NFTs in the hippocampus follows a hierarchical pattern, with the CA1 region being affected early and the CA4 region late. The individual pyramidal neurons go through stages progressing from healthy, unaffected neurons to neurons with iNFTs and then to death of neurons, with eNFTs remaining as the skeletal markers.

In a previous study of PDC cases [10], we found that, in CA4, the combined total of unaffected pyramidal neurons, iNFTs and eNFTs, was remarkably constant in all the cases studied. The density of eNFTs correlated significantly and negatively with the density of surviving neurons, which

Alzheimer's Disease and Related Disorders
Edited by K. Iqbal, D.F. Swaab, B. Winblad and H.M. Wisniewski
© 1999 John Wiley & Sons Ltd

included unaffected neurons and iNFTs. CA1 was more intensely affected than CA4. In advanced cases of PDC, all neurons from CA1 had disappeared, with only eNFTs being observed. The combined total of unaffected pyramidal neurons, iNFTs and eNFTs, was still relatively constant, although greater variability was seen than in CA4. The results indicated that loss of pyramidal neurons was proportional to the appearance of eNFTs, and that eNFTs accumulated without evidence of disappearance through phagocytosis.

We also found that, in very early cases, CA1 was significantly affected, but CA4 was unaffected or minimally affected. We used this observation as the basis for calculating the lifetime of neurons developing intracellular tangles in CA4, since the pathology in this region could be timed from clinical disease onset.

CASES STUDIED AND RESULTS

Eight cases of PDC, age range 60–79 years, cases 4–11, and three neurologically normal controls from Guam, age range 41–79 years, cases 1–3, were studied. Case 3 was a suicide from depression and had a sibling with PDC. It was presumed he may have been an early presymptomatic PDC case. Sections of the hippocampus 30 μm thick were cut on a freezing microtome and stained by various techniques. Cresyl violet staining was used to demonstrate viable neurons. iNFTs were visualized by immunostaining with Alz50 [11–13] and eNFTs with anti-amyloid P (DAKO) [10].

The densities of eNFTs, iNFTs and healthy neurons in the CA4 region were determined by counting populations using an ocular grid at a ×20 objective magnification. A total of five to ten adjacent fields was obtained, corresponding to an area of at least 1.065 mm² for each brain. The number of unaffected neurons was determined by subtracting the number of Alz50-immunolabeled iNFTs from the number of neurons counted in cresyl violet sections. The numbers of viable neurons and eNFTs were added to obtain a value for the total population density. The data for density and total number were corrected according to the formula of Floderus [14]. Correction factors were calculated after measuring the size of 60 neurons and eNFTs in each region (0.837 for neurons and iNFTs and 0.784 for eNFTs). Totals are shown in Table 1.

Neurons with displaced nuclei and a globose shape were abundant in cresyl violet stained sections of severe cases of PDC (Figure 1A, B). When sections were immunostained with Alz50, and then counterstained with cresyl violet, it was observed that all the Alz50 immunostained tangles were intracellular (Figure 1C, D). By contrast, tangles that were strongly immunoreactive with the amyloid P antibody (AP) were all eNFTs (Figure 1E, F). The intensity of staining of NFTs in Bielschowsky silver-impregnated sections varied from light brown to dense black (Figure 1G, H). Counterstaining with cresyl violet, as well as observation of the shape of tangles, indicated that those NFTs heavily stained black were intracellular, while those weakly stained brown

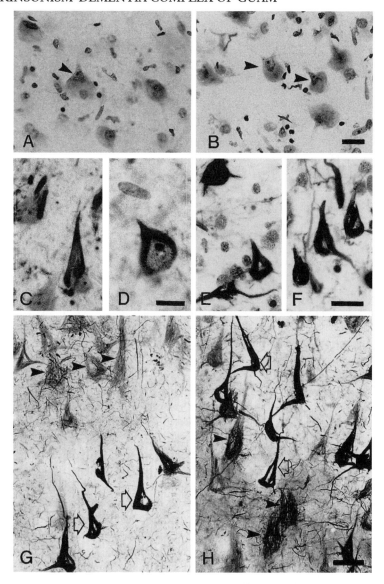

Figure 1. Staining of a severe case of PDC in region CA4. (A, B) Cresyl violet staining in CA4 shows neurons with displaced nuclei and globose neurons (arrowheads). (C, D) Cresyl violet counterstaining of sections immunostained with Alz50 reveals that the tangles immunoreactive for Alz50 are intracellular, having associated neuronal nuclei. (E, F) Amyloid P immunoreactive tangles are extracellular since they are not associated with nuclei, as counterstaining with cresyl violet verifies. (G, H) Staining by the modified Bielschowsky method. Intracellular NFTs are heavily stained (black, arrows), while extracellular NFTs (light brown in the original sections) are only weakly labeled (arrow heads). Calibration bars apply to the section shown and the preceding section. Bars in (B), (F) and (H), 50 μm; calibration bar in (D), 25 μm

Table 1. Density of neurons, iNFTs, eNFTs, duration of disease and mean survival time of tangled neurons*

Case number	Number per mm³ of:*				Duration of disease (years)	Survival time of iNFTs (years)
	N_h	N_i	N_e	N		
1	5257	0	0	5257	0	
2	5414	0	0	5414	0	
3	5597	26	49	5673	0	
4	5414	52	74	5540	5	6.01
5	4760	105	466	5331	5	1.26
6	5264	65	140	5469	3.5	2.55
7	4917	131	466	5514	6	1.44
8	5074	52	172	5298	12	7.98
9	4159	288	1176	5623	3	0.27
10	3531	131	1593	5254	6	0.44
11	759	2066	2842	5667	10	0.13

*N_h = number of healthy neurons; N_i = number of iNFTs; N_e = number of eNTFs; $N = N_h + N_i + N_e$.

were extracellular. Counts on nearby sections demonstrated highly significant correlations between black-stained tangles by the Bielschowsky method and Alz50 immunostained iNFTs (n = 11 slide pairs, r^2 = 0.80, p < 0.0001) and between brown-stained tangles and AP immunostained eNFTs (n = 11 slide pairs, r^2 = 0.97, p < 0.0001).

In the PDC cases (cases 4–11), the number of iNFTs and eNFTs both increased according to the intensity of the disease. This is illustrated in the photomicrographs of Figure 2 and the bar graph of Figure 3. In Figure 2A, B, C, cresyl violet staining is compared in CA4 of a control, a mild case of PDC and a severe case of PDC. High numbers of intact neurons are seen in both the control and mild PDC cases, with the severe PDC case showing a substantial loss of neurons. Alz50 staining (Figure 2D, E, F) showed almost no iNFTs in either the control or mild PDC cases but a substantial number in the severe case. AP staining (Figure 2G, H, I) revealed no eNFTs in the control, a few in the mild PDC case, and many in the severe PDC case.

The sum of the densities of eNFTs, iNFTs and unaffected neurons in CA4 was relatively constant from case to case, with the range being 5254–5673 mm³ (Figure 3; Table 1). Using these data it was possible to derive a series of differential equations to calculate the mean lifetime of tangled neurons for each case. It was assumed for these calculations that iNFT formation in CA4 did not commence prior to disease onset, and that the rate of iNFT formation and the rate of conversion of iNFTs to eNFTs remained constant as the disease progressed. The equations are as follows:

1. $\dfrac{dN_h(t)}{dt} = -R_i N_h(t)$, so that $N_h(t) = N_e^{-R_i t}$

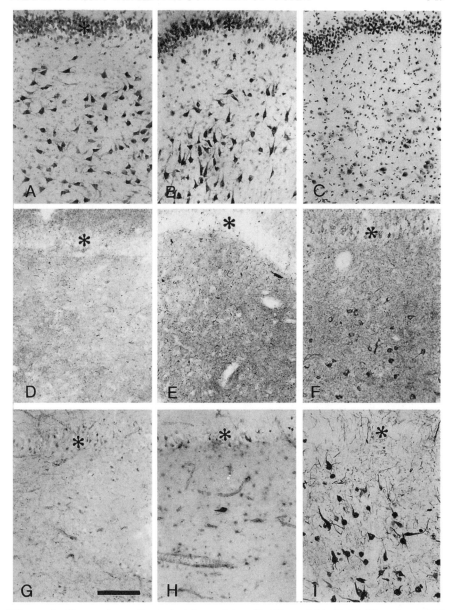

Figure 2. Comparison of cresyl violet staining (A–C), and Alz50 (D–F) and amyloid P (G–I) immunostaining in CA4 of a control (first column), a mild case of PDC (second column) and a severe case of PDC (third column). No iNFTs (D) or eNTFs (G) are present in the control CA4. The mild PDC case demonstrates a few iNTFs (E) and eNFTs (H). In the severe PDC case, many CA4 neurons are lost (C), and moderate numbers of iNFTs (F) and eNFTs (I) can be seen. The granule cell layer is identified by asterisks in all photographs. Calibration bar in G = 200 μm and applies to all photographs

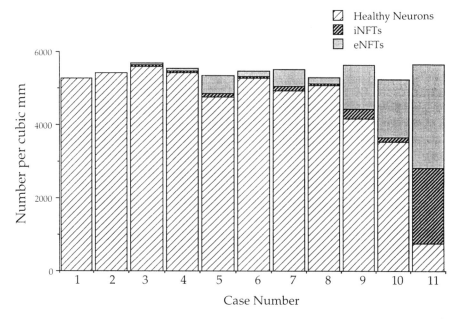

Figure 3. Density of unaffected neurons, iNFTs and eNFTs in all cases. Case numbers as in Table 1, with 1–3 being controls and 4–11 cases of PDC

2. $\dfrac{dN_e(t)}{dt} = -R_e N_i(t)$, so that $N_e(t) = e^{-R_i t} (N + 1) - (N + 1) e^{-R_i t} + N$

3. $\therefore$ Density function in state h: $f(t) = R_i e^{-R_i t}$; $t > 0$
   Mean time in state h: R_i^{-1}

4. Density function of time to reach state e: $g(t) = (1 + \dfrac{1}{N})R_i(e^{-R_i t} - e^{-R_i t(N+1)})$; $t > 0$
   Mean time to reach state e: $\dfrac{N + 2}{R_i(N + 1)}$

5. Mean time in state i: $\dfrac{N + 2}{R_i(N + 1)} - \dfrac{1}{R_i} = \dfrac{1}{R_i(N + 1)} = R_e^{-1}$

where N_h = number of healthy pyramidal neurons per mm³; N_i = number of pyramidal neurons with intracellular tangles per mm³; N_e = number of extracellular (ghost) tangles per mm³; $N = N(t) = N_h(t) + N_i(t) + N_e(t)$ = total population; R_i = rate of formation of intracellular tangles; R_e = rate of conversion of intracellular tangles to extracellular tangles; t = time in years. For a more detailed derivation of these equations, see [15].

The calculations gave mean lifetimes varying between 0.13 years in case 11 and 7.98 years in case 8, with an average of 2.51 years (Table 1).

DISCUSSION

The small variability in total number of neurons plus eNFTs (Table 1 and Figure 3) indicated that there was little phagocytosis of the eNFTs. These appear to remain as fairly permanent markers of degenerated neurons.

Based on our previous observations that PDC cases coming to autopsy at the preclinical or very early clinical stages had significant tangles in CA1 but none in CA4 [10], we assumed that the time of onset of clinical PDC could be taken as the time of onset of degeneration in CA4. We therefore derived differential equations based on this assumption to calculate the lifetime of tangled neurons, assuming a constant rate of intracellular tangle formation and a constant rate of conversion of intracellular tangles to extracellular tangles. Solving these equations yielded lifetimes of CA4 tangled neurons varying from 0.13 years in the most rapidly developing case to 7.98 years in the most slowly developing case. The average for eight cases was 2.51 years.

ACKNOWLEDGEMENTS

Supported by grants from the Alzheimer Society of British Columbia, the Medical Research Council of Canada and the Jack Brown and Family AD Research Fund, as well as donations from individual British Columbians.

REFERENCES

1. Bancher C, Brunner C, Lassman H, Budka H, Jellinger K, Wiche G, Seitelberger F, Grundke-Iqbal K, Wisniewski HM. Accumulation of abnormally phosphory-lated tau precedes the formation of neurofibrillary tangles in Alzheimer's disease. Brain Res 1989; 477: 90–99.
2. Dickson DW, Ksiezak RH, Liu WK, Davies P, Crowe A, Yen SH. Immuno-cytochemistry of neurofibrillary tangles with antibodies to subregions of tau pro-tein: identification of hidden and cleaved tau epitopes and a new phosphorylation site. Acta Neuropathol 1992; 84: 596–605.
3. Goedert M, Jakes R, Crowther RA, Six J, Lubke U, Vandermeeren M, Cras P, Trojanowski JQ, Lee VM. The abnormal phosphorylation of tau protein at Ser-202 in Alzheimer disease recapitulates phosphorylation during development. Proc Natl Acad Sci USA 1993; 5066–70.
4. Kosi, KS. Tau protein and neurodegeneration [review]. Mol Neurobiol 1990; 4: 171–9.
5. Buee-Scherrer V, Buee L, Hof PR, Leveugle B, Gilles C, Loerzel AJ, Perl DP, Delacourte A. Neurofibrillary degeneration in amyotrophic lateral sclerosis/parkinsonism–dementia complex of Guam. Am J Pathol 1995; 68: 924–32.
6. Mawal-Dewan M, Schmidt M, Balin B, Perl D, Lee V, Trojanowski J. Identifica-tion of phosphorylation sites in PHF-tau from patients with Guam amyotrophic lateral sclerosis parkinsonism–dementia comples. J Neuropath Exp Neurol 1996; 55: 1051–59.

7. Bondareff W, Harrington C, Wischik CM, Hauser DL, Roth M. Immuno-histochemical staging of neurofibrillary degeneration in Alzheimer's disease. J Neuropath Exp Neurol 1994; 53: 158–64.
8. Braak E, Braak H, Mandlekow E-M. A sequence of cytoskeleton changes related to the formation of neurofibrillary tangles and neuropil threads. Acta Neuropathol 1994; 87: 554–7.
9. Hof PR, Perl DP, Loerzel AJ, Morrison JH. Neurofibrillary tangle distribution in the cerebral cortex of parkinsonism–dementia cases from Guam: differences with Alzheimer's disease. Brain Res 1991; 564: 306–13.
10. Schwab C, Steele JC, McGeer PL. Pyramidal neuron loss is matched by ghost tangle increase in Guam parkinsonism–dementia hippocampus. Acta Neuropathol 1998; 96: 409–16.
11. Bouras C, Hof PR, Morrison JH. Neurofibrillary tangle densities in the hippocampal formation in a non-demented population define subgroups of patients with differential early pathological changes. Neurosci Lett 1993; 153: 131–5.
12. Cras P, Smith MA, Richey PL, Siedlak SL, Mulvihill P, Perry G. Extracellular neurofibrillary tangles reflect neuronal loss and provide further evidence of extensive protein cross-linking in Alzheimer's disease. Acta Neuropathol 1995; 89: 291–5.
13. Wolozin B, Pruchnicki A, Dickson DW, Davies P. A neuronal antigen in the brains of Alzheimer's disease patients. Science 1986; 232: 648–50.
14. Haug H. History of neuromorphometry. J Neurosci Meth 1986; 18: 1–17.
15. Schwab C, Schulzer M, Steele JC, McGeer PL. On the survival time of a tangled neuron in the hippocampal CA4 region in parkinsonism dementia complex of Guam. Neurobiol Aging 1999 (in press).

Address for correspondence:
Dr Patrick L. McGeer,
Kinsmen Laboratory of Neurological Research,
University of British Columbia,
2255 Wesbrook Mall, Vancouver, BC V6T 1Z3, Canada
Tel: 604 822 7377; fax: 604 822 7086; e-mail: mcgeerpl@unixg.ubc.ca

62 Comparison of the Biological Characteristics of BSE and CJD in Mice

M.E. BRUCE, R.G. WILL, J.W. IRONSIDE AND H. FRASER

INTRODUCTION

There are many phenotypically distinct strains of the agents that cause transmissible spongiform encephalopathies (TSEs) or 'prion' diseases [1, 2]. These strains differ in their incubation periods in panels of inbred mouse strains and in their targeting of pathological changes within the brains of these mice, features that have been developed into formal strain-typing protocols. Extensive studies of mouse-passaged laboratory TSE strains have shown that TSE agents carry some form of strain-specific information that is independent of the host [2], but the molecular basis of this informational component is still a matter for speculation. In recent years, transmission and strain-typing studies in mice have been used to investigate the relationships between TSEs occurring naturally in different animal species. We have now extended these studies to include transmissions of CJD from patients where there was a suspected dietary or occupational link with BSE [3].

TSE STRAIN DISCRIMINATION IN MICE

In mice experimentally infected with TSE isolates, the incubation period of the disease, although long, is remarkably precise and repeatable. This incubation period depends on a precise interaction between the strain of the TSE agent and genetic factors in the challenged mice [4]. The mouse *Sinc* (*s*crapie *inc*ubation) gene has long been known to exert a major influence on the incubation period [5]. The two alleles of *Sinc* (s7 and p7) can account for differences in incubation periods of hundreds of days when mice are infected with a single TSE strain. It is now established that the *Sinc* gene encodes the

Alzheimer's Disease and Related Disorders
Edited by K. Iqbal, D.F. Swaab, B. Winblad and H.M. Wisniewski
© 1999 John Wiley & Sons Ltd

'prion protein', PrP [6, 7]. The s7 and p7 alleles of *Sinc* correspond to the a and b alleles of the PrP gene, encoding proteins that differ in their sequence by two amino acids [8]. It is also known that other host genes influence the incubation period, particularly when TSEs are transmitted to mice from another species.

As a routine, TSE strains are characterized by injection of a panel of inbred mouse strains, differing in their *Sinc* (or PrP) genotypes and also in respect to other genes. Each TSE strain has a characteristic and highly reproducible pattern of incubation periods in these mouse strains [1]. TSE strains also show dramatic and reproducible differences in the type, severity and distribution of pathological changes that they produce in the brains of infected mice. The most prominent change seen in routine histological sections is a vacuolation of the neuropil, which is targeted to different parts of the brain, depending mainly on the strain of TSE, but also to some extent on *Sinc* and other mouse genes. The distribution of vacuolar degeneration is the basis of a semiquantitative method of strain discrimination in which the severity of pathology is scored from coded sections in nine grey matter and three white matter brain areas to construct a 'lesion profile' [9]. Each combination of TSE strain and mouse strain has a characteristic lesion profile [1].

These strain-typing methods were developed originally for mouse-passaged laboratory strains of scrapie and have been used extensively in fundamental studies exploring the basis of agent strain variation. It is now clear that these methods can also be used at the primary transmission to mice of a TSE from another species, making it possible to type the TSE strain present in a naturally infected host.

TRANSMISSIONS OF ANIMAL TSEs TO MICE

BSE has been transmitted to mice from eight unrelated cattle sources, collected at different times during the epidemic and from widely separated geographical locations within the UK. All eight BSE sources produced a similar pattern of incubation periods in a standard panel of mouse strains (Figure 1) [10, 11]. There were large and consistent differences in incubation period between mouse strains of different *Sinc* genotypes and also between mouse strains of the same *Sinc* genotype. For example, the incubation period in RIII mice was consistently shorter than that in C57BL mice by about 100 days, even though these mouse strains have the same *Sinc* genotype. This shows that genes other than that encoding PrP can have a major influence on the progression of the disease. The eight BSE sources also produced a closely similar pattern of pathology in infected mice, as represented by the lesion profile (Figure 2) [10, 11]. This uniformity of transmission results suggests that each cow was infected with the same major strain of agent. The consistency of the pathology reported in cattle with BSE [12] also suggests that a single or a limited number of strains has been involved in the epidemic.

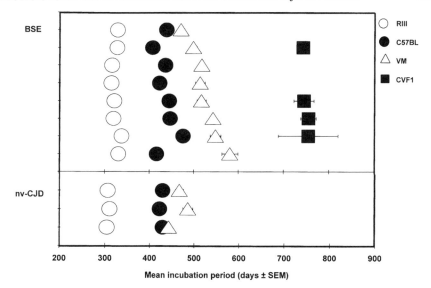

Figure 1. Incubation periods in a panel of mouse strains challenged, by intracerebral and intraperitoneal injection, with brain homogenates from eight sources of BSE and three sources of nvCJD. Based on [3]

More recently, transmissions to mice have been achieved from other species with novel TSEs, which were suspected to be related to the BSE epidemic; the sources were three domestic cats, a greater kudu and a nyala. The results of all five transmissions were strikingly similar to results from cattle sources, indicating that these species were infected with the BSE strain and providing the first clear evidence for the natural spread of a TSE between species [11, 13]. BSE from cattle has also been transmitted experimentally to sheep, goats and pigs and then from each of these species to mice. Again, the results of these mouse transmissions were closely similar to direct transmissions of BSE [11, 14]. These studies show, firstly, that the BSE agent is unchanged when passaged through a range of species and, secondly, that the donor species has had little influence on the disease characteristics of BSE on transmission to mice. In contrast to this uniformity, the incubation periods and lesion profiles in transmissions of natural scrapie from sheep to mice have varied widely between sources, with none resembling BSE [11, 3]. It is likely that this variation reflects scrapie strain variation in the natural host.

TRANSMISSIONS OF 'NEW VARIANT' AND SPORADIC CJD TO MICE

Over 30 cases of a clinically and pathologically atypical form of Creutzfeldt–Jakob disease ('new variant' or nvCJD) [15] have recently been recognized in

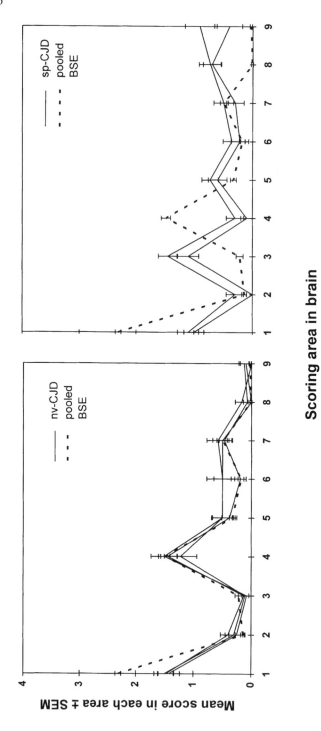

Figure 2. Lesion profiles in RIII mice for transmissions of nvCJD from three sources and spCJD from two sources (a dairy farmer and a contemporary case), compared with a standard lesion profile for BSE, based on pooled data from four transmissions. Based on [3]

unusually young people in the UK and a further case has been reported in France [16]. This raised serious concerns that BSE may have spread to humans, possibly by dietary exposure. Circumstantial evidence that this was the case came from the observation of 'florid' amyloid plaques, identical to those seen in nvCJD, in the brains of rhesus macaques experimentally infected with BSE [17]. Also, nvCJD resembled BSE but differed from typical sporadic CJD (spCJD) in the molecular characteristics of the disease-specific isoform of PrP in brain extracts: in the relative prominence of three different glycoforms of the protein and in the size of the unglycosylated form [18, 19].

To investigate the possible link between nvCJD and BSE further, transmissions to mice were set up from the brains of three patients with nvCJD, using an identical protocol to that used in the series of animal TSE transmissions described above [3]. For comparison, transmissions were also set up from six typical cases of spCJD, with no unusual clinical or neuropathological features. These included two dairy farmers who had had BSE in their herds and had therefore been potentially exposed to BSE-infected cattle or contaminated animal feed [20]; two 'contemporary' cases with no known occupational exposure to BSE; and two 'historical' cases who had died before the onset of the BSE outbreak. All nine individuals were homozygous for methionine at codon 129 of the PrP gene and none had any of the PrP gene mutations associated with familial disease.

The nvCJD transmission experiments are incomplete, but results so far for all three sources are closely similar to those seen in transmissions of BSE from cattle and other species [3]. As in BSE transmissions, the shortest incubation periods of about 300 days were seen in mice of the RIII strain, which were 100% susceptible to the disease (Figure 1). The incubation periods in C57BL and VM mice were also consistent with the BSE pattern. Mean incubation periods are not yet available for the remaining group (C57BL × VM), but are known to be very long. The neuropathology in mice with nvCJD was also closely similar to that seen in mice with BSE. For example, the lesion profiles in RIII mice for the three sources were almost superimposable and also closely similar to those in RIII mice with BSE (Figure 2). As with BSE, a characteristic feature in all mouse strains with nvCJD was a prominent involvement of the cochlear nucleus (an area that is not included in the lesion profile). In general, amyloid plaques were not a prominent feature of this pathology, except in periventricular areas in VM mice, as is also the case for BSE in this mouse strain [10]. These plaques were not of the 'florid' type seen in patients with nvCJD. Overall, the striking similarity between nvCJD and BSE in mice, in terms of both incubation periods and pathology, is strong evidence that the same strain of agent is involved in the two species.

In contrast to the results with the nvCJD sources, no clinical neurological disease was seen in any mice challenged with spCJD, up to 800 days after injection. However, evidence for transmission from all six spCJD sources came from the presence of vacuolar degeneration typical of TSE infection in the brains of most mice dying with intercurrent disease, from about 400 days following challenge [3]. This diagnosis was confirmed by the presence of the disease-associated form of PrP, demonstrated by Western blotting and immunocytochemistry. No such changes were seen in saline-injected control mice housed alongside the challenged groups, or in mice injected with human brain homogenates from patients with amyotrophic lateral sclerosis or laryngeal carcinoma [21]. The neuropathological changes in mice with spCJD differed in severity between individual mice, but showed a consistent pattern between mouse strains and between sources. The distribution of vacuolar degeneration, as illustrated by the lesion profile, was strikingly different from that seen in BSE or nvCJD transmissions to mice (e.g. Figure 2). These transmission results indicate that spCJD is associated with a different TSE strain from that causing nvCJD or BSE. There is therefore no evidence from this study of a link between CJD in dairy farmers and BSE.

CONCLUSIONS

Even though the molecular basis of TSE strain variation is unknown, biological strain-typing can be used to answer pressing questions about the naturally occurring diseases. Most importantly, these methods have shown that the BSE strain has infected several different species, including humans. At the more fundamental level, these studies have important implications for the molecular nature of TSE agents. The BSE strain has been shown to retain its phenotype after passage through eight different species, reinforcing previous evidence for an infection-specific informational component that is independent of the PrP amino acid sequence of the host. A crucial question is whether the host PrP protein alone can carry this information in the form of specific post-translational modifications, as proposed in the 'prion' hypothesis [22], or whether a separate informational molecule is required, such as a nucleic acid.

ACKNOWLEDGEMENTS

The authors would like to thank Irene McConnell, Dawn Drummond, Aileen Chree, Anne Suttie and Linda McCardle for their invaluable technical assistance. This work was supported by DoH, MRC, BBSRC and MAFF.

REFERENCES

1. Bruce ME, McConnell I, Fraser H, Dickinson AG. The disease characteristics of different strains of scrapie in *Sinc* congenic mouse lines: implications for the nature of the agent and host control of pathogenesis. J Gen Virol 1991; 72: 595–603.

2. Bruce ME. Scrapie strain variation and mutation. Br Med Bull 1993; 49: 822–38.
3. Bruce ME, Will RG, Ironside JW, McConnell I, Drummond D, Suttie A, McCardle L, Chree A, Hope J, Birkett C, Cousens S, Fraser H, Bostock CJ. Transmissions to mice indicate that 'new variant' CJD is caused by the BSE agent. Nature 1997; 389: 498–501.
4. Dickinson AG, Meikle VMH. Host-genotype and agent effects in scrapie incubation: change in allelic interaction with different strains of agent. Mol Gen Genet 1971; 112: 73–9.
5. Dickinson AG, Meikle VMH, Fraser H. Identification of a gene which controls the incubation period of some strains of scrapie agent in mice. J Comp Pathol 1968; 78: 293–9.
6. Hunter N, Dann JC, Bennett AD, Somerville RA, McConnell I, Hope J. Are *Sinc* and the PrP gene congruent? Evidence from PrP gene analysis in *Sinc* congenic mice. J Gen Virol 1992; 73: 2751–5.
7. Moore RC, Hope J, McBride PA, McConnell I, Selfridge J, Melton DW, Manson JC. Mice with gene targeted prion protein alterations show that *Prnp, Sinc* and *Prni* are congruent. Nature Genet 1998; 18: 118–25.
8. Westaway D, Goodman PA, Mirenda CA, McKinley MP, Carlson GA, Prusiner SB. Distinct prion proteins in short and long scrapie incubation period mice. Cell 1987; 51: 651–62.
9. Fraser H, Dickinson AG. The sequential development of the brain lesions of scrapie in three strains of mice. J Comp Pathol 1968; 78: 301–11.
10. Fraser H, Bruce ME, Chree A, McConnell I, Wells GAH. Transmission of bovine spongiform encephalopathy and scrapie to mice. J Gen Virol 1992; 73: 1891–7.
11. Bruce M, Chree A, McConnell I, Foster J, Pearson G, Fraser H. Transmission of bovine spongiform encephalopathy and scrapie to mice—strain variation and the species barrier. Phil Trans R Soc Lond B 1994; 343: 405–11.
12. Wells GAH, Hawkins SAC, Hadlow WJ, Spencer YI. The discovery of bovine spongiform encephalopathy and observations on the vacuolar changes. In: Prusiner SB, Collinge J, Powell J, Anderton B (eds) Prion Diseases of Humans and Animals. Chichester: Ellis Horwood, 1992; 256–74.
13. Fraser H, Pearson GR, McConnell I, Bruce ME, Wyatt JM, Gruffydd-Jones TJ. Transmission of feline spongiform encephalopathy to mice. Vet Rec 1994; 134: 449.
14. Foster JD, Bruce M, McConnell I, Chree A, Fraser H. Detection of BSE infectivity in brain and spleen of experimentally infected sheep. Vet Rec 1996; 138: 546–8.
15. Will RG, Ironside JW, Zeidler M, Cousens SN, Estibeiro K, Alperovitch A, Poser S, Pocchiari M, Hofman A, Smith PG. A new variant of Creutzfeldt–Jakob disease in the UK. Lancet 1996; 347: 921–5.
16. Chazot G, Broussolle E, Lapras CI, Blattler T, Aguzzi A, Kopp N. New variant of Creutzfeldt–Jakob disease in a 26-year-old French man. Lancet 1996; 347: 1181.
17. Lasmezas CI, Deslys J-P, Demaimay R, Adjou KT, Lamoury F, Dormont D, Robain O, Ironside J, Hauw J-J. BSE transmission to macaques. Nature 1996; 381: 743–4.
18. Collinge J, Sidle KCL, Meads J, Ironside J, Hill AF. Molecular analysis of prion strain variation and the aetiology of 'new variant' CJD. Nature 1996; 383: 685–90.
19. Hill AF, Will RG, Ironside J, Collinge J. Type of prion protein in UK farmers with Creutzfeldt–Jakob disease. Lancet 1997; 350: 188.
20. Cousens SN, Zeidler M, Esmonde TF, DeSilva R, Wilesmith JW, Smith PG, Will RG. Sporadic Creutzfeldt–Jakob disease in the United Kingdom: analysis of epidemiological surveillance data for 1970–96. Br Med J 1997; 315: 389–95.

21. Fraser H, Behan W, Chree A, Crossland G, Behan P. Mouse inoculation studies reveal no transmissible agent in amyotrophic lateral sclerosis. Br J Pathol 1996; 6: 89–99.
22. Telling GC, Parchi P, DeArmond SJ, Cortelli P, Montagna P, Gabizon R, Mastrianni J, Lugaresi E, Gambetti P, Prusiner SB. Evidence for the conformation of the pathological isoform of the prion protein enciphering and propagating prion diversity. Science 1996; 274: 2079–82.

Address for correspondence:
Dr Moira E. Bruce,
Institute for Animal Health, Neuropathogenesis Unit,
Ogston Building, West Mains Road,
Edinburgh EH9 3JF, UK
Tel: +44 (0) 131 667 5204; fax: +44 (0) 131 668 3872;
e-mail: moira.bruce@bbsrc.ac.uk

63 Agent Strain Variation in Human Prion Diseases: Insight from Transmission to Primates

PIERO PARCHI, PAUL BROWN,
SABINA CAPELLARI, CLARENCE J. GIBBS JR
AND PIERLUIGI GAMBETTI

INTRODUCTION

Prion diseases, also called transmissible spongiform encephalopathies (TSEs), are fatal neurodegenerative disorders that affect most species of mammals. They are caused by an as yet incompletely characterized infectious agent that shows strain variation [1, 2]. The pathogenesis of these disorders is strictly related to a host-encoded glycoprotein of unknown function, designated prion protein [3]. The 'prion', as the infectious agent is commonly named, does not replicate or transmit in the absence of prion protein expression [4]. In addition, an abnormal, partially protease-resistant isoform (PrP-res) of the normal cellular prion protein (PrP-C) specifically accumulates in the nervous system during prion infection and represents the hallmark of these disorders [5]. The conversion of PrP-C to PrP-res is a post-translational event, and involves a conformational change of the protein [6]. The molecular events leading to this conversion, however, remain largely unknown.

In humans, prion diseases comprise a broad spectrum of clinico-pathological variants that show heterogeneity in disease duration, symptoms at onset, relative severity and distribution of brain lesions such as spongiosis, neuronal loss and gliosis, as well as the presence and morphology of amyloid

Alzheimer's Disease and Related Disorders
Edited by K. Iqbal, D.F. Swaab, B. Winblad and H.M. Wisniewski
© 1999 John Wiley & Sons Ltd

plaques [7]. According to broad differences in these phenotypic features, human prion diseases are usually classified into four major groups: Creutzfeldt–Jakob disease (CJD), Gertsmann–Sträussler–Scheinker disease (GSS), kuru and fatal familial insomnia (FFI) [7].

In scrapie transmitted to mice, the strain of the agent, the host genotype and, to a lesser extent, the route of infection have been shown to modulate the disease phenotype [1, 2]. Agent strain variation has also been demonstrated in humans [8, 9]. However, to what extent phenotypic variability of human prion diseases depends on the strain of the agent rather than on host genetic factors remain largely unknown.

Recent studies have shown that there are properties of PrP-res, such as fragment size and ratio of di-, mono- and unglycosylated forms of the protein, that may allow the molecular identification of prion strains [10–15]. Distinct PrP-res profiles correlate with different phenotypes of the disease, even in subjects with the same *PRNP* genotype [12, 15]. Furthermore, PrP-res properties may be largely maintained after inter-species transmission, although changes may occur in certain genotypes of recipients [8, 16]. Thus, whether the different PrP-res types represent indeed the molecular basis of prion strains or just a molecular signature, possibly imparted by another informational molecule, is unknown.

In order to determine the relative contribution of agent strain variation and host genotype in the phenotypic expression of human prion diseases, and further assess the strain specificity of the physicochemical properties of PrP-res after transmission to animal species with different genetic background, we characterized molecular mass and glycoform ratio of PrP-res in 85 cases of human prion diseases that have been transmitted to primates, and compared these characteristics to those of the PrP-res extracted from their correspondent animal recipient/s.

RESULTS

Human and primate brain samples were obtained from the National Institutes of Health series of experimentally transmitted prion disease [17]. Immunoblot analysis of the human samples confirmed previously published results [11,

15]: after deglycosylation, PrP-res consisted of one or more of three N-terminally truncated protein fragments with molecular weights of ~21 kDa (type 1), ~19 kDa (type 2) and ~8 kDa (provisionally designated as type 3). Type 1 was found in most sCJD cases, in all fCJD cases (E200K mutation) and in the three GSS cases (P102L mutation), and was largely associated with the methionine (M) allele at codon 129. Type 2, seen in about 25% of sCJD cases, was usually associated with the valine (V) allele at codon 129. Type 3 was found only in the three GSS cases, exclusively in association with type 1 and methionine at codon 129.

Types 1 and 2 were comprised of diglycosylated, monoglycosylated and unglycosylated protein isoforms, whereas type 3 consisted only of the unglycosylated isoform. Based on the ratio amounts of these differently glycosylated peptides, two subtypes could be identified for type 1 PrP-res. In sCJD, the most abundant isoform was monoglycosylated, whereas in fCJD and GSS, the diglycosylated isoform was more abundant.

Surprisingly, PrP-res from the brains of spider monkeys (Figure 1) and squirrel monkeys (Figure 2) inoculated with these human specimens uniformly showed a molecular weight pattern within the range of type 1. However, analysis of glycoform ratios in the primates revealed a significant overall difference in pattern, resulting from the type of inoculum: type 2 from sCJD subjects (codon 129 VV or MV) produced a predominantly monoglycosylated isoform, whereas type 1 from sporadic (codon 129 MM or MV) and familial CJD or type 1 and 3 from the GSS cases usually produced a nearly equal mix of diglycosylated and monoglycosylated isoforms (Figures 1 and 2). The human type 2 PrP-res inocula also produced a significantly prolonged incubation period in both squirrel and spider monkeys, compared to human type 1 or types 1 and 3.

CONCLUSIONS

The observation of two distinct sCJD phenotypes in *PRNP* syngenic subjects, which correlate with two types of PrP-res with distinct physicochemical characteristics, led us to propose that two major strains of prions are associated with sCJD [12]. In strong support of this hypothesis, the present data show

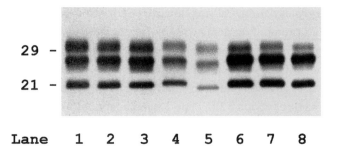

Figure 1. Immunoblot analysis of PrP-res extracted from brains of spider monkeys (lanes 1–3 and 6–8) or sporadic CJD with PrP-res type 1 or 2 (lanes 4 and 5, respectively). Primates were inoculated with brain suspensions from patients with sCJD, M129M, PrP-res type 1 (lane 1), fCJD, E200K–M129M, PrP-res type 1 (lane 2), GSS P102L–M129M, PrP-res types 1 and 3 (lane 3), V129 V, PrP-res type 2 (lanes 6–8)

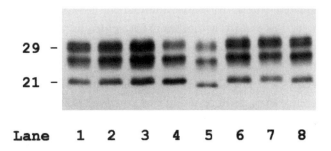

Figure 2. Immunoblot analysis of PrP-res extracted from brains of squirrel monkeys (lanes 1–3 and 6–8) or sporadic CJD with PrP-res type 1 or 2 (lanes 4 and 5, respectively). Primates were inoculated with brain suspensions from patients with sCJD, M129M, PrP-res type 1 (lane 1), fCJD, E200K–M129M, PrP-res type 1 (lane 2), GSS P102L–M129M, PrP-res types 1 and 2 (lane 3), V129 V, PrP-res type 2 (lanes 6–8)

that two significantly different glycoform profiles of PrP-res, which correlate with distinct incubation times of the disease, are found in primates injected with a variety of human sCJD inocula. These findings strongly suggest that two distinct strains of agent are linked to the most common sCJD variants, which account for about 80% of all human prion diseases.

The finding that at least two prion strains are associated with sCJD also has important implications for the understanding of the familial and so-called 'acquired' forms of prion diseases. We previously showed that type 1 and type 2 PrP-res are present in all subtypes of CJD, as well as in kuru, independent of the etiology of the disease, i.e. sporadic, inherited or acquired, by infection [13, 14]. Taken together, these observations raise the critical question whether the same strains of agent causing sCJD are also associated with the familial and acquired forms of the human disease, and, if this is the case, whether the unique phenotypic features of some familial prion diseases, such as GSS, can be only explained by variation in the host *PRNP* genotype. The present data on the transmission of fCJD and GSS to primates are consistent with this hypothesis. No significant differences in incubation time or PrP-res profile were found among the primates inoculated with the homogenates containing PrP-res type 1, irrespective of the form (sporadic or familial) or type (CJD vs. GSS) of disease. This finding strongly suggests that the same strain of agent is involved in these disorders. Furthermore, no type 3 PrP-res and multicentric amyloid plaques, two distinct phenotypic features of GSS [15], were found in the primates injected with the GSS inocula. This finding is consistent with the notion that type 3 PrP-res and multicentric plaque formation are specified by the interaction of one 'CJD' strain of the agent with the mutated PrP expressed by a 'GSS'-specific *PRNP* haplotype. Thus, overall, our data indicate that a limited number of prion strains affect humans and that phenotypic variation of human prion diseases largely depend on host genetic factors.

It is currently highly debated whether the study of the fragment size and glycoform ratio of PrP-res provide distinctive molecular markers that are specific enough to allow the intra- or inter-species identification of prion strains. Overall our data indicate that human PrP-res type 1 and type 2 largely represent strain-specific markers. However, both size and glycoform pattern may change after inter-species transmission. Therefore, our data indicate that PrP-res typing provides a molecular signature for certain prion strains within a certain host genotype, but is of limited value for tracing their passage among different animal species.

ACKNOWLEDGEMENTS

This work was supported by NIH Grants AG08155, AG08992, AG14359 and the Britton Fund.

REFERENCES

1. Fraser H, Dickinson AG. Scrapie in mice. Agent-strain differences in the distribution and intensity of grey matter vacuolation. J Comp Path 1973; 83: 23–40.
2. Bruce ME. Strain typing studies on scrapie and BSE. In: Baker H, Ridley RM (eds) Methods in Molecular Medicine: Prion Diseases. New York: Humana, 1996; 223–36.
3. Oesch B, Westaway D, Walchli M, McKinley MP, Kent SBH, Aebersold R et al. A cellular gene encodes scrapie PrP 27–30 protein. Cell 1985; 40: 735–46.
4. Büeler H, Aguzzi A, Sailer A, Greiner RA, Autenried P, Aguet M, Weissmann C. Mice devoid of PrP are resistant to scrapie. Cell 1993; 73: 1339–47.
5. Bolton DC, McKinley MP, Prusiner SB. Identification of a protein that purifies with the scrapie prion. Science 1982; 218: 1309–11.
6. Caughey BW, Dong A, Bhat KS, Ernst D, Hayes SF, Caughey WS. Secondary structure analysis of the scrapie associated protein PrP 27–30 in water by infrared spectroscopy. Biochemistry 1991; 30: 7672–80.
7. Parchi P, Gambetti P, Piccardo P, Ghetti B. Human prion diseases. In: Kirkham N, Lemoine NR (eds) Progress in Pathology 4. Edinburgh: Churchill Livingstone, 1998; 39–77.
8. Telling GC, Parchi P, DeArmond SJ, Cortelli P, Montagna P, Gabizon R et al. Evidence for the conformation of the pathologic isoform of the prion protein enciphering and propagating prion diversity. Science 1996; 274: 2079–82.
9. Bruce ME, Will RG, Ironside JW, McConnel I, Drummond D, Suttie A et al. Transmissions to mice indicate that 'new variant' CJD is caused by the BSE agent. Nature 1997; 389: 498–501.
10. Bessen RA, Marsh RF. Biochemical and physical properties of the prion protein from two strains of the transmissible mink encephalopathy agent. J Virol 1992; 66: 2096–101.
11. Monari L, Chen SG, Brown P, Parchi P, Petersen RB, Mikol J et al. Fatal familial insomnia and familial Creutzfeldt–Jakob disease: different prion proteins determined by a DNA polymorphism. Proc Natl Acad Sci USA 1994; 91: 2839–42.
12. Parchi P, Castellani R, Capellari S, Ghetti B, Young K, Chen SG et al. Molecular basis of phenotypic variability in sporadic Creutzfeldt–Jakob disease. Ann Neurol 1996; 39: 767–78.
13. Parchi P, Capellari S, Chen SG, Ghetti B, Mikol J, Vital C et al. Similar post-translational modifications of the prion protein in familial, sporadic and iatrogenic Creutzfeldt–Jakob disease. Soc Neurosci Abstr 1996; 711.
14. Parchi P, Capellari S, Chen SG, Petersen RB, Gambetti P, Kopp N et al. Typing prion isoforms. Nature 1997; 386: 232–4.
15. Parchi P, Chen SG, Brown P, Zou W, Capellari S, Budka H et al. Different patterns of truncated prion protein fragments correlate with distinct phenotypes in P102L Gerstmann–Sträussler–Scheinker disease. Proc Natl Acad Sci USA 1998; 95: 8322–7.

16. Hill FA, Desbruslais M, Joiner S, Sidle CL, Gowland I, Collinge J. The same prion strain causes vCJD and BSE. Nature 1997; 389: 448–50.

17. Brown P, Gibbs CJ, Rodgers-Johnson P, Asher DM, Sulima MP, Bacote A et al. Human spongiform encephalopathy: the National Institutes of Health series of 300 cases of experimentally transmitted disease. Ann Neurol 1994; 35: 513–29.

Address for correspondence:

   Piero Parchi,

   Division of Neuropathology, Institute of Pathology,

   Case Western Reserve University,

   2085 Adelbert Road, Cleveland, Ohio 44106, USA

   Tel: (216) 368 0822; fax: (216) 368 2546; e-mail: pxp21@po.cwru.edu

64 A Transgenic Mouse Model of a Familial Prion Disease with an Insertional Mutation

ROBERTO CHIESA, PEDRO PICCARDO,
BERNARDINO GHETTI AND DAVID A. HARRIS

INTRODUCTION

Prion diseases are fatal neurodegenerative disorders that are attributable to the conformational conversion of a normal, cell-surface glycoprotein (PrP^C) into a pathogenic isoform (PrP^{Sc}) that is infectious in the apparent absence of nucleic acid [1]. Familial prion diseases, which include 10% of the cases of Creutzfeldt–Jakob disease and all cases of Gerstmann–Sträussler syndrome and fatal familial insomnia, are linked to dominantly inherited point and insertional mutations in the PrP gene on chromosome 20 [2]. The mutations are presumed to favor conversion of the protein to the PrP^{Sc} state without the necessity for contact with exogenous infectious agent [3].

Familial prion diseases can be modeled by expression of mutant PrPs in cultured cells and transgenic mice. We have previously established a cell culture model by constructing stably transfected lines of CHO cells that express mutant mouse PrP (moPrP) molecules whose human homologues are associated with each of the three familial prion diseases of humans [4–9]. We describe here the construction and analysis of mice expressing a moPrP transgene containing a nine-octapeptide insertional mutation. The human homologue of this mutation, which is the largest insertion thus far described in the PrP gene, has been found in two patients (one British and one German) who were afflicted with an illness characterized by progressive dementia and ataxia, and in the one autopsied case by the presence of PrP-containing amyloid plaques in the cerebellum and basal ganglia [10–12]. We find that these transgenic mice model key clinical and neuropathological features of human familial prion diseases and, unlike other mice bearing PrP transgenes, they spontaneously produce PrP^{Sc} in their brains. A full account of this work has recently been published [13].

Alzheimer's Disease and Related Disorders
Edited by K. Iqbal, D.F. Swaab, B. Winblad and H.M. Wisniewski
© 1999 John Wiley & Sons Ltd

GENERATION OF TRANSGENIC MICE

We have generated transgenic mice that express a moPrP molecule containing a nine-octapeptide insertion, which we will refer to as PG14 since it contains a total of 14 peptide repeats that are rich in proline and glycine (when this work was previously reported in abstract form [14], the mutation was referred to as PG11, although re-sequencing of mouse tail DNA now reveals that the transgene encodes 14 and not 11 octapeptide repeats). For control purposes, we have also produced mice that express a wild-type moPrP transgene. Both wild-type and PG14 molecules carry an epitope tag for the monoclonal antibody 3F4 [15], which makes it possible to distinguish transgene-encoded PrP from endogenous PrP. Wild-type and PG14 PrP cDNAs were cloned in the transgenic vector MoPrP.Xho, which contains the promoter and intron 1 of the moPrP gene, and that has been shown to produce strong expression of foreign genes in a tissue pattern similar to that of endogenous PrP [16]. Transgenic founder mice were bred back to the C57BL/6J × CBA/J parental line, as well as to *Prn-p*[0/0] mice, in which both copies of the endogenous PrP gene have been disrupted [17]. A summary of the transgenic lines is given in Table 1.

Table 1. Characteristics of transgenic mouse lines expressing wild-type and PG14 PrP

Transgene	Line	Transgene copy no.[1]	Tg PrP protein[2]
PG14 PrP	Tg(PG14-A1)	28	4.0
(3F4-tagged)	Tg(PG14-A2)	5	1.0
	Tg(PG14-A3)	33	1.0
	Tg(PG14-B)	2	0.15
	Tg(PG14-C)	4	0.15
Wild-type PrP	Tg(WT-D)	92	ND[3]
(3F4-tagged)	Tg(WT-E1)	9	1.8
	Tg(WT-E2)	1	0.25
	Tg(WT-E3)	59	3.6
	Tg(WT-E4)	15	3.0

[1] Determined by quantitative Southern blotting of tail DNA. Data are for mice that are hemizygous for the transgene array.
[2] Determined relative to endogenous hamster PrP by quantitative Western blotting of brain homogenates using 3F4 antibody. Data are for mice that are hemizygous for the transgene array.
[3] Not determined (the founder did not breed and is still alive).
Reproduced with permission from reference [13], © 1998 Cell Press.

Tg(PG14) MICE DEVELOP NEUROLOGICAL SYMPTOMS

A slowly progressive neurological disorder was observed in Tg(PG14) mice that have the highest expression levels of the mutant protein. Included in this group are the non-breeding A1 founder, which expressed PG14 PrP at 4 × the endogenous PrP level, and mice of the A2 and A3 lines which express 1 × the endogenous level. The primary symptoms of the disorder, which are observable throughout the course of illness, include ataxia (lack of coordination), kyphosis (hunchback posture) and clasping of the hind limbs when the mice are held by their tails (normal mice splay their hind limbs apart). As the disease progresses, affected mice show hypokinesia (decreased spontaneous movement), waddling gait, difficulty righting from a supine position, weight loss, and a ruffled appearance of their coats that may be attributable to deficient grooming. As a general rule Tg(PG14-A2) and Tg(PG14-A3) mice of both sexes breed poorly, and nursing mothers often neglect their litters.

We scored the presence of symptoms in mice of different ages and genotypes, by evaluating all the animals in our colony at a single point in time (Table 2). No mice younger than 71 days old were sick, while 73% of mice between 108 and 188 days old and 100% of mice over 214 days old were sick. These results indicate that the onset of symptoms is between ~100–200 days in Tg(PG14-A2) and Tg(PG14-A3) mice on the C57BL/6J × CBA/J background. In contrast, none of 102 Tg(PG14) mice of the low-expressing B and

Table 2. Analysis of neurological symptoms in transgenic mice. Data are for mice on the C57BL/6J × CBA/J background

	Age (days)	Neurological symptoms (No. of ill mice[1]/total no. of mice)	
Tg(PG14-A2)[2]	28–36		0/9
and Tg(PG14-A3)[2]	46–71		0/4
	108–188		8/11
	214–368		10/10
		Total	18/34
Tg(PG14-B)[3]	42–45		0/6
and Tg(PG14–C)[3]	99–188		0/45
	195–366		0/51
		Total[4]	0/102
Tg(WT)[3], all lines	25–42		0/6
	44–75		0/16
	95–175		0/74
	196–305		0/22
		Total[4]	0/118

[1] Mice are categorized as ill if they display at least two of the four symptoms listed in reference [13].
[2] Data are for mice that are hemizygous for the transgene array (mice on the C57BL/6J × CBA/J background that are homozygous for the transgene array are not available).
[3] Data are for mice that are either hemizygous or homozygous for the transgene array.
[4] One Tg(PG14-B) mouse and one Tg(WT-E1) mouse were excluded from the analysis because they suffered from an unrelated illness.

C lines (the oldest of which is now 532 days of age), and none of 118 Tg(WT) mice (the oldest of which is now 463 days of age) were scored as ill. Taken together, our results indicate that over-expression of wild-type PrP does not produce neurological dysfunction, and that development of the disease is related to the expression level of the mutant protein.

Our preliminary observations indicate that onset and progression of the disease are accelerated by eliminating expression of endogenous wild-type PrP. Symptoms appeared at ~100 days old in Tg(PG14-A2)/*Prn-p*$^{0/0}$ and Tg(PG14-A3)/*Prn-p*$^{0/0}$ mice that were hemizygous for the transgene array, and at ~60 days old in mice that were homozygous for the transgene array. Elimination of endogenous PrP also shortened the clinical phase of the disease from over 7 months to less than 2 months.

Tg(PG14) MICE DISPLAY NEUROPATHOLOGICAL CHANGES

Several abnormalities were observed in the A1, A2 and A3 lines. The most obvious pathological change was atrophy of the cerebellum, with marked reduction in the number of granule cells and a decrease in the thickness of the molecular layer (Figure 1A–D). Loss of granule cells appeared to become more severe as the disease progressed. Neuronal loss was not apparent in other areas of the brain, neither was there evidence of spongiform change in any region. Immunohistochemical staining using anti-GFAP antibody demonstrated gliosis and astrocytic hypertrophy. These changes were most prominent in the cerebellar cortex, particularly the molecular layer, which displayed markedly hypertrophied Bergmann glial fibers (Figure 1E). Staining was performed with anti-PrP antibodies after guanidine thiocyanate treatment and hydrolytic autoclaving of sections to enhance reactivity of PrP^{Sc} and abolish reactivity of PrP^{C}. Tg(PG14) mice showed deposits of PrP that were distributed in a fine, punctate pattern which has been described as 'synaptic-like' [18]. These deposits were most prominent in the cerebellum (molecular and granule cell layers), hippocampal formation (especially the perforant pathway), and olfactory bulb. No pathologic changes were observed in Tg(PG14-B), Tg(PG14-C), or Tg(WT) mice (Figure 1A, B).

DETERGENT-INSOLUBLE AND PROTEASE-RESISTANT PrP IS PRESENT IN THE BRAINS OF Tg(PG14) MICE

PrP^{Sc} can be recognized by several distinctive biochemical properties, including detergent-insolubility, protease-resistance, and resistance to the action of phosphatidylinositol-specific phospholipase C (PIPLC) [5]. We have assayed PrP in the brains of transgenic mice for each of these characteristics.

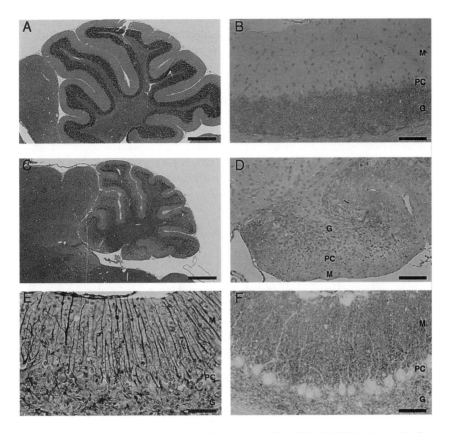

Figure 1. Neuropathological findings in the cerebella of Tg(PG14) mice. (A) Cerebellum of a healthy Tg(WT-E1)/*Prn-p*⁰/⁰ mouse, 184 days old, appears normal after staining with hematoxylin and eosin. (B) Cerebellar cortex of the same mouse shown in panel (A), stained with antibody 3F4, shows no deposits of PrP, and normal appearance of the molecular (M), Purkinje cell (PC) and granule cell (G) layers. (C) Cerebellum of a terminally ill Tg(PG14-A3)/*Prn-p*⁰/⁰ mouse, 183 days old, after staining with hematoxylin and eosin. There is marked atrophy of the cerebellum, with reduction in the thickness of the granule cell and molecular layers. (D) Cerebellar cortex of the same mouse shown in panel (C), stained with antibody 3F4. There is a dramatic reduction in the density of granule cells, and mild staining for PrP. (E) Cerebellar cortex of the symptomatic Tg(PG14-A1) founder, 319 days old, stained for GFAP. There is marked hypertrophy of Bergmann glial fibers in the molecular layer and increased numbers of astrocytes in the granule cell layer. (F) Cerebellar cortex of a moderately symptomatic Tg(PG14-A3)/*Prn-p*⁰/⁰ mouse, 71 days old, stained with antibody 3F4. There is heavy PrP deposition in a synaptic-like pattern in the molecular layer and less prominent staining in the granule cell layer. Purkinje cells are unstained, consistent with the fact that the transgenic vector does not drive expression in these cells [27]. Cerebellar atrophy is less severe in this mouse compared to the older animal shown in panel (D). Scale bars are 556 μm (A, C), 97 μm (B, D), 44 μm (E), and 62 μm (F). Reproduced with permission from reference [13], © 1998 Cell Press

We determined the amount of PrP that is detergent-insoluble by subjecting Triton-deoxycholate extracts of brain to ultracentrifugation under conditions that sediment PrPSc but leave PrPC in the supernatant. As shown in Figure 2, PG14 PrP from all lines was partially detergent-insoluble. Between 50% and 90% of the mutant protein from Tg(PG14-A1), Tg(PG14-A2) and Tg(PG14-A3) mice was found in the pellet. In mice from the low-expressing Tg(PG14-B) and Tg(PG14-C) lines, a lesser proportion of the mutant protein (10–20%) was detergent-insoluble, suggesting a correlation between expression level and acquisition of this PrPSc property, and also demonstrating that PrPSc formation precedes development of clinical symptoms. No detergent-insoluble PrP was detected in the brains of normal hamsters, or of Tg(WT) mice from any of the four lines examined.

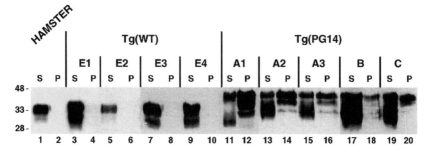

Figure 2. PG14 PrP in the brains of transgenic mice is detergent-insoluble. Detergent lysates of brain (containing 100 µg of protein) from transgenic mice and from Syrian hamsters were centrifuged at 260 000 × g for 40 min. Proteins in supernatants (S lanes) and pellets (P lanes) were then separated by SDS–PAGE and immunoblotted using antibody 3F4. A quarter of each sample (lanes 1–16), or the whole sample (lanes 17–20), was run on the gel. Mice were of the following ages and clinical status at the time of sacrifice: E1–E4, 203 days old (all healthy); A1, 319 days old (severely symptomatic); A2, 71 days old (healthy); A3, 205 days old (mildly symptomatic); B, 169 days old (healthy); C, 226 days old (healthy). Reproduced with permission from reference [13], © 1998 Cell Press

To assess the protease-resistance of PG14 PrP expressed in the brains of transgenic mice, we digested detergent extracts of brain with proteinase K for 30 min at 37 °C (Figure 3). We found PG14 PrP from all five lines yielded a protease-resistant core fragment of 27–30 kDa (PrP 27–30). The fragment from the A1, A2 and A3 lines was observed after digestion with 2–4 µg/ml of proteinase K, and the one from the B and C lines was seen after digestion with 0.5–1.0 µg/ml of protease. In contrast, wild-type hamster PrP and moPrP from all four Tg(WT) lines was completely degraded at proteinase K concentrations as low as 0.5 µg/ml. Mapping of the immunoreactive epitopes present in PrP 27–30 from Tg(PG14) mice suggests that this fragment is produced by cleavage between the end of the octapeptide repeats and amino acid 94, the same region where authentic PrPSc is cut.

A

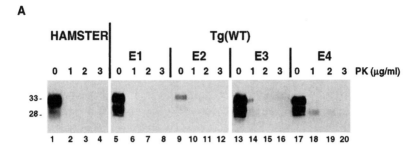

B

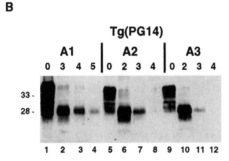

C.

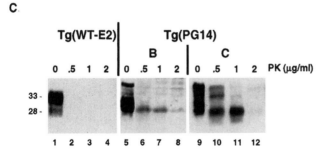

Figure 3. PG14 PrP in the brains of transgenic mice is protease-resistant. Detergent lysates of brain from transgenic mice and Syrian hamsters were incubated with the indicated amounts of proteinase K (PK) for 30 min at 37 °C. Digestion was terminated by addition of PMSF, and methanol-precipitated proteins were separated by SDS–PAGE and immunoblotted using antibody 3F4. 200 μg (A, B) or 800 μg (C) of initial protein was subjected to digestion. The lanes containing undigested samples (0 μg/ml PK) represent 50 μg (A, B) or 200 μg (C) of protein. Age and clinical status of mice at the time of sacrifice are given in the legend to Figure 2. Modified with permission from reference [13], © 1998 Cell Press

PrP IN THE BRAINS OF Tg(PG14) MICE IS PIPLC-RESISTANT

PrP[C] can be released from cell membranes by treatment with the bacterial enzyme PIPLC, which cleaves the C-terminal glycosyl-phosphatidylinositol (GPI) anchor [19]. In contrast, PrP[Sc] remains tightly associated with membranes after PIPLC treatment, a property that can be observed in scrapie-infected brain tissue [20], scrapie-infected cells in culture [5] and transfected cells expressing moPrPs with pathogenic mutations [4]. This abnormal behavior of PrP[Sc] is likely to be due to physical inaccessibility of the GPI anchor as a result of conformational alteration of the protein. Consistent with this proposed mechanism, the GPI anchor of mutant PrP in cultured cells is resistant to PIPLC cleavage after the protein is solubilized in non-denaturing detergents, but it becomes completely susceptible to cleavage after denaturation in SDS (Narwa and Harris, unpublished data).

We used two different assays to determine whether the property of PIPLC-resistance was displayed by PG14 PrP molecules expressed in the brains of transgenic mice. First, suspensions of microsomal membranes were treated with PIPLC, and the amount of PrP released in the medium was determined by immunoblotting pellet and supernatant fractions obtained after sedimenting the membranes by centrifugation. Figure 4A shows that, while ~50% of the wild-type PrP from hamsters and Tg(WT-E1) mice was releasable by PIPLC, none of the PG14 PrP from A1, A2 or A3 mice was releasable.

In the second assay, we measured whether PG14 PrP molecules were rendered hydrophilic by treatment with PIPLC, a change which registers removal of the diacylglycerol portion of the anchor. The hydrophobicity of the protein was determined by Triton X-114 phase partitioning. Figure 4B shows that before treatment with PIPLC, both wild-type and PG14 PrPs partitioned almost exclusively into the detergent phase, as would be expected for molecules carrying an intact GPI anchor. After PIPLC treatment, about 40% of wild-type PrP from hamsters and Tg(WT-E1) mice was shifted into the aqueous phase, indicating that the protein had been rendered hydrophilic by removal of the GPI anchor. In contrast, PG14 PrP from the A1, A2 and A3 lines remained in the detergent phase.

CONCLUSIONS

We have produced a mouse model of a familial prion disorder by introduction of a transgene that encodes the moPrP homologue of a nine-octapeptide insertional mutant associated with an inherited dementia in humans. These mice develop progressive neurological symptoms, display neuropathological changes, and synthesize PrP[Sc] that is recognizable by four different biochemical criteria. Since these abnormalities are not observed in mice expressing a

A.

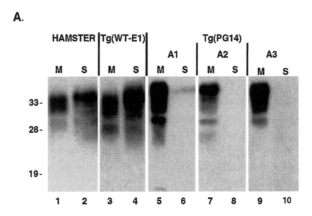

B.

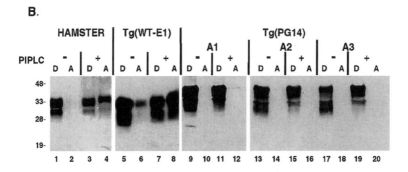

Figure 4. PG14 PrP in the brains of transgenic mice is not released from membranes and remains hydrophobic after treatment with PIPLC. (A) Suspensions of brain membranes from transgenic mice and Syrian hamsters were incubated with PIPLC for 2 h at 4 °C, and membranes collected by centrifugation. PrP in the supernatant (S) and membrane (M) fractions was then visualized by immunoblotting using 3F4 antibody. (B) Brain homogenates were solubilized in a buffer containing 1% Triton X-114 at 4 °C, and then phase separation was induced by raising the temperature to 37 °C. The detergent phase was recovered and diluted to the original volume. One half was incubated with PIPLC at 4 °C for 2 h (+ lanes), and the other half was left untreated (– lanes). Phase separation was repeated, and PrP in the detergent (D lanes) and aqueous (A lanes) phases was analyzed by immunoblotting using 3F4 antibody. Age and clinical status of mice at the time of sacrifice are given in the legend to Figure 2. Reproduced with permission from reference [13], © 1998 Cell Press

wild-type PrP transgene, the phenotype in Tg(PG14) mice results specifically from the presence of the octapeptide insertion.

Several different kinds of PrP transgenic mice have been described which spontaneously develop a neurological illness [21–27], but Tg(PG14) mice are the only animals currently available that spontaneously synthesize PrP^{Sc}. These mice will therefore be extremely valuable for a number of future studies, including analysis of PrP^{Sc} metabolism in differentiated neurons, correlation of PrP^{Sc} production with the clinical and neuropathological features of the disease, and testing the efficacy of therapeutic interventions. Tg(PG14) mice with low expression levels of the mutant protein will also be useful hosts for testing the infectivity of PG14 molecules that are generated in transgenic lines with higher expression levels, and in cell culture and *in vitro* systems.

ACKNOWLEDGEMENTS

We thank David Borchelt for providing the MoPrP.Xho vector, Charles Weissmann for *Prn-p$^{0/0}$* mice, and Richard Kascsak for 3F4 antibody. We also acknowledge David Wozniak for advice on clinical testing of mice, Angie Purvis for help with maintenance of the mouse colony, Constance Alyea and Tatyana Verina for carrying out animal perfusions, Rosemarie Richardson for assistance with histology, and Josh Sanes and Bill Snider for making the transgenic facility available. This work was supported by grants from the American Health Assistance Foundation and the Alzheimer's Association to D.A.H., and by the Indiana Alzheimer Core Center grant to B.G. (P30 AG10133). R.C. was the recipient of a fellowship from Comitato Telethon Fondazione Onlus.

REFERENCES

1. Prusiner SB, Scott MR, DeArmond SJ, Cohen FE. Prion protein biology. Cell 1998; 93: 337–48.
2. Young K, Piccardo P, Dlouhy S, Bugiani O, Tagliavini F, Ghetti B. The human genetic prion diseases. In: Harris DA (ed) Prions: Molecular and Cellular Biology. Wymondham, UK: Horizon Scientific Press, 1999; pp 139–75.
3. Cohen FE, Pan KM, Huang Z, Baldwin M, Fletterick RJ, Prusiner SB. Structural clues to prion replication. Science 1994; 264: 530–31.
4. Lehmann S, Harris DA. A mutant prion protein displays an aberrant membrane association when expressed in cultured cells. J Biol Chem 1995; 270: 24589–97.
5. Lehmann S, Harris DA. Mutant and infectious prion protein display common biochemical properties in cultured cells. J Biol Chem 1996; 271: 1633–7.
6. Lehmann S, Harris DA. Two mutant prion proteins expressed in cultured cells acquire biochemical properties reminiscent of the scrapie isoform. Proc Natl Acad Sci USA 1996; 93: 5610–14.

7. Lehmann S, Harris DA. Blockade of glycosylation promotes acquisition of scrapie-like properties by the prion protein in cultured cells. J Biol Chem 1997; 272: 21479–87.

8. Lehmann S, Daude N, Harris DA. A wild-type prion protein does not acquire properties of the scrapie isoform when co-expressed with a mutant prion protein in cultured cells. Mol Brain Res 1997; 52: 139–45.

9. Daude N, Lehmann S, Harris DA. Identification of intermediate steps in the conversion of a mutant prion protein to a scrapie-like form in cultured cells. J Biol Chem 1997; 272: 11604–12.

10. Owen F, Poulter M, Collinge J, Leach M, Lofthouse R, Crow TJ, Harding AE. A dementing illness associated with a novel insertion in the prion protein gene. Mol Brain Res 1992; 13: 155–7.

11. Duchen LW, Poulter M, Harding AE. Dementia associated with a 216 base pair insertion in the prion protein gene: clinical and neuropathological features. Brain 1993; 116: 555–67.

12. Krasemann S, Zerr I, Weber T, Poser S, Kretzschmar H, Hunsmann G, Bodemer W. Prion disease associated with a novel nine octapeptide repeat insertion in the PRNP gene. Mol Brain Res 1995; 34: 173–6.

13. Chiesa R, Piccardo P, Ghetti B, Harris DA. Neurological illness in transgenic mice expressing a prion protein with an insertional mutation. Neuron 1998; 21: 1339–1351.

14. Chiesa R, Piccardo P, Ghetti B, Harris DA. A transgenic mouse model of a familial prion disease with an insertional mutation. Neurobiol Aging 1998; 19: S300.

15. Bolton DC, Seligman SJ, Bablanian G, Windsor D, Scala LJ, Kim K-S, Chen CM, Kascsak RJ, Bendheim PE. Molecular location of a species-specific epitope on the hamster scrapie agent protein. J Virol 1991; 65: 3667–75.

16. Borchelt DR, Davis J, Fischer M, Lee MK, Slunt HH, Ratovitsky T, Regard J, Copeland NG, Jenkins NA, Sisodia SS, Price DL. A vector for expressing foreign genes in the brains and hearts of transgenic mice. Genet Anal Biomol Eng 1996; 13: 159–63.

17. Büeler H, Fischer M, Lang Y, Fluethmann H, Lipp H-P, DeArmond SJ, Prusiner SB, Aguet M, Weissmann C. Normal development and behavior of mice lacking the neuronal cell-surface PrP protein. Nature 1992; 356: 577–82.

18. Kitamoto T, Shin R-W, Doh-ura K, Tomokane N, Miyazono M, Muramoto T, Tateishi J. Abnormal isoform of prion proteins accumulates in the synaptic structures of the central nervous system in patients with Creutzfeldt–Jakob disease. Am J Pathol 1992; 140: 1285–94.

19. Stahl N, Borchelt DR, Hsiao K, Prusiner SB. Scrapie prion protein contains a phosphatidylinositol glycolipid. Cell 1987; 51: 229–49.

20. Stahl N, Borchelt DR, Prusiner SB. Differential release of cellular and scrapie prion proteins from cellular membranes by phosphatidylinositol-specific phospholipase C. Biochemistry 1990; 29: 5405–12.

21. Hsiao KK, Scott M, Foster D, Groth DF, DeArmond SJ, Prusiner SB. Spontaneous neurodegeneration in transgenic mice with mutant prion protein. Science 1990; 250: 1587–90.

22. Telling GC, Haga T, Torchia M, Tremblay P, DeArmond SJ, Prusiner SB. Interactions between wild-type and mutant prion proteins modulate neurodegeneration in transgenic mice. Genes Develop 1996; 10: 1736–50.

23. Westaway D, DeArmond SJ, Cayetano-Canlas J, Groth D, Foster D, Yang S-L, Torchia M, Carlson GA, Prusiner SB. Degeneraiton of skeletal muscle, peripheral nerves, and the central nervous system in transgenic mice overexpressing wild-type prion proteins. Cell 1994; 76: 117–29.

24. Muramoto T, DeArmond SJ, Scott M, Telling GC, Cohen FE, Prusiner SB. Heritable disorder resembling neuronal storage disease in mice expressing prion protein with deletion of an α-helix. Nature Med 1997; 3: 750–55.

25. Hegde RS, Mastrianni JA, Scott MR, Defea KA, Tremblay P, Torchia M, DeArmond SJ, Prusiner SB, Lingappa VR. A transmembrane form of the prion protein in neurodegenerative disease. Science 1998; 279: 827–34.

26. Shmerling D, Hegyi I, Fischer M, Blättler T, Brandner S, Götz J, Rülicke T, Flechsig E, Cozzio A, von Mering C, Hangartner C, Aguzzi A, Weissmann C. Expression of amino-terminally truncated PrP in the mouse leading to ataxia and specific cerebellar lesions. Cell 1998; 93: 203–14.

27. Fischer M, Rülicke T, Raeber A, Sailer A, Moser M, Oesch B, Brandner S, Aguzzi A, Weissmann C. Prion protein (PrP) with amino-proximal deletions restoring susceptibility of PrP knockout mice to scrapie. EMBO J 1996; 15: 1255–64.

Address for correspondence:
   David A. Harris,
   Department of Cell Biology and Physiology,
   Washington University School of Medicine,
   660 South Euclid Avenue, St. Louis, MO 63130, USA.
   Tel: 314 362 4690; fax: 314 362 7463;
   e-mail: dharris@cellbio.wustl.edu

65 Formation of Protease-resistant Prion Protein *In Vitro*: Stimulation and Inhibition

B. CAUGHEY, J. CHABRY, R. DEMAIMAY,
L.M. HERRMANN, M. HORIUCHI, L.D. RAYMOND,
G.J. RAYMOND, W.S. CAUGHEY, S.K. DebBURMAN,
S. LINDQUIST AND B. CHESEBRO

INTRODUCTION

Transmissible spongiform encephalopathies (TSE) or prion diseases are fatal neurodegenerative diseases which include bovine spongiform encephalopathy (BSE or 'mad cow disease'), Creutzfeldt–Jakob disease (CJD) in humans, scrapie in sheep and chronic wasting disease (CWD) in deer and elk. TSE diseases remain rare in humans; however, the recent BSE epidemic in the UK and Europe has been estimated to have affected more than 1 million cattle. Recent evidence that BSE has been transmitted to humans is troubling, since it has been estimated that approximately 1 million infected cattle entered the human food supply. There is no direct evidence of BSE in the USA, but scrapie is on the rise in sheep and CWD has a high incidence in some wild herds of deer and elk in Colorado and Wyoming.

A central and defining event in the pathogenesis of TSE diseases is the posttranslational conversion of normal protease-sensitive prion protein (PrP-sen or PrP^C) to an abnormal protease-resistant form (PrP-res or PrP^{Sc}) (reviewed in [1]). This conversion involves changes in conformation and aggregation state of PrP-sen. One popular hypothesis is that TSE infectious agents might be composed solely of PrP-res and that it propagates itself by inducing host-derived PrP-sen to convert to PrP-res. In this article, we will summarize selected studies of PrP-res formation in *in vitro* systems with a focus on factors that stimulate or inhibit this reaction.

SELF-INDUCTION OF PrP-res FORMATION

When PrP-res is incubated with ^{35}S-PrP-sen, a portion of the ^{35}S-PrP attains the specific partial protease-resistance that is characteristic of PrP-res [2]. ^{35}S-

Alzheimer's Disease and Related Disorders
Edited by K. Iqbal, D.F. Swaab, B. Winblad and H.M. Wisniewski
© 1999 John Wiley & Sons Ltd

PrP-sen has not been converted to PrP-res on its own, but can readily be induced to do so by the addition of pre-existing PrP-res in largely purified form [2], crude brain fractions or brain slices [3]. This induced conversion reaction occurs with species and strain specificities that correlate with, and might help to explain, TSE species barrier effects and strain differences *in vivo* [4–7].

MECHANISM OF PrP-res FORMATION

Both converting activity and scrapie infectivity are associated with partially protease-resistant multimers of PrP-res [8–10]. After PrP-res is added to the cell-free reaction, the conversion proceeds in a time-dependent manner for a day or more, with the resultant PrP-res conversion product becoming associated with the input PrP-res polymers [3, 11]. These results are consistent with a nucleated polymerization mechanism of PrP-res formation akin to that observed in fibril formation by small synthetic PrP peptides and other amyloidogenic peptides and proteins [8, 12]. Nonetheless, cell-free PrP-res formation has not been found to be as continuous as fibril formation in many other *in vitro* examples of amyloid formation, and the yield of new PrP-res is usually less than the amount of PrP-res used to induce the reaction. It is not clear whether this is due to imperfections in the current *in vitro* reaction conditions, to depletion of an unidentified reaction co-factor/component, or to some other poorly understood aspect of the reaction mechanism.

STIMULATION OF PrP-res FORMATION BY CHAPERONES

Since PrP-res formation appears to involve changes in the conformation and aggregation state of PrP-sen, the influence of chaperone proteins on the conversion reaction was investigated [11]. A large panel of chaperone proteins was tested and none induce conversion in the absence of PrP-res. However, in its presence, the bacterial chaperone protein GroEL promoted conversion without requiring a pretreatment of PrP-res with a partial denaturant. The yeast chaperone Hsp104 also promoted PrP-res induced conversion, but only after pretreatment of PrP-res with urea (optimally 3–4 M). Kinetic analyses indicated that the binding of ^{35}S-PrP-sen to the pre-existing PrP-res aggregate occurred first and was followed by the slower conversion to ^{35}S-PrP-res. GroEL accelerated the initial association of ^{35}S-PrP-sen with PrP-res, but the rate of conversion to ^{35}S-PrP-res was similar to that in our more conventional reactions seeded by guanidine pretreated PrP-res. Although GroEL and Hsp104 cannot be regarded as physiological mediators of the PrP conversion reaction, these observations provide a 'proof-of-principle' that chaperone proteins can be important co-factors in the PrP conversion process. This conclusion is also supported by studies showing that Hsp104 can induce conformational changes in recombinant PrP-sen [13].

INHIBITION OF CONVERSION REACTION BY DISULFIDE REDUCING AGENTS

One prominent feature of the PrP-sen structure that influences its conformation is the disulfide linkage between cysteine residues at positions 179 and 214 [14–16]. Thus, the effects of reduction of the disulfide bond on the cell-free conversion of PrP-sen to PrP-res were examined [17]. The addition of the disulfide reducing agent dithiothreitol inhibited the conversion reaction with an IC_{50} of ~2 mM. Separate pretreatment of either PrP-sen or PrP-res with dithiothreitol and an alkylating agent also inhibited conversion. These results show that preservation of the disulfide bond is important in the conversion of PrP-sen to PrP-res.

INHIBITION OF PrP-res FORMATION BY SYNTHETIC PEPTIDES

Since PrP-res formation involves interactions between PrP molecules, the possibility that peptide fragments of PrP could interfere with PrP-res formation in the cell-free system was investigated [18]. Although peptides corresponding to most regions of the PrP sequence did not inhibit the conversion reaction, those containing residues 119–141 were strong inhibitors. FTIR analysis indicated that the inhibitory peptides were capable of forming aggregates with high β-sheet content but this was also true of some non-inhibitory peptides. These results suggested that the 119–141 region of PrP is important in the specific intermolecular interactions that lead to PrP-res formation.

INHIBITION OF PrP-res FORMATION BY CONGO RED, SULFATED GLYCANS AND ANALOGS THEREOF

Certain polyanions have long been known to have therapeutic value against scrapie if administered early after infection. It was subsequently shown that these compounds are potent inhibitors of PrP-res formation in scrapie-infected cell cultures [19, 20]. We also used these cell cultures and the cell-free PrP conversion reaction to identify new inhibitors and to gain insight into their structural requirements and mechanism(s) of action [21]. For instance, Congo red and several of its analogs inhibit PrP-res formation in both these systems, whereas closely related analogs were much less effective [22]. These results, in combination with molecular modeling, suggested that planarity and/or torsional mobility of the central aromatic ring(s) are important structural features of this type of inhibitor of PrP-res formation and that wide variations in intersulfonate distance can be tolerated.

INHIBITION OF PrP-res FORMATION BY PORPHYRINS AND PHTHALOCYANINES

Since polyanionic inhibitors are only effective therapeutically if given near the time of infection, other types of inhibitors with therapeutic potential have been sought [23–25]. In this effort, certain porphyrins and phthalocyanines were found to selectively inhibit PrP-res formation in both scrapie-infected cell cultures and the cell-free systems [32]. Several features make such tetrapyrroles attractive drug candidates: many are non-toxic; some have been widely used for clinical applications in humans; and, unlike most polyanions, certain tetrapyrroles appear to cross the blood–brain barrier.

CONNECTIONS TO ALZHEIMER'S DISEASE AND OTHER AMYLOIDOSES

Since TSE diseases and Alzheimer's disease all result in the accumulation of amyloid or other abnormal protein deposits in the brain, it is possible that the pathogenic processes of the abnormal protein/peptide deposition have features in common. Thus, stimulators and inhibitors of one system may have interesting activities and therapeutic applications in the other [26]. Indeed, Congo red [27–29], polyanions [30] and tetrapyrroles [31] have been shown to have effects on β-amyloid formation.

CONCLUSIONS

Pathogenesis in the transmissible spongiform encephalopathies (TSE) or prion diseases such as scrapie, BSE and CJD appears to be driven by the accumulation of an abnormal, protease-resistant form of prion protein (PrP-res). Cell-free studies have shown that PrP-res itself can induce the conversion of normal, protease-sensitive PrP to PrP-res. Using this cell-free model of PrP-res formation and scrapie-infected tissue culture cells, a number of factors have been identified that either stimulate or inhibit PrP-res formation. Among the factors that stimulate cell-free PrP-res formation are chaperone proteins (GroEL and Hsp104), detergents and salts. Such stimulating factors have aided in the development of non-denaturing conditions for the cell-free PrP-res formation. Inhibitors of PrP-res formation include certain synthetic peptide fragments of the PrP molecule, sulfated glycans, Congo red, porphyrins, phthalocyanines and analogs thereof. Studies of these compounds have revealed structure–function relationships for inhibitors of PrP-res formation which may aid in the development of therapeutic agents for TSE diseases and other amyloidoses, such as Alzheimer's disease.

ACKNOWLEDGEMENTS

S.K.D. is a Howard Hughes Medical Institute Fellow of the Life Sciences Research Foundation.

REFERENCES

1. Caughey B, Chesebro B. Prion protein and the transmissible spongiform encephalopathies. Trends Cell Biol 1997; 7: 56–62.
2. Kocisko DA, Come JH, Priola SA, Chesebro B, Raymond GJ, Lansbury PT, Caughey B. Cell-free formation of protease-resistant prion protein. Nature 1994; 370: 471–4.
3. Bessen RA, Raymond GJ, Caughey B. *In situ* formation of protease-resistant prion protein in transmissible spongiform encephalopathy-infected brain slices. J Biol Chem 1997; 272: 15227–31.
4. Kocisko DA, Priola SA, Raymond GJ, Chesebro B, Lansbury PT Jr, Caughey B. Species specificity in the cell-free conversion of prion protein to protease-resistant forms: a model for the scrapie species barrier. Proc Natl Acad Sci USA 1995; 92: 3923–7.
5. Bossers A, Belt PBGM, Raymond GJ, Caughey B, de Vries R, Smits MA. Scrapie susceptibility-linked polymorphisms modulate the *in vitro* conversion of sheep prion protein to protease-resistant forms. Proc Natl Acad Sci USA 1997; 94: 4931–6.
6. Raymond GJ, Hope J, Kocisko DA, Priola SA, Raymond LD, Bossers A, Ironside J, Will RG, Chen SG, Petersen RB, Gambetti P, Rubinstein R, Smits MA, Lansbury PT Jr, Caughey B. Molecular assessment of the potential transmissibilities of BSE and scrapie to humans. Nature 1997; 388: 285–8.
7. Bessen RA, Kocisko DA, Raymond GJ, Nandan S, Lansbury PT Jr, Caughey B. Non-genetic propagation of strain-specific phenotypes of scrapie prion protein. Nature 1995; 375: 698–700.
8. Caughey B, Kocisko DA, Raymond GJ, Lansbury PT Jr. Aggregates of scrapie-associated prion protein induce the cell-free conversion of protease-sensitive prion protein to the protease-resistant state. Chem Biol 1995; 2: 807–17.
9. Kocisko DA, Lansbury PT Jr, Caughey B. Partial unfolding and refolding of scrapie-associated prion protein: evidence for a critical 16 kDa C-terminal domain. Biochemistry 1996; 35: 13434–42.
10. Caughey B, Raymond GJ, Kocisko DA, Lansbury PT Jr. Scrapie infectivity correlates with converting activity, protease resistance, and aggregation of scrapie-associated prion protein in guanidine denaturation studies. J Virol 1997; 71: 4107–10.

11. DebBurman SK, Raymond GJ, Caughey B, Lindquist S. Chaperone-supervised conversion of prion protein to its protease-resistant form. Proc Natl Acad Sci USA 1997; 94: 13938–43.

12. Glover JR, Kowal AS, Schirmer EC, Patino MM, Liu J, Lindquist S. Self-seeded fibers formed by sup35, the protein determinant of [PSI⁺], a heritable prion-like factor of S. cerevisiae. Cell 1997; 89: 811–19.

13. Schirmer EC, Lindquist S. Interactions of the chaperone Hsp104 with yeast Sup35 and mammalian PrP. Proc Natl Acad Sci USA 1997; 94: 13932–7.

14. Turk E, Teplow DB, Hood LE, Prusiner SB. Purification and properties of the cellular and scrapie hamster prion proteins. Eur J Biochem 1988; 176: 21–30.

15. Riek R, Hornemann S, Wider G, Glockshuber R, Wuthrich K. NMR characterization of the full-length recombinant murine prion protein, mPrP(23–21). FEBS Lett 1997; 413: 282–8.

16. Zhang H, Stockel J, Mehlhorn I, Groth D, Baldwin MA, Prusiner SB, James TL, Cohen FE. Physical studies of conformational plasticity in a recombinant prion protein. Biochemistry 1997; 36; 3543–53.

17. Herrmann LM, Caughey B. The importance of the disulfide bond in prion protein conversion. NeuroReport 1998; 9.

18. Chabry J, Caughey B, Chesebro B. Specific inhibition of in vitro formation of protease-resistant prion protein by synthetic peptides. J Biol Chem 1998; 273: 13203–7.

19. Caughey B, Race RE. Potent inhibition of scrapie-associated PrP accumulation by Congo red. J Neurochem 1992; 59: 768–71.

20. Caughey B, Raymond GJ. Sulfated polyanion inhibition of scrapie-associated PrP accumulation cultured cells. J Viron 1993; 67: 643–50.

21. Caughey B, Brown K, Raymond GJ, Katzenstien GE, Thresher W. Binding of the protease-sensitive form of PrP (prion protein) to sulfated glycosaminoglycan and Congo red. J Virol 1994; 68: 2135–41.

22. Demaimay R, Harper J, Gordon H, Weaver D, Chesebro B, Caughey B. Structural aspects of Congo red as an inhibitor of protease-resistant PrP formation. J Neurochem 1998; 71: 2534–41.

23. Amyx H, Salazar AM, Gajdusek DC, Gibbs CJ. Chemotherapeutic trials in experimental slow virus disease. Neurology 1984; 34: 149.

24. Demaimay R, Adjou KT, Beringue V, Demart S, Lasmezas CI, Deslys J-P, Seman M, Dormont D. Late treatment with polyene antibiotics can prolong the survival time of scrapie-infected animals. J Virol 1997; 71: 9685–9.

25. Tagliavini F, McArthur RA, Canciani B, Giaccone G, Porro M, Bugiani M, Lievens PM-J, Bugiani O, Peri E, Dall'Ara P, Rocchi M, Poli G, Forloni G, Bandiera T, Varasi M, Suarato A, Cassutti P, Cervini MA, Lansen J, Salmona M, Post C. Effectiveness of anthracycline against experimental prion disease in Syrian hamsters. Science 1998; 276: 1119–22.

26. Caughey B. Scrapie-associated PrP accumulation and its prevention: insights from cell culture. Br Med Bull 1993; 49: 860–72.

27. Lorenzo A, Yankner BA. β-amyloid neurotoxicity requires fibril formation and is inhibited by Congo red. Proc Natl Acad Sci USA 1994; 91: 12243–7.

28. Watson DJ, Lander AD, Selkoe DJ. Heparin-binding properties of the amyloidogenic peptides Aβ and amylin. Dependence on aggregation state and inhibition by Congo red. J Biol Chem 1997; 272: 31617–24.

29. Pollack SJ, Sadler IIJ, Hawtin SR, Tailor VJ, Shearman MS. Sulphated glycosaminoglycans and dyes attenuate the neurotoxic effects of β-amyloid in rat PC12 cells. Neurosci Lett 1995; 184: 113–16.

30. Snow AD, Wight TN, Nochlin D, Koike Y, Kimata K, DeArmond SJ, Prusiner SB. Immunolocalization of heparan sulfate proteoglycans to the prion protein amyloid plaques of Gerstmann–Sträussler syndrome, Creutzfeldt–Jakob disease and scrapie. Lab Invest 1990; 63: 601–11.
31. Howlett D, Crutler P, Heales S, Camilleri P. Hemin and related porphyrins inhibit β-amyloid aggregation. FEBS Lett 1997; 417: 249–51.
32. Caughey WS, Raymond LD, Horiuchi M, Caughey B. Inhibition of protease-resistant prion protein formation by porphyrins and phthalocyanines. Proc Natl Acad Sci USA 1998; 95: 12117–12122.

Address for correspondence:
Dr B. Caughey
NIAID, NIH, Rocky Mountain Laboratories,
Hamilton, MT 59840, USA
Fax: +1 406 363 9371

VII   Cellular and Animal Models

66 hFE65L Over-expression Enhances β-Amyloid Precursor Protein Maturation and Processing

SUZANNE Y. GUÉNETTE, JING CHEN,
AMBER FERLAND AND RUDOLPH E. TANZI

INTRODUCTION

APP processing leads to the generation of the β-amyloid peptide (Aβ) in both the secretory and endocytic pathways. While Aβ40 production occurs in the late Golgi and endosomal compartments [1–4], Aβ42 is generated in the early Golgi and endoplasmic reticulum [3–6]. Events that modulate APP trafficking have a profound impact on APP processing and ultimately on Aβ production. For example, deletion of the YENPTY clathrin-coated pit internalization sequence decreases Aβ production and increases APP ectodomain (APPs) secretion [1]. Furthermore, this deletion is sufficient to shift the processing of APPSwe from β-secretase to α-secretase cleavage and alter the trafficking of APP in MDCK cells [7–11]. To date, the molecular components involved in APP processing and trafficking are poorly understood.

We previously identified hFE65L as a protein that interacts with the carboxy-terminal region of APP and APLP2 using a two-hybrid-based screen [12]. hFE65L is a member of the human FE65 family of proteins [12, 13]. All three known FE65 family members, hFE65, hFE65L and hFE65L2, are binding partners [13–16] for the 43 carboxy-terminal amino acids of APP, which bear a clathrin-coated pit internalization sequence, NPXY, that targets cell surface APP to the endocytic compartment [17]. Deletion or mutagenesis of the NPTY sequence of APP lead to increased secretion of APPs [18–21]. The FE65 proteins share protein–protein interaction motifs that are found in proteins of diverse function, a WW domain and two phosphotyrosine interaction domains (PID1 and PID2). The PID2 mediates the interaction of the FE65 proteins with the NPTY internalization motif of APP [12, 22–23] in the absence of tyrosine phosphorylation [17, 22]. It is for this reason that we

Alzheimer's Disease and Related Disorders
Edited by K. Iqbal, D.F. Swaab, B. Winblad and H.M. Wisniewski
© 1999 John Wiley & Sons Ltd

examined the effect of hFE65L over-expression on APP processing. In this study, we show that hFE65L over-expression increases the proportion of mature to immature APP maturation and produces an increase in APPsα secretion.

MATERIALS AND METHODS

ANTIBODIES AND cDNA CONSTRUCTS

Commercially available anti-hemagglutinin (HA) antibody (Boehringer-Mannheim) was used for Western blot analysis and immunoprecipitations of the HA–hFE65L fusion protein. The APP antibodies used were 22C11 and 6E10, raised against Aβ1–17 (Senetek), and 369W, directed against APP645–694. An HA epitope tag was inserted into the hFE65L gene at a unique *HpaI* restriction enzyme site located between the WW domain and PID1. Northern blot analysis was performed as previously described [12].

CELL CULTURE AND GENERATION OF CELL LINES

H4 neuroglioma founder cell lines for a tetracycline-repressible expression system were established by Kim et al. [24] and cultured in DMEM media supplemented with gentamycin 418 (200 μg/ml) and tetracycline (1 μg/ml). We selected hygromycin-resistant colonies in the presence of tetracycline after transfection of H4 tetracycline-repressible founder cells with lipofectamine (Gibco BRL, Inc.), 10 μg of pHA–FE65L and 1 μg of pCNH2hygro.

METABOLIC LABELING AND IMMUNOPRECIPITATIONS

The H4 neuroglioma clones expressing HA–hFE65L were grown to confluency in either the presence or absence of tetracycline. Cells were trypsinized and resuspended in the respective culture media, pelleted by centrifugation (1000 rpm, 10 min), resuspended in methionine-free DMEM and incubated for 20 min at 37 °C. Cells were pelleted by brief centrifugation and resuspended in 1 ml of methionine-free DMEM containing 250 μCi of [^{35}S]methionine (>1000 Ci/mmol; NEN Research Products) and labeled for 20 min at 37 °C. The chase period was initiated using DMEM containing a five-fold excess of unlabeled methionine after washing the cells once with methionine-free media. Cell extract preparation, immunoprecipitations, and Western blot analyses were performed as previously described [12], with the exception that immunocomplexes were collected with either protein A or goat anti-mouse IgG magnetic beads (PerSeptive Diagnostics). Chase media were collected and treated as described by Caporaso et al. [25]. APPs was immunoprecipitated using 6E10 from chase media volumes normalized using total cell lysate protein values estimated by the BCA protein assay (Pierce).

Immunoprecipitates were separated on SDS–polyacrylamide gradient gels (4–20%) and the gels were dried and subjected to autoradiography.

RESULTS

Of the three known family members of the human FE65 gene family, the expression patterns for two of these genes, hFE65L [12] and hFE65 [13], have been described in human tissues. In contrast to tissues where the hFE65L gene produces two major transcripts of 7.5 and 3.7 kb [12], the expression pattern of the hFE65L gene differs in cell lines of different lineages. We found that the hFE65L 3.7 kb message is transcribed in human H4 neuroglioma, human 238 neuroblastoma cells and African green monkey COS7 cells, while the 7.5 kb message is abundant in primary neurons, H4 neuroglioma and COS7 cells. No hFe65L message is detected in primary astrocytes (Figure 1).

To characterize the function of hFE65L we established a stable hFE65L-inducible H4 neuroglioma cell line using the tetracycline-repressible system described by Gossen and Bujard (1992) [27]. In this system the presence of tetracycline in the culture medium suppresses hFE65L expression while the removal of tetracycline induces the expression of an HA-tagged version of hFE65L. The expression of an 80 kDa anti-HA immunoreactive protein

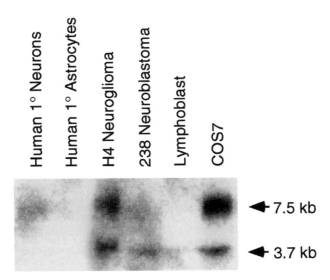

Figure 1. Expression of the hFE65L gene in human primary cells and cultured cells. Total RNA (10 μg) was subjected to gel electrophoresis and transferred to nylon. The membrane was hybridized with a ^{32}P-labeled 400 bp hFE65L cDNA fragment. Total RNA from human primary neurons and astrocytes was a generous gift from Dr Andrea LeBlanc

(Figure 2A) roughly corresponds to the predicted molecular weight of HA–hFE65L. The data show an absence of HA-tagged hFE65L in uninduced cells and significant over-expression of hFE65L at 72 h post-induction. Over-expression of hFE65L does not appear to have any gross detrimental effects on cell growth or viability (data not shown). Using this cell line we also confirmed that endogenous APP can be co-immunoprecipitated with the 80 kDa HA-tagged hFE65L protein, as detected by Western blot analysis of anti-HA immunoprecipitates using the 22C11 antibody (Figure 2B). This finding supports our earlier studies showing the co-immunoprecipitation of a 203 amino acid C-terminal fusion protein of hFE65L with APP [12].

We examined the effect of hFE65L over-expression of APP processing using 35S-Met pulse-chase labeling, followed by immunoprecipitation of APP from cell lysates and conditioned media recovered from H4 neuroglioma cells cultured for 72 h in the presence or absence of tetracycline (Figure 3). We noted an increase in the ratio of mature to immature isoforms of APP for cells over-expressing hFE65L (Figure 3, 72 h induction). The observed increase in the amount of mature APP was accompanied by an increase in APPsα secretion (Figure 3). The amount of label incorporated in H4 neuroglioma cells cultured in the presence or absence of tetracycline did not differ significantly (data not shown). Since hFE65L expression increases over 72 h, the increase in APP secretion over this time course suggests a dosage-dependent effect of hFE65L on the amount of APPsα secreted (Figure 3).

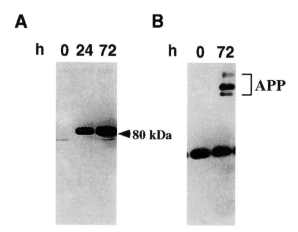

Figure 2. Co-immunoprecipitation of APP with hFE65L. (A) Western blot analysis of cellular extracts obtained from a tetracycline-repressible H4 neuroglioma cell line stably transfected with an HA–hFE65L construct using an anti-HA antibody. Cells were cultured in the absence of tetracycline for 24 and 72 h. (B) Western blot analysis using 22C11 for detection of APP performed on immunoprecipitates obtained with an anti-HA antibody from cells expressing HA–hFE65L for 72 h. APP was detected with the 22C11 antibody

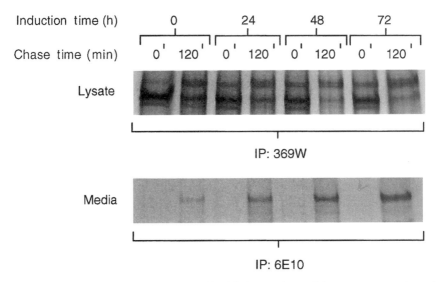

Figure 3. Maturation and secretion of APP is accelerated by over-expression of hFE65L. APP species were immunoprecipitated with 369W antisera from cell lysates (100 μg) of [³⁵S] methionine pulse-labeled H4 cells (clone 32–6), either uninduced or induced, for 24, 48 or 72 h by removal of tetracycline from the media and chased for 2 h (top panel). APPsα was immunoprecipitated from chase media normalized for equal amounts of cell lysate total protein with the 6E10 monoclonal antibody (bottom panel)

DISCUSSION

We have shown that over-expression of hFE65L accelerates APP maturation and increases the rate of APPsα secretion. These data provide the first physiological evidence that members of the family of FE65 proteins modulate APP processing.

The FE65 protein may be mediating its effect on APP processing through its binding to the NPXY reinternalization sequence. This may block access of the APP NPXY sequence to the reinternalization machinery. However, we also noted an increase in the proportion of mature to immature APP, suggesting that hFE65L modulates APP processing at an earlier step in the secretory pathway, especially since H4 cells have been reported to express low levels of cell-surface APP [26]. Given that only 20–30% of newly synthesized APP is transported from the ER to the Golgi apparatus, decreased exposure of improperly folded APP to proteolytic enzymes may be one mechanism by which the cell achieves a rapid increase in relative levels of mature APP and APPsα secretion. It remains to be determined whether hFE65L over-expression has an impact on Aβ generation, which requires over-expression of APP. The data in this study pertain solely to the effects of hFE65L over-expression on endogenous APP processing and not to those that might be observed under less physiological conditions resulting from excess accumulation of APP in intracellular membranes. The exact cellular site of the hFE65L–APP interaction accounting for the observed effect on APP maturation will be important to determine in future studies.

ACKNOWLEDGEMENTS

We thank Tae-Wan Kim for providing the H4 32neo founder cell line for tetracycline repression, Colin Masters for the 22C11 antibody, Sam Gandy for the 369W antisera and Andrea LeBlanc for Total RNA from human 1° neurons and astrocytes. This research was supported by grants from the American Health Assistance Foundation and the NIH.

REFERENCES

1. Koo EH, Squazzo SL. Evidence that production and release of amyloid β-protein involves the endocytic pathway. J Biol Chem 1994; 269: 17386–9.
2. Martin BL, Schrader-Fischer G, Busciglio J, Duke M, Paganetti P, Yankner BA. Intracellular accumulation of β-amyloid in cells expressing the Swedish mutant amyloid precursor protein. J Biol Chem 1995; 270: 26727–30.
3. Hartmann T, Bieger SC, Brühl B, Tienari PJ, Ida N, Allsop D, Roberts GW, Masters CL, Dotti CG, Unsicker K, Beyreuther K. Distinct sites of intracellular production for Alzheimer's disease Aβ40/42 amyloid peptides. Nature Med 1997; 3: 1016–20.
4. Cook DG, Forman MS, Sung JC, Leight S, Kolson DL, Iwatsubo T, Lee VM-Y, Doms RW. Alzheimer's Aβ(1–42) is generated in the endoplasmic reticulum/ intermediate compartment of NT2N cells. Nature Med 1997; 3: 1021–3.
5. Wild-Bode C, Yamazaki T, Capell A, Leimer U, Steiner H, Ihara Y, Haass C. Intracellular generation and accumulation of amyloid β-peptide terminating at amino acid 42. J Biol Chem 1997; 272: 16085–8.
6. Tienari PJ, Ida N, Ikonen E, Simons M, Weidemann S, Multhaup G, Masters CL, Dotti CG, Beyreuther K. Intracellular and secreted Alzheimer β-amyloid species are generated by distinct mechanisms in cultured hippocampal neurons. Proc Natl Acad Sci USA 1997; 94: 4125–30.
7. Felsenstein KM, Ingalls KM, Hunihan LW, Roberts SB. Reversal of Swedish familial Alzheimer's disease mutant phenotype in cultured cells treated with phorbol 12,13-dibutyrate. Neurosci Lett 1994; 174: 173–6.
8. Haass C, Lemer CA, Capell A, Citron M, Seubert P, Schenk D, Lannfelt L, Selkoe D. The Swedish mutation causes early-onset Alzheimer's disease by β-secretase cleavage within the secretory pathway. Nature Med 1995; 1: 1291–6.
9. Essalmani R, Macq A-F, Mercken L, Octave J-N. Missense mutations associated with familial Alzheimer's disease in Sweden lead to the production of the amyloid peptide without internalization of its precursor. Biochem Biophys Res Commun 1996; 218: 89–96.

10. Mellman I, Matter K, Yamamoto E, Pollack N, Roome J, Felsenstein K, Roberts S. Mechanisms of molecular sorting in polarized cells: relevance to Alzheimer's disease. In: Kosik KS et al. (eds) Alzheimer's Disease: Lessons from Cell Biology. Berlin/New York: Springer-Verlag, 1995; 14–26.

11. De Strooper B, Craessaerts K, Dewachter I, Moechars D, Greenberg B, Van Leuven F, Van Den Berghe H. Basolateral secretion of amyloid precursor protein in Madin–Darby canine kidney cells is disturbed by alterations of intracellular pH and by introducing a mutation associated with familial Alzheimer's disease. J Biol Chem 1995; 270: 4058–65.

12. Guénette SY, Chen J, Jondro PD, Tanzi RE. Association of a novel human FE65-like protein with the cytoplasmic domain of the β-amyloid precursor protein. Proc Natl Acad Sci USA 1996; 93: 10832–7.

13. Bressler SL, Gray MD, Sopher BL, Hu Q, Hearn MG, Pham DG, Dinulos MB, Fukuchi K-I, Sisodia SS, Miller MA, Disteche CM, Martin GM. cDNA cloning and chromosome mapping of the human Fe65 gene. Interaction of the conserved cytoplasmic domains of the human β-amyloid precursor protein and its homologues with the mouse Fe65 protein. Hum Mol Gen 1996; 5: 1589–98.

14. Fiore F, Zambrano N, Minopoli G, Donini V, Duilio A, Russo T. The regions of FE65 protein homologous to the phosphotyrosine interaction/phosphotyrosine binding domain of Shc bind the intracellular domain of the Alzheimer's amyloid precursor protein. J Biol Chem 1995; 270: 30853–6.

15. Borg J-P, Ooi J, Levy E, Margolis B. The phosphotyrosine interaction domains of X11 and FE65 bind to distinct sites on the YENPTY motif of amyloid precursor protein. Mol Cell Biol 1996; 16: 6229–41.

16. Duilio A, Faraonio R, Minopoli G, Zambrano N, Russo T. Fe65L2: a new member of the FE65 protein family interacting with the intracellular domain of the Alzheimer's β-amyloid precursor protein. Biochem J 1998; 330: 513–19.

17. Lai A, Sisodia SS, Trowbridge IS. Characterization of sorting signals in the β-amyloid precursor protein cytoplasmic domain. J Biol Chem 1995; 270: 3565–73.

18. Haass C, Hung AY, Schlossmacher MG, Teplow DB, Selkoe DJ. β-amyloid peptide and 3-kDa fragment are derived by distinct cellular mechanisms. J Biol Chem 1993; 75: 1039–42.

19. Koo EH, Squazzo SL, Selkoe DJ, Koo CH. Trafficking of cell surface amyloid β-protein precursor. I. Secretion, endocytosis and recycling as detected by labeled monoclonal antibody. J Cell Sci 1996; 109: 991–6.

20. De Strooper B, Umans L, Van Leuven F, Van Den Berghe H. Study of the synthesis and secretion of normal and artificial mutants of murine amyloid precursor protein (APP): cleavage of APP occurs in a late compartment of the default secretory pathway. J Cell Biol 1993; 121: 295–304.

21. Jacobsen SJ, Spruy MA, Brown AM, Sahasrabudhe SR, Blume AJ, Vitek MP, Muenkel HA, Sonnenberg-Reines J. The release of Alzheimer's disease β amyloid peptide is reduced by phorbol treatment. J Biol Chem 1994; 269: 8376–82.

22. Borg J-P, Ooi J, Levy E, Margolis B. The phosphotyrosine interaction domains of X11 and FE65 bind to distinct sites on the YENPTY motif of amyloid precursor protein. Mol Cell Biol 1996; 16: 6229–41.

23. Zambrano N, Buxbaum JD, Minopoli G, Fiore F, De Candia P, De Renzis S, Faraonio R, Sabo S, Cheetham J, Sudol M, Russo T. Interaction of the phosphotyrosine interaction/phosphotyrosine binding-related domains of FE65 with wild-type and mutant Alzheimer's β-amyloid precursor proteins. J Biol Chem 1997; 272: 6399–405.

24. Kim T-W, Pettingell W, Hallmark OG, Moir RD, Wasco W, Tanzi RE. Endo-proteolytic cleavage and proteasomal degradation of presenilin 2 in transfected cells. J Biol Chem 1997; 272: 11006–10.
25. Caporaso GL, Gandy SE, Buxbaum J, Greengard P. Chloroquine inhibits intra-cellular degradation but not secretion of Alzheimer β/A4 amyloid precursor protein. Proc Natl Acad Sci USA 1992; 89: 2252–6.
26. Kuentzel SL, Ali SM, Altman RA, Greenberg BD, Raub TJ. The Alzheimer β-amyloid protein precursor/protease nexin-II is cleaved by secretase in a *trans*-Golgi secretory compartment in human neuroglioma cells. Biochem J 1993; 295: 367–78.
27. Gossen M, Bujard H. Tight control of gene expression in mammalian cells by tetracycline-responsive promoters. Proc Natl Acad Sci USA 1992; 89: 5547–51.

Address for correspondence:
    Rudolph E. Tanzi,
    Department of Neurology,
    Harvard Medical School, Massachusetts General Hospital—East,
    149 13th St, Charlestown, MA 02129, USA
    e-mail: guenette@helix.mgh.harvard.edu

67 Molecular Genetics and Mutational Analysis of the *Drosophila Presenilin* Gene

IZHAR LIVNE BAR, YIQUAN GUO AND
GABRIELLE L. BOULIANNE

INTRODUCTION

Alzheimer's disease (AD) is a degenerative disorder of the central nervous system that causes progressive memory and cognitive decline during mid- to late adult life. This disease is currently the fourth leading cause of death and a major cause of disability amongst adults in Western societies. Despite the prevalence and the huge emotional and financial burdens imposed by this disease, no effective therapy exists. This therapeutic void in part reflects an incomplete understanding of the biochemical pathogenesis of this disease. One approach which can be used to understand the important pathological events associated with the disease is to identify cases of AD which are inherited as an autosomal dominant trait. This search has led to the identification of three human genes, *amyloid precursor protein (APP), presenilin 1* and *presenilin 2 (PS1* and *PS2)*, for which in-frame, missense mutations have been associated with early onset familial Alzheimer's disease (FAD) (reviewed in [1]). A complete understanding of the role of these genes in the etiology of AD will, however, require that the normal function of these gene products be determined. Recently, a homologue of the *presenilins* has been identified in the nematode, *Caenorhabditis elegans*, in a genetic screen to identify suppressors of a well-characterized signaling molecule (*Notch/lin-12*) involved in specifying cell fate in most complex organisms [2]. This demonstrated that presenilins were conserved through evolution and that they may play a role (direct or indirect) within the Notch signaling cascade. Recently, we have identified and characterized the *Drosophila* homologue of presenilin (*Dps*) [3]. The analysis of presenilin in *Drosophila*, combined with the extensive knowledge of the Notch signaling pathway in that organism, will provide a comprehensive view of presenilin gene function. Here, we describe the molecular and cellular characterization of Dps and the generation of several *Dps*

Alzheimer's Disease and Related Disorders
Edited by K. Iqbal, D.F. Swaab, B. Winblad and H.M. Wisniewski
© 1999 John Wiley & Sons Ltd

mutations and transgenics which provide insights into its role during normal development and pathogenesis.

MOLECULAR CHARACTERIZATION OF THE *DROSOPHILA PRESENILIN* GENE

To date, a single presenilin gene called *Dps* has been identified in *Drosophila* and mapped by chromosome *in situ* hybridization to position 77B-C on the left arm of the third chromosome [3]. The structure of the *Dps* gene is remarkably similar to that of *C. elegans* and human *presenilin* genes, with many of the intron–exon boundaries and splicing sites conserved between species (Figure 1). Overall, the *Dps* gene consists of a total of nine exons, eight of which comprise the coding sequence. Compared to *C. elegans* and human presenilins, this represents an intermediate number of exons and is consistent with the idea that presenilin derives from a common ancestral gene.

Like its vertebrate counterparts [1], the *Drosophila presenilin* gene produces multiple transcripts. Several transcripts ranging from 2 to 5 kb were detected at all developmental stages, with a major transcript (2 kb) most abundant in adults and a minor transcript (approximately 4 kb) most abundant in

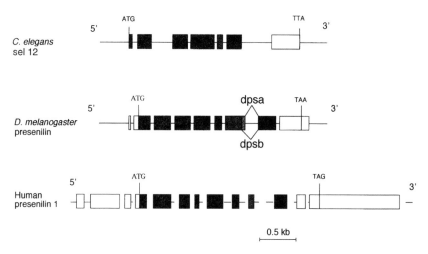

Figure 1. Comparison of presenilin genomic structures. The genomic structures of presenilins were generated by comparing the cDNA and corresponding genomic DNA from *Caenorhabditis elegans*, *Drosophila melanogaster* and human PS1. The *Dps* gene is alternatively spliced and gives rise to at least two splice forms called *dpsa* and *dpsb*. *dpsb* gives rise to a slightly longer protein consisting of an additional 14 amino acids within the large hydrophilic loop. The overall structure of the genes is highly conserved, including the intron–exon boundaries. The sequences were obtained from Genbank, with Accession Numbers U35660, U41540 (*C. elegans*), L42110, 1479972 (human) and U77934 (*D. melanogaster*)

embryos, but detected at all stages. In addition we observed stage-specific transcripts, including a 5 kb transcript in embryos and a 3.5 kb transcript in adults [3]. While several of these transcripts may result from alternative transcript initiation or termination, at least one of these arises from an alternative splicing event, creating a gene product with an additional 14 amino acids (Figure 1).

Presenilins have been identified from numerous species (Figure 2). Comparison of the predicted amino acid sequence of Dps with that of human

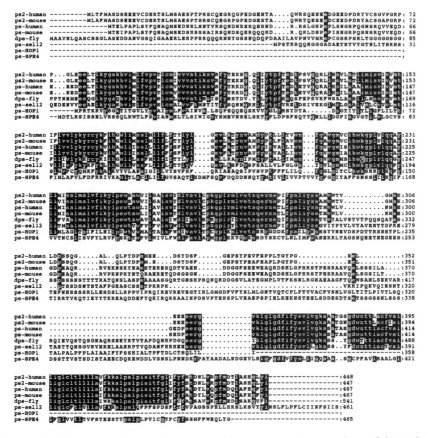

Figure 2. Alignment of presenilin amino acid sequences. A comparison of the amino acid sequence from presenilins of various species is presented. The highest degree of conservation between presenilins is in the transmembrane domains and the C-terminal domain. All sequences are deduced from published cDNAs. Amino acid identities are highlighted. The sources and Accession Numbers for each sequence are listed: dps-fly, *Drosophila melanogaster* presenilin isoform A, U77934, U78084; ps1-human, *Homo sapiens* Presenilin 1, L42110; ps2-human, *Homo sapiens* Presenilin 2, L44577; ps1-mouse, *Mus musculus* Presenilin 1, L42177; ps2-mouse, *Mus musculus* Presenilin 2, AF038935; ps-sell2, *Caenorhabditis elegans* presenilin homologue, U35660; ps-SPE4, *C. elegans* presenilin homologue, Z14067; ps-Hop, *C. elegans* presenilin homologue, AF021905

presenilins reveals 53% overall sequence identity. However, residues predicted to compose transmembrane domains or membrane-associated domains
showed a much higher level of sequence identity. In addition, the C-terminal
portion of the protein is also highly conserved, in contrast to the large hydrophilic loop between TM6 and TM7, which is poorly conserved amongst all
species. Interestingly, many of the residues mutated in human *PS1* or *PS2* and
giving rise to human FAD are conserved in Dps. In addition, the cysteine
residue, which is mutated in the *C. elegans sel-12* gene, is also conserved. This
suggests that these residues form an important functional or structural domain
of the presenilins.

Although full-length Dps protein (~57 kDa) can be detected in transgenic
lines which over-express a full-length Dps cDNA, the majority of the endogenous protein appears to be proteolytically cleaved to generate two polypeptides (Figure 3A). The N-terminal fragment is ~32 kDa and the C-terminal
fragment is ~25 kDa. Using immunocytochemical techniques we have found
that Dps is broadly expressed during development. However, some tissues,
such as the larval CNS, express higher levels of Dps. In this tissue, Dps is
primarily associated with neurons rather than glia. Like its vertebrate counterparts [1], Dps is primarily located in the cytoplasm in a perinuclear location
consistent with the endoplasmic reticulum and Golgi (Figure 3B).

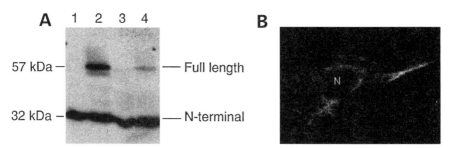

Figure 3. (A) Western blot of Dps. Dps protein was detected from third instar larval
extracts by Western blotting using an N-terminal-specific antibody. The majority of the
endogenous protein is cleaved and detected as an ~32 kDa N-terminal peptide. When
Dps is over-expressed in transgenic flies, using either a heatshock driver or specific
GAL4 drivers, full-length protein can be detected. 1, Wild-type larvae. No full-length
protein is detected. 2, Wild-type larvae containing a heatshock-driven *Dps* transgene.
Note the presence of the full-length Dps protein in addition to the N-terminal peptide.
3, Wild-type larvae containing a UAS-driven *Dps* transgene expressed from the elav-
GAL4 driver, whose expression is restricted to neurons. Very little full-length protein is
produced using this particular GAL4 driver. 4, Wild-type larvae containing a UAS-
driven *Dps* transgene expressed from the C41-GAL4 driver, with high levels of expression in the larval CNS. As in lane 2, when *Dps* is expressed at high levels, full-length
protein can be detected. (B) Immunocytochemistry of third instar larval neurons. High
levels of Dps expression in larval CNS were obtained by expressing a full-length *Dps*
transgene from a ubiquitous GAL4 driver. Dps protein accumulates throughout the
cytoplasm and in a perinuclear location consistent with endoplasmic reticulum and
Golgi. The nucleus is indicated by (N)

FUNCTIONAL ANALYSIS OF *DROSOPHILA PRESENILIN*

The function of presenilin in *Drosophila* is still unclear. However, we have recently identified two mutations in the gene based on their ability to interact genetically with *Notch* (Guo Y, Livne Bar I, Boulianne GL, submitted). This is consistent with a role for presenilin in the *Notch* signaling pathway first suggested by studies in *C. elegans* [2]. Sequence analysis has revealed that one of these mutations corresponds to a single missense mutation within the highly conserved C-terminal domain of the protein, suggesting that this domain plays an important role in presenilin function. We have also generated a series of overlapping deletions in *Dps* by imprecise excision of a nearby P-element insertion. Deletions which completely remove the *Dps* coding region make no presenilin protein and die at second instar larval stages. The fact that null mutations in *Dps* give rise to a larval lethal phenotype is likely due to the presence of high levels of maternal *Dps* which is deposited in the embryo and sufficient to support early development. To confirm this, germ-line clones which remove maternal *Dps* are now being generated. Interestingly, deletions which remove only the C-terminal portion of *Dps* also behave as null mutations and die as second instar larval lethals, despite the fact that the N-terminal portion of the protein is made. This provides further evidence that the C-terminal portion of the presenilin protein plays an important functional role.

To further investigate the function of presenilin we have also generated transgenic flies which express either wild-type or mutant forms of *Dps*. Specifically, we have used the GAL4/UAS system [4] to target expression of presenilins during third instar larval development. The wild-type presenilin cDNA used in these experiments is full-length and corresponds to the shorter *Dpsa* splice form. To generate mutant *Dps* we introduced FAD-linked mutations associated with *PS1* or *PS2* as well as the mutations originally identified in *sel-12* into a wild-type presenilin cDNA by *in vitro* mutagenesis techniques. All of the transgenic lines gave rise to supernumerary sensory bristles in the adult notum and eye when over-expressed in third instar larval imaginal discs. However, the severity of the phenotype correlated with the type of mutation expressed with *WT* > *PS2* > *sel-12* > *PS1*. Shown is the adult notum phenotype produced by over-expression of a wild-type *Dps* transgene (Figure 4B).

We have also taken advantage of the adult phenotypes generated by misexpression of presenilins to carry out genome wide screens for genetic modifiers. An example of such a genetic modifier is illustrated in Figure 4C. Modifiers could correspond to genes which interact in a common pathway with *Dps* during development and provide insight into its normal biological function. More importantly, genetic modifiers could themselves be candidate genes in AD which have yet to be identified, and such genes may provide novel targets for therapeutic intervention.

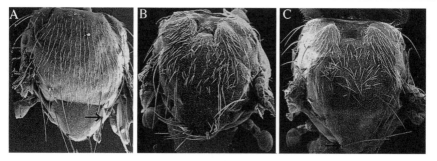

Figure 4. Transgenic lines expressing Dps give rise to distinct phenotypes in the adult notum. Scanning electron microscopy was used to examine the phenotypes of *Dps* over-expression in the adult notum. Adult phenotypes were obtained using a GAL4 driver, which is expressed in third instar wing imaginal discs to drive a wild-type UAS–*Dps* transgene. (A) Wild-type adult notum. Note the regular array of microchaetes (small bristles) on the notum and the presence of macrochaetes (large bristles) on the scutellum (arrow). (B) Adult notum from a transgenic line which expresses a wild-type *Dps* transgene under the transcriptional control of a specific GAL4 driver. Note the general disorganization of microchaetes (small bristles) on the notum and the presence of supernumerary bristles on the scutellum (arrow). (C) Adult notum of transgenic lines carrying a *Dps* transgene under the transcriptional control of a specific GAL4 driver, shown in (B) in the presence of a genetic modifier. Note that although the microchaetes on the notum are still disorganized, there is a marked reduction in the number of supernumerary bristles on the scutellum (arrow)

CONCLUSION

We have described the identification and characterization of the *Drosophila* presenilin gene. This provides us with a unique opportunity to establish an invertebrate model to gain insight into the normal and pathological function of presenilins. Molecular characterization has demonstrated that the *Dps* gene structure is highly conserved when compared to presenilin genes of both vertebrates and *C. elegans*. In addition, the predicted amino acid sequence suggests that presenilins belong to a highly conserved novel family of proteins which are broadly expressed throughout development. Mutational analysis of *Dps* further demonstrates that this gene is required for normal development in flies, since null mutations are lethal as second instar larvae. The fact that mutations which completely remove *Dps* do not cause lethality at earlier stages likely reflects the large maternal contribution of *Dps* which we have previously observed by Northern blot and *in situ* hybridization studies. Interestingly, we find that mutations which remove only portions of the C-terminal domain of *Dps* behave like null mutations despite the fact that a functional N-terminal peptide is produced. This suggests that the C-terminal domain of presenilin is functionally important. This observation is supported by the fact that this domain is highly conserved between all species, in contrast to the hydrophilic loop between TM6 and TM7 which is highly variable and poorly conserved. Interestingly, the majority of FAD mutations are excluded from the C terminus and many are found within the hydrophilic TM6-TM7 loop. It is important to note that over-expression of Dps containing FAD-associated mutations in flies produces weaker phenotypes than those obtained when using a wild-type *Dps* transgene. This indicates that the FAD mutations produce a functional presenilin protein which has reduced activity. This observation is consistent with the hypothesis that the FAD mutations in humans are functionally 'weak' or hypomorphic with respect to protein function, and may explain why pathological effects appear only after prolonged periods of time. The fact that mutations in the C-terminal portion of presenilins are rarely associated with AD suggests that these mutations might affect protein function much more severely and would therefore be lethal during embryogenesis. This hypothesis is supported by the fact that, as in flies, knock-out mutations in *PS1* in mice are embryonic lethal, while over-expression of mutant presenilins causes no overt pathology and only alters levels of Aβ.

Mutational analysis of *Dps* has also revealed that presenilins can interact with the *Notch* signaling pathway. Specifically, we find that a point mutation in the C-terminal domain of Dps can enhance the phenotype of a *Notch* mutant. This is consistent with previous studies in *C. elegans*, whereby the presenilin homologue *sel-12* was identified in a genetic screen looking to identify modifiers of an activated *lin-12/Notch* mutation [2] and the observation that null mutations in *PS1* give rise to a similar phenotype in mice as 'knock-out' mutations in *Notch* [5, 6]. Whether the interaction between *Notch* and presenilins is direct or indirect has yet to be determined. However, the subcellular location of presenilins in the endoplasmic reticulum and Golgi together would suggest that presenilins are likely to be involved in some aspect of protein processing or trafficking within the cell.

Finally, we have begun to exploit the powerful genetic techniques which are available in *Drosophila* to identify and characterize genetic modifiers of *Dps*. By generating transgenic flies which express wild-type and mutant *Dps* we have obtained adult phenotypes which are easily scorable and can be used as the basis to search for mutations in other genes which can enhance or suppress the *Dps* phenotypes. These genetic modifiers could correspond to genes which interact in a common pathway with presenilins during development and provide insight into their normal biological functions. More importantly, genetic modifiers could themselves be candidate genes in AD which have yet to be identified or provide novel targets for therapeutic intervention.

ACKNOWLEDGEMENTS

We thank Lily Zhou for expert technical assistance and Dr W.S. Trimble for helpful discussions and comments on the manuscript. Work in the laboratory of G.L.B. is supported from the American Health Assistance Foundation, the American Alzheimer's Association and the Medical Research Council of Canada.

REFERENCES

1. Hutton M, Hardy J. The presenilins and Alzheimer's disease. Hum Mol Genet 1997; 6: 1639–46.
2. Levitan D, Greenwald I. Facilitation of *lin-12*-mediated signalling by *sel-12*, a *Caenorhabditis elegans* S182 Alzheimer's disease gene. Nature 1995; 377: 351–4.
3. Boulianne GL, Livne Bar I, Humphreys JM, Liang Y, Lin C, Rogaev E, St George-Hyslop P. Cloning and characterization of the *Drosophila* presenilin homologue. NeuroReport 1997; 8: 1025–9.
4. Brand AH, Perrimon N. Targeted gene expression as a means of altering cell fates and generating dominant phenotypes. Development 1993; 118: 401–15.
5. Wong PC, Zheng H, Chen H, Becher MW, Sirinathsinghji DJ, Trumbauer ME, Chen HY et al. Presenilin 1 is required for Notch 1 and DII 1 expression in the paraxial mesoderm. Nature 1997; 387: 288–92.
6. Qian S, Jiang P, Guan X-M, Singh G, Trumbauer ME, Yu H, Chen HY et al. Mutant human presenilin 1 protects presenilin 1 null mouse against embryonic lethality and elevates Ab1–42/43 expression. Neuron 1998; 20: 611–17.

Address for correspondence:
Gabrielle L. Boulianne,
Program in Developmental Biology,
Hospital for Sick Children, 555 University Avenue, Toronto, Ontario,
Canada M5G 1X8
Tel: 416 813 8701; fax: 416 813 5086; e-mail: gboul@sickkids.on.ca

68 Familial Alzheimer's Disease Mutations Enhance Apoptotic Effects of Presenilin-1

DORA M. KOVACS, RONALD MANCINI, SANG NA,
TAE-WAN KIM AND RUDOLPH E. TANZI

INTRODUCTION

The mechanism by which mutations in the presenilin genes lead to neuro-degeneration is not clear. The most widely studied pathogenic effect of presenilin mutations is an increase in the generation of the Aβ42 peptide. However, both presenilins have also been shown to play a role in apoptotic cell death. PS2, when highly over-expressed, increases sensitivity to apoptosis in PC-12 and HeLa cells [1, 2, 3]. Conversely, transfection with an antisense PS2 construct has been shown to inhibit the apoptotic pathway. The N141I mutation appears to potentiate the apoptotic effect of trans-fected cells [1, 3]. Somewhat unexpectedly, the C-terminal portion of mouse PS2 has been reported to protect cells undergoing Fas-mediated apoptosis [4]. The role of PS1 in the apoptotic process is less clear. It has been shown that one mutation, the familial Alzheimer's disease (FAD) L286V mutation, sensitizes neuronal cells to apoptosis induced by trophic factor withdrawal and by Aβ [5]. Over-expression of PS1 itself has been shown to induce apoptosis [6]. However, although a consensus sequence for caspase cleavage has been identified in both presenilins, recombinant caspase-3 (CPP-32) appears to cleave only PS2 [7, 8]. Therefore, the direct involvement of PS1 in apoptotic cell death and the identity of the enzyme cleaving the potential caspase site of PS1 are not as well understood as they are for PS2. The effect of FAD mutations on constitutive and alternative cleavage of PS1 is also not well characterized. In transgenic animals, PS1 FAD mutations have been reported to increase the absolute amount of fragments generated by con-stitutive endoproteolytic cleavage of the protein [9]. The rate of accumula-tion of the alternative C-terminal fragment (CTF) of PS2 has been reported

Alzheimer's Disease and Related Disorders
Edited by K. Iqbal, D.F. Swaab, B. Winblad and H.M. Wisniewski
© 1999 John Wiley & Sons Ltd

to increase roughly three-fold due to the presence of the N141I mutation in PS2-transfected cells [10].

To study the effect of PS1 FAD mutations on apoptotic cell death and on the rate of cleavage at the PS1 alternative endoproteolytic cleavage site, we induced apoptosis by staurosporine (STS) treatment of human H4 neuroglioma cell lines stably transfected with wild-type and FAD mutant PS1 constructs and immortalized lymphocyte cell lines from FAD patients and from age-matched controls. As shown in Figure 1, STS activates the caspase pathway upstream from caspase-3. Although caspase-3 may not be the, or the only, caspase enzyme cleaving PS1 at the alternative site, it is one of the last enzymes being induced before the final, execution phase of the apoptotic process. We therefore chose to not only measure the effect of PS1 FAD mutations on cell death, but also to correlate the activation of caspase-3 (as measured by cleavage of caspase-3 itself and of its substrate, PARP) with decreased cell viability and with cleavage of PS1 itself.

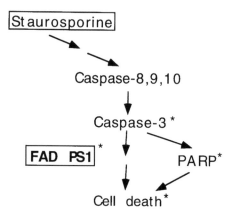

Figure 1. Experimental model for assessment of response to an apoptotic stimulus in stably transfected cells expressing relatively low levels of mutant FAD vs. wild-type PS1. *Cellular response assessed in this report

MATERIALS AND METHODS

CELL LINES AND CONSTRUCTS

Human H4 neuroglioma cells were stably transfected with wild-type (wt), A246E and L286V PS1–FLAG constructs in pcDNA3 [11] and wt and ΔE10 PS1-pcDNA3 constructs (gift of Dr J. Hardy, Mayo Clinic, Florida). H4 clones with comparable expression levels were used. Immortalized lymphocyte cell lines were generated from blood drawn from members of FAD kindreds. Staurosporine was used at a concentration of 1 μM.

IMMUNOBLOT AND CELL DEATH ANALYSES

Detergent lysates and total cellular extracts were quantitated and resolved on 4–20% gradient Tris–glycine gels under reducing conditions. Blotting was performed as described by Kim et al. [12]. A Bio-Rad phosphorimager was used to quantitate the intensity of the signals. Cell viability was assessed with the Live/Dead assay kit (Molecular Probes).

RESULTS AND DISCUSSION

CELL VIABILITY DECREASES AS AN EFFECT OF FAD PS1 MUTATIONS

Stably transfected cell lines expressing wt or FAD mutant (A246E, L286V and Δ10) PS1 were subjected to immunoblot analysis to ensure low and comparable expression levels of the transgenes. Low levels of full-length protein were detected in each cell line, but not the high molecular weight aggregates seen with very high expression of PS1 or PS2 [11]. In addition, the level of PS1 expression in these cells did not induce spontaneous apoptosis.

The effect of transfected FAD mutant relative to wt PS1 on cell viability was assessed when cells were treated with 1 μM staurosporine (STS). Cell viability was measured by decreased intracellular esterase activity (decreased calcein AM fluorescence) and by increased membrane damage (ethidium bromide staining of nuclear DNA). As expected, the rate of cell death was elevated in all mutant vs. wt PS1-transfected cell lines (Figure 2). The ΔE10 mutation resulted in approximately 75% of non-viable cells, while the A246E and the L286V mutations caused a lower, but comparable decrease in viability (40–50%) over 9 h of STS treatment. The A246E and the L286V mutation-

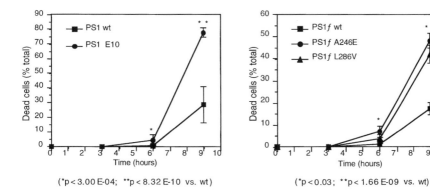

(*p < 3.00 E-04; **p < 8.32 E-10 vs. wt)   (*p < 0.03; **p < 1.66 E-09 vs. wt)

Figure 2. Assessment of cell death in H4 cells expressing wild-type vs. FAD mutant forms of PS1 and induced to undergo apoptosis with staurosporine. During the time course, mutant PS1-expressing cells die more quickly than the wild-type PS1 cells

containing PS1 constructs also expressed a FLAG epitope-tag at the C-terminal end of the molecules. The FLAG epitope-tag did not interfere visibly with cell viability levels when wt constructs with and without the epitope-tag were compared. The FLAG-tag, however, did induce a higher rate of caspase activation and possibly interfered with PS1 aCTF generation (data not shown). Therefore, we only compared wt and FAD mutant cell lines of the same kind (with or without the epitope-tag, as indicated in Figure 2).

EFFECT OF FAD MUTANT PS1 ON ITS ALTERNATIVE
CLEAVAGE AND ON CASPASE ACTIVATION

We then correlated the rate of cell viability with increased generation of the alternative 14 kDa C-terminal fragment (CTFa) and with caspase-3 activation. The alternative cleavage fragment first became detectable 3–9 h after apoptotic stimulation, depending on the transfected cell line used, and then steadily accumulated through 24 h of STS treatment. We determined the effect of FAD mutations on the accumulation of PS1–CTFa relative to constitutive or normal CTF (CTFn). Quantitation of the ratio of PS1–CTFa to PS1–CTFn (or PS1–CTFa to full-length molecule, in the case of the Δ10 FAD mutant protein) revealed a marked increase of the ratio in mutant vs. wt transfected cells. At 24 h of STS treatment, the ΔE10 PS1 mutation (without the FLAG epitope-tag) resulted in the highest increase, a 5.6-fold increase in C-terminal alternative fragment relative to the full-length protein (data not shown). All FAD mutations tested resulted in elevated ratios of PS1–CTFa to PS1–CTFn in transfected H4 cells.

Because the ΔE10 PS1 mutation resulted in the biggest decrease in cell viability and in the highest rate of aCTF generation, we correlated these two effects of the mutation with caspase activation. Caspase-3 activation is a very specific feature of apoptotic cell death, widely used to assess apoptosis levels. Figure 3 shows increased cleavage of caspase-3 itself (indicating activation), and of a very sensitive apoptotic substrate, PARP, at 9 h of treatment with STS in a cell line expressing ΔE10 PS1. When the same two lanes were also stained for PS1 aCTF, the aCTF was clearly increased in the ΔE10 PS1 cells. When this effect was quantitated over a larger number of samples (n = 6), caspase-3 was activated 2–3-fold more in the ΔE10 PS1 cells at 6 and 9 h of STS treatment when compared to wt. From these experiments we conclude that FAD mutant PS1 potentiates STS-induced apoptosis, and the specific mechanism by which FAD mutant PS1 contributes to caspase activation remains to be determined.

Endogenous heterozygous expression of A246E and L286V mutant PS1 in seven immortalized lymphocyte cell lines from FAD patients result in a small, but not significant, increase in the ratio of CTFa:CTFn relative to six age-matched controls. Very low levels of endogenous PS1 in these cells or the nature of this cell type may explain this result.

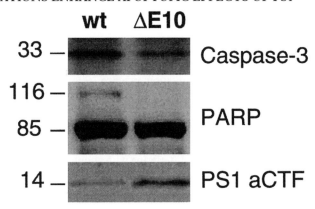

Figure 3. Analysis at the molecular level of apoptosis in wt PS1 vs. mutant ΔE10 PS1-expressing cells. In the mutant cells, caspase-3 is activated more robustly, PARP is cleaved more rapidly, and generation of the PS1-aCTF is enhanced

CONCLUSIONS

In this study, we compared cell viability, caspase activation and corresponding ratios of alternative:normal PS1 CTFs in wt vs. FAD mutant PS1-expressing human H4 neuroglioma cells. FAD mutations correlated with a decrease in cell viability, an increase in caspase activation and in the amount of PS1–CTFa relative to PS1–CTFn during STS-induced apoptosis. Although heterozygous expression of endogenous FAD mutant PS1 in the immortalized lymphocyte cell lines led only to a small, but non-significant, increase in alternative cleavage, the effect of the mutation may be below the level of detection. Elevated caspase activation in the transfected cell lines by the presence of FAD mutant PS1 suggests that either the mutant form is pro-apoptotic, or that it obliterates the beneficial effects of wt PS1 by replacement or by interaction. Either way, our data confirm previous results on apoptotic effects of the presenilins and point future research towards study of the effect of FAD mutant presenilins on the caspase pathway.

ACKNOWLEDGEMENTS

We thank Sam Sisodia and Gopal Thinakaran for providing the PS1-Loop antibody, and Sam Gandy and Mary Seeger for the Ab-14. This research was supported by grants from the NINDS, NIA and the Alzheimer Association.

REFERENCES

1. Wolozin B, Iwasaki K, Vito P, Ganjei K, Lacana E, Sunderland T, Zhao B, Kusiak JW, Wasco W, D'Adamio L. PS2 participates in cellular apoptosis: constitutive activity conferred by Alzheimer mutation. Science 1996; 274: 1710–13.
2. Deng G, Pike CJ, Cotman CW. Alzheimer-associated presenilin-2 confers increased sensitivity to apoptosis in PC12 cells. FEBS Lett 1996; 397: 50–54.
3. Janicki S, Monteiro MJ. Increased apoptosis arising from increased expression of the Alzheimer's disease-associated presenilin-2 mutation (N141I). J Cell Biol 1997; 139: 485–95.
4. Vito P, Lancana E, D'Adamio L. Interfering with apoptosis: Ca^{2+}-binding protein ALG-2 and Alzheimer's disease gene ALG-3. Science 1996; 271: 521–4.
5. Guo Q, Furukawa K, Sopher BL, Pham DG, Xie J, Robinson N, Martin GM, Mattson MP. Alzheimer's PS-1 mutation perturbs calcium homeostasis and sensitizes PC12 cells to death induced by amyloid β-peptide. NeuroReport 1996; 8: 379–83.
6. Guo Q, Sopher BL, Furukawa K, Pham DG, Robinson N, Martin GM, Mattson MP. Alzheimer's presenilin mutation sensitizes neural cells to apoptosis induced by trophic factor withdrawal and amyloid β-peptide: involvement of calcium and oxyradicals. J Neuroscience 1997; 17: 4212–22.
7. Loetscher H, Deuschle U, Brockhaus M, Reinhardt D, Nelboeck P, Mous J, Grunberg J, Haass C, Jacobsen H. Presenilins are processed by caspase-type proteases. J Biol Chem 1997; 33: 20655–9.
8. Vito P, Ghayurt T, D'Adamio L. Generation of anti-apoptotic presenilin-2 polypeptides by alternative transcription, proteolysis, and caspase-3 cleavage. J Biol Chem 1997; 272: 28315–20.
9. Lee MK, Borchelt DR, Kim G, Thinakaran G, Slunt HH, Ratovitski TR, Martin LJ, Kittur A, Gandy S, Levey AI, Jenkins N, Copeland N, Price DL, Sisodia SS. Hyperaccumulation of FAD-linked presenilin 1 variants *in vivo*. Nature Med 1997; 3: 756–60.
10. Kim T-W, Pettingell WH, Jung Y-K, Kovacs DM, Tanzi RE. Alternative cleavage of Alzheimer-associated presenilins during apoptosis by caspase-3 family protease. Science 1997; 277: 373–6.
11. Kovacs DM, Fausett HJ, Page KJ, Kim T-W, Mori RD, Merriam DE, Hoillister RD, Hallmark OG, Mancini R, Felsenstein KM, Hyman BT, Tanzi RE, Wasco W. Alzheimer associated presenilins 1 and 2: neuronal expression in brain and localization to intracellular membranes in mammalian cells. Nature Med 1996; 2: 224–9.
12. Kim T-W, Pettingell WH, Hallmark OG, Moir RD, Wasco W, Tanzi RE. Endoproteolytic processing and proteasomal degradation of presenilin 2 in transfected cells. J Biol Chem 1997; 272: 11006–10.

Address for correspondence:
Dora M. Kovacs,
Genetics and Aging Unit, Department of Neurology,
Harvard Medical School, Massachusetts General Hospital—East,
149 13th St, Charlestown, MA 02129, USA
Tel: 617 726 3668; fax: 617 726 5677;
e-mail: kovacs@helix.mgh.harvard.edu

69 Monoamine Oxidase Activities in Murine Neuroblastoma Cells upon Acute or Chronic Treatment with Aluminum or Tacrine

PAOLO ZATTA AND PAMELA ZAMBENEDETTI

INTRODUCTION

Aluminum (Al) is a known neurotoxic agent, and its proposed link to Alzheimer's disease (AD) etiopathogenesis has been discussed for more than 20 years. In the murine neuroblastoma cell line N2A, Al is able to produce several biological effects, including the formation of extended cytoplasmatic processes with many filaments in a metal speciation-dependent manner [1], accumulation of neurofilaments in the cell perykaria [2], activation of metal ion channels [3], activation of acetylcholinesterase activity [4], inhibition of muscarinic agonist inositol derivatives [5], interference with signal transduction [6], modification of the electrical response to a short hypertonic pulse due to the rigidification of the plasma membrane [7] and alteration of the electrophoretic properties of neurofilament tau proteins, a reflection of modifications in their phosphorylation state [8].

Treatment with tacrine (THA) can improve cognitive deficits in subpopulations of AD patients, especially those affected by mild dementia [9–11]. In addition, THA is able to influence various biochemical processes: it antagonizes morphine, inhibits AMP_c phosphodiesterase, inactivates Na^+ and K^+ channels, downregulates type I muscarinic receptors, alters intracellular phosphorylation and stimulates cholinergic firing [12]. In addition, THA increases the release of serotonin, noradrenalin, dopamine and GABA [13]. Recently, we have also observed encouraging results on the ability of THA to reduce the hyperphosphorylation of tau proteins in neuroblastoma cells [14].

Monoamine oxidase (MAO) catalyses the oxidative-deamination of various amines, an activity that increases as the brain ages [15]. In particular, the

Alzheimer's Disease and Related Disorders
Edited by K. Iqbal, D.F. Swaab, B. Winblad and H.M. Wisniewski
© 1999 John Wiley & Sons Ltd

activity of the isoform MAO-B was found to be significantly elevated in the hippocampus and cortex gyrus cinguli of AD patients [16, 17]. Although the basis for this higher MAO-B activity is still to be fully clarified, it is most likely associated with a proliferation of glial cells that accompanies the neuronal loss characterizing AD [18].

The present paper reports data regarding the changes in MAO-A and MAO-B activities in N2A cells after acute treatment or after adaptation for several months to either Al(III) or THA. The clinical implication of our preliminary findings must be further explored to extrapolate possible therapeutic implications. Results suggest that Al has a clear stimulatory effect on both isoforms, suggesting that the metal may be responsible for elevated MAO activity observed in some neuropathologies and with aging.

MATERIALS AND METHODS

The murine neuroblastoma cell line C1300 (clone N2A) was obtained from the American Type Culture Collection (Rockville, MD, USA). Cells were adapted for 7 months to 1 μM tacrine (9-amino-1,2,3,4-tetrahydroacridine), which represents a pharmacological dose, or to 1.3 mM aluminum lactate (AlLac$_3$). After adaptation to Al and THA, all cells survived, as ascertained by Trypan blue vital staining. MAO-A and MAO-B [monoamine oxidase (monoamine:oxygen-oxidoreductase (deaminating) EC1.4.3.4)] activities were assayed radiochemically [19] by using [2-^{14}C]hydroxytryptamine binoxalate (58 mCi/mmol) (NEN) as a substrate for MAO-A and β-[ethyl-^{14}C]-phenylethylamine-HCl (50 mCi/mmol, PEA) (Du Pont) as a substrate for MAO-B [20]. Al solutions were prepared from aluminum lactate (AlLac$_3$), as described elsewhere [21]. Statistical analysis was carried out using Macintosh Statwork^{TM} software. Data are presented as mean $\pm$ SEM (standard error of mean). Each experiment was carried out at least three times with the SEM representing the mean of these experiments. For multiple observations, data were evaluated by ANOVA and statistical differences were evaluated as the Fisher's least-significant difference (LSD). Differences were assumed to be significant for $p < 0.05$.

RESULTS

N2A cells treated for 72 h with 1 μM THA did not show variations in radioactive leucine [Leu] and thymidine [Thy] incorporation (Figure 1A, B). In contrast, cells adapted for 7 months to THA showed an increase in the incorporation of both radioisotopes (Figure 1A, B). Al-adapted cells also showed a marked increase in [Leu] and [Thy] incorporation (Figure 1C, D), while acute treatment with the metal ion reduced the incorporation of both radio-isotopes, indicating an adaptation mechanism when the toxicant is applied for a long period of time. Figure 2 shows that N2A cells chronically exposed to Al exhibit markedly increased MAO-A and MAO-B enzymatic activities. In contrast, chronic treatment with THA produces a clear inhibitory effect on MAO-A and no discernible effect on MAO-B. All experiments were statistically significant ($p < 0.01$). The great majority of the metal ions in the cell medium are complexed to transferrin; in this form they appear to lose the toxicity associated with the free metal ion species. When fetal calf serum is omitted from the medium, the cells show greatly increased mortality in the presence of lower concentration of Al^{3+} (μM range), which is present in toxic form, such as $Al(OH)^{4-}$ at physiological pH.

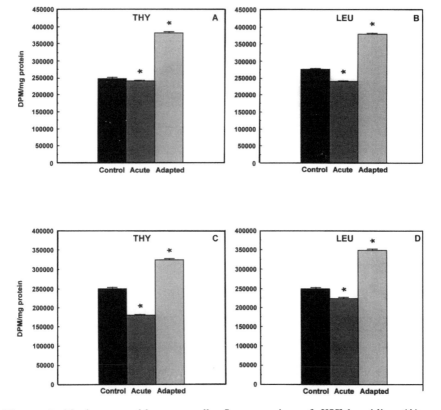

Figure 1. Murine neuroblastoma cells. Incorporation of [³H]thymidine (A) or [¹⁴C]leucine (B) (DPM/mg protein) after acute or long-term adaptation to 1 μM THA. *$p < 0.01$. Bars = SEM. Incorporation of [³H]thymidine (C) or [¹⁴C]leucine (D) (DPM/mg protein) after acute or long-term adaptation to 1.3 mM (nominal) AlLac₃. *$p < 0.01$. Bars = SEM

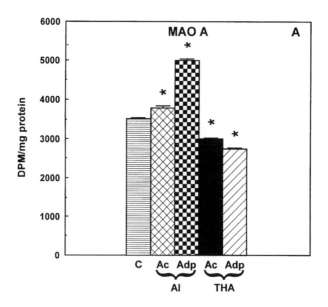

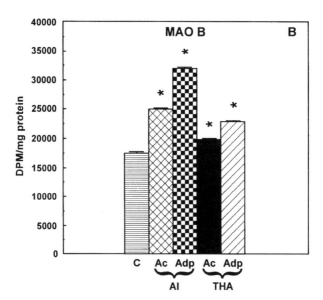

Figure 2. Murine neuroblastoma cells. MAO-A (A) and MAO-B (B) activity (DPM/ mg protein) evaluated after acute or prolonged treatment to (nominal) 1.3 mM AlLac$_3$ or to 1 μM THA. * p < 0.01. Bars = SEM

DISCUSSION

Our data show that N2A cells adapted to THA exhibit reduced MAO-A activity with respect to the controls, while MAO-B activity is similar to that of untreated cells. In contrast, N2A cells adapted to Al show elevated activity of both enzyme isotypes compared to the controls. In terms of THA concentration and extent of inhibition, these observations confirm those previously reported by Adem et al. [22] for MAO-A, but differ for those regarding the activity of MAO-B. This apparent discrepancy could be due to the lower concentration of THA used in our experiments (10^{-6} M), which corresponds to a therapeutic dose, compared to the higher THA concentrations used by Adem et al. [22].

The strong activating effect of Al on both MAO-A and MAO-B may provide further evidence that faulty Al metabolism, for instance its abnormal accumulation inside neuronal cells, could potentially interfere with the activities of these enzymes. Interestingly MAO-B activity in the human brain increases with age, and in a more pronounced way, in some neuropathologies such as AD and Parkinson's disease. The abnormal accumulation of Al in senile plaques and neurofibrillary tangles reported in several studies suggests a potential role of the metal ion as a co-factor involved in the etiology of AD, or at least as an aggravating factor.

The mechanism by which Al is internalized into the cell is yet to be fully understood and could be quite complicated, based on our knowledge of the complex system governing iron import [23]. It was recently reported that patients affected by AD possess elevated levels of transferrin C2 subtype [24]. Such a genetic phenotype has been hypothesized to be implicated in the etiology of AD, with this type of transferrin acting as a Trojan Horse carrying toxic metal ions such as aluminum into cells. Other authors reported an abnormal concentration of transferrin in AD [25] as well as abnormal iron metabolism as a cause of neurodegenerative disorders [26]. Thus, once inside the cell, Al could exhibit several detrimental activities such as those described in this paper and in the vast body of literature on Al biochemistry.

CONCLUSIONS

In summary, MAO catalyses the oxidative deamination of several primary amines. This paper reports a study of the activity of the two MAO isoforms (A and B) in murine neuroblastoma cells upon acute treatment or after adaptation for several months to aluminum (Al) and tacrine (THA). While Al has a pronounced activating effect on both MAO-A and B, THA shows an inhibitory action on MAO-A, and an insignificant effect on MAO-B. Data are discussed in terms of neurotoxicological implications for Al and the neuropharmacological aspects for THA.

REFERENCES

1. Zatta P, Perazzolo M, Facci L, Skaper SD, Corain B, Favarato M. Effects of aluminum speciation on murine neuroblastoma cells. Mol Chem Neuropathol 1992; 16: 11–22.
2. Shea TB, Clarke JF, Wheelock TR, Pakevich PA, Nixon RA. Aluminum salts induce accumulation of neurofilaments in perikarya of N2Ba/dl neuroblastoma. Brain Res 1989; 92: 53–64.
3. Oortgiesen M, Van Kleef RG, Vjiverberg HP. Novel type of ion channel activated by Pb^{2+}, Cd^{2+} and Al^{3+} in cultured mouse neuroblastoma cells. J Membr Biol 1990; 113: 261–8.
4. Zatta P, Zambenedetti P, Bruna V, Filippi B. Activation of acetylcholinesterase by aluminum(III): the relevance of the metal speciation. NeuroReport 1994; 5: 1777–8.
5. Wood PC, Wojcikiewicz RJ, Burgess J, Castleden CM, Nahorski SR. Aluminum inhibits muscarinic agonist-induced inositol 1,4,5-triphosphate production and calcium mobilisation in permeabilized SH-SY5Y human neuroblastoma cells. J Neurochem 1994; 62: 2219–23.
6. Shi B, Haug A. Aluminium interferes with signal transduction in neuroblastoma cells. Pharmacol Toxicol 1992; 71: 308–13.
7. Sorek N, Meiri H. Aluminium modifies electrical response of neuroblastoma cells to a short hypertonic pulse. Arch Toxicol 1992; 66: 90–94.
8. Shea TS, Beermann ML, Nixon RA. Aluminum alters the electrophoretic properties of neurofilament proteins: role of phosphorylation state. J Neurochem 1992; 55: 542–7.
9. Davis KL, Thal LJ, Gamzu ER, Davis CS, Woolson RF, Gracon SI, Drachman DA, Schneider LS, Whitehouse PJ, Hoover TM, Moris JC, Kawas CH, Knopman DS, Eari NL, Kumar V, Doody RS. A double-blind, placebo, controlled multicenter study of tacrine in Alzheimer's disease. N Engl J Med 1992; 327: 1253–9.
10. Eagger SA, Levy R, Sahakian BJ. Tacrine in Alzheimer's disease. Lancet 1991; 337: 989–92.
11. Knapp MJ, Knopman DS, Solomon PR, Pendlebury WW, Davis CS, Gracon SI. A 30 week randomized controlled trial of high dose tacrine in patients with Alzheimer's disease. JAMA 1994; 271: 985–91.
12. Thorton JE, Gersham S. The history of THA. In: Giacobini E, Becker S (eds) Current Research in Alzheimer's Disease Therapy. New York: Taylor & Francis, 1988; 267–78.
13. DeBelleroche J, Gardiner IM. Inhibitory effect of 1,2,3,4-tetrahydro-9-aminoacridine on the depolarisation-induced GABA from cerebral cortex. Br J Pharmacol 1988; 94: 1017–19.
14. Zatta P, Zambenedetti P, Marturano B, Palumbo M, Nicolini M. Effects of tacrine upon neuroblastoma cells. J Neuron Transm 1995; 102: 113–23.
15. Robinson DS. Changes in monoamine oxidase and monoamines with human development and aging. Fed Proc 1979; 4: 103–7.
16. Adolfsson R, Gottfries C, Roos R, Winblad B. Changes in brain catecholamines in patients with dementia of Alzheimer's type. Br J Psychiat 1979; 135: 216–23.
17. Reinikainen KJ, Paljarvi L, Halonen T, Malminen O, Kosma V-M, Laakso M, Riekkinen PJ. Dopaminergic system and monoaminergic oxidase-B activity in Alzheimer's disease. Neurobiol Aging 1988; 9: 245–52.
18. Zatta P, Giordano R, Zambenedetti P. Glycosylation and microglial activation in Alzheimer's disease. In: Seve A-P, Caron M (eds) Lectins and Pathology. Amsterdam: Harwood Academy (in press).

19. Eckert B, Gottfries CG, Von Knorring L, Oreland L, Wiberg A, Winblad B. Brain and platelet monoamine oxidase in mental disorders.1. Schizophrenics and cycloid psychotics. Progr Neuro-Psychopharmacol 1980; 4: 57–68.
20. Kitahama K, Maeda T, Denney RM, Jouvet M. Monoamine oxidase: distribution in the cat brain studied by enzyme and immunohistochemistry: recent progress. Progr Neurobiol 1996; 42: 53–78.
21. Zatta P, Zambenedetti P, Pizziuti A, Perazzolo M. Different effects of aluminum upon carbonic anhydrases and Na^+/K^+-ATPase activities in rat. Neurosci Lett 1995; 197: 65–8.
22. Adem A, Jossa SS, Oreland L. Tetrahydroaminoacridine inhibits human rat and brain monoamine oxidase. Neurosci Lett 1989; 107: 313–17.
23. Qian ZM, Tang PL. Mechanisms of iron uptake by mammalian cells. Biochim Biophys Acta 1995; 1269: 205–14.
24. Van Rensburg SJ, Carstens ME, Potocnik FCV, Taljaard JFH. Increased frequency of the transferrin C2 subtype in Alzheimer's disease. NeuroReport 1993; 1269–71.
25. Kalaria RN, Sromek SM, Grahovac I, Harik SI. Transferrin receptors of rat and human brain and cerebral microvessels and their status in Alzheimer's disease. Brain Res 1992; 585: 87–93.
26. Gerlach M, Ben-Shachar D, Riederer P, Youdim MBH. Altered brain metabolism of iron as a cause of neurodegenerative diseases. J Neurochem 1994; 63: 793–807.

Address for correspondence:
    Paolo Zatta,
    CNR-Center on Metalloproteins, University of Padova,
    Via G. Colombo 3, 35131 Padova, Italy
    e-mail: zatta@cribi1.bio.unipd.it;
    www.bio.unipd.it/zatta/aluminum.html

VIII   Therapeutics

70 Trends in Alzheimer's Disease Treatment and Prevention

FRANÇOISE FORETTE AND FRANÇOIS BOLLER

INTRODUCTION

In the past 10 years or so, there have been several advances in the therapy of Alzheimer's disease (AD) and some medications are already available to produce symptomatic improvements in selected patients. These medications have clear limitations in terms of time and efficacy, but recent data on the genetics and the molecular biology of AD should provide the premise for more rational and physiopathologically orientated treatments of the disease in the not-too-distant future [1].

SUBSTITUTION THERAPIES

CHOLINERGIC TREATMENTS

Even though it has been known for years that other neurotransmitters are involved in AD, the cholinergic theory raised hopes that replacement, or at least increased availability, of ACh might improve memory in the aged and in patients affected by AD, analogously to the effect of L-dopa in Parkinson's disease. On the basis of the cholinergic theory, several potential pharmacological strategies are available. The most successful has been the use of cholinesterase inhibitors.

Because physostigmine is relatively safe, crosses the blood–brain barrier easily and is available in oral form (even though its absorption is poor [2]), many researchers have used it. In their review, Becker and Giacobini [3] found that 20 of 31 studies reported some improvement in memory using physostigmine. In most cases, however (see e.g. [4]), improvements have been modest and short-lived, even when physostigmine was combined with ACh precursors such as lecithine [5]. Tacrine was introduced because it was felt to be a less potent but longer-acting centrally active cholinesterase inhibitor than physostigmine.

Alzheimer's Disease and Related Disorders
Edited by K. Iqbal, D.F. Swaab, B. Winblad and H.M. Wisniewski
© 1999 John Wiley & Sons Ltd

Tacrine (tetrahydroaminoacridine) was first used in AD in the early 1980s [6, 7], with what were considered 'modest results'. However, in an article published by the prestigious *New England Journal of Medicine* in November 1986 [8], Summers et al. reported having treated 17 patients with a diagnosis of AD, 12 of whom had entered Phase III (long-term administration of oral THA). The degree of improvement, they wrote, 'had often been dramatic'. At least some improvement had been observed in all subjects and 'no serious side effects attributable to THA had been observed'.

Several studies conducted subsequently provided results that were sometimes equivocal. The 'final' word was given only recently, thanks to the results of trials of larger sample size. Two studies conducted respectively in North America and in France [9, 10] found a significant clinical benefit on the ADAS–Cog, the ADAS–Total and, less so, on the IADL and the 'Progressive Deterioration Scale', but not on the 'Clinical Global Impression' (CGI). The study by Knapp et al. [11] demonstrated dose-related clinical efficacy, as judged on the ADAS–Cog, the Clinician-Based Impression of Change (CIBI) and the Final Comprehensive Consensus Assessment (FCCA).

The introduction of tacrine has prompted the development of other replacement drugs. The following are now, or are soon going to be, on the market:

- *Donepezil or E2020*, known commercially as Aricept E2020, is a piperidine cholinesterase inhibitor (ChEI) which is structurally distinct from other compounds currently under study for the treatment of AD. It has been studied extensively in animals [12]. Phase III studies performed in the USA have shown good efficacy and tolerability in patients with mild to moderate AD [13]. The drug is now available in the USA, Canada and many other countries.
- *ENA 713* (Exelon, Sandoz) is a CNS-selective, pseudo-irreversible cholinesterase inhibitor also showing brain region selectivity. It is not metabolized by the hepatic microsome system. Its duration of cholinesterase inhibition is 10 h. Phase II trials using doses of 6–12 mg/day have suggested efficacy and reasonably low levels of side effects. Phase III trials suggest an efficacy comparable to that of other, newer cholinesterase inhibitors [14]. The drug has recently been released in Switzerland and in many other European countries.
- *Metrifonate*, on the other hand, is an organophosphate which, through the action of its metabolite diclorvinyl dimethyl phosphate (DDVP or dichlorvos), produces an irreversible CAT enzyme inhibition and increases local cerebral glucose utilization in young and aged rats [15]. A recent study [16] has shown a mean of 52.3% decrease in red blood cell acetylcholinesterase activity. During up to 18 months of subsequent open metrifonate treatment, there was a deterioration of 1.68 points/year in MMSE performance. Adverse effects were uncommon and did not require adjustment of the dose of metrifonate or discontinuation of treatment.

There are many other cholinergic agents currently under development. A probably incomplete list is provided by Tariot [17] and includes the following:

Cholinesterase inhibitors
  Eptastigmine (Mediolanum)
  Sustained-release physostigmine (Synapton, Forest)
  Huperzine (Chinese Academy of Science)
  NX-066 (Astra Arcus)
  KA-672 (Schwabe)
  Galanthamine (Janssen)
Cholinergic receptor agents
  Milameline (Warner-Lambert)
  AF102B (Forest/Snow Brand Products)
  SB202026 (SmithKline Beecham)
  Xanomeline (Lilly)
  ENS 163 (Sandoz)
Indirect cholinergic enhancers
  ABT 418 (Abbott)
  ABT 089 (Abbott)

OTHER REPLACEMENT TREATMENTS

As mentioned above, AD affects several neurotransmitter systems. This has been the rationale for several therapeutic trials involving systems other than the cholinergic system.

Even though the adrenergic system is known to be implied in memory storage, in recall and in selective attention, the efficacy of biogenic amines has never been proved: trials with L-dopa, amantadine, bromocriptine and pirebidil have given contradictory, but on the whole negative, results [18]. Similarly, despite the known involvement of the serotonergic system, block of 5-HT recapture has been without effect.

Neuropeptides have been studied extensively. Despite the known somatostatinergic deficit [19], somatostatine analogues have not shown impressive results. This applies also to vasopressin analogues, ACTH and other neuropeptides such as TRH, VIP and neuropeptide Y. Excitatory amino acids, such as glutamate or aspartate, are implicated in synaptic mechanisms and play a major role in the potentiation of neurotransmission. The NMDA and AMPA receptors which are implicated in memory mechanisms are the subject of recent research [20] but the therapeutic trials have not yet produced practical results.

Despite their limitations, replacement therapies must be given credit for having taken AD out of the mould of diseases totally inaccessible to pharmacological treatment. Clearly, however, they cannot durably modify the course of the disease and even less prevent it. Therapies of the future must therefore be based on an aetiological approach.

AETIOLOGICAL APPROACHES

There is general agreement that AD is highly heterogeneous and that several different processes may lead to β-amyloid deposits (for review, see [21, 22]). It is natural, therefore, that some therapeutic trials have been based on these processes, whether definite or only hypothetical.

TRANSMISSIBLE AGENT

Comparison of AD with spongiform encephalopathies, such as Kuru and Creutzfeldt–Jakob disease, has led to the hypothesis of a slow virus or prion-related aetiology for AD. The total absence, so far, of demonstration of infectious transmission has very much reduced hopes for an anti-infectious treatment [23, 24]. However, the 'transmissible agent hypothesis' may have taken an unexpected turn: recent findings suggest that the combination of HSV-1 in brain and carriage of an APOE ε4 allele is a strong risk factor for AD [25]. It is far from certain that this finding, if confirmed, will lead to new therapeutic possibilities.

IMMUNOLOGICAL THEORY

There are some data in favour of an immunological hyper-reactivity in AD. These include microglial reaction around the senile plaques (SP), astrocytosis, production of inflammatory cytokines, some of which (IL-1 and IL-2) are said to increase the synthesis of a precursor of the amyloid protein [26]. Several studies have shown a reverse correlation between the occurrence of AD [27] or cognitive deterioration [28] and use of non-steroidal anti-inflammatory agents (NSAIDs). A therapeutic trial using indomethacine is in favour of this hypothesis [29].

NEUROPROTECTION: CALCIUM CHANNEL BLOCKERS

The limited effect of substitution treatments may perhaps be explained by neuronal death. Calcium channel blockers might have a neuroprotective role by opposing intracellular influx of calcium responsible for enzymatic activation and cell destruction. Several therapeutic trials use nimodipine to confirm the results of a short study which has shown that this treatment tends to slow the rate of deterioration [30].

NERVE GROWTH FACTORS

It has been known for some time that nerve growth factors (NGFs) may have a trophic action at the level of nerve cells and particularly of cholinergic neurons. It is therefore natural to explore the possible therapeutic action of NGFs, even though NGF decrease has not been postulated as an aetiological agent of AD. The future of NGF is, however, quite uncertain because of doubts about its efficacy, difficulty of delivery to the CNS and possible long-term toxicity.

THERAPIES FOR THE FUTURE

AGENTS ACTING ON THE AMYLOID PROTEIN

The production and the deposit of β-amyloid A4 by abnormal cleavage of the precursor (APP) seems to be the principal element of the pathological process which, in turn, is the final common pathway of many potential mechanisms [31].

Abnormal APP function may lead to neurodegeneration in AD by several mechanisms: direct toxicity of aggregated amyloid protein, disruption of synaptic function and deficient neuroprotective activity of soluble proteins.

The logical therapeutic approach is to attempt to intervene in the production, the deposit or the neurotoxicity of the protein at the earliest possible stage of the disease in subjects at risk. Several directions are being pursued. They include the inhibition of proteolytic enzymes capable of splitting APP in an inappropriate or excessive fashion. The goal would be to inhibit β- or γ-secretases in favour of α-secretases, which allow the production of soluble non-amyloidogenic proteins; the inhibition of neurotoxicity; the reduction of APP synthesis; the inhibition of the inflammatory reaction at the level of SPs; and the prevention or slowing down of polymerization of soluble proteins into amyloid fibrils [32].

GENETIC PREDISPOSITION AND TREATMENT

In the last 10 years, the genetic determination of familial diseases and the genetic predisposition of sporadic cases have made enormous advances (for review, see [33]). In 1993, the group led by Allan Roses provided a fundamental advance by showing an excessive representation of the ε4 allele of apolipoprotein E (ApoE4) in patients with late familial or sporadic AD. This cholesterol-carrying protein plays an important trophic role at the level of the brain and the gene coding for its production is located on chromosome 19 under the form of three main alleles, ε2, ε3 and ε4 [34]. Furthermore, this protein shows a high affinity for amyloid protein [35].

The presence of ApoE4, especially in its homozygotic form (ε4-ε4), increases the risk of AD and probably plays a role in the age of onset and the rate of progression of the disease. Its role in the pathogenesis of senile plaques (SP) and neurofibrillary tangles (NFT) formation, if confirmed, could lead to new therapeutic advances [36, 37]. If the effects of ApoE4 on the promotion and neurotoxicity of the A4 amyloid protein and destabilization of microtubules are confirmed, one might conceive of molecules able to reproduce or potentiate the action of ApoE3 in patients who carry the ε4 allele. One study has shown that the ApoE4 genotype is associated with a lower probability of cognitive improvement following therapy with tacrine [38].

Finally, the characterization of gene PS-1 (or S-182) on chromosome 14 (early AD) [39] and of gene PS-2 (or STM2) on chromosome 1 (AD of varying age of onset; one of the families was Volga German) [40] marks the entry of AD genetics in the area of presenilins which might play a major role in intracellular 'traffic' of APP. Major advances may derive from this approach.

OESTROGENS

The favourable effects of oestrogen therapy on cognitive functions, the prevention of AD and its treatment represent a new area of investigation [41]. This hypothesis is based on the beneficial effects of this therapy on memory functions and other cognitive skills of post-menopausal or aged women [42–44], the increased risk of AD in women with oestrogen deficiencies [45] and the increased response to cholinergic treatment of women receiving replacement oestrogen treatment [46]. Large therapeutic trials are currently under way to verify this hypothesis. Recent results show that oestrogens may regulate APP metabolism, favouring non-amyloidogenic pathways [47] and preventing the action of free radicals [41]. A reduced risk of AD for women having reported use of oestrogens has been recently reported in the Baltimore Longitudinal Study of Aging [48].

ANTI-RADICAL THERAPIES

It is generally recognized that the brain is particularly vulnerable to oxidative stress. Recent research suggests an important role of free radicals in the development of the toxicity of the amyloid protein [49], the formation of NFT and eventually neuronal death. The ties between trisomy 21, characterized by an excess of the gene for superoxide dismutase 1 (SOD1), and AD are in keeping with this hypothesis [50]. Oxidative stress may play a role in all stages of the disease, hence the idea of a possible protective role of antioxidant agents [51]. In a more recent trial [52], a total of 341 patients received the selective monoamine oxidase inhibitor selegiline, α-tocopherol, both selegiline and α-tocopherol or placebo for two years. There were significant delays in the time to the primary outcome (defined as time to the occurrence of death, institutionalization, loss of the ability to perform basic ADL, or severe dementia) for the patients treated with selegiline, α-tocopherol or combination therapy, as compared with the placebo group.

CONCLUSIONS

Recent years have witnessed the appearance of many pharmacological agents with definite or probable action on a disease which, until recently, was considered totally beyond therapeutic reach. Following the palliative agents already available, one can foresee the development of more aetiologically orientated drugs. Physiopathological and genetic approaches are not mutually exclusive and could indeed be complementary. Preventive or early treatment in subjects with measurably high levels of risk factors could be with us in the relatively near future.

REFERENCES

1. Aisen P, Davis K. The search for disease-modifying treatment for Alzheimer's disease. Neurology 1997; 48: S35–41.
2. Becker R, Giacobini E, Elble R, McIlhany M, Sherman K. Potential pharmacotherapy of Alzheimer disease. A comparison of various forms of physostigmine administration. Acta Neurol Scand 1988; 77: 19–32.
3. Becker R, Giacobini E. Mechanisms of cholinesterase inhibition in senile dementia of the Alzheimer type: clinical, pharmacological and therapeutic aspects. Drug Dev Res 1988; 12: 163.
4. Beller S, Overall J, Rhodes H, Swann A. Long-term outpatient treatment of senile dementia with physostigmine. J Clin Psychiat 1988; 49: 400–404.
5. Thal L, Fuld P, Masur M, Sharples N. Oral physostigmine and lecithin improve memory in Alzheimer's disease. Ann Neurol 1983; 13: 491–6.
6. Kaye W, Sitaram N, Weingartner H, Ebert M, Smallberg S, Gillin J. Modest facilitation of memory in dementia with combined lecithin and anticholinesterase treatment. Biol Psychiat 1982; 17: 275–80.
7. Summers W, Viesselman J, Marsh G, Candelora K. Use of THA in treatment of Alzheimer-like dementia: pilot study in twelve patients. Biol Psychiat 1981; 16: 145–53.
8. Summers W, Majovski V, Marsh G, Tachiki K, Kling A. Oral tetrahydroaminoacridine in long-term treatment of senile dementia. N Engl J Med 1986; 315: 1241–5.
9. Davis KL, Thal LJ, Gamzu ER et al. A double-blind, placebo-controlled multicenter study of tacrine for Alzheimer's disease. N Engl J Med 1992; 327: 1253–9.
10. Forette F, Hoover T, Gracon S et al. A double-blind, placebo-controlled, enriched population study of tacrine in patients with Alzheimer's disease. Eur J Neurol 1995; 2: 229–38.
11. Knapp MJ, Knopman DS, Solomon PR, Pendlebury WW, Davis CS, Gracon SI. A 30-week randomized controlled trial of high-dose tacrine in patients with Alzheimer's disease. JAMA 1994; 271(13): 985–91.
12. Giacobini E, Zhu XD, Williams E, Sherman K. The effect of the selective reversible acetylcholinesterase inhibitor E2020 on extracellular acetylcholine and biogenic amine levels in rat cortex. Neuropharmacology 1996; 35: 205–11.
13. Rogers S, Farlow M, Mohs R, Friedhoff L and the Donezepil study group. A 24-week double-blind placebo-controlled trial of donezepil in patients with Alzheimer's disease. Neurology 1998; 50: 136–45.
14. Anand R, Gharabawi G. Efficacy and safety results of the early phase studies with Exelon (ENA 713) in Alzheimer's disease: an overview. J Drug Develop Clin Prac 1996; 8: 1–14.

15. Bassant M, Jazat-Poindessous F, Lamour Y. Effects of metrifonate, a cholinesterase inhibitor, on local cerebral glucose utilization in young and aged rats. J Cereb Blood Flow Metab 1996; 16: 1014–25.

16. Becker R, Colliver J, Markwell S, Moriarty P, Unni L, Vicari S. Double-blind, placebo-controlled study of metrifonate, an acetylcholinesterase inhibitor, for Alzheimer disease. Alzheimer Dis Assoc Disord 1996; 10: 124–31.

17. Tariot P, Schneider L. Clinical reviews: contemporary treatment approaches to Alzheimer's disease. Consult Pharm 1996; 11 (suppl E): 16–24.

18. Coull JT. Pharmacological manipulations of the α2 noradrenergic system. Effect on cognition. Drugs Aging 1994; 5: 116–26.

19. Bissette G, Myers B. Mini-review. Somatostatin in Alzheimer's disease and depression. Life Sci 1992; 51: 1389–410.

20. Izquierdo I. Role of NMDA receptors in memory. Trends Pharmacol Sci 1991; 12: 128–9.

21. Boller F, Forette F, Khatchaturian Z, Poncet M, Christen Y. Heterogeneity of Alzheimer's disease. In Research and Perspectives in Alzheimer's Disease. Berlin: Springer-Verlag, 1992.

22. Shvaloff A, Neuman E, Guez D. Lines of therapeutics research in Alzheimer's disease. Psychopharmacol Bull 1996; 32: 343–52.

23. Prusiner SB. Prions and neurodegenerative diseases. N Eng J Med 1987; 317: 1571–81.

24. Friedland R, May C, Dahlberg G. The viral hypothesis of Alzheimer's disease. Arch Neurol 1990; 47: 177–8.

25. Itzhaki R, Lin W, Shang D, Wilcock G, Faragher B, Jamieson G. Herpes simplex virus type 1 in brain and risk of Alzheimer's disease. Lancet 1997; 349: 241–4.

26. McGeer P, McGeer E. The inflammatory response system of the brain: implications for therapy of Alzheimer and other neurodegenerative disease. Brain Res Rev 1995; 21: 195–218.

27. Breitner JCS, Gau MSW, Welsh KA, Plassman BL, McDonald WM, Helms MJ, Anthony JC. Inverse association of anti-inflammatory treatments and Alzheimer's disease. Neurology 1994; 44: 227–32.

28. Rich JB, Rasmusson DX, Folstein MF, Carson KA, Kawas C, Brandt J. Non-steroidal anti-inflammatory drugs in Alzheimer's disease. Neurology 1995; 45: 51–5.

29. Rogers J, Kirby LC, Hempelman SR et al. Clinical trial of indomethacine in Alzheimer's disease. Neurology 1993; 43: 1609–11.

30. Tollefson GD. Short term effect on the calcium blocker nimodipine in the management of primary degenerative dementia. Biol Psychiat 1990; 27: 1133–42.

31. Hardy J, Allsop D. Amyloid deposition as the central event in the aetiology of Alzheimer's disease. Trends Pharmacol Sci 1991; 12(10): 383–8.

32. Maury CPJ. Biology of disease. Molecular pathogenesis of β-amyloidosis in Alzheimer's disease and other cerebral amyloidosis. Lab Invest 1995; 72: 4–16.

33. Mullan M, Crawford F. The molecular genetics of Alzheimer's disease. Molec Biol 1994; 9: 15–22.

34. Saunders AM, Strittmatter WJ, Schmechel DE et al. Association of apolipoprotein E allele ε4 with late-onset familial and sporadic Alzheimer's disease. Neurology 1993; 43: 1467–72.

35. Strittmatter WJ, Saunders AM, Schmechel DE, Pericak-Vance MA, Roses AD. Apolipoprotein E: high affinity binding to βA amyloid and increased frequency of type 4 allele in familial Alzheimer's disease. Proc Natl Acad Sci USA 1993; 90: 1977–81.

36. Hardy J. Apolipoprotein E in the genetics and epidemiology of Alzheimer's disease. Am J Med Genet 1995; 60: 456–60.
37. Roses A. Perspective. On the metabolism of apolipoprotein E and the Alzheimer disease. Exp Neurol 1995; 132: 149–56.
38. Farlow M, Lahiri D, Poirier J, Davignon J, Hui S. Apolipoprotein E genotype and gender influence response to tacrine therapy. Ann NY Acad Sci 1996; 802: 101–10.
39. Sherrington R, Rogaev EI, Liang Y et al. Cloning of a gene bearing missense mutations in early onset familial Alzheimer's disease. Nature 1995; 375: 754–60.
40. Levy-Lahad E, Wasco W, Poorkaj P et al. Candidate gene for the chromosome 1 familial Alzheimer's disease locus. Science 1995; 269: 973–7.
41. Fillit H. Future therapeutic developments of estrogen use. J Clin Pharmacol 1995; 35: S25–8.
42. Robinson D, Fireadman L, Marcus R. Estrogen replacement therapy and memory in older women. J Amer Geriat Soc 1994; 42: 919–22.
43. Henderson W, Paganini-Hill A, Emanuel CK, Dunn ME, Galen Buckwalter J. Estrogen replacement therapy in older women. Comparisons between Alzheimer's disease cases and nondemented control subjects. Arch Neurol 1994; 51: 896–900.
44. Henderson V, Watt L, Buckwalter J. Cognitive skills associated with estrogen replacement in women with Alzheimer's disease. Psychoneuroendocrinology 1996; 21: 421–30.
45. Paganini-Hill A, Henderson W. Estrogen deficiency and risk of Alzheimer's disease. Am J Epidemiol 1994; 140: 256–61.
46. Schneider L, Farlow MR. Predicting response to cholinesterase inhibitors. Possible approaches. CNS Drugs 1995; 4: 114–24.
47. Jaffe AB, Toran-Allerand D, Greengard P. Estrogen regulates metabolism of Alzheimer amyloid beta precursor protein. J Biol Chem 1994; 269: 13065–8.
48. Kawas C, Resnick S, Morrison A et al. A prospective study of estrogen replacement therapy and the risk of developing Alzheimer's disease. Neurology 1997; 48: 1517–21.
49. Iversen LL, Mortishire-Smith RJ, Pollack SJ. The toxicity in vitro of β-amyloid protein. Biochem J 1995; 311: 1–16.
50. Sinet PM, Ceballos-Picot I. Role of free radicals in Alzheimer's disease and Down's syndrome. In: Packer L, Prilikpo L, Christen Y (eds) Free Radicals in the Brain. Berlin: Springer-Verlag, 1992; 91–8.
51. Kagan VE, Bakalova RA, Koynova GM. Antioxidant protection of the brain against oxidative stress. In: Packer L, Prilikpo L, Christen Y (eds) Free Radicals in the Brain. Berlin: Springer-Verlag, 1992: 49–61.
52. Sano M, Ernesto C, Thomas R et al. A controlled trial of selegiline, α-tocopherol or both as treatment for Alzheimer's disease. The Alzheimer's Disease Cooperative Study. N Engl J Med 1997; 336: 1216–22.

Address for correspondence:
Dr Françoise Forette,
Service de Gérontologie, Hôpital Broca,
CHU Cochin, Université Paris V,
54–56 rue Pascal, 75 013 Paris, France

71 Clinical Improvement in a Placebo-controlled Trial with Memantine in Care-dependent Patients with Severe Dementia (M-BEST)

BENGT WINBLAD, NILS PORITIS AND
HANS-JÖRG MÖBIUS

INTRODUCTION

Currently approved pharmacotherapeutic approaches to dementia are limited to the mild-to-moderate stages of the disease. However, pharmaco-economic data show that two-thirds of society's costs for demented patients are being caused by the group of patients who are severely demented [1]. Cholinergic drugs were the first to be approved in the indication of Alzheimer's disease. Their clinical treatment effects remain far from being satisfactory and the search for new therapeutic avenues is continued.

In contrast to cholinergic drugs, memantine acts on the glutamatergic system, the most important excitatory neurotransmitter system in the brain [2, 3]. Memantine is an uncompetitive, moderate-affinity, voltage-dependent NMDA receptor antagonist with fast-blocking/unblocking kinetics. Its receptor-binding characteristics are very similar to magnesium, the physiologic cation channel blocker [4]. Therefore, in contrast to competitive NMDA antagonists like MK 801, normal synaptic transmission is not affected by memantine. Thus, over years of marketing in Germany, psychotomimetic side effects have rarely been observed with memantine.

The impairment of cholinergic neurotransmission in Alzheimer's disease has been known for more than a decade. Today, there is growing evidence for the role of glutamatergic neurons and NMDA-receptor-mediated excitotoxicity in the pathogenesis of dementia [5–7]. Preclinical studies show symptomatic effects of memantine on long-term potentiation and learning as well as neuroprotective (anti-excitotoxic) effects *in vitro* and *in vivo* [8–10].

Alzheimer's Disease and Related Disorders
Edited by K. Iqbal, D.F. Swaab, B. Winblad and H.M. Wisniewski
© 1999 John Wiley & Sons Ltd

METHODS

This trial was designed in a prospective, randomized, placebo-controlled, double-blind way with two parallel treatment groups. It was carried out in seven centers in Latvia, one psychiatric ward and six nursing homes, observing GCP standards and the Declaration of Helsinki, including amendments. The treatment period was 12 weeks. Efficacy assessments were carried out at baseline, week 4 and week 12.

The study population were care-dependent in-patients aged between 60 and 80 years. The diagnosis of primary dementia had to be established according to DSM-IIIR criteria. Severity of dementia was rated by MMSE [11]; for inclusion in the study, the MMSE total score had to be below 10. The second criterion for severity of dementia was GDS stages 5, 6 or 7 [12]. Exclusion criteria included secondary dementia (as assessed by medical history, clinical and neurological examination and laboratory findings), such as major depression, schizophrenia, alcoholism, epilepsy, cerebral tumor or Parkinson's disease. Patients with clinically relevant pathologic changes in blood chemistry and hematology and decompensated systemic disease or renal dysfunction (defined as serum creatine levels > 2 mg/100 ml) were also excluded. Concomitant psychotropic medication was not allowed with the exception of chloral hydrate and short-acting benzodiazepines. There was a 2 week wash-out period prior to randomization.

Patients were randomly allocated to two treatment groups. One group received 5 mg/day memantine during the first week and 10 mg/day for the rest of the treatment period, while the other group received matching placebo treatment. Regimen was once daily.

The primary efficacy criteria in this trial focused on clinical global and functional endpoints: Clinical Global Impression of Change [13] and the BGP subscale 'Care dependence' were assessed at baseline, after 4 weeks and after 12 weeks of treatment. The BGP is an observer-rated scale for the assessment of geriatric patients performed by the nursing staff. This scale has been adapted from the Stockton Geriatric Rating Scale and has been used and validated in The Netherlands (called BOP) since 1971 [14, 15]. The scale consists of 35 items in 4 subscales, 'Care dependence' being the largest subscale, containing 23 items focusing on functional aspects. Each item is rated on a three-step ordinal scale (0, 1, 2).

Among other secondary efficacy variables, the G2 scale (a modification of the D-test by Ferm) was used [16]. This test was designed to evaluate descriptively behavioral activities and functioning in demented geriatric patients. Thirty behavioural variables were assessed by the staff, including activities of daily living. The extent of the patient's impairment was rated on a six-point ordinary scale.

RESULTS

The intent to treat (ITT) population consisted of 166 patients (see Table 1). There were no major differences in demographic data between treatment groups at baseline. Severity of dementia, as measured by the MMSE total score, was comparable between the two groups as well as the mean HIS sum score. According to the modified HIS (Rosen version [17]), about 50% of the patients included were classified as having a diagnosis of Alzheimer's disease and 50% as vascular dementia or dementia of mixed type. This was confirmed by a subgroup analysis of patients with available CT scans (89 patients). Patients with radiological signs of Alzheimer's disease and patients with vascular dementia were nearly equally distributed.

The statistical analysis of efficacy variables was performed in the ITT population (n = 166) as well as in the treated-per-protocol (TPP; n = 151) group (Fischer's exact test and Wilcoxon rank sum test). A total of 15 patients was not included in the TPP sample because of violation of inclusion or exclusion criteria (memantine = 0, placebo = 1), discontinuation (M = 4, p = 4), or noncompliance (M = 3, p = 3). As this was a trial in nursing homes, the dropout rate was very low, all dropouts being patients who died during the trial. None of the deaths was causally related to memantine medication.

In conclusion, there were no significant differences between memantine and placebo with regard to safety and tolerability. The number of adverse events

Table 1. Patient characteristics at baseline (ITT analysis, n = 166)

		Memantine	Placebo	Total
Sex (male/female)		33/49	37/47	70/96
Age (years) (mean ± SD)	male	67.7 ± 5.1	69.1 ± 5.8	68.4 ± 5.5
	female	73.6 ± 5.8	74.2 ± 5.3	73.9 ± 5.6
BMI (kg/qm) (mean ± SD)	male	25.1 ± 3.9	25.8 ± 3.0	25.5 ± 3.5
	female	25.9 ± 4.7	25.2 ± 3.7	25.6 ± 4.3
Smokers (%)		22.0	15.5	18.7
Patients with antidementia premedication (%)		39.0	39.3	39.2
Patients with concomitant diseases (%)		87.8	90.5	89.2
Patients with concomitant medication (%)		41.5	42.9	42.2
GDS (cognitive decline) (%)	moderately severe	3.7	3.6	3.6
	severe	91.5	89.3	90.4
	very severe	4.9	7.1	6.0
MMSE total score (mean ± SD)		6.6 ± 2.7	6.1 ± 2.8	6.3 ± 2.7
HIS sum score (mean ± SD)		5.2 ± 2.9	5.7 ± 3.2	5.5 ± 3.1
HAM-D total score (mean ± SD)		8.5 ± 2.0	8.9 ± 2.1	8.7 ± 2.1
CGI-S (%)	markedly ill	63	47	55
	severely ill	32	39	36
	extremely ill	5	13	9
BGP subscore 'Care dependence' (mean ± SD)		21.3 ± 7.6	21.8 ± 7.7	21.5 ± 7.6

ITT = intent to treat.
SD = standard deviation.

and serious adverse events was equally distributed (AEs, $M = 18$, p = 18; SAEs, $M = 4$, p = 5). There was a small number of abnormal laboratory values of clinical relevance, showing no specific pattern with regard to trial medication or time course of the trial. Common side effects of memantine— already known from previous trials and postmarketing experience in Germany—include dizziness and vertigo, fatigue or insomnia, and restlessness.

The clinical global endpoint CGI-C rating showed superiority of memantine treatment at week 4 and at week 12 on a 0.006 and 0.001 level of significance, respectively (Figure 1). Also, in the other primary endpoint BGP, subscore 'Care dependence' (Figure 2), ITT and TPP analysis showed improvement in both treatment groups (lower scores represent improvement). There was a statistically significant difference (p < 0.05) between the treatment groups in favor of memantine.

On both the clinical global and the functional endpoint, a subgroup analysis was performed, separating treatment groups by means of the patients' scores on the ischemic scale (HIS). Descriptively, memantine treatment benefit was apparent in the subgroup of patients with a low ischemic score (probably representing Alzheimer's disease patients or dementia of mixed type) as well as in the subgroup of patients with vascular dementia (as defined by a HIS score of ≥ 5).

The relevance of clinical improvement by memantine is further supported by a single item analysis of the secondary parameter, the G2 scale (modified Ferm scale). Figure 3 shows the pre–post improvement (baseline 3 months) in selected G2 items.

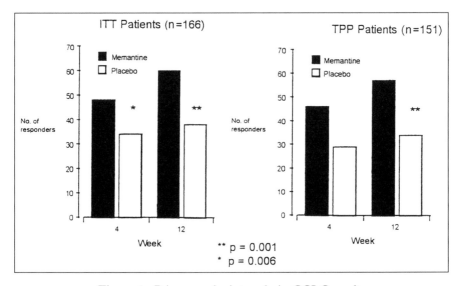

Figure 1. Primary endpoint analysis: CGI-C results

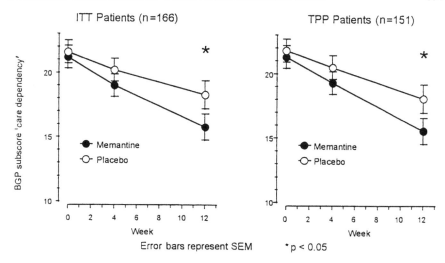

Figure 2. Primary endpoint analysis: BGP subscore 'Care dependence'

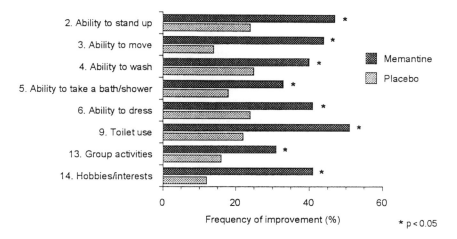

Figure 3. Secondary endpoint G2 scale (selected items)

In addition, a descriptive responder analysis was performed, by combining two independent criteria for individual response. In the CGI-C, any form of individual improvement (score 1–3) was defined as response. On the BGP subscale 'Care dependence', improvement of more than 15% as compared to baseline was defined as individual treatment response. Non-responders were included in the analysis. According to this definition, in CGI-C ratings, 76% of the memantine-treated patients were responders, compared to 45% in the placebo group. In the BGP subscore 'Care dependence', 65% of the patients treated with memantine were responders, compared to 39% in the placebo group. There was a strong coincidence of response in the two primary out-come parameters; 61.3% of patients in the memantine group were coincident responders, compared to 31.6% of the patients in the placebo group.

DISCUSSION

In contrast to most reported trials in dementia, this study was conducted in a target population of patients with severe dementia. In this patient group, changes in cognitive test scores may be clinically less relevant as compared to improvement of functional parameters [18, 19]. This is also reflected in the latest European anti-dementia drug development guidelines. Functional and clinical global endpoints were therefore selected as primary efficacy parameters.

At a 10 mg daily dose, confirmatory analysis revealed statistically significant differences between the treatment groups in both primary efficacy parameters. Applying even stricter responder analysis procedures, the results confirm the hypothesis that memantine treatment significantly improves functional capa-cities in severely demented patients and that this improvement is of clinical relevance. This memantine treatment benefit appears to extend to Alzheimer's patients as well as to patients with dementia of vascular or mixed type etiology.

In the clinical global rating as well as in the functional assessment, there was a remarkable improvement also in the placebo group. This observation confirms the importance of non-pharmacological intervention, especially improved caregiving, also for severely demented nursing home patients.

No unexpected side effects occurred during this first-ever reported well-controlled trial in severely demented patients. The safety and tolerability pro-file observed in this advanced stage of dementia matches the pharmaco-vigilance data obtained in Germany, where memantine has been marketed for years. Given this aged, multi-morbid population, the death rate observed was within expected limits.

CONCLUSIONS

Memantine was well tolerated in severely demented patients over a treatment period of 3 months. The results of this trial indicate that memantine treatment leads to remarkable improvement in clinical global and functional endpoints and reduces care dependence in patients with advanced stages of primary dementia. This benefit appears to be independent of the etiology of primary dementia. Considering the social and health-economic burden brought about by severe dementia, these results warrant further confirmation of the thera-peutic potential of the uncompetitive NMDA-antagonist memantine, includ-ing assessment of its potential health–economic impact.

REFERENCES

1. Wimo A, Karlsson G, Sandman PO, Corder L, Winblad B. Cost of illness due to dementia in Sweden. Int J Geriat Psychiatry 1997; 12: 857–61.
2. Müller WE, Mutschler E, Riederer P. Noncompetitive NMDA receptor antagonists with fast open-channel blocking kinetics and strong voltage-dependency as potential therapeutic agents for Alzheimer's dementia. Pharmacopsychiatry 1995; 28: 113–24.
3. Greenamyre JT, Maragos EF, Albin RL, Penney JB, Young AB. Glutamate transmission and toxicity in Alzheimer's disease. Prog Neuro-Psych Biol Psych 1988; 12: 421–30.
4. Parsons CG, Gruner R, Rosental J, Millar J, Lodge D. Patch clamp studies on the kinetics and selectivity of N-methyl-D-aspartate receptor antagonism by memantine (1-amino-3,5-dimethyl-adamantan). Neuropharmacology 1993; 32: 1337–50.
5. Francis PT, Sims NR, Procter AW, Bowen DM. Cortical pyramidal neurone loss may cause glutamatergic hypoactivity and cognitive impairment in Alzheimer's disease—investigative and therapeutic perspectives. J Neurochem 1993; 60: 1589–604.
6. Li S, Mallory M, Alford M, Tanaka S, Masliah E. Glutamate transporter alterations in Alzheimer disease are possibly associated with abnormal APP expression. J Neuropathol Exp Neurol 1997; 56: 901–11.
7. Palmer AM, Gershon S. Is the neuronal basis of Alzheimer's disease cholinergic or glutamatergic? FASEB J 1990; 4: 2745–52.
8. Misztal M, Frankiewicz T, Parsons CG, Danysz W. Learning deficits induced by chronic intraventricular infusion of quinolinic acid—protection by MK-801 and memantine. Eur J Pharmacol 1996; 296: 1–8.
9. Zajaczkowski W, Frankiewicz T, Parsons CG, Danysz W. Uncompetitive NMDA receptor antagonists attenuate NMDA-induced impairment of passive avoidance learning and LTP. Neuropharmacology 1997; 36: 961–71.
10. Zajaczkowski W, Quack G, Danysz W. Infusion of (+)-MK-801 and memantine—contrasting effects on radial maze learning in rats with entorhinal cortex lesion. Eur J Pharmacol 1996; 296: 239–46.
11. Folstein MF, Folstein SE, McHugh PR. Mini-Mental State: a practical method for grading the cognitive state of patients for the clinician. J Psychiat Res 1975; 12: 189–98.
12. Reisberg B, Ferris SH, de Leon MJ, Crook T. The global deterioration scale (GDS): an instrument for the assessment of primary degenerative dementia (PDD). Am J Psychiat 1982; 139: 1136–9.
13. National Institute of Mental Health: 028 CGI. Clinical global impressions. In: Guy W (ed) ECDEU Assessment Manual for Psychopharmacology, revised edn. Rockville, MD: NIMH, 1986; 217–22.
14. van der Kam P, Mol F, Wimmers MMC. Beoordelingsschaal voor ondere patienten (BOP). Van Loghum Slaterus, The Netherlands, 1971.
15. van der Kam P, Hoeksma BH. The usefulness of BOP and SIVIS (ADL and behavior rating scales) for the estimation of workload in a psychogeriatric nursing home. Results of a time-standard study. Tijdschr Gerontol Geriatr 1989; 20(4): 159–66.
16. Ferm L. Behavioural activities in demented geriatric patients. Gerontol Clin 1974; 16: 185–94.
17. Rosen WG, Terry RD, Fuid PA, Katzmann R, Peck A. Pathological verification of ischaemic score in differentiation of dementias. Ann Neurol 1980; 7: 486–8.

18. Franssen EH, Reisberg B, Kluger A, Sinaiko E, Boja C. Cognition-independent neurologic symptoms in normal ageing and probable Alzheimer's disease. Arch Neurol 1991; 48: 148–54.
19. Souren LEM, Franssen EH, Reisberg B. Contractures and loss of function in patients with Alzheimer's disease. JAGS 1995; 43: 650–55.

Address for correspondence:
  Bengt Winblad,
  Stockholm Gerontology Research Center,
  Box 6401, SE–113 82 Stockholm, Sweden.

72 Clonidine Impairs Sustained Attention in Alzheimer's Disease

M. RIEKKINEN, M.P. LAAKSO, P. JÄKÄLÄ AND P. RIEKKINEN JR

INTRODUCTION

Neurochemical and neuropathological studies conducted with post-mortem brain samples from patients with Alzheimer's disease (AD) have revealed a degeneration of the noradrenaline-containing neurons of the locus coeruleus (LC) [1]. Several experimental studies have shown that the noradrenergic LC system and drugs acting via noradrenergic receptors may modulate attention capacity [2]. Dysfunction of the frontal cortex may play a major role in the impaired accuracy of attention in AD patients [3]. Therefore, it is possible that noradrenergic dysfunction in AD patients may disrupt activity of the attention mechanisms of the frontal areas.

The function of the ascending LC projections of the dorsal noradrenergic bundle (DNAB) in the modulation of attention has been characterized in animal models of cognition and also in humans [2, 4]. First, studies conducted with animal cognition models suggested that the noradrenergic DNAB system is selectively involved in effortful or controlled information processing taking place in a novel situation or in those situations which place an additional load on attention-processing resources [4]. However, automatic processing and well-trained performance may be mediated independently of the noradrenergic DNAB systems [4, 5]. Second, there is evidence also for a role for the LC and the α_2-adrenoceptors in the modulation of attention functions in humans. In healthy volunteers, administration of an α_2-adrenoceptor agonist, clonidine, decreases the activity of the LC neurons and disrupts attention accuracy. For example, orally administered clonidine 5 µg/kg, but not 0.5 and 2 µg/kg, impaired accuracy at the most difficult level of simple and choice reaction test in healthy volunteers (Jäkälä, unpublished). Furthermore, clonidine impairs performance in a sustained attention task, such as a rapid visual information processing task [6].

The present study was designed to investigate whether decreased activity of the LC induced by treatment with clonidine disrupts attention in AD patients.

Alzheimer's Disease and Related Disorders
Edited by K. Iqbal, D.F. Swaab, B. Winblad and H.M. Wisniewski
© 1999 John Wiley & Sons Ltd

METHODS

PATIENTS

Twenty-eight patients fulfilling the NINCDS–ADRDA criteria of probable AD were selected for the study. The assessment of clinical severity of dementia, MRI, quantitative EEG and SPECT (ECD retention) and neuropsychological (verbal, visuoconstructive, praxis, executive and immediate and delayed memory recall) studies were made to support the clinical diagnosis of AD. Three to four days after the baseline neuropsychological examinations, the drug study was started. Routine laboratory tests were made to exclude secondary dementia. Hamilton and Hachinski scales were used to exclude depression and vascular pathology, respectively. The local ethical committee and the national drug regulatory authorities had reviewed and approved the study plan. The patients, their caregivers and the controls gave written informed consent for participation in the study.

During the study period, 19 patients were free of any CNS active medication. Five AD patients were receiving a low-dose neuroleptic medication and 6 AD patients were using a serotonin selective uptake inhibitor medication at a stable dose level for a minimum of 2 months before the initiation of the study.

CLONIDINE TREATMENT

A double-blind, placebo-controlled study design was used. Clonidine (0, 0.5 and 2 µg/kg) (Catapressan^R) was administered orally 90 min before the initiation of the neuropsychological testing. Placebo tablets were of equal size and appearance as the clonidine tablets. An interval of 6–7 days was allowed between the dose levels. A Latin square design was used.

ANALYSIS OF CLONIDINE TREATMENT ON ATTENTION

A computerized system with a touch-sensitive video screen that measures visual memory was used. The tests utilize non-verbal stimuli and record responses using the touch-sensitive screen. The baseline accuracy in neuropsychological tests was measured during the first visit and subsequently the three stages of the drug treatment were conducted (placebo, clonidine 0.5 and 2 µg/kg).

FOLLOWING A SIMPLE RULE AND ITS REVERSAL TEST

Subjects were presented with a large and a small dot and required to point as quickly as possible at first to the smaller dot for 20 trials and then to the larger dot for the following 20 trials. The number and the latency to correct responses were recorded.

SIMPLE AND CHOICE REACTION TIME TEST

There were five ascending levels of difficulty in this test, the first four of which acted as training exercises to prepare the subjects for the final level. In the first stage, subjects simply had to touch the screen when a yellow dot appeared in the centre, being neither too early nor too late. The choice reaction was introduced at the second stage, with the dot now appearing in one of five locations. Subjects were introduced to the use of a touch pad at the third level. They were required to release their hand from a touch pad as quickly as possible after a dot appeared in a single location on a screen. The requirement to release the pad was then combined with the requirement to touch the screen at the fourth level. Subjects were required to hold down the touch pad until a single dot appeared in the centre of the screen and then to touch the position of the dot as quickly as possible (Simple Reaction Time Test). Subjects were then considered as being adequately trained for the fifth and final level, a Choice Reaction Time Test. They were required to hold down the touch pad until the dot appeared at one of five locations on the screen, and then point as quickly as possible to the position on the screen where the dot had been presented. Stimulus display time was 250 ms for all the stages, and the response was considered correct if the subject touched the dot when it was displayed on the screen or the correct position of the dot within 5000 ms after the dot had disappeared from the screen (limited hold). The intertrial interval was 1000 ms for all the stages. At the first three stages, the subjects were required to reach a criterion of five out of six correct responses within 18 trials to go on to the next stage. At the fourth stage, the subjects continued until a criterion of five out of six correct responses was reached or 18 trials had been completed. Then, at the fifth stage, the subjects were required to reach a criterion of five out of six correct within a maximum of 40 trials. Both accuracy (the number of correct responses and the number of total moves at each stage) and speed of response were recorded. For stages 4 (Simple Reaction Time Test) and 5 (Choice Reaction Time Test), the speed of response was divided into reaction latency (latency to release the touch pad) and movement latency (from release of touch pad to touch of the screen). The baseline accuracy of the patients was tested before the drug study was initiated. During the drug study, the patients were tested only at those stages that they could perform adequately (reached criterion) at the baseline.

MONITORING OF BLOOD PRESSURE

Blood pressure of the subjects was measured before the patients received the study drugs or matching placebo tablets, 90 min afterwards (i.e. just before beginning of the test session), and after completion of the test session, which lasted for 60–90 min.

STATISTICAL ANALYSIS

The repeated measures ANOVA was used to analyze the treatment and group effects, and the interaction of treatment with group.

RESULTS

At the baseline, we observed that 12 AD patients could attain the final and most difficult stage 5 (Best group), 10 AD patients only reached the penultimate stage 4 (Medium group) and six of them only managed to stage 3 (Worst group). The effect of clonidine was analyzed using these three groups.

FOLLOWING A SIMPLE RULE AND ITS REVERSAL TEST

Clonidine decreased the number of correct responses in the Worst group at 2 μg/kg, but not at 0.5 μg/kg (treatment effect: $F(2,50) = 6.8$, $p < 0.01$; treatment × group interaction: $F(4,50) = 3.8$, $p < 0.01$) and accuracy of the Medium and Best groups remained unaffected by clonidine 0.5 or 2 μg/kg (data not shown).

SIMPLE AND CHOICE REACTION TIME TEST

Again, clonidine 2 μg/kg, but not 0.5 μg/kg, decreased the percentage of correct responses at stages 1–3 only in the Worst group (treatment effect: $F(2,50) = 7.8$, $p < 0.01$; treatment × group interaction: $F(4,50) = 4.8$, $p = 0.01$) (Figure 1). No effect of clonidine treatment on movement time was found (treatment effect: $F(2,50) = 0.3$, $p > 0.5$) (data not shown).

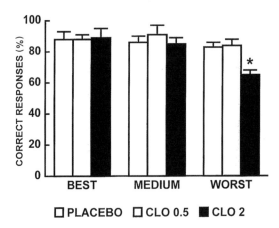

Figure 1. Clonidine-reduced accuracy at the easiest level of a Simple and Choice Reaction Time Test measuring attention only in those Alzheimer's disease patients that suffered from the most severe attention defect at the baseline (Worst group: 6 out of 28 patients). Clonidine 2 μg/kg, but not 0.5 μg/kg, retarded accuracy in those Alzheimer's disease patients. * $p < 0.05$ group treatment interaction

The Medium and the Best groups were tested at stage 4 and performance of these groups was equally impaired by clonidine 2 µg/kg (treatment effect: $F(2,40) = 29.6$, $p < 0.01$; treatment × group interaction: $F(2,40) = 0.44$, $p > 0.1$) (Figure 2).

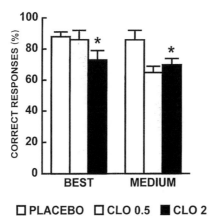

Figure 2. Clonidine-reduced accuracy at the penultimate stage of Simple and Choice Reaction Time Test measuring attention in those Alzheimer's disease patients that could reach this stage at the baseline (Medium and Best groups: 10 and 12 out of 28 patients). Clonidine 2 µg/kg, but not 0.5 µg/kg, retarded accuracy in those Alzheimer's disease patients. * $p < 0.05$ group treatment interaction

The accuracy of the Best group was reduced at the final stage 5 by clonidine 2 µg/kg (treatment effect: $F(2,22) = 9.25$, $p < 0.01$) (Figure 3). Clonidine failed to increase reaction and movement time at stage 4 in the Medium group and at stage 4 and 5 in the Best group (treatment effect: $F(2,40)/(2,22) < 0.2$, $p > 0.5$, for both comparisons).

DISCUSSION

We observed that clonidine disrupted attention in AD patients, but the effect was dependent on the attention capacity of the patients. Clonidine impaired performance only at the most difficult stages that the patients could complete at baseline, but failed to affect the accuracy at those stages that were easy for the patients. The effects of clonidine may be explained within the context of the distinction between automatic and controlled (or effortful) information processing [7]. Automatic information processing may be characterized by its involuntary nature, and lack of susceptibility to interference from activities involving attention [7]. Effortful processing, on the other hand, occurs in a novel situation when a new behavioral strategy is needed. This requires effort, is slower than automatic processing, and is resource-limited. The role of the

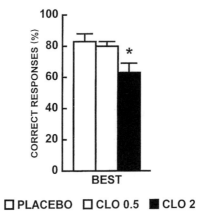

Figure 3. Clonidine-reduced accuracy at the final stage of Simple and Choice Reaction Time Test measuring attention in those Alzheimer's disease patients that could reach this stage at the baseline (Best group: 12 out of 28 patients). Clonidine 2 µg/kg, but not 0.5 µg/kg, retarded accuracy in those Alzheimer's disease patients. * $p < 0.05$ group treatment interaction

DNAB has been shown to be important only in demanding attention tasks requiring effortful processing [2, 4]. Indeed, DNAB lesion induced by 6-hydroxydopamine infusion failed to impair baseline accuracy in a Five Choice Reaction Time Test, which is a test analogous to the Simple and Choice Reaction Time Test employed in this study [2, 4]. However, under more difficult conditions, the accuracy of attention in DNAB-lesioned rats was disrupted more severely than in the controls [2, 4]. Furthermore, we have previously investigated the effect of clonidine on attention in healthy volunteers using a similar test battery as in this study, observing that only at the most difficult stage did clonidine 5 µg/kg retard accuracy (Jäkälä et al., unpublished). Therefore, the present result suggests that AD patients, irrespective of the changes in their baseline attention capacity, also suffer selective impairment of only controlled or effortful information-processing capacity after diminished activation of the DNAB system [4, 5, 7].

EFFECT OF CLONIDINE VS. TETRAHYDROAMINOACRIDINE ON ATTENTION

In rats, excitatory amino acid lesioning of the cholinergic cells in the nucleus basalis (NB) decreases cortical cholinergic activity and impairs accuracy of attention [8]. Unlike the DNAB-lesioned rats, which showed impairment only at the most demanding stage of performance, the attention accuracy of NB-lesioned rats was disrupted also at easy, baseline task conditions [8]. This result points to a more general role for the NB-to-frontal-cortex projection in attention and cortical arousal. A comparison of the effect of an anticholinesterase, tetrahydroaminoacridine (THA), on attention in AD patients, at doses that alleviate the severity of clinical dementia, with that of clonidine is also warranted [9]. Sahakian et al. (1993) [9] observed that THA facilitated attention at easy and difficult levels and this action may be mediated via the frontal areas [3]. Therefore, drugs acting via the LC DNAB projection selectively disrupt effortful attentional performance, and modulation of the cholinergic NB affects overall attention and cortical arousal in AD patients.

REFERENCES

1. Mann DMA, Yates PO, Hawkes J. The pathology of the human locus coeruleus. Clin Neuropathol 1983; 2: 1–7.
2. Cole BJ, Robbins TW. Forebrain norepinephrine: role in controlled information processing in the rat. Neuropsychopharmacology 1982; 7: 129–42.
3. Riekkinen PJ Jr, Riekkinen M, Soininen H, Kuikka J, Laakso M, Riekkinen P Sr. Frontal dysfunction blocks the therapeutic effect of THA on attention in Alzheimer's disease. NeuroReport 1997; 8: 1845–9.
4. Carli M, Robbins TW, Evenden JL, Everitt BJ. Effects of lesions to ascending noradrenergic neurons on performance of a 5-choice serial reaction time task in rats: implications for theories of dorsal noradrenergic bundle function based on selective attention and arousal. Behav Brain Sci 1983; 9: 361–80.
5. Schneider W, Shriffin RM. Controlled and automatic information processing: 1. Detection, search and attention. Psychol Rev 1977; 84: 1–66.
6. Coull JT, Middleton HC, Robbins TW, Sahakian BJ, Clonidine and diazepam have differential effects on tests of attention and learning. Psychopharmacology (Berl) 1995; 120: 322–32.
7. Kahneman D, Treisman A. Changing views of the attention and automaticity. In: Parasuraman R, Davies DR (eds) Varieties of Attention. Orlando, FL: Academic Press, 1984; 29–61.
8. Muir JL, Everitt BJ, Robbins TW. AMPA-induced excitotoxic lesions of the basal forebrain: a significant role for the cortical cholinergic system in attentional function. Neurosci 1994; 14: 2313–26.
9. Sahakian BJ, Owen AM, Morant NJ, Eagger SA, Boddington S, Crayton L, Crockford HA, Crooks M, Hill K, Levy R. Further analysis of the cognitive effects of tetrahydroaminoacridine (THA) in Alzheimer's disease: assessment of attentional and mnemonic function using CANTAB. Psychopharmacology (Berl) 1993; 110: 395–401.
10. Scheinin H, Kallio A, Koulu M, Scheinin M. Pharmacological effects of medetomidine in humans. Acta Vet Scand 1989; 85: 145–7.

Address for correspondence:
  Paavo Riekkinen Jr, MD PhD,
  Department of Neuroscience and Neurology,
  University and University Hospital of Kuopio,
  PO Box 1627, FIN-70211, Kuopio, Finland
  Tel: 358 17 163446; fax: 358 17 162048;
  e-mail: PaavoJr.Riekkinen@uku.fi

73 Olfactory Route: A New Pathway to Deliver Nerve Growth Factor to the Brain

XUE-QING CHEN, JOHN R. FAWCETT,
YUEH-ERH RAHMAN, THOMAS A. ALA AND
WILLIAM H. FREY II

INTRODUCTION

Neurotrophic factors are important for the survival, growth and differentiation of nerve cells. In recent years, these trophic factors have gained much attention as promising therapeutic agents for neurodegenerative diseases. The potential use of nerve growth factor (NGF) for the treatment of Alzheimer's disease (AD) has been proposed by many researchers [1–3]. NGF exhibits trophic effects primarily on cholinergic neurons in the basal forebrain of the central nervous system (CNS). It elevates choline acetyltransferase activity both *in vitro* and *in vivo* [4, 5]. It also prevents degeneration of cholinergic neurons following fimbria–fornix lesion in both rats and monkeys [6, 7]. Further, NGF ameliorates learning impairment in aged animals [8]. Although it remains unknown whether NGF is directly involved in the pathogenesis of AD, treatment with exogenous NGF may still prevent neuronal atrophy and improve memory and cognition, as has been demonstrated in animal studies.

However, as a 26.5 kDa protein, NGF is unable to cross the blood–brain barrier (BBB), making its delivery to the brain difficult. While delivery methods such as intracerebroventricular infusion and transplantation of NGF-releasing cells have been developed, associated surgical risks and high cost may limit the use of these methods in humans [9]. The development of a less invasive, lower-cost delivery method for NGF may therefore significantly improve the prospects of using NGF clinically. Delivery of NGF to the brain via the olfactory pathway is a novel, non-invasive drug delivery strategy in which the BBB is bypassed [10].

The rationale for olfactory delivery of NGF derives from the unique anatomic connection between the brain and the nasal cavity. The olfactory

Alzheimer's Disease and Related Disorders
Edited by K. Iqbal, D.F. Swaab, B. Winblad and H.M. Wisniewski
© 1999 John Wiley & Sons Ltd

receptor cells in the olfactory epithelium are bipolar sensory neurons and are the only known nerve cells to be directly connected with both the CNS and the external environment [11]. The axons of these neurons project to the olfactory bulb, which has connections with various brain regions, including the horizontal limb of the diagonal band, anterior olfactory nucleus, entorhinal cortex, locus coeruleus, raphe nucleus and amygdala, all of which are affected in AD. Also, drug delivery via the olfactory pathway may be particularly beneficial for AD patients, since the olfactory system is involved in the disease. One of the early symptoms in AD is loss of the sense of smell [12]. Pathologic changes have been found in the olfactory mucosa, olfactory bulb and brain regions interconnected with the olfactory bulb, suggesting that the disease may extend from the olfactory epithelium to the brain along the connecting fibers [13].

MATERIALS AND METHODS

Male Sprague–Dawley rats (200–280 g) were used in the study. Recombinant human NGF (rhNGF, 9.15 nM, generously provided by Genentech, Inc.), diluted in 40 mM potassium phosphate buffer (pH 7.0), was given by either olfactory pathway (O.P.) or intravenous (I.V.) administration. In some studies, ^{125}I-NGF (25 μCi, Dupont NEN), mixed with 500-fold excess of unlabeled NGF (Harlan Bioproduct), was administered to the rat with a total dose of 4.5 nM.

The femoral vein was cannulated for I.V. injection. For O.P. administration, the anaesthetized rats were placed on their backs, and 100 μl NGF solution was given as nose drops over 30 min. During the administration, the mouth and the opposite naris were closed in order for the drops to be inhaled with sufficient force to reach the roof of the nasal cavity. Saline (50 ml) was perfused via the descending aorta immediately after completing the administration in order to remove blood from the brain. In radiolabel studies, the rat brain was also perfused with 500 ml fixative containing 1.25% glutaraldehyde and 1% paraformaldehyde in 0.1 M Sorenson's phosphate buffer. The rat brain was then dissected into olfactory bulb, cerebellum, brainstem, and four approximately equal coronal brain sections labeled as B1, B2, B3 and B4. In addition, selected interior regions of the brain, including the frontal cortex, parietal cortex, olfactory tubercle, septal nucleus, hippocampus and amygdala, were also dissected out. In some studies, the olfactory epithelium was collected at 0, 2, 5 and 20 h after O.P. administration, and the time course of NGF uptake was determined.

A two-site enzyme-linked immunosorbent assay (ELISA) was utilized to determine the concentration of rhNGF in rat brains. For NGF extraction, brain tissue homogenates were freeze-thawed three times followed by centrifugation at $10\ 000 \times g$ for 10 min. The rhNGF in the supernatant fractions was then assayed by ELISA [14]. In radiolabel studies, the concentration of ^{125}I-NGF was determined by gamma counting.

RESULTS

As shown in Figure 1, following O.P. administration, high rhNGF levels were found in the olfactory epithelium up to 2 h. The highest rhNGF concentration of 4.5 mM at the time immediately after O.P. administration decreased rapidly with time to 7 μM at 20 h. Within 30–45 min following O.P. administration, a significant amount of rhNGF was delivered to the brain, achieving a concentration of 3.4 nM in the olfactory bulb and 0.66–2.2 nM in other brain regions. In contrast, significantly lower rhNGF was found in the brain after I.V. injection (Table 1). The distribution of NGF in the brain was also studied

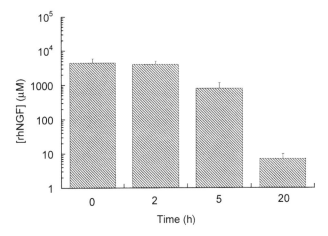

Figure 1. Concentration of rhNGF (mean ± SEM, n = 3–5) in olfactory epithelium at 0, 2, 5 and 20 h after the end of the olfactory pathway administration. Adapted from reference [14]

Table 1. Concentration of delivered rhNGF in different brain regions following O.P. and I.V. administration*

Brain regions	O.P. (nM)[a, b] (mean ± SEM, n = 5)	I.V. (nM)[a, b] (mean ± SEM, n = 6)
Olfactory bulb	3.4 ± 1.0	0.11 ± 0.017[c]
B1[d]	0.73 ± 0.23	0.042 ± 0.014[c]
B2	1.3 ± 0.62	0.075 ± 0.017[c]
B3	0.66 ± 0.24	0.065 ± 0.019[c]
B4	0.74 ± 0.30	0.060 ± 0.015[c]
Cerebellum	1.8 ± 1.0	0.12 ± 0.010[c]
Brainstem	2.2 ± 1.5	0.049 ± 0.011[c]

[a] The dose given to each rat was 9.15 nM.
[b] The endogenous levels of NGF were subtracted; all data represented rhNGF delivered to the brain 30–45 min after O.P. administration.
[c] $p < 0.0005$.
[d] B1–B4 are four coronal sections of the cerebral hemisphere taken from anterior to posterior.
* Adapted from reference [14], with modifications.

following O.P. administration of a lower dose of ^{125}I-NGF. Relatively high levels of NGF, ranging from 150 to 450 pM, were found in selected brain regions such as the frontal cortex, parietal cortex, olfactory tubercle, septal nucleus, hippocampus and amygdala (Table 2).

Table 2. Distribution of ^{125}I-NGF in selected brain regions following O.P. administration

	Brain regions					
	Frontal cortex	Olfactory tubercle	Septal nucleus	Parietal cortex	Hippo-campus	Amyg-dala
[NGF] (pM)*	240 ± 60	390 ± 80	450 ± 210	200 ± 30	150 ± 20	220 ± 100

* ^{125}I-NGF (25 μCi) was mixed with 500-fold excess of unlabeled NGF. The total dose given to each rat was 4.5 nM. All values represent mean ± SEM, n = 4.

DISCUSSION

Following O.P. administration, rhNGF was found to decrease with time in the olfactory epithelium. This decrease may not result from enzymatic degradation, since rhNGF was found to be fairly stable in olfactory epithelium *in vitro* [14]. Rather, the olfactory epithelium may serve as a depot from which O.P.-delivered NGF can be further transported to the olfactory bulb and other brain regions. Some NGF may be lost from the olfactory epithelium due to turnover and ciliary clearance of the mucous layer and lymphatic drainage from the submucosa. Within 1 h following O.P. but not I.V. administration, high levels of NGF were obtained in the olfactory bulb and, to a lesser extent, in other brain regions. Moreover, NGF was not simply present on the surface of the brain, but indeed, relatively high levels of NGF were also found in the frontal cortex, parietal cortex, olfactory tubercle, septal nucleus, hippocampus and amygdala. Some of these regions are known to be severely affected in AD. It has been shown that NGF as low as 38 pM is effective in elevating choline acetyltransferase activity in septal cholinergic cell cultures [4]. The ability to achieve NGF concentrations above 100 pM in selected target brain regions following O.P. administration is therefore very encouraging for the treatment of AD.

The detection of rhNGF by ELISA indicates that the rhNGF delivered to the brain is relatively intact. This is consistent with our previous results, in which about 80% of the radiolabel in the brain could be precipitated by trichloroacetic acid following O.P. administration of ^{125}I-NGF [10]. The rapid appearance of NGF in the brain following O.P. administration suggests a direct transport pathway between the nasal passage and the brain. While the underlying mechanism is still unclear, a variety of substances, including metals [15, 16], dyes [17], viruses [18], peptides [19, 20], proteins [21–24] and drugs [25, 26], have all been reported to reach the brain from the nasal cavity, without having to cross the BBB. Shipley [23] has found that, following intranasal administration, wheat germ agglutinin–horseradish peroxidase is endocytosed and transported within olfactory neurons to the olfactory bulb, where trans-synaptic transfer of the molecule occurs. On the other hand, horseradish peroxidase (HRP) has been found in intercellular openings of the olfactory epithelium as well as on the pial surface and nerve fiber layer of the olfactory bulb shortly (within 1 h) after intranasal administration [22]. Balin et al. have suggested that the rapid turnover of the olfactory sensory neurons, with the coexistence of mature and developing neurons in the olfactory epithelium, may explain the lack of tight junctions in some areas of the epithelium and the 'leakiness' of the epithelium to intranasally administered HRP [22]. Moreover, the distribution of NGF to interior brain areas in the present study also suggests that some transport or distribution mechanisms other than diffusion may be involved in the movement of NGF, since simple diffusion of macromolecules in the brain parenchyma is very limited. Further studies are under way to elucidate the mechanism of NGF transport to the brain following olfactory pathway delivery.

In conclusion, the olfactory pathway appears to be a promising route for the delivery of potent drugs to the CNS. This method, which is less expensive, more convenient to use and less prone to systemic side effects than other methods currently in use, may be of particular benefit for the long-term treatment of neurodegenerative diseases.

ACKNOWLEDGEMENTS

This work was supported by the Health Partners Research Foundation (St. Paul, MN) and the Pharmaceutical Research Fund. We thank Genentech Inc. for generously providing rhNGF. We also thank Herb Crandall, Joel Frandson and Terrie Grove-Bebow for their technical assistance.

REFERENCES

1. Hefti F, Schneider LS. Rationale for the planned clinical trials with nerve growth factor in Alzheimer's disease. Psychiat Dev 1989; 4: 297–315.
2. Lapchak PA. Nerve growth factor pharmacology: application to the treatment of cholinergic neurodegeneration in Alzheimer's disease. Exp Neurol 1993; 124: 16–20.
3. Olson L. NGF and the treatment of Alzheimer's disease. Exp Neurol 1993; 124: 5–15.

4. Knusel B, Michel PP, Schwaber JS, Hefti F. Selective and nonselective stimulation of central cholinergic and dopaminergic development *in vitro* by nerve growth factor, basic fibroblast growth factor, epidermal growth factor, insulin and the insulin-like growth factors I and II. J Neurosci 1990; 10: 558–70.

5. Mobley WC, Rutkowski JL, Tennekoon GI, Buchanan K, Johnston MV. Choline acetyltransferase activity in striatum of neonatal rats increased by nerve growth factor. Science 1985; 229: 284–7.

6. Kromer LF. Nerve growth factor treatment after brain injury prevents neuronal death. Science 1987; 235: 214–16.

7. Kordower JH, Winn SR, Liu Y-T, Mufson EJ, Sladek JR Jr, Hammang JP, Baetge EE, Emerich DF. The aged monkey basal forebrain: rescue and sprouting of axotomized basal forebrain neurons after grafts of encapsulated cells secreting human nerve growth factor. Proc Natl Acad Sci USA 1994; 91: 10898–902.

8. Gage FH, Bjorklund A, Stenevi U. Intrahippocampal septal grafts ameliorate learning impairments in aged rats. Science 1984; 225: 533–6.

9. Kordower JH, Mufson EJ, Granholm A, Hoffer B, Friden PM. Delivery of trophic factors to the primate brain. Exp Neurol 1993; 124: 21–30.

10. Frey WH II, Liu J, Chen X-Q, Thorne RG, Fawcett JR, Ala TA, Rahman Y-E. Delivery of ^{125}I-NGF to the brain via the olfactory route. Drug Delivery 1997; 4: 87–92.

11. Lewis JL, Dahl AR. Olfactory mucosa: composition, enzymatic localization, and metabolism. In: Doty RL (ed). Handbook of Olfaction and Gustation. New York: Marcel Dekker, 1995; 33–52.

12. Murphy C, Gilmore MM, Seery CS, Salmon DP, Lasker BR. Olfactory thresholds are associated with degree of dementia in Alzheimer's disease. Neurobiol Aging 1990; 11: 465–9.

13. Pearson RCA, Esiri MM, Hiorns RW, Wilcock GK, Powell TPS. Anatomical correlates of the distribution of the pathological changes in the neocortex in Alzheimer disease. Proc Natl Acad Sci USA 1985; 82: 4531–4.

14. Chen X-Q, Fawcett JR, Rahman Y-E, Ala TA, Frey WH II. Delivery of nerve growth factor to the brain via the olfactory pathway. J Alzheimer's Dis 1998; 1: 35–44.

15. de Lorenzo AJD. The olfactory neuron and the blood–brain barrier. In: Wolstenholme JEW (ed) Taste and Smell in Vertebrates. London: Churchill, 1970; 151–76.

16. Hastings L, Evans JE. Olfactory primary neurons as a route of entry for toxic agents into the CNS. Neurotoxicology 1991; 12: 707–14.

17. Suzuki N. Anterograde fluorescent labeling of olfactory receptor neurons by procion and lucifer dyes. Brain Res 1984; 311: 181–5.

18. Perlman S, Sun N, Barnett EM. Spread of MHV-JHM from nasal cavity to white matter of spinal cord—transneuronal movement and involvement of astrocytes. In: Talbot PJ, Levy GA (eds) Corona- and Related Viruses. New York: Plenum, 1995; 73–8.

19. Pietrowsky R, Struben C, Molle M, Fehm HL, Born J. Brain potential changes after intranasal vs. intravenous administration of vasopressin: evidence for a direct nose–brain pathway for peptide effects in humans. Biol Psychiat 1996; 39: 332–40.

20. Pietrowsky R, Thiemann A, Kern W, Fehm H, Born J. A nose–brain pathway for psychotropic peptides: evidence from a brain-evoked potential study with cholecystokinin. Psychoneuroendocrinology 1996; 21: 559–72.

21. Baker H, Spencer RF. Transneuronal transport of peroxidase-conjugated wheat germ agglutinin (WGA–HRP) from the olfactory epithelium to the brain of the adult rat. Exp Brain Res 1986; 63: 461–73.
22. Balin BJ, Broadwell RD, Salcman M, El-Kalliny M. Avenues for entry of peripherally administered protein to the central nervous system in mouse, rat, and squirrel monkey. J Comp Neurol 1986; 251: 260–80.
23. Shipley MT. Transport of molecules from nose to brain: transneuronal anterograde and retrograde labeling in the rat olfactory system by wheat germ agglutinin–horseradish peroxidase applied to the nasal epithelium. Brain Res Bull 1985; 15: 129–42.
24. Thorne RG, Emory CR, Ala TA, Frey WH II. Quantitative analysis of the olfactory pathway for drug delivery to the brain. Brain Res 1995; 692: 278–82.
25. Chou K-J, Donovan MD. Distribution of antihistamines into the CSF following intranasal delivery. Biopharmaceut Drug Disposition 1997; 18: 335–46.
26. Sakane T, Akizuki M, Yoshida M, Yamashita S, Nadai T, Hashida M, Sezaki H. Transport of cephalexin to the cerebrospinal fluid directly from the nasal cavity. J Pharm Pharmacol 1991; 43: 449–51.

Address for correspondence:
Xue-Qing Chen,
Department of Pharmaceutics, College of Pharmacy,
University of Minnesota, 308 Harvard Street SE,
Minneapolis, MN 55455, USA

74 Propantheline Enhances Tolerability of Tacrine

RAYMOND A. FABER AND PAULO J. NEGRO

Since 1993 tacrine has been available for the treatment of Alzheimer's disease (AD). Tacrine is a reversible cholinesterase inhibitor which slows the metabolism of acetycholine and thus elevates acetylcholine concentrations. Only a minority of patients in whom tacrine is initiated are able to tolerate the recommended dosage increases, with a target of 160 mg daily [1]. This is most often accounted for by the development of gastrointestinal side effects, including cramping, nausea, vomiting and diarrhea. These are predictable consequences of the cholinomimetic properties of tacrine, mediated by vagotonic effects. We have been able to overcome such gastrointestinal side effects with the use of the peripherally-acting anticholinergic medication, propantheline. We describe below four patients for whom adjunctive propantheline has allowed treatment with tacrine to continue.

PATIENT 1

A 49 year-old man was referred for memory difficulties and executive dysfunction. The patient was a high school mathematics teacher and reported initial difficulties remembering the names of students, difficulties in geometry classes and, eventually, algebra classes. He was diagnosed with probable AD. The initial Mini-Mental State Examination (MMSE) score was 23 and Executive Interview Scale (EXIT) score was 16, consistent with mild executive dysfunction [2]. A brain SPECT scan showed deceased uptake bilaterally in the parietal and occipital regions and left temporal region. The same findings, with additional decrease of uptake in the right temporal region, were found on a repeat scan 6 months later. The patient was already receiving tacrine 160 mg/day and paroxetine 20 mg/day at the referral date, but complained of nausea, gas and an ill-defined GI upset, mainly related to use of medication taken on an empty stomach. He had been skipping the last dose of the day due to this problem. Propantheline was added to the regimen, initially 7.5 mg 30 min

Alzheimer's Disease and Related Disorders
Edited by K. Iqbal, D.F. Swaab, B. Winblad and H.M. Wisniewski
© 1999 John Wiley & Sons Ltd

before each tacrine dose, with eventual increase to 15 mg 30 min before each tacrine dose, with satisfactory control of nausea and 'GI upset'.

PATIENT 2

A 75 year-old man was referred due to a noticeable decrease of cognitive abilities for 1 year, with confusion and anxiety. He was managed with PRN benzodiazepines and buspirone. Cognitive assessment revealed an MMSE of 20 and an EXIT of 21. A work-up for dementia was unrevealing, with exception of a magnetic resonance image (MRI), which showed diffuse prominence of ventricles and sulci, diffuse small foci of abnormal signal intensity within the periventricular deep white matter, and a brain SPECT that showed mild decrease uptake in the temporoparietal regions bilaterally. He was diagnosed with probable AD. The patient received tacrine 20 mg QID and propantheline in addition to buspirone 10 mg TID.

The response to the medication was excellent. The patient has been socializing in a day hospital and resumed playing cards with his wife and friends. Buspirone was eventually decreased to 15 mg/day, but attempts to increase the dose of tacrine were refused by the patient and his wife due to the robust response with the 80 mg/day dose and exacerbation of nausea and vomiting with increased attempts. The patient has received propantheline 15 mg 30 min before each tacrine dose and denies significant GI side effects at current tacrine dosage. If the propantheline is omitted, there is significant nausea and vomiting with each 20 mg tacrine dose.

PATIENT 3

A 72 year-old man was referred due to a 4–5 year history of memory disturbance, losing objects at home and neglecting his hygiene and grooming. The patient showed prominent executive dysfunction and memory losses, with an MMSE of 15, tangential thinking and inappropriate jocularity. Medical work-up was unremarkable, except for a CT scan that revealed 'age-related' atrophy and bilateral carotid calcification. A brain SPECT showed decreased uptake in the temporoparietal regions bilaterally, extending to posterior frontal regions, and in the right side of the cerebellum. He was diagnosed with probable AD. The patient received tacrine up to 120 mg/day and risperidone 0.5 mg at bedtime for paranoid ideation and insomnia. He denied GI upset until the tacrine dose was increased to 160 mg/day and risperidone to 1 mg/day for persistent paranoid ideation. At that point the patient complained of significant nausea, which resolved with the addition of propantheline 7.5 mg before each tacrine dose. The patient was then comfortable taking 160 mg of tacrine daily.

PATIENT 4

A 49 year-old man with amnestic syndrome was responsive to tacrine 80 mg/day. He presented with severe memory disturbance, reflected in his performance on short story passages of the Wechsler Memory Scale—Revised as well as impairing digit span (score 4) and digit symbol subtest (score 6) in WAIS-R testing. His medical work-up was unremarkable, including an MRI of the brain, and there was no history of alcohol abuse or specific insults which explained the memory problems. He was diagnosed with probable AD. He had a robust response to tacrine up to 80 mg/day, without any noticeable side effects. When a dosage increase to 120 mg/day was attempted, there was a sudden onset of severe nausea, vomiting and GI upset; the patient requested to resume the 80 mg/day dose of medication. Several months later, propantheline (7.5 mg 30 min before tacrine doses) was started and the patient could then tolerate the same tacrine dose of 120 mg/day without any noticeable GI side effects.

DISCUSSION

Since tacrine has a fairly linear dose response curve, it is recommended that all patients treated with tacrine reach the target dose of 160 mg daily to afford the maximum chance of a positive response. Only a minority of patients are able to tolerate this dosage target, hence most patients started on tacrine are non-responders and have the drug discontinued altogether. Propantheline is a potent quaternary ammonium muscarinic receptor antagonist that does not readily cross the blood–brain barrier and is devoid of CNS effects [3]. Thus, propantheline should not antagonize the therapeutic effects of tacrine. In the four cases described above, we found propantheline to be a simple adjunctive treatment which neutralized the gastrointestinal problems caused by tacrine and allowed tacrine treatment to continue in relative comfort.

This report should be regarded as preliminary, with the following cautions kept in mind. It is possible that propantheline reduced the absorption of tacrine, resulting in reduced tacrine blood levels and reduced GI side effects. Since we did not measure tacrine blood levels, we cannot rule out this possibility. Although propantheline has little CNS penetration, any CNS penetration by an anticholinergic might offset tacrine's positive effects. As we did not quantitate cognitive or behavioral status, such a diminution of benefit is possible. A controlled trail of propantheline with appropriate cognitive and behavioral measures could answer the above questions.

With the availability of cholinesterase inhibitors, such as donepezil, having less peripheral activity, GI side effects should become less problematic in the treatment of AD. Nonetheless, with the cautions noted, we suggest propantheline be considered for adjunctive use in patients experiencing untoward GI discomforts from any cholinesterase inhibitor.

REFERENCES

1. Farlow M, Gracon SI, Hershey LA, Lewis KW, Sadowsky CH, Dolan-Ureno J. A controlled trial of tacrine in Alzheimer's disease. JAMA 1992; 268: 2523–9.
2. Royall DR, Mahurin RK, Gray KF. Bedside assessment of executive dyscontrol: the Executive Interview (EXIT). J Am Ger Soc 1992; 40: 1221–6.
3. Brown JG, Taylor P. Muscarinic receptor agonists and antagonists. In: Hardman JG (ed) Goodman and Gilman's The Pharmacological Basis of Therapeutics, 9th edn. New York: McGraw-Hill, 1996; 141–60.

Address for correspondence:
    Raymond A. Faber,
    South Texas Veterans Health Care Systems, Department of Psychiatry,
    University of Texas Health Science Center at San Antonio, 116A,
       7400 Merton Minter,
    San Antonio, TX 78284, USA
    Tel: 210 617 5130; fax: 210 949 3306; e-mail: faber@uthscsa.edu

75 Dual Anti-amyloidogenic and Antioxidant Properties of Melatonin: A New Therapy for Alzheimer's Disease?

M.A. PAPPOLLA, Y.-J. CHYAN, P. BOZNER, C. SOTO,
H. SHAO, R.J. REITER, G. BREWER, N.K. ROBAKIS,
M.G. ZAGORSKI, B. FRANGIONE AND J. GHISO

INTRODUCTION

It has recently been reported that melatonin, a hormone with a proposed role in the aging process, prevents death and oxidative damage of neuronal cells exposed to Aβ [1, 2]. Because of the relationship between oxidative stress and Alzheimer's disease (AD) [3] and the recently established antioxidant properties of melatonin [4, 5], we had initially interpreted that the observed neuroprotective effects were simply a reflection of such antioxidant activities [1]. While investigating various possible mechanisms of action, however, we found that melatonin inhibited spontaneous formation of β-sheets and of amyloid fibrils. These interactions between melatonin and the Aβ peptides were demonstrated by circular dichroism and electron microscopy and further corroborated by nuclear magnetic resonance spectroscopy [6]. Inhibition of β-sheets and fibrils could not be accomplished in control experiments when a free-radical scavenger or a melatonin analog were substituted for melatonin under otherwise identical conditions. These properties may thus be synergistic with the powerful antioxidant activities of this hormone and suggest a novel anti-amyloidogenic activity for a physiologic substance. In sharp contrast with conventional anti-oxidants and synthetic anti-amyloidogenic compounds, melatonin crosses the blood–brain barrier, is relatively devoid of toxicity and thus constitutes a potential new therapeutic agent for AD.

Alzheimer's Disease and Related Disorders
Edited by K. Iqbal, D.F. Swaab, B. Winblad and H.M. Wisniewski
© 1999 John Wiley & Sons Ltd

METHODS AND RESULTS

CIRCULAR DICHROISM (CD) STUDIES

CD was performed as noted in Figure 1. As reported by several investigators [7, 8], the amount of β-sheets Aβ1–40 incubated alone increased spontaneously over time. With the batch of peptide employed we observed an increase from 52% at time zero, to 66% after 24 h at 37 °C (Figure 1A). The relative proportion of the structures dramatically changed by addition of melatonin to sister tubes. At time zero, the original β-sheet content markedly diminished (Figure 1A, left panel) at the expense of increases in the random coil configuration. *This effect was not observed with NAT or PBN.* The amount of β-sheet structures for Aβ1–40 plus melatonin decreased over time, reaching 24% after 24 h incubation (Figure 1A, right panel). At 24 h, no structural changes were again detected in control experiments with the melatonin analog NAT and only small effects were observed with PBN. Experiments with the Aβ1–42 showed qualitatively similar results (Figure 1B).

TRANSMISSION ELECTRON MICROSCOPY

Ultrastructural studies were done by conventional methods, as described in the legend to Figure 2. These studies reflected the conformational changes observed by CD and supported the hypothesis that increased formation of β-sheet structures precedes fibrillogenesis [7, 9]. In three independent experiments, fibrils were abundant in the tubes containing Aβ1–40 alone incubated for 36 h. By contrast, no fibrils were detected for solutions of Aβ1–40 plus melatonin up to 48 h (Figure 2). In the experiments with Aβ1–42, fibrils were identified in the tubes containing the peptide alone incubated after 2 and 6 h (no fibrils were seen at time zero). In contrast, only amorphous material was identified in the tubes containing Aβ1–42 plus melatonin at these time points (not shown).

NUCLEAR MAGNETIC RESONANCE SPECTROSCOPY

We used the NMR approach because it has the distinct advantage of being able to specifically locate the amino acid side chains that bind to a particular ligand. Shown in Figure 3 are the downfield spectral regions for the Aβ1–40 peptide, melatonin (Figure 3) and the Aβ1–40 with 0.4, 0.8 and 1.2 molar equivalents of melatonin (Figure 3B, C, D). The three well-resolved His-2H and His-4H signals are consistent with the Aβ1–40 peptide being partly folded into an ordered structure which, according to the CD studies, should be β-sheet and random coil. If only random coil structure were present, then degenerate signals should be present for His6, His13 and His14 [10]. The NMR spectra of the mixtures of melatonin and Aβ1–40 show changes in chemical shifts indicative of binding and local conformational changes. The

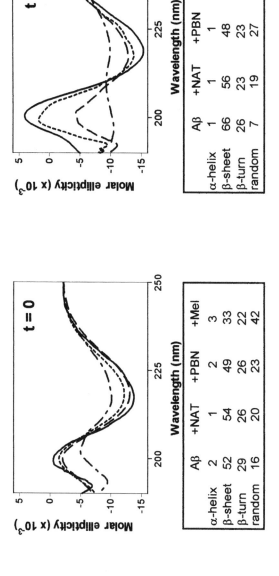

Figure 1. Circular dichroism studies of Aβ1–40 in the presence and absence of melatonin. The peptide (250 μM in 5 mM Tris–HCl, pH 7.4) was incubated at room temperature with and without 100 μM of either melatonin or the melatonin analog 5-methoxy-N-acetyl-tryptamine (NAT) or N-t-butyl-α-phenylnitrone (PBN), a powerful free-radical scavenger structurally unrelated to melatonin. Circular dichroism was performed with a Jasco-720 spectropolarimeter, as previously described [6]. The curves designate the spectra of Aβ alone (solid line), Aβ + NAT (short dashes), Aβ + PBN (long dashes) or Aβ + melatonin (short and long dashes). The corresponding percentages of different structure motifs are shown in the tables below each respective tracing. Experiments using Aβ1–42 yielded qualitatively similar data following 4 h incubation [6]

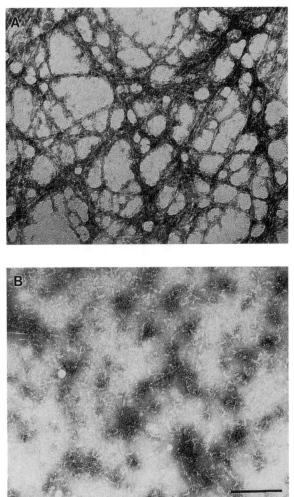

Figure 2. Electron microscopy studies of Aβ1–40 in the presence and absence of melatonin. Aβ1–40 was incubated at the same concentrations as noted in the legend to Figure 1 in the presence or absence of melatonin, and fibril formation was monitored at 0, 12, 24, 36 and 48 h in three independent experiments. Additional controls containing Aβ + NAT and Aβ + PBN were incubated in parallel for 48 h. The minimal inhibitory concentration of melatonin on fibril formation was performed with melatonin concentrations (1 nM–200 μM) in tubes containing 250 μM Aβ1–40, incubated for 48 h and then examined. Illustrated are typical areas from a representative experiment showing of Aβ1–40 incubated for 48 h, either alone (A) or with melatonin (B) (bar = 200 nm). EM grids were extensively and carefully examined and a negative result was only documented when fibrils were *totally* absent from the grids. No inhibition of fibril formation was seen under the conditions tested with NAT or PBN (not shown). These results were reproduced three times on different days. Electron microscopy experiments using Aβ1–42 show qualitatively similar data following 2 h and 6 h incubations. Scale bar = 200 nm

His-2H and His-4H signals shift downfield 0.05 and 0.02 ppm, respectively, while the aromatic peaks of melatonin also shift downfield. In addition, careful analysis of the upfield spectral region (spectra not shown) revealed downfield shifts for the Asp βCH_2 groups. Control NMR experiments with NAT showed only minor chemical shift perturbations (± 0.01 ppm), suggesting a specificity for the interaction of melatonin with Aβ.

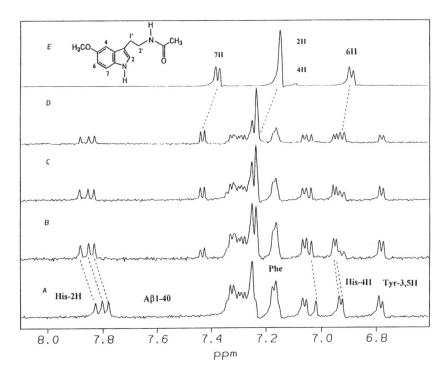

Figure 3. Nuclear magnetic resonance spectroscopy studies. Downfield ^{1}H NMR spectral region (600 MHz) of 0.25 mM Aβ1–40 peptide (A) and 5.0 mM melatonin (E), with the chemical structure of melatonin provided above the upper plot. The spectra in (B), (C) and (D) contain 0.25 mM Aβ1–40 plus 0.1 mM, 0.2 mM and 0.3 mM melatonin, respectively. Assignments for the aromatic signals of melatonin and the Aβ1–40 peptide are shown and those resonances exhibiting changes in shifts are connected by dotted lines. All ^{1}H NMR spectra were obtained at 600 MHz using a Varian Unity Plus-600 spectrometer and the data processed using the FELIX program (version 95.0, Biosym Inc.). The NMR measurements were performed at 10 °C and the residual protium absorption of D_2O was suppressed by low-power irradiation during the recycle delay. For all spectra, 128 scans were required with a total recycle delay of 4.2 s, which included an acquisition time and recycle delay of 2.2 and 2.0 s, respectively. The digital resolution of the acquired data was 0.24 Hz/pt, which was reduced to 0.12 Hz/pt by zero-filling the data once before processing. To further improve the resolution, before Fourier transformation spectra were multiplied by a Lorentzian-to-Gaussian weighting factor. This experiment was duplicated on two different days. Reproduced with permission from reference [6]

CELL VIABILITY STUDIES

Neurotoxicity was assessed in several cell types (see Figure 4 for methologic details). As expected, addition of melatonin along with Aβ peptides to rat primary hippocampal neurons and neuronally derived cells (Figure 4) showed *complete* protection against the neurotoxic effects of the peptides (Figure 4).

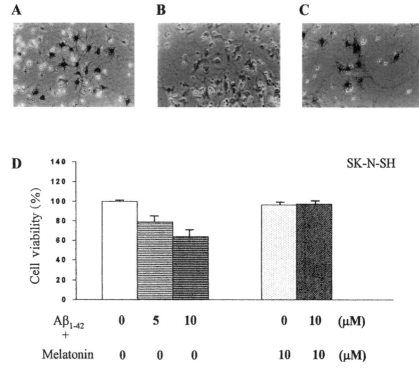

Figure 4. Cell viability studies. The neurotoxic properties of the peptides as well as the neuroprotective effects of melatonin were verified in primary rat hippocampal neurons [24]. Cell survival experiments were also performed in human neuroblastoma SK-N-SH cells and PC12 rat pheochromocytoma following previously described methods [1]. Cell survival was quantified by the MTT technique [25] and by Trypan blue exclusion. The neurotoxic effects of the peptides were readily detectable following 24 h incubations with either Aβ1–40 or Aβ1–42. In (A–C), representative microscopic fields of typical responses are illustrated from one of the experiments conducted with primary hippocampal neurons exposed to Aβ1–42, as visualized by a modified MTT method. Untreated control cells (A) show dark cytoplasmic staining, reflecting normal levels of cell viability. More than 95% of the control cells exhibit marked cytoplasmic staining. After exposure to Aβ1–42 (2.5 μM) for 24 h, virtually every cell in the culture plates showed markedly reduced staining intensity (B). Addition of melatonin along with Aβ1–42 resulted in staining intensity comparable to control cells (C). The measurements were also verified by spectroscopic absorbance measurements of cell lysates as described (not shown, [25]) and by Trypan blue exclusion (D). The results are reproducible across various cell lines, including human neuroblastomas SK-N-SH (D) and PC12 rat pheochromocytoma (not shown, see [1])

DISCUSSION

The secondary structure determines several important properties of Aβ that may be relevant to the pathogenesis of AD. First, it has been demonstrated that the amyloid peptide is neurotoxic [11–13] and that this characteristic is associated with formation of β-sheets [14–19] or amyloid fibrils [19]. Second, the ability of Aβ to form fibrils is directly correlated with the content of β-sheet structures adopted by the peptide [7]. In this regard, it has been proposed that peptides with high contents of β-sheets can act as seeds for nucleation and fibril formation [8, 9]. Finally, Aβ peptides with high contents of β-sheets become partially resistant to proteolytic degradation and this may be a crucial mechanism in amyloid deposition [20]. Such protease resistance and insolubility features, shared by all known forms of amyloidoses, prevent amyloid removal from tissue deposits. Thus, by preventing the formation of β-sheets one could not only reduce neurotoxicity but also facilitate clearance of Aβ via increased proteolytic degradation. As determined by circular dichroism (CD), electron microscopy and [1]H-nuclear magnetic resonance spectroscopy (^{1}H-NMR), melatonin interacted with Aβ and had a profound inhibitory effect on the formation of β-sheets and fibrils. While the molecular bases of Aβ-mediated neurotoxicity are not totally understood, it appears that oxygen-free radicals play a major role in this process [21, 22]. In this regard, earlier studies showed that melatonin also prevented Aβ-induced lipid peroxidation [1] and Aβ-induced oxidation of mitochondrial DNA [2]. Since melatonin is also effective in preventing injury produced by other forms of oxidative neurotoxicity [1, 23], it is likely that the powerful neuroprotective activity against Aβ reflects a unique combination of anti-oxidant *and* anti-amyloidogenic properties, rather than a single mechanism of action.

At this time, no information is available about the possible therapeutic or preventive values of melatonin or of its potential efficacy at physiologic or pharmacologic dosages. It would be premature to conclude that a subgroup of AD is caused by an age-related deficiency of this hormone, although such a possibility is nonetheless intriguing. The results reported here suggest that melatonin can provide a combination of antioxidant and anti-amyloidogenic features that can be explored, either as a preventive or therapeutic treatment for AD or as a model for development of anti-amyloidogenic indole analogs.

ACKNOWLEDGEMENTS

Supported by NIH Grants Nos AG11130, AR02594, AG08992, AG14363.

REFERENCES

1. Pappolla MA, Sos M, Omar RA, Bick RJ, Hickson-Bick DLM, Reiter RJ, Efthimiopoulos S, Robakis NK. Melatonin prevents death of neuroblastoma cells exposed to the Alzheimer amyloid peptide. J Neurosci 1997; 17: 1683–90.

2. Bozner P, Grishko V, LeDoux SP, Wilson GL, Chyan Y-J, Pappolla MA. The amyloid β protein induces oxidative damage of mitochondrial DNA. J Neuropathol Exp Neurol 1997; 563: 1356–62.

3. Pappolla MA, Sos M, Omar RA, Sambumurti K. The heat shock/oxidative stress connection: reference to Alzheimer's disease. Mol Chem Nueropathol 1996; 28: 21–34.

4. Tan DX, Chen DL, Poeggeler B, Manchester LC, Reiter RJ. Melatonin: a potent, endogenous hydroxyl radical scavenger. Endocrinol J 1993; 1: 57–60.

5. Reiter RJ, Poeggeler B, Tan DX, Chen DL, Manchester LC. Antioxidant capacity of melatonin: a novel function not requiring a receptor. Neuroendocrinol Lett 1993; 15: 103–16.

6. Pappolla M, Bozner P, Soto C, Shao B, Robakis N, Zagorski M, Frangione B, Ghiso J. Inhibition of Alzheimer β-fibrillogenesis by melatonin. J Biol Chem 1998; 273: 7185–8.

7. Soto C, Castaño EM, Kumar RA, Beavis RC, Frangione B. Fibrillogenesis of synthetic amyloid-beta peptides is dependent on their initial secondary structure. Neurosci Lett 1995; 200: 105–8.

8. Terzi E, Holzemann G, Seelig J. Self-association of beta-amyloid peptide (1–40) in solution and binding to lipid membranes. J Mol Biol 1995; 252: 633–42.

9. Jarrett JT, Berger EP, Lansbury PT Jr. The carboxyl terminus of the beta amyloid protein is critical for the seeding of amyloid formation: implications for the pathogenesis of Alzheimer's disease. Biochemistry 1993; 32: 4693–7.

10. Zagorski MG, Barrow CJ. NMR studies of amyloid beta-peptides: proton assignments, secondary structure, and mechanism of an alpha-helix–beta-sheet conversion for a homologous, 28-residue, N-terminal fragment. Biochemistry 1992; 31: 5621–31.

11. Yankner DA, Duffy LK, Kirschner DA. Neurotrophic and neurotoxic effects of amyloid β protein: reversal by tachykinin neuropeptides. Science 1990; 250: 279–82

12. Pappolla MA, Chyan Y-J, Omar RA, Hsiao K, Perry G, Smith MA, Bozner P. Evidence of oxidative stress and in vivo neurotoxicity of β-amyloid in a transgenic mouse model of Alzheimer's disease: a chronic oxidative paradigm for testing antioxidant therapies in vivo. Am J Pathol 1998; 152: 871–7.

13. Harris ME, Hensley K, Butterfield DA, Leedle RA, Carney JM. Direct evidence of oxidative injury produced by the Alzheimer's beta-amyloid peptide (1–40) in cultured hippocampal neurons. Exp Neurol 1995; 131: 193–202.

14. Buchet R, Tavitian E, Ristig D, Swoboda R, Stauss U, Gremlich HU, de La Fourniere L, Staufenbiel M, Frey P, Lowe DA. Conformations of synthetic beta peptides in solid state and in aqueous solution: relation to toxicity in PC12 cells. Biochim Biophys Acta 1996; 1315: 40–46.

15. Simmons LK, May PC, Tomaselli KJ, Rydel RE, Fuson KS, Brigham FF, Wright S, Lioberburg I, Becker GW, Brems DN, Li W. Secondary structure of amyloid beta peptide correlates with neurotoxic activity in vitro. Mol Pharmacol 1994; 45: 373–9.

16. Greenfield NJ, Fasman GD. Computed circular dichroism spectra for the evaluation of protein conformations. Biochemistry 1969; 8: 4108–16.

17. Tomski S, Murphy RM. Kinetics of aggregation of synthetic beta-amyloid peptide. Arch Biochem Biophys 1992; 294: 630–38.
18. Pike CJ, Walencewicz-Wasserman AJ, Kosmoski J, Cribbs DH, Glabe CG, Cotman CW. Structure–activity analyses of beta-amyloid peptides: contributions of the beta 25–35 region to aggregation and neurotoxicity. J Neurochem 1995; 64: 253–65.
19. Lorenzo A, Yankner BA. Beta-amyloid neurotoxicity requires fibril formation and is inhibited by Congo red. Proc Natl Acad Sci USA 1994; 91: 12243–7.
20. Soto C, Castaño EM. The conformation of Alzheimer's β peptide determines the rate of amyloid formation and its resistance to proteolysis. Biochem J 1996; 314: 701–7.
21. Behl C, David JB, Cole GM, Schubert D. Vitamin E protects nerve cells from amyloid protein toxicity. Biochem Biophys Res Commun 1992; 186: 944–50.
22. Behl C, David JB, Lesley R, Schubert D. Hydrogen peroxide mediates amyloid protein toxicity. Cell 1994; 77: 817–27.
23. Reiter RJ, Guerrero JM, Escames G, Pappolla MA, Acuna-Castroviejo D. Prophylactic actions of melatonin in oxidative neurotoxicity. Ann NY Acad Sci 1997; 825: 70–78.
24. Brewer GJ, Torricelli JR, Evege EK, Price PJ. Optimized survival of hippocampal neurons in B27-supplemented Neurobasal™, a new serum-free medium combination. J Neurosci Res 1993; 35: 567–76.
25. Hansen MB, Neilsen SE, Berg K. Re-examination and further development of a precise and rapid dye method for measuring cell growth/cell kill. J Immunol Methods 1989; 119: 203–10.

Address for correspondence:
Dr M.A. Pappolla,
University of South Alabama College of Medicine,
Mobile, AL, USA

76 Novel 17α-Estradiol Analogues as Potent Radical Scavengers

DORIS BLUM-DEGEN AND MARIO E. GÖTZ

INTRODUCTION

A role for estrogens in the prevention of dementia of the Alzheimer type (DAT) has been implicated by retrospective epidemiological studies, showing a dose- and duration-dependent correlation between estrogen replacement therapy and a reduction in the incidence of DAT [1, 2]. Estrogen use may delay the onset and decrease the risk of DAT in postmenopausal women [3] and long-term, low-dose treatment with 17β-estradiol is reported to improve cognitive functions, dementia symptoms and daily activity skills in women with mild to moderate DAT [4]. One explanation for these positive effects of estrogens is their antioxidative capacity, either by directly scavenging reactive oxygen species (ROS) or triggering protective mechanisms inside the cell, resulting in an improved defense against ROS. Oxidative stress, a cellular imbalance between production and elimination of ROS, is considered to be of major pathophysiological relevance for neurodegenerative disorders [5].

In our studies we used the so-called 'scav(enger)estrogens' J811 and J861, two $\Delta^{8,9}$-dehydro homologs of 17α-estradiol, first described by Oettel et al. in 1996 [6]. Scavestrogens are known to exhibit anti-oxidative activity by altering iron redox state and inhibiting the formation of superoxide anion radicals *in vitro* [7]. Furthermore, these compounds possess more potent radical-scavenging activities than the naturally occurring 17β-estradiol [7]. *In vitro*, prolonged exposure of cells to hydrogen peroxide and/or iron leads to cell death. We have studied the protective potential of these scavestrogens, compared with 17α-estradiol and 17β-estradiol, against Fenton reagent-mediated cell death (50 μM $FeSO_4$ plus 200 μM H_2O_2) using cell culture.

MATERIALS AND METHODS

J811 (Estra-1,3,5(10),8-tetraene-3,17α-diol) and J861 (14α,15α-methylene-estra-1,3,5(10),8-tetraene-3,17α-diol) were synthesized by Professor Dr S.

Alzheimer's Disease and Related Disorders
Edited by K. Iqbal, D.F. Swaab, B. Winblad and H.M. Wisniewski
© 1999 John Wiley & Sons Ltd

Schwarz (Department of Chemistry, Jenapharm GmbH & Co. KG, Jena, Germany) with HPLC purity > 99%. 17α-estradiol and 17β-estradiol, glutathione (GSH) and Trypan blue stain (0.4%) were purchased from Sigma (Deisenhofen, Germany). 1,1,3,3-Tetramethoxypropan was obtained from Fluka (Buchs, Switzerland). All other chemicals were obtained from Merck (Darmstadt, Germany). All methods (IMR32 cell culture, Trypan blue staining, TBARS assay, HPLC-based measurement of GSH) were performed as described in [8].

PROTECTIVE DESIGN

The steroidal compounds, freshly diluted in ethanol (0.1 μM, 1 μM and 10 μM), were added to cell cultures simultaneously with Fenton reagent in fresh DMEM containing dialysed FCS (10%). The vehicle volume of ethanol did not exceed 2 μl in 1 ml of medium and was also added to the control and Fenton reagent dishes, which contained no other additives. Following a 24 h incubation, cells were subsequently harvested for the various assays.

RESCUE DESIGN

Drugs were added to the cultures in DMEM containing 10% dialysed FCS 6 h after the exposure to Fenton reagent. Following incubation for 18 h, cells were harvested.

STATISTICS

Data are displayed as means ± SEM (standard error of the mean). Statistical differences in our model were calculated using one-way ANOVA Fisher's PLSD test (analysis of variance, Protected Least Significant Difference). The accepted significance level was $p < 0.05$.

RESULTS

To optimize Fenton-mediated cell death in our cell culture system, we investigated cell survival in pilot studies with varying concentrations of $FeSO_4$ (10–150 μM) and H_2O_2 (100–500 μM) for different incubation times (6, 24, 30 or 48 h) (data not shown). In the experiment reported here, cells were exposed to Fenton reagent (50 μM $FeSO_4$ + 200 μM H_2O_2) for 24 h in DMEM containing 10% dialysed fetal calf serum, which consistently reduced the amount of viable cells to 20–30% of controls ($p < 0.001$, ANOVA).

The steroidal compounds were added either simultaneously (protective design) or 6 h after the toxic stimulus (rescue design). J811, J861, 17α- and 17β-estradiol significantly increased cell viability in a dose-dependent manner (Figure 1). Furthermore, even when added 6 h after the Fenton reagent, J811 and J861 (each 1 and 10 μM) were able to rescue IMR32 cells from death, whereas estradiols were ineffective (Figure 2).

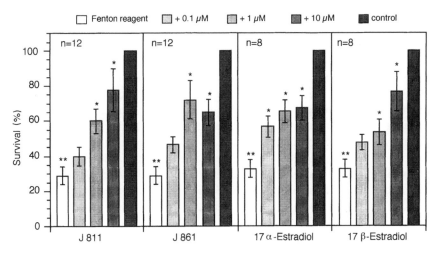

Figure 1. Protective design. Cells were treated simultaneously with Fenton reagent (50 μM FeSO4 + 200 μM H$_2$O$_2$) and the compounds at the concentrations indicated. Values (percentage of control) are expressed as means ± SEM. The absolute mean ± SEM control value in experiments involving J811 and J861 was 816.625 ± 63.713. The absolute mean ± SEM control value in experiments involving 17α- and 17β-estradiol was 813.919 ± 69.137. Analyses were performed after 24 h treatments. * p ≤ 0.05 vs. Fenton reagent. ** p ≤ 0.001 vs. control

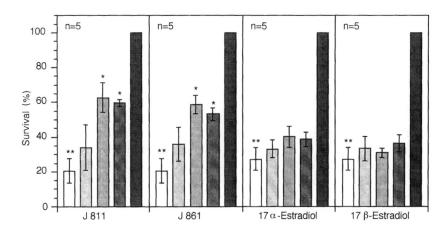

Figure 2. Rescue design. Cell viability expressed as a percentage of control (100%). The absolute mean ± SEM control value in experiments involving J811 and J861 was 935.685 ± 91.900. The absolute mean ± SEM control value in experiments involving 17α- and 17β-estradiol was 788.130 ± 40.167. Six hours after addition of Fenton reagent (50 μM FeSO$_4$ + 200 μM H$_2$O$_2$), cells were treated with the compounds at the concentrations indicated. Analyses were performed 24 h following the toxic stimulus. Values are expressed as means ± SEM; * p ≤ 0.05 vs. Fenton reagent. ** p ≤ 0.001 vs. control

Due to the production of ROS, cellular membrane components are very likely to undergo oxidation. Thus, we investigated the formation of lipid peroxides using a highly sensitive and improved assay for the determination of TBARS. Since the yield of TBARS was the same irrespective of the presence of air or inert gas (argon) all assays were performed under air. Addition of Fenton reagent resulted in a 30–40% increase of TBARS compared to that of controls. The protective activity of the steroidal compounds tested varied, although all substances demonstrated some protective effect (data not shown). Among the compounds tested, J811 and 17α-estradiol were the most effective inhibitors of TBARS formation, significantly reducing the TBARS values in all three dosages. Even when the compounds were added 6 h following Fenton reagent exposure, TBARS concentrations were significantly reduced to control levels by J811 (0.1 and 1 μM), followed by J861 (0.1 μM) and 17α-estradiol (1 μM) (data not shown).

Since the important intracellular antioxidant GSH scavenges radicals directly, complexes iron and serves as a co-substrate for GSH-peroxidases, we investigated the cellular levels of GSH in surviving cells after 24 h exposure to the Fenton reagent, a treatment which resulted in an increase of GSH concentrations of 50–150%. A dose-dependent normalization of GSH concentrations was shown by J811, J861 and 17α-estradiol, but significant reductions only occurred following the addition of J811 (10 μM) and J861 (10 μM) (data not shown). Also, in the rescue design only J811 and J861 (all three dosages) were able to significantly reduce GSH values. 17α-estradiol and 17β-estradiol did not change GSH levels (data not shown).

DISCUSSION

IMR32 neuroblastoma cells are of human origin and upon differentiation express most of the proteins of cholinergic neurons [9]. Since the cholinergic system is predominantly affected in DAT, these cells are appropriate to study oxidative stress-related death suggested to occur in DAT.

Based on the phenolic unit, estrogens are potent radical scavengers [10]. Their lipophilic character is a prerequisite for a possible membrane interaction, while to demonstrate protective properties at least three rings of the steroid structure, such as that shown for 17β-estradiol, the naturally occurring estrogen, are required.

The $\Delta^{8,9}$-dehydro derivatives of 17α-estradiol, J811 and J861, so-called scavestrogens [6, 7], both increased IMR32 cell viability, even at doses 200-fold lower than the toxic stimulus hydrogen peroxide. Estradiols also increased cell viability when given simultaneously with the toxic stimulus. However, the rescue effect mediated by natural estrogens was less pronounced than that mediated by the scavestrogens, particularly when these were given 6 h after the Fenton reagent.

In the rescue design, 0.1 μM J811 decreased the amount of TBARS to control levels, while there was no significant increase in cell survival (Figure 2). This suggests that inhibition of lipid peroxidation might not be the only cause for increased cell viability. At present, we cannot explain why J811, but not J861, is effective in lowering TBARS levels, since the only structural difference between the two compounds is a methylene group in the 14α,15α-position in J861. Differential interactions with lipids might be a possible reason for this phenomenon.

These results evoked our interest in determining post-treatment GSH content to characterize the status of the intracellular defences against $FeSO_4$ plus H_2O_2. Following treatment with Fenton reagent in combination with J811 or J861, the concentration of GSH per cell is approximately equal to that found in the control condition in both designs. This suggests that there is either no requirement for a pronounced upregulation of GSH in the presence of scavestrogens or that GSH-upregulation occurs early and transitionally and is no longer elevated at the time of measurement. Interestingly, the scavestrogens are more potent at normalizing GSH levels in the rescue design than in the protective condition. We assume that the compounds investigated are, in part, inactivated by a direct reaction with the Fenton reagent when added simultaneously to the culture medium. After 6 h the death process is most likely completed and the H_2O_2 is largely metabolized. Thus, viable cells at the 6 h time point probably face a higher effective dose than with the simultaneous addition.

In our experiments, 1 μM of the protective agent appeared to be sufficient to rescue IMR32 cells from Fenton reagent-induced cell death. That scavestrogens are able to rescue cells from death and prevent major changes in GSH content, even when given 6 h after the toxic stimulus, is suggestive of a different mechanism of action in addition to the direct scavenging of radicals, chelation of iron and extra- and intracellular reaction with hydrogen peroxide [7].

Estrogens attenuate neuronal injury caused by haemaglobin, chemical hypoxia and excitatory amino acids in murine cortical cultures [11], increase dendritic spine density by reducing GABA neurotransmission in hippocampal neurons [12] and enhance the outgrowth and survival of neocortical neurons in culture (17β-estradiol at 1 nM). Increasing the antioxidant capacity of cells by providing estrogens protects cells from Aβ(25–35)-toxicity [13]. Recent results by Green et al. [14] demonstrate that activation of the nuclear estrogen receptor is not necessary for the neuroprotective action of estrogens against amyloid peptide.

Such findings, together with our current demonstration of protective activities of J811 and J861 *in vitro*, suggest that estrogens and some of their derivatives may be useful in the development of novel therapeutic strategies for chronic progressive neurodegenerative disorders and other pathophysiological conditions where reactive oxygen species are operative in accelerating the disease, such as Alzheimer's and Parkinson's diseases, stroke, atherosclerosis or neurotrauma. Further studies are required to define the endocrinological profile, the protective efficacy and safety of these compounds in different experimental conditions *in vivo*.

CONCLUSIONS

In summary, oxidative stress is considered an important pathophysiological mechanism contributing to the promotion of cell death in a broad variety of diseases, including Alzheimer's disease. The so-called 'scavestrogens' J811 and J861, structurally derived from 17α-estradiol, are potent radical scavengers and inhibitors of iron-induced cell damage *in vitro*. In this study the potential cytoprotective effects of the scavestrogens J811 and J861 against Fenton reagent-induced cell damage (50 μM $FeSO_4$ plus 200 μM H_2O_2) have been compared with those of 17α- and 17β-estradiol. Cell viability studies investigated by Trypan blue staining showed that estradiols and scavestrogens at concentrations ranging from 0.1 μM to 10 μM are able to protect IMR32 neuroblastoma cells from Fenton-mediated death. In addition, these compounds decrease lipid peroxidation, measured as thiobarbituric acid reactive substances (TBARS), and normalize intracellular glutathione levels. J811 and J861 rescued 60% of cells, even given 6 h after the toxic stimulus, whereas 17α- and 17β-estradiol were ineffective. These results suggest that the scavestrogens J811 and J861 are powerful antioxidants capable of interfering with radical-mediated cell death in diseases known to be aggravated by reactive oxygen species. Such compounds may be useful in the development of novel treatments for stroke or neurodegenerative disorders, such as Alzheimer's and Parkinson's diseases, because of their non-hormonal mode of action.

ACKNOWLEDGEMENTS

We are indebted to the Jenapharm GmbH & Co. KG for supplying J811 and J861 and financially supporting this work. We also want to thank Maximiliane Haas, Sabine Pohli and Roland Harth for their contributions to this study.

REFERENCES

1. Paganini-Hill A, Henderson VW. Estrogen deficiency and risk of Alzheimer's disease in women. Am J Epidemiol 1994; 140; 256–61.
2. Kawas C, Resnick S, Morrison A, Brookmeyer R, Corrada M, Zonderman A, Bacal C, Donnell-Lingle D, Metter E. A prospective study of estrogen replacement therapy and the risk of developing Alzheimer's disease: The Baltimore Longitudinal Study of Aging. Neurology 1997; 48: 1517–21.

3. Tang MX, Jacobs D, Stern Y, Merder K, Schofield P, Gurland B, Andrews H, Mayeux R. Effect of estrogen during menopause on risk and age at onset of Alzheimer's disease. Lancet 1996; 348: 429–32.
4. Ohkura T, Isse K, Akazawa K, Hamamoto M, Yaoi Y, Hagino N. Long-term estrogen replacement therapy in female patients with dementia of the Alzheimer type: seven case reports. Dementia 1995; 6: 99–107.
5. Götz ME, Künig G, Riederer P, Youdim MBH. Oxidative stress: free radical production in neural degeneration. Pharmacol Ther 1994; 63: 37–122.
6. Oettel M, Römer W, Heller R. The therapeutic potential of scavestrogens. Eur J Obstet Gynecol 1996; 65: 153.
7. Römer W, Oettel M, Droescher P, Schwarz S. Novel scavestrogens and their radical scavenging effects, iron-chelating, and total antioxidative activities: $\Delta^{8,9}$-dehydro derivatives of 17α-estradiol and 17β-estradiol. Steroids 1997; 62: 304–10.
8. Blum-Degen D, Haas M, Pohli S, Harth R, Römer W, Oettel M, Riederer P, Götz ME. Scavestrogens protect IMR32 cells from oxidative stress-induced cell death. Toxicol Apply Pharmacol 1998 (in press).
9. Neill D, Hughes D, Edwardson JA, Rima BK, Allsop D. Human IMR32 neuroblastoma cells as a model cell line in Alzheimer's disease research. J. Neurosci Res 1994; 39: 482–93.
10. Mooradian AD. Antioxidant properties of steroids. J Steroid Biochem Molec Biol 1993; 45: 509–11.
11. Regan RF, Gua Y. Estrogens attenuate neuronal injury due to hemoglobin, chemical hypoxia, and excitatory amino acids in murine cortical cultures. Brain Res 1997; 764: 133–40.
12. Murphy DD, Cole NB, Greenberger V, Segal M. Estradiol increases dendritic spine density by reducing GABA neurotransmission in hippocampal neurons. J Neurosci 1998; 18: 2550–59.
13. Goodman Y, Bruce A, Cheng B, Mattson MP. Estrogens attenuate and corticosterone exacerbates excitotoxicity, oxidative injury, and amyloid-β-peptide toxicity in hippocampal neurons. J Neurochem 1996; 66: 1836–44.
14. Green PS, Gridley KE, Simpkins JW. Nuclear estrogen receptor-independent neuroprotection by estratrienes—a novel interaction with glutathione. Neuroscience 1998; 84: 7–10.

Address for correspondence:
Dr Doris Blum-Degen,
Clinical Neurochemistry, Department of Psychiatry,
University of Würzburg,
Füchsleinstrasse 15, 97080 Würzburg, Germany
Tel: +49 931 203323; fax: +49 931 203356

77 Treatment with Metrifonate Promotes Soluble Amyloid Precursor Protein Release from SH–SY5Y Neuroblastoma Cells

MARCO RACCHI, BERNARD SCHMIDT,
GERHARD KOENIG AND STEFANO GOVONI

INTRODUCTION

β-amyloid (Aβ) is derived from a large precursor protein called amyloid precursor protein (APP) [1, 2]. The precursor protein can be processed by various protease activities, among which α-secretase cleaves APP extracellularly within the amyloidogenic portion, leading to a large secreted fragment [3, 4]. β- and α-secretase instead cleave at the N and C termini of Aβ, respectively, releasing the amyloidogenic peptide. Both amyloidogenic and non-amyloidogenic metabolism appear to occur normally [5, 6]. In Alzheimer's disease (AD), mutations of APP, presenilins and non-genetic factors lead to increased Aβ production and subsequent extracellular deposition of these peptides. Since these gene mutations lead to autosomal dominant early (40s–60s) onset of AD, it is assumed that Aβ may play an active role in the pathogenesis of the disease, possibly by exerting neurotoxic activities [7]. One of the most important aspects of AD-related neurodegeneration is the loss of brain cholinergic cell bodies, therefore one current intervention strategy is focused on the enhancement of cholinergic neurotransmission.

The mechanism of action of metrifonate is the inhibition of acetylcholinesterase (AChE), thus increasing the availability of the transmitter at cholinergic synapses, thereby ameliorating some of the key symptoms of AD. Metrifonate itself is not an inhibitor of AChE but acts through its hydrolytic degradation product, dichlorvos (DDVP) [8]. AChE inhibition by DDVP is derived from a competitive interaction with the catalytic site of the enzyme, leading to irreversible inhibition within minutes. It is an intriguing possibility that neurotransmitters, including acetylcholine and muscarinic cholinergic receptors, may modulate APP metabolism. In that case, AChE inhibition

Alzheimer's Disease and Related Disorders
Edited by K. Iqbal, D.F. Swaab, B. Winblad and H.M. Wisniewski
© 1999 John Wiley & Sons Ltd

would have additional advantages in correcting such defects, possibly modifying the biological progression of the illness in addition to delaying the symptomatic progression of the disease [9, 10]. The purpose of our study was to establish whether metrifonate has major effects on APP metabolism, exploring the response to the drug in the SH–SY5Y neuroblastoma cell line.

METHODS

SH–SY5Y NEUROBLASTOMA CELLS

Cells were cultured in minimum essential medium (MEM) supplemented with 10% FCS, penicillin (100 U/ml), streptomycin (100 µg/ml), Na Pyruvate (1 mM) at 37 °C in a 5% CO_2 incubator. Cells were seeded at a density of 1.5 × 10⁶/dish (60 mm) and used 48 h after plating.

EXPERIMENTAL TREATMENTS

Cells were treated for 2 h at 37 °C in serum-free MEM in the presence of vehicle alone or in the presence of increasing concentrations of dichlorvos (DDVP) or metrifonate (MTF). The compounds were dissolved and diluted to working concentrations (see Results) at the time of use. Other treatments included carbachol and phorbol-12,13-dibutyrate (PdBu) at the concentrations detailed in the Results section. Following the recovery of conditioned media, cells were washed and collected with phosphate buffer, pH 8.0, and used for the determination of AChE activity according to Ellman [11].

ANALYSIS OF BASAL AND STIMULATED sAPP RELEASE

Proteins from conditioned media were prepared by deoxycholate/TCA precipitation [12] and loaded onto 10% SDS–PAGE gels. The separated proteins were transferred electrophoretically onto PVDF membranes. The membranes were saturated with 5% non-fat dry milk in 20 mM Tris–HCl (pH 7.5), 500 mM NaCl, Tween-20 (1%) for 1 h. The blots were incubated overnight with the monoclonal antibody 22C11 at 2 µg/ml. After incubation with the secondary antibody conjugated to HRP, the blots were developed by chemiluminescence.

DENSITOMETRIC AND STATISTICAL ANALYSIS

Quantitation of bands on Western blots was performed by gel imaging analysis, as described [13]. Data were analyzed using the analysis of variance test (ANOVA) followed, when significant, by an appropriate *post hoc* comparison, such as the Tukey test; a p value < 0.05 was considered significant. The data in the figures are expressed as mean ± SD of triplicate/quadruplicate samples in two/three independent experiments.

RESULTS

CHARACTERIZATION OF sAPP RELEASE FROM SH–SY5Y CELLS

The SH–SY5Y human neuroblastoma cell line expresses and secrete sAPP in response to both PdBu stimulation and carbachol (Figure 1). sAPP was identified on Western blots as a doublet band, consistent with other reports and also consistent with the pattern of expression of the three major APP

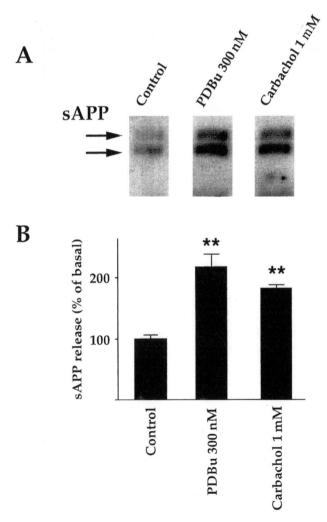

Figure 1. (A) Effect of carbachol and phorbol esters on sAPP release from SH–SY5Y cells. Cells were treated for 2 h, as indicated. (B) Semiquantitative evaluation of Western blots. ** $p < 0.001$ compared to basal release

isoforms in this cell line [14–15] (M. Racchi, unpublished observations). Cells were treated with PdBu 300 nM for 2 h, resulting in a significant increase of sAPP released (2.3-fold of basal release). Equally 1 mM carbachol elicited an increase of sAPP in the conditioned medium at levels 1.8-fold above basal.

CHARACTERIZATION OF THE EFFECT OF METRIFONATE ON THE RELEASE OF sAPP

We evaluated the effect of AChE inhibition on sAPP release following the release of the protein into the conditioned medium of cells treated with anti-cholinesterase agents. The reference molecule used was metrifonate (1–100 μM), a long-acting and well-tolerated cholinesterase inhibitor currently in clinical trials for the treatment of AD. Metrifonate is a prodrug that decomposes in aqueous solution and releases the true anticholinesterase drug DDVP.

Figure 2(A) shows an example of Western blot demonstrating that treatment with metrifonate induced a concentration-dependent increase in sAPP release. On the same set of cells we evaluated the AChE activity. Cumulative results of these experiments are shown in panel (B). The increase in sAPP release following metrifonate treatment was associated with increasing levels of inhibition of AChE.

CHARACTERIZATION OF THE EFFECT OF DDVP ON THE RELEASE OF sAPP FROM SH–SY5Y CELLS

Figure 3 shows that the treatment with DDVP (10 nM–1 μM), similarly to what was observed with metrifonate, elicited an increase in the release of sAPP above basal that was concentration-dependent. Comparison with a typical secretory stimulus, such as the direct activation of PKC by PdBu, showed that using the maximally active concentration of DDVP the effects of the two types of treatments were comparable.

DISCUSSION

The rationale for using anticholinesterase agents in AD relies on the possibility of increasing the cholinergic transmission by increasing the availability of acetylcholine in the synaptic cleft. Some major limitations to the use of AChE inhibitors are posed by the possibility of inducing severe cholinergic side effects. These adverse events are, however, correlated with the intrinsic pharmacological and pharmacokinetic properties of the drug used [16], rather than the actual level of AChE inhibition.

Metrifonate is unique among ChE inhibitors since it acts as a prodrug, slowly releasing, by non-enzymatic hydrolysis, the active compound DDVP

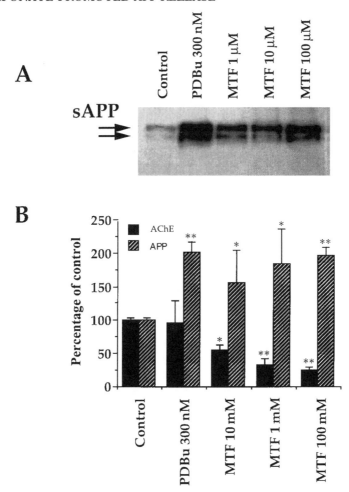

Figure 2. (A) Effect of MTF treatment on sAPP release from SH–SY5Y cells. Cells were treated for 2 h, as indicated. (B) Effect of MTF treatment on sAPP release and on AChE activity. Data are expressed as a percentage of control (basal release if referred to sAPP). * p < 0.05; ** p < 0.01 compared to control (basal)

[8]. This results in a slow onset of AChE inhibition that reduces the occurrence of side effects.

An added value element to cholinergic therapy for AD is the possibility that drugs taken with the purpose of increasing cholinergic transmission may improve or correct APP metabolism imbalance. Such an effect was first suggested using transfected cells expressing various subtypes of cholinergic receptors [17]. The effect of cholinergic activity in the regulation of sAPP release has also been inferred from studies conducted in *ex vivo* rat brain slices, electrically stimulated or following depolarization with KCl [18].

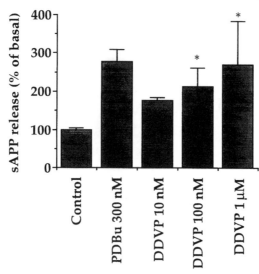

Figure 3. Effect of DDVP treatment on sAPP release. Data expressed as a percentage of control (basal) release. *$p < 0.05$ compared to basal release

Cultured cells offer a convenient model for studying the pharmacological modulation of APP metabolism. In particular, in the present investigation we chose to work with the neuroblastoma cell line SH–SY5Y because these cells express endogenously various subtypes of muscarinic receptors, mainly m1, m2 and m3, as well as choline acetyltransferase and AChE [19, 20] activities. The cells respond to carbachol stimulation with a release of sAPP quantitatively similar to that obtained with direct PKC stimulation with phorbol esters.

Treatment with metrifonate elicited a concentration-dependent increase in sAPP release, reaching a maximal response of approximately two-fold above basal release. This was somewhat reminiscent of the increase in sAPP obtained with carbachol or PdBu. Because metrifonate in aqueous solution is rapidly converted to DDVP, which has a longer half-life and therefore represents the active drug, we expected that the results could be replicated by using DDVP instead of metrifonate. Treatment with DDVP elicited a concentration-dependent increase of sAPP release at concentrations two orders of magnitude lower compared with the active concentration of metrifonate. This effect matches with the 100-fold more potent inhibition of AChE by DDVP compared to the parent drug [8], suggesting that the activity of metrifonate on APP processing and secretion is dependent on its metabolic conversion to DDVP.

While in most cell types the activation of sAPP secretion is often associated with a reduction in Aβ release, the levels of Aβ are very low in untransfected SH–SY5Y cells and could not be detected in the same experimental paradigm we used for the detection of sAPP. The effect of acute treatment with metrifonate/DDVP on the levels of Aβ still remains to be investigated when an appropriate experimental approach has been designed.

Recent work by Mori et al. [21] has shown that superfused rat cortical slices release sAPP in response to stimulation by heptylphysostigmine, physostigmine and DDVP. The effect of a single concentration of DDVP of 20 nM was consistent with our present results. By contrast, the work of Lahiri et al., showing inhibition of sAPP release using tacrine as an AChE inhibitor [15], can lead to confounding interpretations in this context, since tacrine is not only an AChE inhibitor, but also has an effect on multiple neurotransmitter systems.

Parallel measurements of AChE activity in the presence of metrifonate revealed an inverse relationship between the levels of AChE inhibition achieved and the levels of sAPP released into the medium of SH–SY5Y cells. Moreover, the difference in potency observed for DDVP and metrifonate is an indication for AChE being mechanistically involved in sAPP release stimulation by these two agents, as is the apparent inverse correlation between AChE activity and sAPP release. These data strongly suggest that the anti-AChE activity of metrifonate through its metabolite DDVP is directly correlated with an increase in sAPP release through the non-amyloidogenic pathway and supports the possibility of an influence of AChE-targeted cholinergic therapy on other molecular aspects of AD pathogenesis.

CONCLUSIONS

In summary, we wanted to establish whether metrifonate, a long-acting and well-tolerated cholinesterase inhibitor currently in clinical trials for the treatment of Alzheimer's disease, has major effects on amyloid precursor protein (APP) metabolism in the SH–SY5Y human neuroblastoma cell line. Treatment with dichlorvos (DDVP), the active metabolite of metrifonate, for 2 h, elicited a concentration-dependent increase in the release of sAPP above basal levels. The maximal effect was observed using 1 μM DDVP, producing a mean increase 2.7-fold above basal. The same effect was obtained with 100-fold higher concentrations of metrifonate. Parallel experiments measuring acetylcholinesterase activity demonstrated that the increase in sAPP release was inversely related to the levels of AChE activity. An inhibition of AChE activity by 75% (at 100 μM metrifonate) was associated with a doubling in sAPP release. These data suggest that AChE inhibition may contribute to the regulation of APP metabolism, possibly via an indirect agonist effect on cholinergic muscarinic receptors.

REFERENCES

1. Sandbrink R, Masters CL, Beyreuther K. APP gene family. Alternative splicing generates functionally related isoforms. Ann NY Acad Sci 1996; 777: 281–7.

2. Konig G, Monning U, Czech C, Prior R, Banati R, Schreiter-Gasser U, Bauer J, Masters CL, Beyreuther K. Identification and differential expression of a novel alternative splice isoform of the beta A4 amyloid precursor protein (APP) mRNA in leukocytes and brain microglial cells. J Biol Chem 1992; 267(15): 10804–9.

3. Esch FS, Keim PS, Beattie EC, Blacher RW, Culwell AR, Oltersdorf T, McClure D, Ward PJ. Cleavage of amyloid β-peptide during constitutive processing of its precursor. Science 1990; 248: 1122–4.

4. Anderson JP, Esch FS, Keim PS, Sambamurti K, Lieberburg I, Robakis NK. Exact cleavage site of Alzheimer precursor protein in neuronal PC 12 cells. Neurosci Lett 1991; 128: 126–8.

5. Haass C, Schlossmacher MG, Hung AY, Vigo-Pelfrey C, Mellon A, Ostaszewski BL, Lieberburg I, Koo EH, Schenk D, Teplow DB, Selkoe DJ. Amyloid β-peptide is produced by cells during normal metabolism. Nature 1992; 359: 322–5.

6. Busciglio J, Gabuzda DH, Matsudaria P, Yankner BA. Generation of β-amyloid in the secretory pathways in neuronal and non-neuronal cells. Proc Natl Acad Sci USA 1993; 90: 2092–6.

7. Yankner BA. Mechanisms of neuronal degeneration in Alzheimer's disease. Neuron 1996; 16: 921–32.

8. Hinz VC, Grewing S, Schmidt BH. Metrifonate induces cholinesterase inhibition exclusively via slow release of dichlorvos. Neurochem Res 1996; 21(3): 331–7.

9. Cummings JL, Cyrus PA, Bieber F, Mas J, Orazem J, Gulanski B. Metrifonate treatment of the cognitive deficits of Alzheimer's disease Neurology 1998; 50(5): 1214–21.

10. Morris JC, Cyrus PA, Orazem J, Mas J, Bieber F, Ruzicka BB, Gulanski B. Metrifonate benefits cognitive, behavioral, and global function in patients with Alzheimer's disease. Neurology 1998; 50(5): 1222–30.

11. Ellman GL, Courtney KD, Andres VJ, Featherstone RM. A new, rapid colorimetric determination of acetylcholinesterase activity. Biochem Pharmacol 1961; 7: 88–95.

12. Loffler J, Huber G. Modulation of β-amyloid precursor protein secretion in differentiated and non-differentiated cells. Biochem Biophys Res Comm 1993; 195: 97–103.

13. Racchi M, Ianna P, Binetti G, Trabucchi M, Govoni S. Bradykinin-induced amyloid precursor protein secretion: a protein Kinase C-independent mechanism that is not altered in fibroblasts from patients with sporadic Alzheimer's disease. Biochem J 1998; 330: 1271–5.

14. Ganter U, Strauss S, Jonas U, Weidemann A, Beyreuther K, Volk B, Berger M, Bauer J. Alpha 2-macroglobulin synthesis in interleukin-6 stimulated human neuronal (SH–SY5Y neuroblastoma) cells. Potential significance for the processing of Alzheimer beta amyloid precursor protein. FEBS Lett 1991; 282: 127–31.

15. Lahiri DK, Lewis S, Farlow MR. Tacrine alters the secretion of the beta-amyloid precursor protein in cell lines. J Neurosci Res 1994; 37: 777–87.

16. Schmidt BH, Roland Heinig R. The pharmacological basis for metrifonate's favourable tolerability in the treatment of Alzheimer's disease. Dementia Geriat Cogn Dis 1998; 9 (suppl 2): 15–19.

17. Nitsch RM, Slack BE, Wurtman RJ, Growdon JH. Release of Alzheimer amyloid precursor derivatives stimulated by activation of muscarinic acetylcholine receptors. Science 1992; 258: 304–7.

18. Nitsch RM, Farber SA, Growdon JH, Wurtman RJ. Release of amyloid beta-protein precursor derivatives by electrical depolarization of rat hippocampal slices. Proc Natl Acad Sci USA 1993; 90: 5191–3.

19. Lambert DG, Ghattore AS, Nahorski SR. Muscarinic receptor binding charac-
    teristics of a human neuroblastoma cell, SK-N-SH, and its clones SH–SY5Y and
    SH–EP1. Eur J Pharmacol 1989; 165: 71–7.
20. Serra ML, Mei WR, Roeske GK, Lui M, Watson M, Yamamura HI. The intact
    human neuroblastoma cell (SH–SY5Y) exhibits high affinity ^{3}H-pirenzepine bind-
    ing associated with hydrolysis of phosphatidylinositols. J Neurochem 1988; 50:
    1513–21.
21. Mori F, Lai CC, Fusi F, Giacobini E. Cholinesterase inhibitors increase secretion
    of APPs in rat brain cortex. NeuroReport 1995; 6: 633–6.

Address for correspondence:
    Marco Racchi,
    Institute of Pharmacology,
    Viale Taramelli 14, I-27100 Pavia, Italy
    Tel: +39 0382 507738; fax: +39 0382 507405; e-mail: racchi@unipv.it

78 Cholinesterase Inhibitory Activity of New Geneserine Derivatives

C. PIETRA, G. VILLETTI, P.T. BOLZONI,
M. DELCANALE, G. AMARI, P. CARUSO AND
M. CIVELLI

INTRODUCTION

Physostigmine (PHY) and geneserine (GEN) are the two major alkaloids found in Calabar beans and show different degrees of cholinesterase (ChE) inhibitory activity [1]. Chemical manipulation of the PHY moiety has generated compounds with different profiles of ChE inhibitory activity, duration of action and also of selectivity upon the two forms of ChE, i.e. acetyl-cholinesterase (AChE) and butyrylcholinesterase (BuChE) [2, 3]. Although the pharmacology of this class of compounds has been extensively studied, ChE inhibitory activity of GEN-derivatives has not been fully described. Indeed, GEN was reported as a weak AChE inhibitor on *in vitro* studies when compared to PHY [4], whereas a significant inhibition of plasmatic ChE was demonstrated in a study performed in healthy volunteers [5]. The aim of this study was therefore to evaluate the *in vitro* inhibition of ChE in human erythrocytes and plasma, and *ex vivo* AChE inhibition in rat brain and heart of GEN and new chemical entities derived from manipulation of its chemical structure (Figure 1). In particular, alkyl and aryl GEN-derivatives were considered. Activities of these compounds in both experimental paradigms were then correlated.

MATERIALS AND METHODS

INHIBITION OF ChE IN HUMAN PLASMA AND ERYTHROCYTES

A sample of 10 ml human blood was collected in a heparinized tube and then centrifuged at $4000 \times g$ for 10 min. After separation of plasma, the pellet containing the erythrocytes was rinsed three times in isotonic saline. The

Alzheimer's Disease and Related Disorders
Edited by K. Iqbal, D.F. Swaab, B. Winblad and H.M. Wisniewski
© 1999 John Wiley & Sons Ltd

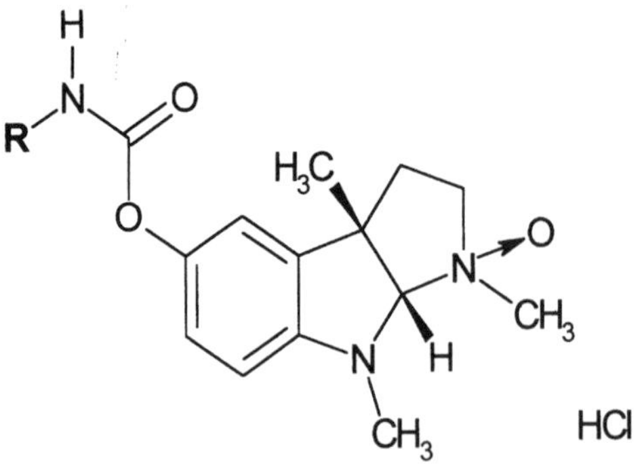

R

	R	
	-methyl	Geneserine
	-heptyl	CHF2060
	2-ethylphenyl	CHF2819
	2-methylphenyl	CHF2822
	3-methylphenyl	CHF2957

Figure 1. Chemical structures of GEN derivatives

erythrocytes were then suspended and haemolysed in 9 volumes of 0.1 M sodium phosphate buffer, pH 7.4, containing 0.5% Triton X-100. All enzyme preparations were diluted immediately before use with 0.1 M sodium phosphate buffer to reach a final dilution of 1:100. ChE activity was determined at 25 °C by the photometric method of Ellman et al. [6], using acetylthiocoline (0.5 mM) and butyrylthiocoline (0.5 mM) as substrates for the assay of AChE and BuChE, respectively. Compounds under investigation were dissolved in dimethylsulphoxide (DMSO) and preincubated with the enzyme preparation for 30 min before the reaction was initiated by the addiction of the substrate. Control samples received in parallel the same addition of DMSO (30 µl). To correct for non-specific substrate hydrolysis, aliquots of each ChE preparation were incubated under the condition of complete inhibition of either AChE (+100 µM BW254c51) or BuChE (+100 µM iso-OMPA), and the change in absorbance under these conditions was subtracted from that observed with the test compounds or only in the presence of the vehicle.

INHIBITION OF *EX VIVO* AChE IN RAT BRAIN AND HEART HOMOGENATES

Male Sprague–Dawley rats weighing 200–250 g were treated orally by gavage with test substances at different dose levels in an application volume of 2 ml/kg. Owing to low bioavailability, PHY was administered S.C. in a volume of 2 ml/kg. Control rats received the vehicle (distilled water) under identical conditions. At selected times after treatment, groups of at least eight animals were sacrificed by decapitation and brains and hearts were rapidly removed. The whole brain separated from the cerebellum and 100 mg of ventricular cardiac muscle were homogenized in 1 and 0.5 ml phosphate buffer (pH 8.0), respectively, with 1% Triton X-100. The homogenates were centrifuged at 19 943 $\times$ g for 15 min at 4 °C and aliquots of the clear supernatant used as the enzyme source. Assessment of the ChE activity was performed according to the method of Ellman et al. [6], as previously described.

STATISTICS

In the *in vitro* ChE evaluation, the percentage inhibition of the enzyme activity at each test compound concentration was evaluated. IC_{50} values were then calculated by non-linear least square curve fitting, using Allfit computer program. In the *ex vivo* study, data were analysed by Students' t-test for comparison between means of treated and control groups at each time interval. Compounds were compared at the time of their peak effect. Analyses of dose–response data were performed by using linear regression analysis and ED_{50}s with 95% confidence limits were calculated accordingly. Data are presented as mean ± SE.

RESULTS

INHIBITION OF ChE IN HUMAN PLASMA AND ERYTHROCYTES

Potencies of PHY, GEN and GEN-related compounds in inhibiting erythrocyte AChE and plasma BuChE are reported in Table 1. The compounds under investigation inhibited AChE with IC_{50} values at the μM level. GEN was 45-fold less potent than PHY in inhibiting AChE. GEN-derivatives exhibited an almost similar activity, the compounds 2-ethylphenyl-GEN (CHF2819) and heptyl-GEN (CHF2060) being more potent. A different pattern of activity was observed in inhibiting BuChE. In fact, CHF2060

Table 1. Potencies of PHY, GEN and GEN-related compounds in inhibiting erythrocytes AChE and plasmatic BuChE

Compound	IC_{50} (μM ± SE)		Ratio (AChE:BuChE)
	AChE	BuChE	
PHY	0.179 ± 0.014	0.053 ± 0.004	1:3
GEN	8.16 ± 0.634	0.680 ± 0.055	1:12
CHF2060	0.852 ± 0.085	0.005 ± 0.0007	1:170
CHF2819	0.477 ± 0.063	55.17 ± 6.43	115:1
CHF2822	2.01 ± 0.078	7.19 ± 0.282	3.5:1
CHF2957	4.20 ± 0.298	133.8 ± 9.70	32:1

n = 2–4 in duplicate/triplicate.

was 10-fold more potent than PHY. Conversely, both GEN and aryl GEN-derivatives showed a significantly lower activity in comparison to PHY. Comparing the effect on the two enzymes, CHF2819 appeared a selective inhibitor of AChE. This selectivity was less evident for 3-methylphenyl-GEN (CHF2957), while it was almost completely lost for 2-methylphenyl-GEN (CHF2822). Also, PHY and GEN appeared to be non-selective inhibitors of ChE, but with a slight preference for BuChE. By contrast, CHF2060 was a selective inhibitor of BuChE, being 170 times more potent against this enzyme than AChE.

INHIBITION OF *EX VIVO* ChE IN RAT BRAIN AND HEART HOMOGENATES

The time course of *ex vivo* AChE inhibitory activity was further investigated in rat brain after oral administration of the compounds at doses one-fifth of their LD_{50} values. In these experimental conditions compounds had similar symptoms of cholinergic stimulation. Drugs showed differences in time of peak inhibition and duration of action (Figure 2).

GEN-derivatives exhibited a significant ($p < 0.05$) activity up to 16 h after administration, whereas for PHY and GEN the duration of action was shorter (up to 2–4 h after administration). Peak AChE inhibition was 34%, 67%, 41% and 45% for CHF2819, CHF2957, CHF2060 and CHF2822, respectively, whereas for the PHY and GEN peaks AChE inhibition was in the order of 50%.

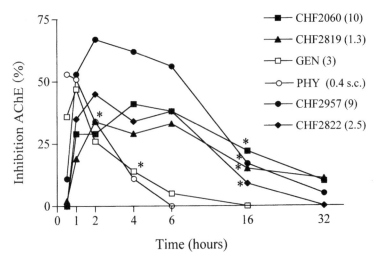

Figure 2. Inhibition of AChE in rat brain. Time course of effect after oral administration of PHY, GEN and related compounds. Doses in brackets are mg/kg; all points at the left of * are $p < 0.05$ vs. controls. SE are omitted for clarity; n = 8

A further analysis with regard to the selective action of the compounds in inhibiting central rather than peripheral AChE was performed by comparing dose–response curves at their time of peak effect on rat brain and heart homogenates (Figures 3 and 4). CHF2819, CHF2957, CHF2822 and CHF2060 inhibited brain AChE, ED_{50}s (with 95% confidence limits), being 1.5 (0.4–3.7), 4.1 (1.5–9.6), 1.6 (0.6–3.1) and 13.1 (5.9–26.6) mg/kg P.O., respectively. PHY and GEN showed ED_{50}s values of 0.09 (0.04–0.11) mg/kg S.C. and 1.6 (0.3–5.1) mg/kg P.O., respectively.

The heart homogenates showed substantial differences in their profiles of AChE activity. CHF2819 was almost inactive, whereas CHF2957 and

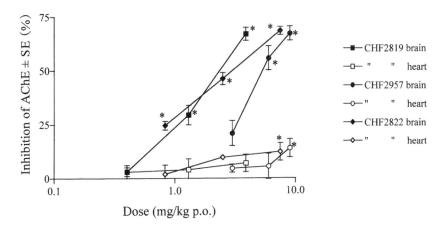

Figure 3. Effect of CHF2819, CHF2957 and CHF2822 on inhibition of rat brain and heart AChE at the time of their peak effect. * p < 0.05 vs. controls; n = 8

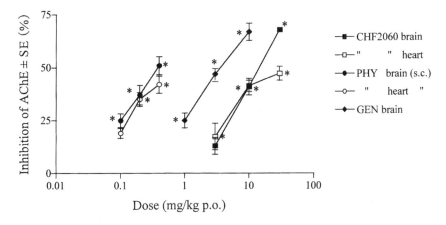

Figure 4. Effect of PHY, GEN and CHF2060 on inhibition of rat brain and heart AChE at the time of their peak effect. * p < 0.05 vs. controls; n = 8

CHF2822 significantly (p < 0.05) inhibited heart AChE by 14% and 12%, respectively, at the higher doses tested. Conversely, PHY significantly (p < 0.05) inhibited heart AChE at the same extent as brain AChE. Moreover, CHF2060 showed a significant (p < 0.05) inhibition of heart AChE by 17%, 41% and 48% at 3, 10 and 30 mg/kg P.O., respectively.

DISCUSSION AND CONCLUSIONS

This study provides an insight into the effects of the introduction of aryl and alkyl substitutes on the GEN chemical structure in inhibiting AChE. Some of the results obtained resemble those obtained in other studies, in which substitution of the carbamate structure of PHY displayed different degrees of selectivity and duration of action in the inhibition of AChE and BuChE [7, 8]. These changes reflect the interaction of this class of compounds with the ester and the anion subsites of the enzyme.

It has been reported that increasing the hydrophobicity of the carbamoyl group (butyl-octyl-carbamoyl eseroline) increased the potency of the compound against human plasma BuChE, whereas the effect on AChE in erythrocytes was augmented only slightly [8]. This suggests that binding of the inhibitor to human BuChE, and to a lesser extent to human AChE, is enhanced by increasing hydrophobic interactions at the ester subsite. In line with this evidence, CHF2060 was 10-fold more potent than GEN in inhibiting AChE, whereas its potency against plasma BuChE was 135-fold higher. However, the aryl GEN-derivatives CHF2819 and CHF2957 were 155- and 32-fold more potent in inhibiting human AChE than BuChE. Surprisingly, CHF2822 was only 3.5-fold more selective for AChE than BuChE. This result indicates that placement of the methyl group at the 2-position of the N-phenyl ring enhanced the binding of the inhibitor to human BuChE, both compared to the 3-methyl (CHF2957) and the 2-ethyl GEN-derivative (CHF2819).

The above results obtained in *in vitro* experiments can be discussed in view of the *ex vivo* data obtained in both rat brain and heart homogenates. All GEN-derivatives were endowed with a significant duration of rat brain AChE inhibitory activity compared with PHY and GEN. Indeed, the alkyl or aryl substitution of the carbamoyl group of PHY resulted in compounds with a long-lasting inhibition of AChE. Prototypes of this class of compounds are eptastigmine (heptyl-PHY) and phenserine (phenyl-PHY). These compounds have been reported to inhibit rat brain and plasma AChE by 8 and 6 h after oral administration, respectively [2, 7]. By contrast, the duration of action of both PHY and GEN was significantly shorter. For PHY this result is correlated with the low bioavailability of the compound and also with the fact that the fast kinetics of carbamylation is counterbalanced by the rise of the decarbamylation process [3]. In this regard further studies are necessary to elucidate the mechanistic interactions between GEN and GEN-derivatives with the enzyme AChE. The observed features of the kinetics of AChE inhibition should have a relevant influence on the therapeutic action of this kind of molecule, since strong and long-lasting inhibitory effects are required for AChE inhibitors to be suitable for AD therapy.

In addition to the kinetic profile, another important aspect of AChE inhibitors is their selective activity in inhibiting the enzyme in the brain, rather than in peripheral organs, thus resulting in a decrease of the peripheral cholinergic effects and toxicity. In this respect, the aryl GEN-derivatives CHF2819, CHF2957 and CHF2822 appeared more selective for inhibiting central (brain) than peripheral (heart) AChE. For CHF2819 and CHF2957 this activity might be correlated with their selective *in vitro* activity in inhibiting AChE rather than BuChE. However, CHF2822 was equipotent on both enzymes. Therefore other factors, such as differences in the distribution or kinetics of brain penetration, could account for the *in vivo* brain selectivity. In accordance with this hypothesis, activity on BuChE would result in a loss of brain selectivity in AChE inhibition. In fact the *in vitro* non-selective AChE inhibitors PHY and CHF2060 were almost not selective in inhibiting brain and heart AChE *ex vivo*. However, the assumption of this correlation between *in vitro* and *in vivo* data is not reported with other new AChE inhibitors structurally different from PHY and GEN, such as SDZ ENA 713 (Exelon), which represents a non-selective *in vitro* carbamate derivative with *in vivo* selectivity for brain AChE [9]. For this compound, a rapid brain penetration and a preferential activity on the G1 isoform of the enzyme could contribute to selective brain AChE inhibitory activity [9].

In summary, the results of the present study demonstrate that GEN is less potent than PHY in inhibiting ChE enzymes in both human plasma and erythrocytes. The aryl GEN derivatives, but not the alkyl-GEN CHF2060, displayed a selectivity in inhibiting AChE more than BuChE, depending upon the substitutions in the phenyl group. In comparison to GEN and PHY, the carbamate-synthetized compounds showed a similar potency but a long-lasting inhibition of *ex vivo* rat brain AChE activity. The aryl GEN-derivatives, but not CHF2060 and PHY, appeared more selective in inhibiting brain than heart AChE. The above *in vitro* profile might be correlated with the specific activity of compounds in inhibiting central (brain) rather than peripheral (heart) AChE.

REFERENCES

1. Robinson B. Alkaloids of the calabar bean. Alkaloids 1971; 13: 213–26.
2. Greig NH, Pei XF, Soncrant TT, Ingram DK, Brossi A. Phenserine and ring C hetero-analogues: drug candidates for the treatment of Alzheimer's disease. Med Res Rew 1995; 15: 3–31.

3. Perola E, Cellai L, Lambda D, Filocamo L, Brufani M. Long chain analogs of physostigmine as potential drugs for Alzheimer's disease: new insights into the mechanism of action in the inhibition of acetylcholinesterase. Biochim Biophys Acta 1997; 1343: 41–50.

4. Robinson B, Robinson JB. The anti-cholinesterase activities of the alkaloids of *Physostigma venenosum* seeds. J Pharm Pharmacol 1968; 20: 213–17.

5. Astier A, Petitjean D. Pharmacokinetics of an anticholinesterasic agent (eserin N-oxide) in humans after administration of two galenic forms. J Pharm Clin 1985; 4: 521–7.

6. Ellman GL, Courtney KD, Andres V, Featherstone RM. A new and rapid colorimetric determination of acetylcholinesterase activity. Biochem Pharmacol 1961; 7: 88–95.

7. De Sarro P, Pomponi M, Giacobini E, Tang XC, Williams E. The effect of heptyl-physostigmine, a new cholinesterase inhibitor, on the central cholinergic system in the rat. Neurochem Res 1989; 14: 971–7.

8. Atack JR, Yu QS, Soncrant TT, Brossi A, Rapoport S. Comparative inhibitory effects of various physostigmine analogs against acetyl- and butyrylcholinesterase. J Pharmacol Exp Ther 1989; 249: 194–202.

9. Enz A, Amstutz R, Boddeke H, Gmelin G, Malanowski J. Brain selective inhibition of acetylcholinesterase: a novel approach to therapy for Alzheimer's disease. In: Cuello AC (ed) Progress in Brain Research. Amsterdam: Elsevier Science, 1993; 431–8.

Address for correspondence:
    C. Pietra,
    Pharmacology Department, Chiesi Pharmaceuticals S.p.A.,
    via Palermo 26/A, 43100 Parma, Italy

79 The Role of Estrogens and NF-κB in Neuroprotection against Oxidative Stress

FRANK LEZOUALC'H AND CHRISTIAN BEHL

OXIDATIVE STRESS IN ALZHEIMER'S DISEASE

The occurrence of reactive oxygen species (ROS) or free radicals is referred to as oxidative stress [1]. Since ROS rapidly react with macromolecules of the cell, their generation can lead to immediate damage of intracellular structures or ultimately to the disintegration of cells in various tissues, including the central nervous system (CNS). Therefore, ROS have been suggested to be implicated in a variety of non-neuronal and neuronal disorders, including atherosclerosis, stroke, cerebral ischemia, amyotrophic lateral sclerosis, Parkinson's disease, and Alzheimer's disease (AD) (for review, see [2]). Since the majority of cases of AD are age-related and age, therefore, is a reliable risk factor for the non-genetic sporadic forms of this disease (85% of all cases), age-associated physiological and pathophysiological alterations have to be taken into account in the investigation of the pathogenesis of AD. Although this deadly neurodegenerative disorder has been known for over 90 years, having first been described by Alois Alzheimer [3], the pathogenetic events leading to the progressive loss of neurons and cognitive decline in AD are not fully understood. Various hypotheses to explain AD's development have been formulated and represent the basis of various current therapeutic approaches. Among these hypotheses is the so-called *oxidative stress hypothesis* of AD (for review, see [2]).

The histopathology of AD shows many signs of oxidative stress, such as the oxidation end-products of proteins, DNA and membrane lipids. One major player in the generation of an overall oxidative micro-environment for neurons is the AD-associated amyloid β-protein (Aβ), which accumulates in the so-called senile plaques in brain areas affected in AD. Aβ can be neurotoxic under certain conditions *in vitro* (for review, see [4]) and this toxicity has been shown to be mediated by peroxides and ultimately by the peroxidation of

Alzheimer's Disease and Related Disorders
Edited by K. Iqbal, D.F. Swaab, B. Winblad and H.M. Wisniewski
© 1999 John Wiley & Sons Ltd

membrane lipids, leading to the lysis of the cell [5]. Besides this direct oxidizing effect of accumulated neurotoxic Aβ, this peptide also attracts and activates inflammatory cells such as microglia, which in turn generate free radicals as well. Therefore, these inflammatory reactions are also believed to add to the oxidative environment during the pathogenesis of the disease [6].

In conformity with the oxidative stress hypothesis, lipophilic free radical scavengers, such as vitamin E, and the recently discovered antioxidant activity of the female sex hormone estrogen, may be used as neuroprotectants against the oxidative events in AD. But besides the exogenous addition of antioxidants to nerve cells under oxidative stress conditions, the activation of intrinsic antioxidants and, therefore, neuroprotective genetic programs may also be a possibility for helping neurons to resist accumulating oxidative events.

ESTROGENS AS NEUROPROTECTIVE ANTIOXIDANTS

Ovarian steroids in general and the female sex hormone estrogen in particular have a variety of functions in the brain. The steroid estrogen binds to cognate intracellular estrogen receptors, which belong to a superfamily of steroid nuclear receptors [7] and, when activated, function as transcription factors. After binding to specific estrogen response elements in the promoter regions of various genes, an estrogen-specific gene transcription is induced [8]. Such a mode of action represents the hormonal receptor-mediated activities of estrogens that modulate various neuronal functions, e.g. the expression of neurotransmitter receptors, membrane excitability, and may regulate synapse formation during nerve system development and regeneration (for review, see [9, 10]). As a direct consequence of such important physiological functions of estrogen in maintaining the normal functions of the brain, a potential role of this hormone in the development of neurodegenerative disorders is discussed. Indeed, there are several links between estrogens and AD: (a) women are twice as likely as men to develop AD [11, 12]; (b) the loss of estrogens during menopause is implicated in degenerative processes leading to cognitive decline [13]; (c) increased incidence of AD in older women may be due to an estrogen deficit [14, 15]. As additional experimental evidence for a link between the hormonal activity of estrogens and AD pathogenesis, it has recently been reported that estrogens enhance the non-amyloidogenic processing of APP and, therefore, reduce the production of potentially neurotoxic Aβ [16].

In addition to their genomic effects, estrogens have also short-term non-genomic effects such as altering neurotransmission and are, for this reason, acting as so-called neuroactive steroids (for review, see [17–19]). Recently, another non-genomic activity of estrogens on neurons has been identified. In

1995, it was reported that 17β-estradiol has a potent neuroprotective activity against oxidative stress as induced by Aβ, peroxides and glutamate employing clonal hippocampal cells [20]. To identify the structural prerequisite of the antioxidant activity of estrogens, employing various oxidative stress toxicity paradigms *in vitro*, several estrogen derivatives were tested, including estriol, estrone, ethinyl-estradiol, 2-hydroxy-estradiol, 4-hydroxy-estradiol, 3-methyl-ether, ethinyl-estradiol and 3-cyclopenthylether. Chemically, estrogen is a steroidal compound with the basic structure of an aromatic alcohol. In summary, it was demonstrated that the structural prerequisite of an antioxidant activity of estrogen and estrogen derivatives is the presence of a hydroxyl group at a mesomeric system [21, 22]. Whenever an intact phenolic group was present, the toxin-induced increase in intracellular peroxides and ultimately neuronal cell death could be blocked (Table 1). As an additional proof of the concept, these studies were extended also to other aromatic alcohols with intact phenolic groups and different phenol derivatives that could all protect neurons against oxidative cell death induced by glutamate and peroxides *in vitro* [23]. This neuroprotective activity was shown to be independent of the estrogen receptor activation and is, therefore, due to a chemical reaction of the

Table 1. Protection of clonal hippocampal cells against oxidative stress-induced cell death by different estrogens

Reagents	Concentration (μM)	MTT		Cell count		Peroxide
Control		100		100		100
Glutamate (or H_2O_2)	1000 (60)	9 ± 7	(15 ± 4)	16 ± 5	(19 ± 4)	168 ± 4
Estrone	10	$91 \pm 6^*$	$(74 \pm 2)^*$	$96 \pm 3^*$	$(91 \pm 6)^*$	$107 \pm 4^{**}$
17α-Estradiol	10	$86 \pm 3^*$	$(63 \pm 6)^*$	$92 \pm 5^*$	$(89 \pm 5)^*$	$105 \pm 3^{**}$
17β-Estradiol	10	$91 \pm 6^*$	$(66 \pm 5)^*$	$90 \pm 6^*$	$(93 \pm 5)^*$	$108 \pm 4^{**}$
Estriol	10	$80 \pm 6^*$	$(80 \pm 2)^*$	$95 \pm 9^*$	$(96 \pm 2)^*$	$103 \pm 2^{**}$
Ethinyl estradiol	10	$85 \pm 2^*$	$(65 \pm 4)^*$	$83 \pm 5^*$	$(90 \pm 5)^*$	$110 \pm 4^{**}$
Mestranol	10	5 ± 3	(21 ± 5)	6 ± 7	(14 ± 4)	164 ± 2
Quinestrol	10	3 ± 5	(10 ± 3)	5 ± 4	(17 ± 5)	165 ± 2
2-OH Estradiol	10	$78 \pm 6^*$	$(85 \pm 5)^*$	$74 \pm 6^*$	$(69 \pm 4)^*$	$105 \pm 4^{**}$
4-OH Estradiol	10	$83 \pm 5^*$	$(46 \pm 4)^*$	$82 \pm 6^*$	$(73 \pm 4)^*$	$107 \pm 4^{**}$

HT22 cells were incubated with various estrogens for 20 h at 10 μM before the indicated toxins were added. After 6 h the intracellular formation of H_2O_2 and related peroxides were determined using DCF fluorescence. Parallel cultures were treated for an additional 14 h. At that time, either the reduction of 3-(4,5-dimethylthiazol-2-yl)-2,5-diphenyl tetrazolium bromide as a measure of cellular viability or Trypan blue exclusion and cell countings as a measure of cell lysis were performed. The data in parentheses refer to the treatment of the cells with H_2O_2. All results were normalized to control values (no addition of reagent) as 100%. The data of the survival assays are presented as means ± SEM of five independent experiments. Peroxide formation as detected with DCF fluorescence is expressed as a percentage of fluorescent cells. Presented data are the means ± SEM of five independent experiments. Comparisons were made by ANOVA followed by a Scheffe's *post hoc* test. The p values of $^*p < 0.01$ and $^{**}p < 0.05$ were considered significant. **Bold** compounds represent estrogen derivatives with an intact phenolic structure. Modified from reference [21].

free radical scavenger estrogens rather than the induction of neuroprotective antioxidant mechanisms.

When comparing the chemical structure of estrogen with the structure of vitamin E (Figure 1), it again appears that the phenolic moiety present in both molecules may be responsible for the free radical scavenging effect of these compounds. Moreover, both molecules also consist of a large lipophilic structure, conferring the ability to permeate and accumulate in the neuronal membrane. Phenolic compounds such as estrogen and vitamin E may act as free radical scavengers by donating a proton from the hydroxyl group to generated hydroxyl radicals or lipid radicals, therefore detoxifying these ROS (Figure 2) [1]. Indeed, it appears that these *in vitro* concepts of a potent neuroprotective activity of antioxidants may perhaps also apply to the clinical situation. According to a recently published study, vitamin E slows down the progression of AD in moderately severe patients [24], and the use of estrogens in postmenopausal women can delay the onset of AD and lowers the overall risk of getting AD [15]. Therefore, the definition of the basic structural requirements for an antioxidant neuroprotective activity may be the basis of the design of novel estrogen derivatives that may act as neuroprotectants in a non-hormonal manner.

In summary, in addition to its receptor-dependent neurotrophic activities, the female sex hormone estrogen may function as a 'chemical shield' to prevent oxidative damage for neurons.

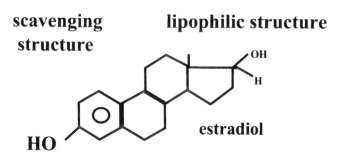

Figure 1. Chemical structures of the antioxidants vitamin E and 17β-estradiol. Chemically, both compounds are aromatic alcohols with an intact phenolic moiety (scavenging structure) and a lipophilic tail (lipophilic structure)

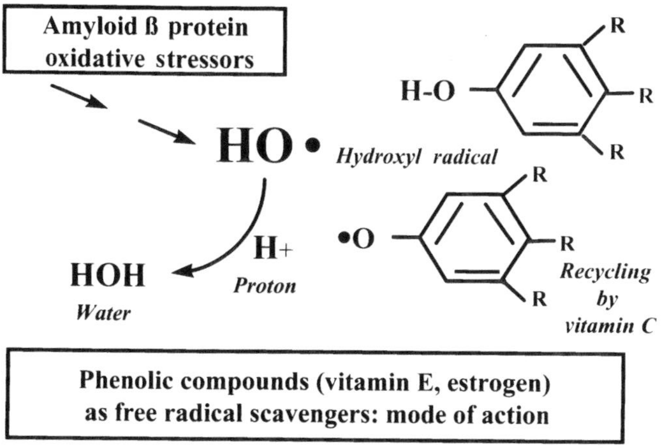

Figure 2. Phenolic compounds as antioxidants

ACTIVATION OF NF-κB IN NEURONAL CELLS

Oxidative challenges may not only lead to immediate detrimental effects, such as the oxidation of membrane lipids, but may also induce secondary effects, such as the activation of transcription factors. Aggregated Aβ induces the activity of the redox-sensitive nuclear transcription factor NF-κB [5, 25]. NF-κB is believed to be one central mediator for gene expression in response to pathogens and inflammatory cytokines in immune cells and for the development of the immune system [26]. Recently, a pivotal role for the activation of NF-κB during neuronal cell survival and neuronal cell death has been under intensive discussion [27–29]. Since reactive oxygen species are powerful inducers of NF-κB [30], whenever oxidative stress challenges neurons, the activation of NF-κB has to be taken into consideration. Several recent papers demonstrated the activation of NF-κB as a central part of a regulatory mechanism preventing cell death via the induction of the expression of anti-apoptotic genes in tumor cells [31].

To investigate the role of NF-κB activation during Aβ-induced oxidative cell death, and to determine whether the activation of NF-κB is pro-apoptotic or anti-apoptotic and, therefore, neuroprotective, neuronal cells were selected for their resistance against the toxic challenges of Aβ [5, 32]. PC12 cell subclones that are resistant to Aβ are also resistant to high concentrations of peroxides. Such Aβ-resistant cells exert an increased expression and activity of the antioxidant enzymes glutathione peroxidase and catalase when compared to their oxidative stress-sensitive PC12 parental counterparts [32]. For this reason, these two antioxidant enzymes may be part of a neuroprotective program mediating the resistance of these cells against Aβ. Interestingly, the combined over-expression of these two protective enzymes in parental sensitive cells does not completely confer resistance [32]. Therefore, various other neuroprotective programs may play a role in the resistance of these particular neuronal cells. In order to find such additional endogenous neuroprotective programs and their molecular trigger, the level of NF-κB was studied in these Aβ-resistant cells. In comparison to the PC12 parental cells, Aβ-resistant cells exert much higher levels of NF-κB activity as found at the expression level and the DNA binding level as well as at the transcriptional activity level [33]. The suppression of this enhanced NF-κB activity by glucocorticoids, such as dexamethasone or corticosterone, or by the over-expression of IκBα, the intracellular inhibitor and regulator of NF-κB, leads to a reversal of the resistance and, therefore, renders these initially oxidative stress-resistant cells vulnerable for exogenous oxidative events [33] (Table 2). These data clearly indicate that, indeed, a constitutively increased NF-κB activity can drive the transcription of neuroprotective target genes in oxidative stress-resistant cells. Consequently, such target genes are also major pharmaceutical targets with respect to prevention and treatment of AD (Figure 3).

In the search for such neuroprotective target genes, it was found that upon suppression of the NF-κB activity in Aβ-resistant cells, the intracellular glutathione content is strongly reduced. Glutathione is known as a central intracellular antioxidant, able to detoxify accumulating peroxides and other ROS. Moreover, following the treatment of resistant cells with dexamethasone, the expression of the glutathione-synthesizing enzyme γ-glutamylcysteine-synthetase is significantly reduced (Lezoualc'h and Behl, unpublished). In conclusion, these studies employing Aβ-resistant neuronal cells suggest that constitutively increased levels of NF-κB activity may mediate the resistance of neurons against oxidative stress and that the suppression of this activity

Table 2. Suppression of NF-κB by dexamethasone (DEX) reverses Aβ-resistance

μM	H_2O_2 alone	+0.1 μM DEX
Control*	100	100
60	94 ± 5	85 ± 8
125	96 ± 6	**56 ± 6*****
250	95 ± 8	**32 ± 4*****
500	36 ± 10	**4 ± 5*****
750	4 ± 3	0

Resistant Cl8 cells were pretreated with 0.1 μM DEX and then challenged with increasing concentrations of H_2O_2 for 20 h. Cell survival was determined by MTT assays and data presented are the means ± SEM for triplicate determinations. The viability of the control cells was defined as 100%. * Control = no addition of reagent. *** p < 0.001 was considered significant (**bold** data). The reversal of the resistance can also be achieved by the over-expression of IκBα super-repressor [33].

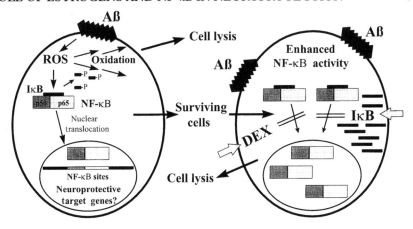

Figure 3. The role of NF-κB in oxidative stress resistance. Neuronal cells resistant against the neurotoxic Aβ aggregates have increased levels of activated NF-κB. The suppression of NF-κB by glucocorticoids (e.g. dexamethasone, DEX) or by the over-expression of NF-κB's inhibitor, IκB, reverses the resistance against oxidative stress. NF-κB may drive the transcription of neuroprotective target genes [33]

increases the vulnerability of neurons for oxidative challenges. The search for NF-κB-driven neuroprotective target genes is under way. The detailed analysis of the glutathione pathways in the oxidative-resistant cells may lead to the identification of possible neuroprotective target genes. Consistent with the developed concept that NF-κB activity may be protective for neurons exposed to Aβ is the *in vivo* finding that living neurons surrounding amyloid-β depositions in the post-mortem AD brain show an increased expression of the active form of NF-κB [25].

CONCLUSIONS

Since oxidative stress has been implicated in neuronal cell degeneration and, therefore, also in neurodegenerative conditions such as AD, antioxidant approaches are important avenues with respect to the prevention and treatment of AD. The addition of antioxidants to neuronal cells in single cell and tissue culture shows a potent neuroprotective effect in the presence of oxidative challenges. This neuroprotection is mediated by the ability of free radical scavengers, such as estrogen or vitamin E, to detoxify generated free radicals and, therefore, to prevent the peroxidation of lipids and, ultimately, the lysis of the cells. On the other hand, neurons exposed to oxidative toxins may react by activating cell defense programs which may be driven by redox-sensitive transcription factors such as NF-κB. An age-dependent accumulation of oxidative stress mediators may overcome the neurons' intrinsic ability to defend themselves in the long run, and may then therefore lead to neuronal cell death. This is consistent with the concept that AD-associated neuronal degeneration is an age-dependent process and age is the major risk factor of AD. In the future, potential neuroprotective target genes of NF-κB transcription will be identified and a specific induction of their transcription may help to strengthen the neurons in their battle against oxidation. In addition, the design of even more effective antioxidants could be further developed on the basis of the structural prerequisites defined so far.

ACKNOWLEDGEMENTS

The authors wish to thank Ms Sandra Rengsberger for the editing of this manuscript.

REFERENCES

1. Halliwell B, Gutteridge JMC. Free Radicals in Biology and Medicine, 2nd edn. Oxford: Oxford University Press, 1989.
2. Behl C. Amyloid β-protein toxicity and oxidative stress in Alzheimer's disease (review). Cell Tiss Res 1997; 296: 471–80.
3. Alzheimer A. Über eine eigenartige Erkrankung der Hirnrinde. Allgem Zeitschr Psychiat Psych Gericht Med 1907; 64: 146–8.
4. Yankner BA. Mechanism of neuronal degeneration in Alzheimer's disease. Neuron 1996; 16: 921–32.
5. Behl C, Davis JB, Lesley R, Schubert D. Hydrogen peroxide mediates amyloid β protein toxicity. Cell 1994, 77: 817–22.
6. McGeer PL, McGeer EG. The inflammatory response system of brain—implications for therapy of Alzheimer and other neurodegenerative diseases. Brain Res Rev 1995; 21: 195–218.
7. Evans RM. The steroid and thyroid hormone receptor superfamily. Science 1988, 240: 889–95.
8. Kumar V, Chambon P. The estrogen receptor binds to its responsive element as a ligand-induced homodimer. Cell 1988; 55: 145–56.
9. Honjo H, Tanak K, Kashiwagi T, Urabe M, Okada H, Hayashi M, Hayashi K. Senile dementia—Alzheimer's type and estrogen. Horm Metab Res 1995; 27: 204–7.
10. Alonso R, Lopezcoviella I. Gonadal steroids and neuronal function. Neurochem Res 1988; 23: 675–88.
11. Aronson MK, Ooi WL, Morgenstern H, Hafner A, Masur D, Crystal H, Frishman WH, Fisher D, Katzman R. Women, myocardial infarction, and dementia in the very old; Behav Neural Biol 1990; 40: 1102–6.
12. Rocca W, Hofman A, Brayne C et al. Frequency and distribution of Alzheimer's disease in Europe: a collaborative study of 1980–1990 prevalence findings. Ann Neurol 1991; 3: 381–90.
13. Simpkins JW, Singh M, Bishop J. The potential role for estrogen replacement therapy in the treatment of the cognitive decline and neurodegeneration associated with Alzheimer's disease. Neurobiol Aging 1994; 15: 195–7 (S).

14. Paganini-Hill A, Henderson VW. Estrogen deficiency and risk of Alzheimer's disease in women. Am J Epidemiol 1994; 140: 256–61.
15. Tang MX, Jacobs D, Stern Y, Marder K, Schofield P, Gurland B, Andrews H, Mayeux R. Effect of oestrogen during menopause on risk and age of onset of Alzheimer's disease. Lancet 1996; 348: 429–32.
16. Xu H et al. Estrogen reduces neuronal generation of Alzheimer β-amyloid peptides. Nature Med 1998; 4: 447–51.
17. McEwen BS. Non-genomic and genomic effects of steroids on neural activity. Trends Pharmacol Sci 1991; 12: 141–7.
18. Paul SM, Purdy RH. Neuroactive steroids. FASEB J 1992; 6: 2311–22.
19. Rupprecht R. The neuropsychopharmacological potential of neuroactive steroids. J Psychiat Res 1997; 31: 297–314.
20. Behl C, Widmann M, Trapp T, Holsboer F. 17β-Estradiol protects from oxidative stress-induced cell death in vitro. Biochem Biophys Res Commun 1995; 216: 473–82.
21. Behl C, Skutella T, Lezoualc'h F, Post A, Widmann M, Newton C, Holsboer F. Neuroprotection against oxidative stress by estrogens: structure–activity relationship. Mol Pharmacol 1997; 51: 535–41.
22. Green PS, Gordon K, Simpkins JW. Phenolic ring for the neuroprotective effects of estrogens. J Steroid Biochem Mol Biol 1997; 63: 229–35.
23. Moosmann B, Uhr M, Behl C. Neuroprotective potential of aromatic alcohols against oxidative cell death. FEBS Lett 1997; 413: 467–72.
24. Sano M, Ernesto C, Thomas RG et al. A controlled trial of selegiline, alpha-tocopherol, or both as treatment for Alzheimer's disease. N Engl J Med 1997; 336: 1216–22.
25. Kaltschmidt B, Uherek M, Volk B, Baeuerle P, Kaltschmidt C. Transcription factor NF-κB is activated in primary neurons by amyloid beta peptides and in neurons surrounding early plaques from patients with Alzheimer disease. Proc Natl Acad Sci USA 1997; 94: 2642–7.
26. Baeuerle PA, Henkel T. Function and activation of NF-kappa B in the immune system. Ann Rev Immunol 1994; 12: 141–79.
27. Barger SW, Mattson MP. Induction of neuroprotective κB-dependent transcription by secreted forms of the Alzheimer's β-amyloid precursor. Mol Brain Res 1996; 40: 116–26.
28. Lipton SA. Janus faces of NF-kappa B: neurodestruction versus neuroprotection. Nature Med 1997; 3: 20–22.
29. Lezoualc'h F, Behl C. Transcription factor NF-κB: friend or foe of neurons? Mol Psychiat 1998; 3: 15–20.
30. Schreck R, Rieber P, Baeuerle PA. Reactive oxygen intermediates are apparently widely used messengers in the activation of the NF-κB transcription factor and HIV-1. EMBO J 1991; 10: 2247–58.
31. Baichwal VR, Baeuerle PA. Apoptosis: activate NF-κB or die? Curr Biol 1997; 7: 94–6.
32. Sagara Y, Dargusch R, Klier FG, Schubert D, Behl C. Increased antioxidant enzyme activity in amyloid β protein resistant cells. J Neurosci 1996; 16: 497–505.

33. Lezoualc'h F, Sagara Y, Holsboer F, Behl C. High constitutive NF-κB activity mediates resistance to oxidative stress in neuronal cells. J Neurosci 1998; 18: 3224–32.

Address for correspondence:
    Christian Behl PhD,
    Max Planck Institute of Psychiatry,
    Kraepelinstrasse 2–16, 80804 Munich, Germany
    Tel: +49 89/30622 246; fax: +49 89/30622 642;
    e-mail: chris@mpipsykl.mpg.de

80 Peptide Derivatives as Potent Neuroprotectants: Relevance to Alzheimer's Disease

ILLANA GOZES, RACHEL ZAMOSTIANO,
MATI FRIDKIN AND DOUGLAS E. BRENNEMAN

VIP

The 28 amino acid peptide, VIP [1], promotes the survival of electrically blocked spinal cord neurons [2] in the presence of glial cells [3, 4]. VIP gene cloning [5] has allowed detection of prominent VIP expression throughout postnatal brain development [6], with a major decrease in the aging brain [7]. Utilizing a neurotensin $_{6-11}$VIP$_{7-28}$ hybrid antagonist [8–16] and transgenic animals under-expressing VIP [17] indicated that VIP is an important mediator of cell division [13, 15] and neuronal survival *in vivo* [12, 16]. Interference with VIP activities resulted in retardation in growth (especially of the brain, during a critical period of embryonic development), retardation in the acquisition of behavioral milestones, neuronal damage and disturbance of the biological clock during postnatal development, and impairments of sexual behavior, learning and memory in adult animals [8, 11].

Given the potential of VIP to inhibit neurodegeneration and promote neuronal survival, VIP-based molecules that could cross barriers such as the blood–brain barrier were sought. To that end, we have utilized lipophilization of peptides for the creation of lipid–peptide hybrids. This led to the discovery of stearyl-Nle^{17}-VIP (SNV), a peptide that is 100-fold more potent than VIP in promoting neuronal survival and protection against electrical blockade [16].

SNV: NOVEL NEUROPROTECTIVE STRATEGY AGAINST ALZHEIMER'S DISEASE: INHALATION OF 'FATTY NEUROPEPTIDES'

With SNV providing potent neuroprotection against electrical blockade, we set out to investigate the efficacy of the lipophilic drug in models relevant to

Alzheimer's Disease and Related Disorders
Edited by K. Iqbal, D.F. Swaab, B. Winblad and H.M. Wisniewski
© 1999 John Wiley & Sons Ltd

Alzheimer's disease. The *in vitro* model included rat cerebral cortical cells treated with the β-amyloid peptide fragment (amino acids 25–35); 50–70% neuronal death was observed in the treated culture and this death was prevented in the presence of SNV. While VIP also provided neuroprotection in the same paradigm, at least 100-fold more VIP was required to obtain the same level of protection. Furthermore, SNV provided protection over a broader range of concentrations.

The *in vitro* results prompted *in vivo* studies. Preliminary results indicated efficacy for SNV against hypoxia [18]. Further studies relevant to Alzheimer's disease included: (a) rats exposed to the cholinotoxin, ethylcholine aziridium (AF64A), a blocker of choline uptake [19, 20]; and (b) apolipoprotein E4 (ApoE4)-deficient mice [21–25]. In the first model, significant impairments in learning and memory were observed in the Morris water maze [20]. Inhalation of SNV prior to the daily test prevented learning and memory deficits. In the second model, not only learning and deficits in short-term memory were apparent, but also developmental retardation in the acquisition of developmental milestones of behavior. Daily subcutaneous injection of SNV to the newborn apolipoprotein E-deficient mice resulted in facilitation of normal development and learning capacities that resembled the control apolipoprotein E-expressing mice.

ADNF

Studies which encompassed techniques in pharmacology, molecular biology, biochemistry and behavior [26] allowed the experiments leading to the discovery of the unique, glial-derived, femtomolar-acting, activity-dependent neurotrophic factor (ADNF) [27]. Thus, it was recently discovered that the neuroprotective actions of VIP are mediated, in part, via a new glial-derived growth factor, ADNF [27]. Femtomolar concentrations of ADNF (mol mass, 14 kDa, and pI, 8.3 ± 0.25) protected neurons from death associated with electrical blockade. Initial studies have identified the potent neuroprotective glial protein, ADNF, and an active peptide of 14 amino acids, ADNF-14, that provide a basis for developing treatments of currently intractable neurodegenerative diseases. Results now show that the active site of ADNF can be shortened to a nine amino acid active core, ADNF-9 [28]. The sequence of ADNF-14, VLGGGSALLRSIPA, and of ADNF-9, SALLRSIPA, correspond to the most conserved sequence of the stress protein, heat shock protein 60 (hsp60), VLGGGCALLRCIPA [29]. In this respect, hsp60 antibodies produced neuronal cell death that was inhibited by ADNF [27]. Similarly, ADNF antibodies produced apoptosis that was inhibited by ADNF [30]. We have now identified the secretion of hsp60-like immunoreactive protein from glia and neurons [31]. It is hypothesized that VIP causes a rapid release of intracellular hsp60 and ADNF, thereby enhancing the protective extracellular milieu.

ADNF AND RELATED PEPTIDES AS NEUROPROTECTANTS *IN VITRO*

Structure–activity studies with over 40 peptides derived from ADNF revealed the structure of ADNF-9: SALLRSIPA, a peptide that captured and exceeded the neurotrophic properties of ADNF-14 and the parent molecule ADNF. The summary of the *in vitro* studies has been recently published [28]. Several pharmacological advantages were apparent in ADNF-9 in comparison to ADNF-14: neurotrophic activity was evident over a broader range of effective concentrations and the molecule was significantly shortened. Mechanistic studies incidated that less than 2 h of treatment with ADNF-9 produced neuroprotection for 4 days in cerebral cortical cultures treated with tetrodotoxin. In addition, pre-incubation with bafilomycin A1 (an inhibitor of receptor-mediated endocytosis) prevented the neuroprotective properties of both ADNF and ADNF-9.

ADNF and ADNF-9 have been shown to interact with neurons and glia. Interactions with glia have apparent influence on the inverted-U shaped dose–response curve to ADNF. The molecules mediating ADNF-9–glial interaction are the subject of future research. ADNF-9 exhibited a protection against a broad array of neurotoxins, including tetrodotoxin, gp120 (the HIV envelope protein), N-methyl-D-aspartate, and the β-amyloid peptide. Against all of these toxins, very low peptide concentrations were effective in preventing deleterious effects in cerebral cortical cultures [28]. These findings were particularly exciting because several of these toxins have been implicated in the etiology of neurodegenerative diseases. Relevant to the protection of Alzheimer's disease, ADNF-9 protected against toxicity associated with the β-amyloid peptide.

CONCLUSIONS AND PERSPECTIVES

ADNF is secreted from astroglial cells in the presence of VIP. Progress has been made in our understanding of the receptor that mediates the survival-promoting actions of VIP. Utilizing a battery of antisense oligodeoxy-nucleotides directed against cloned VIP and the related-peptide pituitary adenylate cyclase activating peptide (PACAP) receptor [32], we found that a specific splice variant of the PACAP receptor produced neuronal cell death [33]. Binding and displacement experiments have shown that the same receptor represented the high-affinity VIP receptor in astroglial cells that was previously implicated in neuronal survival and ADNF secretion. Another VIP receptor was recently implicated in mouse neocortical astrocytogenesis [34]. The chromosomal localization of the VIP receptor genes is in close association with genes responsible for craniofacial defects [35] and cancer growth [36]. Future studies should reveal other genetic traits that may be associated with the inheritance of the VIP-related receptors, VIP and ADNF. Interestingly, VIP can enhance its own expression [37, 38], perhaps leading to increased survival and division, depending on the receptor subtype that is expressed and the signal transduction pathway that is activated [39]. While the VIP literature is vast and growing, ADNF is new and the relationship of ADNF/hsp60 and VIP to neurodegeneration–neuroprotection and neuroglial interaction is the focus of future research years. It is important to add that the Alzheimer's brain shows a reduction in VIP [40]. Given the increased potency of the VIP-based SNV, and the femtomolar activity of ADNF-based peptides, a novel therapeutic approach to combat Alzheimer's neurodegeneration is suggested here.

CONCLUSIONS

In summary, the key neuropeptide, vasoactive intestinal peptide (VIP), has been shown to be tightly regulated during development and aging. Daily rhythms, synaptic activity and hormonal changes contribute to the regulation of VIP gene expression. VIP has been shown to facilitate its own expression as well. The marked reduction in VIP transcription with aging and the activity-dependent regulation of VIP content, coupled with the findings of VIP association with neuronal survival, learning and memory, prompted research into mechanisms of action. These studies led to the discovery of potent lipophilic peptides and the femtomolar-acting activity-dependent neurotrophic factor (ADNF).

ACKNOWLEDGEMENTS

Professor Illana Gozes is the incumbent of the Lily and Avraham Gildor Chair for the Investigation of Growth Factors. Supported, in part, by the US–Israel Binational Science Foundation (BSF).

REFERENCES

1. Gozes I, Brenneman DE. VIP molecular biology and neurobiological function. Mol Neurobiol 1989; 3: 201–36.
2. Brenneman DE, Eiden LE. Vasoactive intestinal peptide and electrical activities influence neuronal survival. Proc Natl Acad Sci USA 1985; 83: 1159–62.
3. Brenneman DE, Neale EA, Foster GA, d'Autremont SW, Westbrook GL. Non-neuronal cells mediate neurotrophic action of vasoactive intestinal peptide. J Cell Biol 1987; 104: 1603–10.

4. Brenneman DE, Nicol T, Warren D, Bowers LM. Vasoactive intestinal peptide: a neurotrophic releasing agent and an astroglial mitogen. J Neurosci Res 1990; 25: 386–94.

5. Bodner M, Fridkin M, Gozes I. VIP and PHM-27 sequences are located on two adjacent exons in the human gnome. Proc Natl Acad Sci USA 1985; 82: 3548–51.

6. Gozes I, Shani Y, Rostene W. Developmental expression of the VIP-gene in brain and intestine. Mol Brain Res 1987; 2: 137–48.

7. Gozes I, Shachter P, Shani Y, Giladi E. Vasoactive intestinal peptide gene expression from embryos of aging rats. Neuroendocrinology 1988; 47: 27–31.

8. Gozes I, Meltzer E, Rubinrout S, Brenneman DE, Fridkin M. Vasoactive intestinal peptide potentiates sexual behavior: inhibition by novel antagonist. Endocrinology 1989; 125: 2945–9.

9. Gozes I, McCune SK, Jacobson L, Warren D, Moody TW, Fridkin M, Brenneman DE. An antagonist to vasoactive intestinal peptide: effect on cellular functions in the central nervous system. J Pharmacol Exp Ther 1991; 257: 959–66.

10. Gozes Y, Brenneman DE, Fridkin M, Asofsky R, Gozes I. A VIP antagonist distinguishes VIP receptors on spinal cord cells and lymphocytes. Brain Res 1991; 540: 319–21.

11. Glowa JR, Panlilio LV, Brenneman DE, Gozes I, Fridkin M, Hill JM. Learning impairment following intracerebral administration of the HIV envelope protein gp120 or a VIP antagonist. Brain Res 1992; 570: 49–53.

12. Hill JM, Gozes I, Hill JL, Fridkin M, Brenneman DE. Vasoactive intestinal antagonist retards the development of neonatal behaviors in the rat. Peptides 1991; 12: 187–92.

13. Gressens P, Hill JM, Gozes I, Fridkin M, Brenneman DE. Growth factor function of vasoactive intestinal peptide in whole cultured mouse embryos. Nature 1993; 362: 155–8.

14. Moody TW, Zia F, Draoui M, Brenneman DE, Fridkin M, Davidson A, Gozes I. A novel antagonist inhibits non-small cell lung cancer growth. Proc Natl Acad Sci USA 1993; 90: 4345–9.

15. Gressen P, Hill JM, Paindaveine B, Gozes I, Fridkin M, Brenneman DE. Severe microcephally induced by blockade of vasoactive intestinal peptide function in the primitive neuroepithelium of the mouse. J Clin Invest 1994; 2020–27.

16. Gozes I, Lilling G, Glazer R, Ticher R, Ashkenasi IE, Davidson A, Rubinraut S, Fridkin M, Brenneman DE. Superactive lipophilic peptides discriminate multiple VIP receptors. J Pharmacol Exper Therap 1995; 273: 161–7.

17. Gozes I, Glowa JR, Brenneman JR, McCune SK, Lee E, Westphal H. Learning and sexual deficiencies in transgenic mice carrying a chimeric vasoactive intestinal peptide gene. J Mol Neurosci 1993; 4: 185–93.

18. Gozes I, Bachar M, Bardea A, Davidson A, Rubinraut S, Fridkin M. Protection against developmental deficiencies by a lipophilic VIP analogue. Neurochem Res 1998; 23: 689–93.

19. Fisher A, Brandeis R, Pittel Z, Karton I, Sapir M, Dachir S, Levy A, Heldman E. (+–)-cis-2-methyl-spiro(1,3-oxathiolane-5,3') quinuclidine (AF102B): a new M1 agonist attenuates cognitive dysfunctions in AF64A-treated rats. Neurosci Lett 1998; 102; 325–31.

20. Gozes I, Bardea A, Reshef A, Zamostiano R, Zhukovsky S, Rubinraut S, Fridkin M, Brenneman DE. Novel neuropeprotective strategy for Alzheimer's disease: inhalation of a fatty neuropeptide. Proc Natl Acad Sci 1996; 93: 427–32.

21. Plump AS, Smith JD, Hayek T, Aalto-Setala K, Walsh A, Verstuyft JG, Rubin EM, Breslow JL. Severe hypercholesterolemia and atherosclerosis in apolipoprotein E-deficient mice created by homologous recombination in ES cells. Cell 1992; 71: 343–53.

22. Gozes I, Bachar M, Bardea A, Davidson A, Rubinraut S, Fridkin M, Giladi E. Protection against developmental retardation in apolipoprotein E-deficient mice by a fatty neuropeptide: implication for early treatment of Alzheimer's disease. J Neurobiol 1997; 33: 329–42.

23. Oitzl MS, Mulder M, Lucassen PJ, Havekes LM, Grootendorst J, de Kloet ER. Severe learning deficits in apolipoprotein E knockout mice in a water maze task. Brain Res 1997; 752: 189–96.

24. Masliah E, Samuel W, Veinbergs I, Mallory M, Mante M, Saito T. Neuro-degeneration and cognitive impairment in apoE-deficient mice is ameliorated by infusion of recombinant apoE. Brain Res 1997; 751: 307–14.

25. Gordon I, Grauer E, Genis I, Sehayek E, Michaelson DM. Memory deficits and cholinergic impairments in apolipoprotein E-deficient mice. Neurosci Lett 1995; 199: 1–4.

26. Brenneman DE, Hill JM, Gressens P, Gozes I. Neurotrophic action of VIP: from CNS ontogony to therapeutic strategy. From: Proinflammatory and Anti-inflammatory Peptide. In: Said SI (ed) Lung Biology in Health and Disease. New York: Marcel Dekker, 1998; 383–408.

27. Brenneman DE, Gozes I. A femtomolar-acting neuroprotective peptide. J Clin Invest 1996; 97: 2299–307.

28. Brenneman DE, Hauser J, Neale E, Rubinraut S, Fridkin M, Davidson A, Gozes I. Activity-dependent neurotrophic factor: structure–activity relationships of femtomolar-acting peptides. J Pharmacol Exp Therap 285, 1998; 619–27. On-line: http://www.jpet.org.

29. Gozes I, Brenneman DE. Activity-dependent neurotrophic factor (ADNF): an extracellular neuroprotective chaperonin? J Molec Neurosci 1996; 7: 235–44.

30. Gozes I, Davidson A, Gozes Y, Mascolo R, Barth R, Warren D, Hauser J, Brenneman DE. Antiserum to activity-dependent neurotrophic factor produces neuronal cell death in CNS cultures: immunological and biological specificity. Dev Brain Res 1997; 99: 167–75.

31. Bassan M, Zamostiano R, Davidson A, Wollman Y, Pitman J, Hauser J, Brenneman DE, Gozes I. The identification of secreted heat shock 60 (hsp60)-like protein from rat glial cells and a human neuroblastoma cell line. Neurosci Lett 1998; 249: 1–4.

32. Harmar AJ, Arimura A, Gozes I, Journot L, Laburthe M, Pisegna JR, Rawlings SR, Robberecht P, Said SI, Sreedharan SP, Wank SA, Waschek JA. International Union of Pharmacology XVIII: nomenclature of receptors for vasoactive intestinal peptide (VIP) and pituitary adenylate cyclase-activating polypeptide (PACAP). Pharmacol Rev 1998; 50: 265–70.

33. Ashur-Fabian O, Giladi E, Brenneman DE, Gozes I. Identification of VIP/PACAP receptors on astrocytes using antisense oligodeoxynucleotides. J Mol Neurosci 1997; 9: 211–22.

34. Zupan V, Hill JM, Brenneman DE, Gozes I, Fridkin M, Robberecht P, Evrard P, Gressens P. Involvement of pituitary adenylate cyclase-activating polypeptide II vasoactive intestinal peptide 2 receptor in mouse neocortical astrocytogenesis. J Neurochem 1998; 70: 2165–73.

35. Mackay M, Fantes J, Scherer S, Boyle S, West K, Tsui LC, Belloni E, Lutz E, Van Heyningen V, Harmar AJ. Chromosomal localization in mouse and human of the vasoactive intestinal peptide receptor type 2 gene: a possible contributor to the holoprosencephaly 3 phenotype. Genomics 1996; 37: 345–53.
36. Sreedharan SP, Huang JX, Cheung MC, Goetzl EJ. Structure, expression, and chromosomal localization of the type I human vasoactive intestinal peptide receptor gene. Proc Natl Acad Sci USA 1995; 92: 2939–43.
37. Lilling G, Wollman Y, Goldstein MN, Rubinraut S, Fridkin M, Brenneman DE, Gozes I. Inhibition of human neuroblastoma growth by a specific VIP antagonist. J Mol Neurosci 1995; 5: 231–9.
38. Mohney RP, Zigmond RE. Vasoactive intestinal peptide enhances its own expression in sympathetic neurons after injury. J Neurosci 1998; 18: 5285–93.
39. Gressens P, Marret S, Martin JL, Laquerriere A, Lombet A, Evrard P. Regulation of neuroprotective action of vasoactive intestinal peptide in the murine developing brain by protein kinase C and mitogen-activated protein kinase cascades: in vivo and in vitro studies. J Neurochem 1998; 70: 2574–84.
40. Zhou JN, Hofman MA, Swaab DF. VIP neurons in the human SCN in relation to sex, age, and Alzheimer's disease. Neurobiol Aging 1995; 16: 571–6.

Address for correspondence:
Professor Illana Gozes,
Department of Clinical Biochemistry,
Sackler School of Medicine, Tel Aviv University, Tel Aviv, Israel
Tel: 972 3 640 7240; fax: 972 3 640 8541;
e-mail: igozes@post.tau.ac.il

81 Nicotinic Receptor Stimulation Protects Neurons against Glutamate- and Amyloid-β-induced Cytotoxicity

T. KIHARA, S. SHIMOHAMA AND A. AKAIKE

INTRODUCTION

Alzheimer's disease (AD) is one of the most common forms of dementia and there are no definitive treatments or prophylactic agents for this neuro-degenerative disease, which is characterized by the presence of two types of abnormal deposits, senile plaques (SP) and neurofibrillary tangles (NFT), and by extensive neuronal loss. Although pathologic changes are found in the brains of AD patients, they can be found in the brains of normal elderly individuals, possibly because early changes may predate development of symptoms. SPs are composed of a core of amyloid-β (Aβ), and it has been hypothesized that accumulation of Aβ precedes other pathologic changes and causes neurodegeneration or neuronal death *in vivo*. On the other hand, glutamate, one of the neurotransmitters in the CNS, can cause intracellular calcium influx, activation of calcium-dependent enzymes such as nitric oxide (NO) synthase, and production of toxic oxygen radicals leading to cell death. In addition, some reports indicated that Aβ causes the reduction of glutamate uptake in cultured astrocytes [1], indicating that Aβ-induced cytotoxicity might be, to some extent, mediated via glutamate cytotoxicity.

There are two strategies for therapies for the neurodegenerative diseases. One is replacement therapy, like L-dopa in Parkinson's disease. The other is protection of cells. In studying the latter strategy, we selected nicotinic receptor agonists because degeneration of cholinergic projections to the cerebral cortex is among the most prominent pathologic changes, while nicotinic receptors are reduced in number in AD [2]. In the present study we examined the protective effect of nicotinic receptor stimulation against Aβ- and glutamate-induced cytotoxicity.

Alzheimer's Disease and Related Disorders
Edited by K. Iqbal, D.F. Swaab, B. Winblad and H.M. Wisniewski
© 1999 John Wiley & Sons Ltd

SUBJECTS AND METHODS

MATERIALS

Eagle's minimum essential medium (EMEM) was purchased from Nissui Pharmaceutical Co. The drugs and sources were as follows: amyloid-β protein (25–35) (Bachem); ionomycin (Calbiochem); (–)-nicotine and dihydro-β-erythroidine (DHβE) (Research Biochemicals International); α-bungarotoxin (Wako); 3-(2,4)-dimethoxybenzylidene anabaseine (DMXB) (Taiho Pharmaceutical Co.); and cytisine (Sigma).

CELL CULTURE

Primary cultures were obtained from the cerebral cortex of fetal rats (17–19 days gestation) by procedures described previously [3–5]. Only mature cultures (10–14 days *in vitro*) were used for the experiments. The animals were treated in accordance with the guidelines published in *The NIH Guide for the Care and Use of Laboratory Animals*.

MEASUREMENT OF NEUROTOXICITY

Neurotoxicity was quantitatively assessed by the methods described previously [3–5]. Cell viability was assessed by Trypan blue exclusion method.

STATISTICS

Data are expressed as the percentage of surviving neurons relative to the number of neurons in control culture and represents the mean ± SE. Statistical significance was determined using one-way analysis of variance (ANOVA) followed by a Tukey–Kramer multiple comparisons test.

RESULTS

GLUTAMATE CYTOTOXICITY

The cell viability was decreased by 10 min treatment with 1 mM glutamate followed by 1 h incubation with glutamate-free medium (Figure 1A). Incubating the cultures with 10 μM nicotine for 24 h prior to glutamate exposure significantly reduced glutamate cytotoxicity (Figure 1A). To investigate whether nicotine-induced neuroprotection is due to a specific effect mediated by nicotinic receptors, the effects of cholinergic antagonists were examined. Dihydro-β-erythroidine (DHβE), an α4β2 nicotinic receptor antagonist, was added to the medium containing nicotine. Figure 1A shows that the protective effect of nicotine was reduced by DHβE. The protective effect of nicotine was also reduced by α-bungarotoxin (α-BTX), an α7 selective nicotinic receptor antagonist.

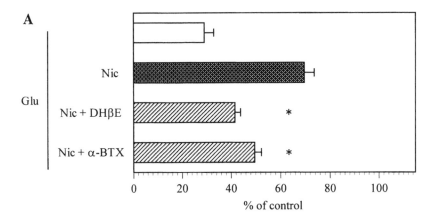

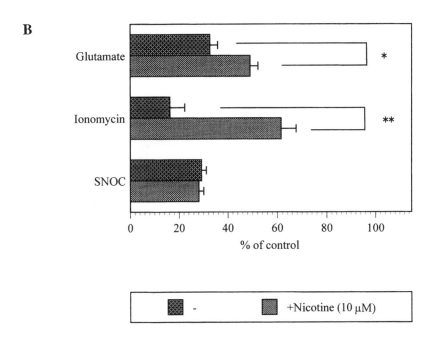

Figure 1. (A) Effects of nicotine (Nic) on glutamate (Glu)-induced neurotoxicity. Cultures were exposed to each 1 mM glutamate for 10 min followed by a 1 h incubation. Nicotine was added to medium for 24 h prior to the exposure to glutamate. Nicotine (10 μM) and α-BTX (1 nM) or DHβE were added simultaneously to medium. n = 5. *p < 0.01 compared with nicotine plus glutamate. (B) Effect of nicotine on glutamate, ionomycin and SNOC toxicity. Cultures were exposed to each neurotoxin for 10 min followed by a 1 h incubation. Nicotine was added for 24 h prior to application of neurotoxins. *p < 0.05, **p < 0.01

To investigate the mechanism of the protective effect of nicotine, we examined the effect of nicotine against ionomycin, a calcium ionophore, and SNOC, an NO-generating agent (Figure 1B). Incubating the cultures for 10 min in either 3 μM ionomycin- or 300 μM SNOC-containing medium markedly reduced viable cells. A 24 h pretreatment of nicotine significantly attenuated the ionomycin cytotoxicity. In contrast, nicotine did not affect SNOC cytotoxicity.

AMYLOID-β CYTOTOXICITY

We used the 25–35 fragment of Aβ peptide because of the reported neurotoxic effects of this fragment. A 48 h exposure to 20 μM Aβ caused a reduction of the neuronal cells significantly. Incubating the cultures with nicotine significantly reduced Aβ-induced cytotoxicity when nicotine was added simultaneously to the medium containing Aβ. Figure 2A shows that the protective effect of nicotine was reduced by DHβE. The protective effect of nicotine was also reduced by α-BTX.

EFFECT OF NICOTINIC RECEPTOR AGONISTS ON Aβ CYTOTOXICITY

The effect of a selective $\alpha4\beta2$ nicotinic receptor agonist, cytisine, against Aβ cytotoxicity was also examined. Figure 3A summarizes the concentration-dependent relationship of cytisine-induced protection against Aβ cytotoxicity. The reduction of Aβ cytotoxicity was statistically significant when cytisine was provided at concentration 10 μM. The effect of a selective $\alpha7$ nicotinic receptor agonist, 3-(2,4)-dimethoxybenzylidene anabaseine (DMXB) [6], against Aβ cytotoxicity was examined. Figure 3B summarizes the concentration-dependent relationship of DMXB-induced protection against Aβ cytotoxicity. The reduction of Aβ cytotoxicity was statistically significant when DMXB was provided at concentrations over 1 μM.

DISCUSSION

There is still controversy over the role of Aβ and glutamate in the pathogenesis of AD. However, evidence is accumulating that Aβ is directly neurotoxic in most culture systems. Likewise, in our culture system, Aβ induced neuronal death. Amyloid accumulation is one of the earliest changes in AD pathology, and this peptide may cause neuronal death in the CNS. The precise mechanism of Aβ-induced cytotoxicity remains unknown, although various hypotheses are now suggested. Oxidative stress or free radical generation is one of the candidates for mediating Aβ-induced cytotoxicity [7]. Recent reports indicated that Aβ stimulates nitric oxide (NO) production in astrocyte culture

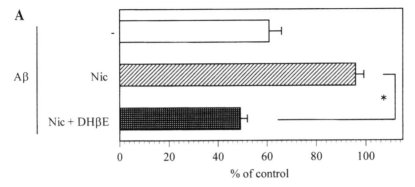

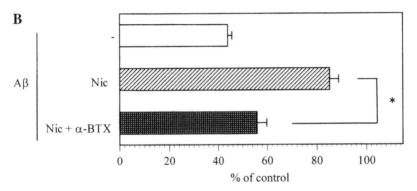

Figure 2. (A) Effect of α4β2 nicotinic receptor antagonist, dihydro-β-erythroidine (DHβE), on nicotine-induced neuroprotection against 20 μM of Aβ cytotoxicity. n = 5. * p < 0.001. (B) Effects of nicotine (Nic) on amyloid-β (Aβ)-induced neurotoxicity. Nicotine was added to medium containing 20 μM Aβ simultaneously and incubated for 48 h. α-Bungarotoxin (α-BTX) is a selective α7 nicotinic receptor antagonist. Nicotine (10 μM) and α-BTX (1 nM) were added simultaneously to medium. n = 5. * p < 0.01

through a NF-κB-dependent mechanism [8], or through Ca^{2+} entry triggered by activated N-methyl-D-aspartate (NMDA)-gated channels in certain cell lines [9]. Other reports have suggested that Aβ inhibits glutamate uptake [10]. These reports imply that Aβ-induced cytotoxicity might be at least in part mediated via glutamate toxicity. Glutamate is thought to induce Ca^{2+} entry, which activates NO synthase (NOS) to form NO, which reacts with superoxide to form peroxynitrite. NO and peroxynitrite exert neurotoxic effects as a result of initiating free radical-mediated lipid peroxidation and sulfhydryl oxidation [11, 12]. Our data indicated that nicotine inhibited the glutamate-induced cytotoxicity by NOS regulation because nicotine inhibited neurotoxicity induced by glutamate and by ionomycin, although NO toxicity was not blocked [12].

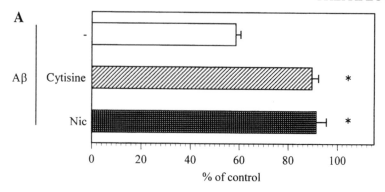

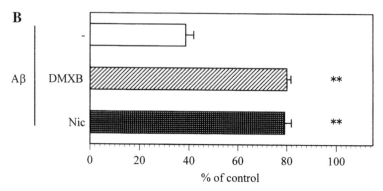

Figure 3. (A) Dose–response relationship of cytisine-induced protection against Aβ (20 μM) cytotoxicity. Cytisine, an α4β2 nicotinic receptor agonist, was added simultaneously with Aβ for 48 h. n = 5. * p < 0.001, compared with Aβ alone. (B) Concentration-dependent neuroprotective effects of DMXB, a selective α7 agonist, against Aβ cytotoxicity. DMXB was added to the medium containing Aβ (20 μM) and incubated for 48 h. Nic, nicotine. n = 5. ** p < 0.01, compared with Aβ alone

In the brain, nicotinic receptors show some receptor subtypes with differing properties and functions. At least six α-subunits (α2–α7, α9 in mammals; α8 in chicks) and three β-subunits (β2–β4) have been identified in the brain. Both α- and β-subunits are required to form functional receptors, with the exception of α7 subunits [13]. In rat brain, over 85% of acetylcholine binding is reported to reflect the presence of the α4 subunit. The α4 subunit is the most widely expressed in rodent CNS. Our present study indicated that stimulation of α4β2 nicotinic receptors, which include α4 subunits, protected neurons from Aβ-induced cytotoxicity. This implies that stimulation of α4β2 nicotinic receptors could protect vast parts of cholinergic neurons.

On the other hand, the abundant presence of α7 receptors in the hippocampus, neocortex and basal ganglia [14], in conjunction with memory-enhancing actions of selective α7 nicotinic agonists such as DMXB, indicate a significant role for α7 receptors in learning and memory. The protective action of nicotine against Aβ cytotoxicity is mediated at least in part through the α7 receptors. Highly permeable to Ca^{2+}, α7 receptors are rapidly desensitized after activation [15]. These channel properties suggest that the receptors modulate neuronal Ca^{2+} homeostasis.

The cholinergic system is affected in dementing disease such as AD, and a reduction of the number of nicotinic receptors is reported [16]. This may be because damage to nicotinic receptors precedes neuronal cell death or neurodegeneration. Nicotine might function not only as a cholinergic agonist but possibly also as a neuroprotective agent. Our present study suggests that nicotinic receptor stimulation may be able to protect neurons from degeneration induced by Aβ or glutamate. Thus, when we make an early diagnosis of AD and start protective therapy with nicotinic receptor stimulation, we could delay the progress of AD.

REFERENCES

1. Harris ME, Wang Y, Pedigo NW Jr, Hensley K, Butterfield DA, Carney JM. Amyloid beta peptide (25–35) inhibits Na^+-dependent glutamate uptake in rat hippocampal astrocyte cultures. J Neurochem 1996; 67: 277–86.

2. Shimohama S, Taniguchi T, Fujiwara M, Kameyama M. Changes in nicotinic and muscarinic cholinergic receptors in Alzheimer-type dementia. J Neurochem 1986; 46: 288–93.

3. Akaike A, Tamura Y, Sato Y, Ozaki K, Matsuoka R, Miura S, Yoshinaga T. Cholecystokinin-induced protection of cultured cortical neurons against glutamate neurotoxicity. Brain Res 1991; 557: 303–7.

4. Tamura Y, Sato Y, Akaike A, Shiomi H. Mechanisms of cholecystokinin-induced protection of cultured cortical neurons against N-methyl-D-aspartate receptor-mediated glutamate cytotoxicity. Brain Res 1992; 592: 317–25.

5. Shimohama S, Ogawa N, Tamura Y, Akaike A, Tsukahara T, Iwata H, Kimura J. Protective effect of nerve growth factor against glutamate-induced neurotoxicity in cultured cortical neurons. Brain Res 1993; 632: 296–302.

6. Hunter BE, de Fiebre CM, Papke RL, Kem WR, Meyer EM. A novel nicotinic agonist facilitates induction of long-term potentiation in the rat hippocampus. Neurosci Lett 1994; 168: 130–34.

7. Behl C, Davis JB, Lesley R, Schubert D. Hydrogen peroxide mediates amyloid beta protein toxicity. Cell 1994; 77: 817–27.

8. Akama KT, Albanese C, Pestell RG, Van Eldik LJ. Amyloid beta-peptide stimulates nitric oxide production in astrocytes through an NF kappa B-dependent mechanism. Proc Natl Acad Sci USA 1998; 95: 5795–800.

9. Le WD, Colom LV, Xie WJ, Smith RG, Alexianu M, Appel SH. Cell death induced by beta-amyloid 1–40 in MES 23.5 hybrid clone: the role of nitric oxide and NMDA-gated channel activation leading to apoptosis. Brain Res 1995; 686: 49–60.

10. Harris ME, Carney JM, Cole PS, Hensley K, Howard BJ, Martin L, Bummer P, Wang Y, Pedigo NW Jr, Butterfield DA. Beta-amyloid peptide-derived, oxygen-dependent free radicals inhibit glutamate uptake in cultured astrocytes: implications for Alzheimer's disease. NeuroReport 1995; 6: 1875–9.

11. Kume T, Kouchiyama H, Kaneko S, Maeda T, Kaneko S, Akaike A, Shimohama S, Kihara T, Kimura J, Wada K, Koizumi S. BDNF prevents NO mediated glutamate cytotoxicity in cultured cortical neurons. Brain Res 1997; 756: 200–204.

12. Shimohama S, Akaike A, Kimura J. Nicotine-induced protection against glutamate cytotoxicity: nicotinic cholinergic receptor-mediated inhibition of nitric oxide formation. Ann NY Acad Sci 1996; 777: 356–61.

13. Seguela P, Wadiche J, Dineley MK, Dani JA, Patrick JW. Molecular cloning, functional properties, and distribution of rat brain alpha 7: a nicotinic cation channel highly permeable to calcium. J Neurosci 1993; 13: 596–604.

14. Clarke PB, Schwartz RD, Paul SM, Pert CB, Pert A. Nicotinic binding in rat brain: autoradiographic comparison of [3H]acetylcholine, [3H]nicotine, and [125I]-alpha-bungarotoxin. J Neurosci 1985; 5: 1307–15.

15. Vijayaraghavan S, Pugh PC, Zhang ZW, Rathouz MM, Berg DK. Nicotinic receptors that bind alpha-bungarotoxin on neurons raise intracellular free Ca^{2+}. Neuron 1992; 8: 353–62.

16. Whitehouse PJ, Kalaria RN. Nicotinic receptors and neurodegenerative dementing diseases: basic research and clinical implications. Alzheimer Dis Assoc Disord 1995; 9: 3–5.

Address for correspondence:
Shun Shimohama MD PhD,
Department of Neurology, Graduate School of Medicine,
Kyoto University,
54 Shogoin-Kawaharacho, Sakyoku, Kyoto 606, Japan
Tel: +81 75 751 3767; fax: +81 75 751 9541;
e-mail: i53367@sakura.kudpc.kyoto-u.ac.jp

82 Biotechnological Production of Aβ Peptides

R.G. VIDAL, X. SHAO, J. GHISO, P. GOREVIC AND B. FRANGIONE

INTRODUCTION

Alzheimer's disease (AD) is the most common form of dementia in elderly people, appearing both sporadically and in an autosomal dominant familial (FAD) form [1]. The defining pathological feature of AD is the presence of an insoluble, fibrous, extracellular deposit of amyloid in the brains of affected patients. The major constituent of these deposits is a hydrophobic 39–43 amino acid peptide named amyloid β peptide (Aβ), a cleavage product of a much larger transmembrane precursor protein (APP) encoded by a single gene on chromosome 21 [2].

Synthetic peptides homologous to Aβ have low solubility and at high concentrations (over μM concentrations) assemble spontaneously into fibrils that are morphologically similar to those found in AD [3]. Aβ peptides can adopt different secondary structures (either mainly α-helical/random coil or β-sheet) when incubated at different pH or solvents [4–6]. Under the conditions in which the peptide adopts the α-helical or random coil structure it aggregates slowly, but when Aβ adopts a β-sheet conformation, it rapidly aggregates. Controversial results have been reported on the effects of Aβ in cell culture and fibril formation (for review, see Neurobiol Aging 1992; 5), perhaps due to variations in the methodology or in peptide preparations. The most important variable seems to be the physical state of the synthetic peptide as a result of the synthesis process, since the peptides were synthesized correctly and were free of contamination. To avoid problems originating from the synthesis process, we have attempted to establish a different system for the production of Aβ peptides by recombinant DNA technology.

Alzheimer's Disease and Related Disorders
Edited by K. Iqbal, D.F. Swaab, B. Winblad and H.M. Wisniewski
© 1999 John Wiley & Sons Ltd

MATERIAL AND METHODS

CLONING STRATEGY

The coding region of Aβ was amplified by PCR with primers, AβF(5'-CATAGCATATGGATGCAGAATTCCGA-3')-NdeI and R(5'-GACAAC-ACCGCCCAC-3') for Aβ40, and R(5'-GCTATGACAACACC-3') for Aβ42 and cloned into vector pCYB1 (New England Biolabs). The 5'-region of the intein and chitin binding domain (CBD) was amplified using oligonucleotides F(5'-TGGGCGGTGTGTCTGCTTTGCCAAGGGT-3') for Aβ40, F(5'-GTGTTGTCATAGCGTGCTTTGCCAAGGGT-3') for Aβ42 and reverse R(5'-CAACAGAAAAGATCT-3')-BglII for both. Equal amounts of both PCR reactions were mixed and amplified with oligonucleotides AβF and reverse R-BglII. The resulting PCR fragments (one for Aβ40 and one for Aβ42) were cloned into the NdeI and BglII site of the pCYB1 expression vector, containing, in addition to an ampicillin resistance gene, a strong P_{tac} promoter and the translation initiation signal of Aβ(Met-1). Aβ peptides were also cloned in-frame with maltose binding protein (MBP) into the pMal-p2 vector (New England Biolabs), introducing the intein and CBD domains from the pCYB1 vector at the C-terminus of the Aβ peptide. Aβ was amplified by PCR with primers (5'-GGGATCGAGGGAAGGGATGCAGAATTCCGA-3') and (5'-GACAACACCGCCCAC-3') for Aβ40 and (5'-CGCTATGACAA-CACC-3') for Aβ42. The intein–CBD domain was amplified using primers F(5'-GTGGGCGGTGTTGTCTGCTTTGCCAAGGGT-3') for Aβ40, F(5'-GGTGTTGTCATAGCGTGCTTTGCCAAGGGT-3') for Aβ42 and R(5'-CTGCAGGTCGACTCATTGAAGCTGCCACAA-3')-Sal I. Double PCRs were performed with both PCR products. PCR was also performed for the malE gene with F(5'-CCGCCACCATGGAAAACGC-3')-NcoI and R(5'-CCTTCCCTCGATCCCGAG-3'). Equal amounts of PCR products were mixed, reamplified using primers malE-F(NcoI) and R(SalI) and the resulting PCR products (one for Aβ40 and one for Aβ42) were cloned into the NcoI and SalI sites of the pMal-p2 vector, which contains an ampicillin resistance gene, a strong P_{tac} promoter and the translation initiation signal of MBP.

PROTEIN EXPRESSION AND PURIFICATION

Bacteria (*Escherichia coli* BL21DE3) carrying the recombinant plasmids were grown containing 100 μg/ml ampicillin with vigorous shaking. When the density of the cultures reached (OD_{600}) 0.5, isopropyl-β-D-thiogalactoside (IPTG) was added to a final concentration of 0.1 mM to induce the production of the recombinant proteins. Aβ–intein–CBD constructs were purified using chitin columns (New England Biolabs) equilibrated with 10 volumes of column buffer (CB: 20 mM HEPES or Tris–HCl (pH 8.0), 500 mM NaCl, 0.1 mM EDTA, 0.1% Triton X-100). Cells were broken by sonication in CB and the lysate clarified by centrifugation. Columns were washed with >10 volumes of CB and flushed with three volumes of cleavage buffer (20 mM HEPES or Tris–HCl (pH 8.0), 50–2000 mM NaCl, 0.1 mM EDTA, 30 mM DTT or 50 mM of 2-mercaptoethanol (β-ME)). Aβ peptides were purified by high performance size exclusion chromatography using a Superdex peptide PC 3.2/30 column (Pharmacia Biotech) in isocratic conditions of 50 mM ammonium bicarbonate (pH 8.0) and rapidly lyophilized. The pMAL-p2 proteins were purified from crude extracts after osmotic shocks or alternatively after sonication. The release of protein was monitored using the Bradford assay. Either supernatant (cold osmotic shock fluid or crude extract) was poured into amylose resin columns. Protein elution was done with CB containing 10 mM maltose. Aβ peptides were released by sequential cleavage with factor Xa (carried out at a w/w ratio of 1% of the amount of fusion protein) and treatment with DTT/βME. Initial expression of the proteins was analyzed by lysing the recovered cells in sodium dodecyl sulfate (SDS)-gel loading buffer and electrophoresis on 16% and 10% SDS–Tris–tricine polyacrylamide gels. After migration, gels were transferred onto PVDF membranes and subjected to Western blotting analysis, using monoclonal antibodies to Aβ (6E10 and 4G8; 1:1000), polyclonal anti-MBP (1:5000) and polyclonal anti-intein (1:500). Fluorograms were prepared with an ECL Western Blotting Kit (Amersham).

RESULTS AND DISCUSSION

The design of the vectors for the expression of Aβ was based on the presence of a fusion protein at the N- and C-terminal regions of Aβ, using a PCR-based cloning strategy (Figure 1).

The expression with IPTG of the fusion gene was done at 37 °C for 2 h in LB with glucose and ampicillin inoculated with 10 ml of an overnight culture of cells containing the Aβ40 or Aβ42 fusion plasmids (variations were tested to find out optimum conditions in pilot experiments). The expression of the fusion plasmids was monitored by Western blotting analysis (Figure 2).

A marked lot-to-lot variability in the secondary structure adopted by synthetic Aβ peptides exists [7], suggesting that slight variations in the synthesis, purification or lyophilization processes may alter significantly the peptide conformation and its fibrillogenic properties. To overcome these problems, recombinant expression of Aβ peptides has been tried in the past [8, 9]. We have developed a different approach to produce recombinant Aβ peptides in *E. coli* that may be used instead of synthetic peptides. Such a peptide will have great advantages over the synthetic ones, and our long-term goal is to use this technology to produce radiolabeled Aβ peptides for studies such as NMR, receptor-binding experiments, and the study of the metabolism, catabolism and blood–brain barrier transport of the Aβ peptide *in vivo*.

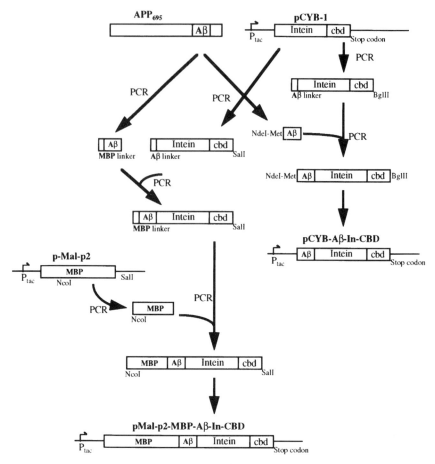

Figure 1. Schematic representation of PCR amplifications and cloning of Aβ peptides into pCYB1 and pMal-p2 vectors

CONCLUSIONS

In summary, synthetic peptides homologous to Aβ have been used to study a variety of processes, including cytotoxicity in cell culture, fibril formation, and blood–brain barrier transport. However, synthetic preparations of Aβ peptide have different secondary structure and a variable degree of physical heterogeneity due to aggregation into inert precipitates and/or fibrils produced during synthesis, purification or labeling. We have designed a new method for producing Aβ peptides fused to maltose binding protein and/or the protein-splicing element named intein in *Escherichia coli*. These fusion proteins can be affinity purified, and the Aβ peptides released by subsequent cleavage with

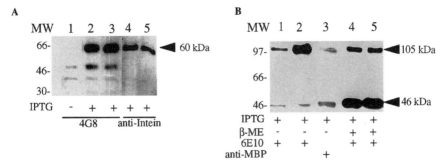

Figure 2. Western blotting analysis of expressed recombinant Aβ peptides. Molecular weights are 60 kDa for Aβ–intein–CBD constructs and 105 kDa for MBP–Aβ–intein–CBD constructs. (A) Cell extracts run on 16% Tris–tricine SDS–PAGE. Lanes 1, 2 and 4 are Aβ40 and lanes 3 and 5 are Aβ42. (B) 10% Tris–tricine SDS–PAGE. Lanes 1, 3 and 4 are MBP–Aβ40–intein–CBD constructs and lanes 2 and 5 are MBP–Aβ42–intein–CBD constructs. The band immunoreactive at 46 kDa is the result of endogenous processing by reductases present in *E. coli*

factor Xa and 2-mercapto-ethanol, which induces a self-cleavage reaction. The Aβ peptides generated by this method are devoid of any residual tag amino acids and they can be radiolabeled *in vivo* using different isotopes without introducing any extra modifications.

ACKNOWLEDGEMENTS

Supported by NIH Grants Nos AG10973 (B.F.) and NS34839 (P.G.) and an Alzheimer's Association Grant (P.G.).

REFERENCES

1. Castaño E, Frangione B. Biology of disease: human amyloidosis, Alzheimer disease and related disorders. Lab Invest 1988; 58: 122–32.
2. Kang J, Lemaire HG, Unterbeck A, Salbaum JM, Masters CL, Grzeschik KH, Multhaup G, Beyreuther K, Muller-Hill B. The precursor of Alzheimer's disease amyloid A4 protein resembles a cell-surface receptor. Nature (Lond) 1987; 325: 733–6.
3. Castaño EM, Ghiso J, Prelli F, Gorevic PD, Migheli A, Frangione B. *In vitro* formation of amyloid fibrils from two synthetic peptides of different lengths homologous to Alzheimer's disease beta-protein. Biochem Biophys Res Commun 1986; 141(2): 782–9.
4. Barrow CJ, Yasuda A, Kenny PT, Zagorski MG. Solution conformations and aggregational properties of synthetic amyloid beta-peptides of Alzheimer's disease. Analysis of circular dichroism spectra. J Mol Biol 1992; 225(4): 1075–93.
5. Burdick D, Soreghan B, Kwon M, Kosmoski J, Knauer M, Henschen A, Yates J, Cotman C, Glabe C. Assembly and aggregation properties of synthetic Alzheimer's A4/beta amyloid peptide analogs. J Biol Chem 1992; 267(1): 546–54.

6. Wood SJ, Wetzel R, Martin JD, Hurle MR. Prolines and amyloidogenicity in fragments of the Alzheimer's peptide β/A4. Biochemistry 1995; 34: 724–30.
7. Simmons LK, May PC, Tomaselli KJ, Rydel RE, Fuson KS, Brigham EF, Wright S, Lieberburg I, Becker GW, Brems DN, Li WY. Secondary structure of amyloid beta peptide correlates with neurotoxic activity *in vitro*. Mol Pharmacol 1994; 45(3): 373–9.
8. Döbeli H, Draeger N, Huber G, Jakob P, Schmidt D, Seilheimer B, Stüber D, Wipf B, Zulauf M. A biotechnological method provides access to aggregation competent monomeric Alzheimer's 1–42 residue amyloid peptide. Biotechnology 1995; 13: 988–93.
9. Seilheimer B, Bohrmann B, Bondolfi L, Müller F, Stüber D, Döbeli H. The toxicity of the Alzheimer's β-amyloid peptide correlates with a distinct fiber morphology. J Struct Biol 1997; 19: 59.

Address for correspondence:
   Ruben G. Vidal PhD,
   Department of Pathology, TH 429 New York University School
      of Medicine,
   550 1st Avenue, New York, NY 10016, USA
   Tel: (212) 263 5775; fax: (212) 263 6751;
   e-mail: vidalr01@popmail.med.nyu.edu

83 β-Sheet Breaker Peptides Prevent the Formation of Fibrillar Amyloid-β Deposits

CLAUDIO SOTO, EINAR M. SIGURDSSON,
LAURA MORELLI, R. ASOK KUMAR,
GABRIELA P. SABORIO, EDUARDO M. CASTAÑO AND
BLAS FRANGIONE

Alzheimer's disease (AD) is neuropathologically characterized by the cerebral deposition of amyloid, an insoluble substance composed mainly of a 39–43 residue peptide, named amyloid β-peptide (Aβ). Genetic, neuropathological and biochemical evidences strongly suggest that amyloid plays an important role in the early pathogenesis of AD. Therefore, inhibiting amyloid deposition in the brain seems a good target for AD therapy. We have postulated that fibrillogenesis can be inhibited by short peptides partially homologous to Aβ that contain residues acting as β-sheet blockers (β-sheet breaker peptides) [1, 2].

In this study we used a five-residue β-sheet breaker peptide, iAβ5 (LPFFD), that was designed using as a template the central hydrophobic region within the N-terminal domain of Aβ (LVFF). Amino acid substitutions in this region of Aβ produce large changes in peptide conformation and its ability to make amyloid fibrils [3–5]. Proline residues, a well-known β-sheet blocker [6, 7], were introduced into the inhibitor to decrease the propensity of the peptide to adopt a β-sheet structure and a charged residue was added at the end of the peptide to increase solubility.

PREVENTION OF Aβ FIBRILLOGENESIS AND NEUROTOXICITY BY iAβ5

iAβ5 partly inhibited in a dose-dependent manner amyloid formation by Aβ1–40 and Aβ1–42 *in vitro*, as studied by thioflavine T binding to amyloid fibrils and by electron microscopy [2]. It has been shown that Aβ is neurotoxic in cell culture and that the toxicity of the peptide is related to the formation of

Alzheimer's Disease and Related Disorders
Edited by K. Iqbal, D.F. Swaab, B. Winblad and H.M. Wisniewski
© 1999 John Wiley & Sons Ltd

oligomeric β-sheet conformation [8]. Therefore, we decided to study the effect of iAβ5 on Aβ-induced toxicity in neuronal culture. For these studies we used human neuroblastoma cells IMR-32. Cells were treated for 2 days with 50 μM aggregated Aβ1–42. Under these conditions a 74% reduction of cell viability was observed, as assessed by DNA/RNA staining with acridine orange-ethidium bromide (AO/EtBr) (Plate III). When Aβ1–42 was co-incubated with a 1.2-fold molar excess of iAβ5 for 48 h prior to addition to the cells, a marked inhibition of Aβ1–42 neurotoxicity (p < 0.01) was observed (Plate III). At 60 μM, iAβ5 was not significantly toxic, as reflected by a cell loss of less than 10% as compared to control cells. The results of this study support the concept that Aβ neurotoxicity is mediated by the formation of a β-pleated sheet structure [8, 9]. However, the relevance of Aβ neurotoxicity *in vitro* to Alzheimer's dementia is unclear at this time [8].

To evaluate the effect of the inhibitor on amyloid deposition *in vivo*, we used a rat model of cerebral Aβ deposition by injecting freshly solubilized Aβ1–42 directly into the amygdala, as described [2, 10]. All the rats injected with Aβ1–42 (5 nmol, 22.5 μg into each amygdala; n = 9) had bilateral Aβ deposits at the injection site, as determined by immunohistochemistry using EM-3, a polyclonal anti-Aβ1–42 antibody [11] (Plate IVA). The deposits were always Congo red-positive, showing the typical apple-green birefringence under polarized light, and were fibrillar as evaluated by electron microscopy analysis (Plate IVB, C). When a 20-fold molar excess of iAβ5 was co-injected with Aβ1–42 (n = 9), smaller Aβ deposits (Plate IVD) were observed that were always Congo red-negative (not shown) and had a punctuate amorphous appearance under electron microscopy (Plate IVE). No deposits were observed in control rats injected with vehicle (n = 6) or iAβ5 alone (n = 6) (data not shown). Image analysis of the brain sections, stained with EM-3, showed that the size of the Aβ deposits was significantly smaller (49% reduction, p = 0.011) in the rats injected with the mixture of Aβ1–42 and iAβ5 than in rats injected with Aβ1–42 alone.

BLOOD–BRAIN BARRIER PERMEABILITY STUDIES

A major drawback with the *in vivo* use of peptides as CNS drugs is that they are subjected to degradation by natural enzymes and exhibit poor blood–brain barrier (BBB) permeability. We have carried out experiments to investigate brain uptake of β-sheet breaker peptides in two different animal species. For those studies we have modified the peptides by introducing a tyrosine residue in order to allow labelling of the peptide with iodine. In a preliminary experiment using the tyrosine-modified 5-residue β-sheet breaker peptide (YiAβ5: LPYFD), Dr B. Zlokovic (personal communication) found that the peptide was mainly retained in the cerebral vessels of guinea pigs without significant brain uptake under the conditions used. However, BBB permeability was observed in rats using an 11-residue tyrosine-modified β-sheet breaker peptide synthesized with D-amino acids (YiAβ11-D: RDLPFYPVPID) [12].

DISCUSSION

This study demonstrates a compound that prevents amyloid neurotoxicity in cell culture, reduces *in vivo* cerebral Aβ deposition and blocks the formation of Congo red-positive amyloid fibrils in the rat brain. The rat model used in this study was developed by intracerebral injections of synthetic Aβ1–42 in solution, which after a certain time aggregates, making fibrillar deposits with staining properties similar to those found in amyloid lesions in Alzheimer's brain. The model is useful as a quick screening tool for Aβ inhibitors. Results on the therapeutic potential of compounds are easily obtained within 1–2 months. The effect of β-sheet breaker peptides on amyloid deposition in APP transgenic mice will be evaluated in the near future when the plasma pharmacokinetics and BBB permeability studies have been completed.

Whether or not amyloid is directly causative to the AD pathogenesis, current data suggest that inhibition of fibril formation is a good target for AD therapy. Moreover, compounds with the capability to prevent and/or revert amyloidosis could be very useful to study the role of amyloid deposition in the histopathological and clinical alterations observed in AD.

ACKNOWLEDGEMENTS

This research was supported by NIH Grants AG05891 (MERIT), AG08721 and AG10953 (LEAD) to B.F. and MH56472 to C.S.

REFERENCES

1. Soto C, Kindy MS, Baumann M, Frangione B. Inhibition of Alzheimer's amyloidosis by peptides that prevent β-sheet conformation. Biochem Biophys Res Commun 1996; 226: 672–80.
2. Soto C, Sigurdsson EM, Morelli L, Kumar RA, Castaño EM, Frangione B. β-sheet breaker peptides inhibit fibrillogenesis in a rat brain model of amyloidosis: implications for Alzheimer's therapy. Nature Med 1998; 4: 822–6.
3. Hilbich C, Kisters-Woike B, Reed J, Masters CL, Beyreuther K. Substitutions of hydrophobic amino acids reduce the amyloidogenicity of Alzheimer's disease βA4 peptides. J Mol Biol 1992; 228: 460–73.
4. Soto C, Castaño EM, Frangione B, Inestrosa NC. The alpha-helical to beta-strand transition in the amino-terminal fragment of the amyloid beta-peptide modulates amyloid formation. J Biol Chem 1995; 270: 3063–7.
5. Tjernberg LO, Naslund J, Lindqvist F, Johansson J, Karlstrom AR, Thyberg J, Terenius L, Nordstedt C. Arrest of β-amyloid fibril formation by a pentapeptide ligand. J Biol Chem 1996; 271: 8545–8.

6. Wood JD, Wetzel R, Martin JD, Hurle MR. Prolines and amyloidogenicity in fragments of the Alzheimer's peptide β/A4. Biochemistry 1995; 34: 724–30.
7. Chou PY, Fasman GD. Empirical predictions of protein conformation. Ann Rev Biochem 1978; 47: 251–76.
8. Yankner BA. Mechanisms of neuronal degeneration in Alzheimer's disease. Neuron 1996; 16: 921–32.
9. Simmons LK et al. Secondary structure of amyloid beta peptide correlates with neurotoxic activity *in vitro*. Mol Pharmacol 1994; 45: 373–9.
10. Sigurdsson EM, Lorens SA, Hejna MJ, Dong XW, Lee JM. Local and distant histopathological effects of unilateral amyloid-β 25–35 injections into the amygdala of young F344 rats. Neurobiol Aging 1996; 17: 893–901.
11. Jimenez-Huete A et al. Antibodies directed to the carboxyl terminus of amyloid beta peptide recognize sequence epitopes and distinct immunoreactive deposits in Alzheimer's disease brain. Alzheimer's Rep 1998; 1: 41–8.
12. Poduslo J, Curran G, Frangione B, Soto C. Polyamine-modified anti-β-sheet peptide inhibitor of Alzheimer's amyloid formation with increased BBB permeability and resistance to proteolytic degradation in plasma. 6th International Conference on Alzheimer's Disease and Related Disorders (Abstract 1069).
13. Duke CR, Cohen JJ, Boehme SA, Lenardo MJ, Surh CD, Kishimoto H, Sprent J, Coligan JE, Kruibeek AM, Margulies DH, Shevach EM, Strober W. Morphological, biochemical and flow cytometric assays of apoptosis. In: Coligan JE, Kruisbeek AM, Margulies DH, Shevach EM, Strober W (eds) Current Protocols in Immunology. New York: Wiley, 1995; 17.1–17.33.

Address for correspondence:
    Dr Claudio Soto,
    New York University Medical Center,
    550 First Avenue, Room TH 427,
    New York, NY 10016, USA
    Tel: 212 2635093; fax: 212 2636751;
    e-mail: Claudio.Soto@mcfpo.med.nyu.edu

84 Modulation of Tau Hyperphosphorylation in apoE-deficient Mice by Muscarinic Activation and Closed Head Injury

I. GENIS, A. FISHER, E. SHOHAMI AND D.M. MICHAELSON

INTRODUCTION

Genetic and epidemiological studies have revealed that the allele E4 of apolipoprotein E (apoE) is a major risk factor for Alzheimer's disease (AD) and suggest that the effects of this apoE allele (apoE4) are mediated by specific impairments in cellular maintenance and repair mechanisms [1, 2]. This assertion is supported by recent studies utilizing apoE-deficient mice, which revealed that apoE deficiency results in memory deficits which are accompanied by specific neurochemical derangements of distinct brain projecting neurons [3, 4]. Furthermore, it was shown that apoE-deficient mice are impaired in their ability to recover neuronal, neurological and cognitive functions following head injury [5].

Tau hyperphosphorylation is a neuropathological hallmark of AD and is presumed to play an important role in the molecular mechanisms underlying its neuropathology [6, 7]. *In vitro* model studies revealed that apoE4, which is the AD risk factor, does not bind effectively to the microtubule binding protein tau and thus, unlike the other apoE isoforms, is unable to block tau phosphorylation [8]. These *in vitro* experiments led to the suggestion that the *in vivo* neuropathological effects of apoE4 in AD are related to its inability to block tau hyperphosphorylation [2, 8, 9]. Accordingly tau phosphorylation in animal models which lack apoE should be more extensive than in normal controls. Indeed, we have previously shown, by use of the anti-phosphorylated tau monoclonal antibody (mAb) AT8, that the epitope recognized by this mAb is hyperphosphorylated in apoE-deficient mice [10].

Alzheimer's Disease and Related Disorders
Edited by K. Iqbal, D.F. Swaab, B. Winblad and H.M. Wisniewski
© 1999 John Wiley & Sons Ltd

It is not yet known whether additional epitopes are hyperphosphorylated in tau of apoE-deficient mice and if any of the neuronal and cognitive deficits of these mice are related to tau hyperphosphorylation. These problems are addressed in this study by immunoblot experiments utilizing a large panel of anti-phosphorylated and non-phosphorylated tau mAbs, and by pharmacological and head injury paradigms in which the known and opposing effects of these treatments on the neuronal and cognitive performances of apoE-deficient and control mice are compared to their effects on tau phosphorylation.

RESULTS

MAPPING OF THE HYPERPHOSPHORYLATED TAU EPITOPES OF apoE-DEFICIENT MICE

This was performed by immunoblot experiments utilizing the following anti-tau mAbs: T46, whose binding to tau is phosphorylation-independent [11, 12]; mAbs RT97 and PHF1, which bind to phosphorylated tau epitopes located on, respectively, the N-terminal and C-terminal of tau [11, 13, 14]; and mAb AT8, which binds to phosphorylated Ser 193, which is situated in the mid-section of tau just N-terminally to its microtubule binding domain [11, 15, 16]. Immunoblots of tau of apoE-deficient and control mice utilizing mAbs T46, AT8 and PHF1 are depicted in Figure 1. As can be seen, the immunoreactivities of the phosphorylation-independent mAb T46 towards tau of apoE-deficient and control mice were similar, suggesting that the total tau levels of the two mice groups are the same. The immunoreactivity of mAb AT8 was markedly higher in tau of apoE-deficient than in control mice

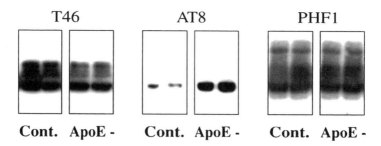

Figure 1. Immunoblots of tau of apoE-deficient (apoE-) and control (Cont.) mice utilizing the phosphorylation-insensitive mAb T46 and the anti-phosphorylated tau mAbs AT8 and PHF1. Results presented correspond to tau of two mice (4 month-old males) from each group. The experiment was performed as previously described [10], utilizing similar amounts of material from each individual mouse. MAbs T46 and AT8 were, respectively, from Zymed Laboratories and Innogenetics, whereas mAb PHF1 was a kind gift from Dr P. Davis

(Figure 1). In contrast, mAbs PHF1 (Figure 1) and RT97 (not shown) re-acted equally with tau of the two mice groups. These findings suggest that tau of apoE-deficient mice is hyperphosphorylated at a selective position which is situated in the mid-section of the molecule.

PHARMACOLOGICAL MANIPULATION OF TAU PHOSPHORYLATION

It has previously been shown [17] that the memory deficits and cholinergic impairments of apoE-deficient mice [3, 4] can both be reversed by chronic treatment with the M_1 muscarinic agonist 1-methyl-piperidine-4-spiro-(2'-methyl-thiazoline) (AF150(S)). We presently examined whether these benefi-cial muscarinic effects are accompanied by diminution or abolition of the difference in tau phosphorylation between the two mice groups. As shown in Figure 2, chronic treatment of the mice with AF150(S) had no effect on the

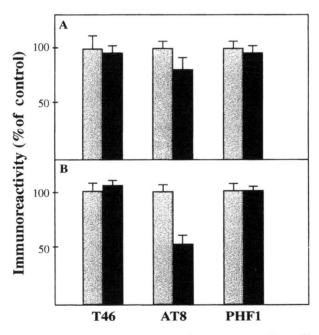

Figure 2. Comparison of the effects of the muscarinic agonist AF150(S) on the mAbs T46, AT8 and PHF1 anti-tau immunoreactivities of control (A) and of apoE-deficient mice (B). The mice were treated orally with AF150(S) (0.5 mg/kg) every day for 3 weeks, after which their brains were removed and rapidly frozen. Results for each of the mAbs were obtained by immunoblot assays and computerized densitometry of three mice in each group which were all run on the same blot. The results (average ± SD) for each of the mAbs and mouse groups (n = 3 in each group) are presented as percentages of the corresponding non-AF150(S)-treated group. The dark bars correspond to AF150(S)-treated mice, whereas the gray-colored bars correspond to sham-treated mice

mAb T46 tau immunoreactivities of the two mice groups, suggesting that this treatment does not affect total tau levels. AF150(S) did, however, cause a marked decrease in the mAb AT8 immunoreactivity of the apoE-deficient mice (p < 0.05) but had a much smaller dephosphorylating effect on the corresponding control tau (Figure 2). In contrast, the PHF1 tau immunoreactivities of the two mice groups (Figure 1) and their mAb RT97 immunoreactivities (not shown) were unaffected by AF150(S). This suggests that AF150(S) has a specific and selective effect on tau of the two mice groups, and that the mAb AT8 epitope, which is hyperphosphorylated in the non-treated apoE-deficient mice (Figure 1), is dephosphorylated in these mice more extensively by AF150(S) than in the controls.

EFFECTS OF HEAD INJURY ON TAU PHOSPHORYLATION

ApoE-deficient mice are particularly susceptible to closed head injury and are impaired in their ability to recover from this insult [5]. We presently examined the effects of closed head injury on the levels of tau phosphorylation of apoE-deficient and control mice and the extent to which this correlates with the increased vulnerability of apoE-deficient mice to head injury. As shown in Figure 3, closed head injury increased the mAb AT8 tau immunoreactivities of the two mice groups. However, the extent of injury-induced hyperphosphorylation of this tau epitope at the time-point examined (e.g. 24 h after injury) was markedly more pronounced in the apoE-deficient mice than in the controls. In contrast, closed head injury had no effect on the tau immunoreactivities of mAbs T46, RT97 and PHF1 of either of the two mice groups (not shown). This suggests that the effect of closed head trauma on tau hyperphosphorylation under these conditions is more pronounced in apoE-deficient than in control mice and is selective for epitopes residing in the mid-section of this molecule.

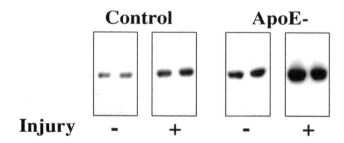

Figure 3. The effects of closed head injury on tau phosphorylation of apoE-deficient and control mice. Two mice from each group were subjected to closed head injury, as previously described [5]. They were sacrificed 24 h following injury, after which tau immunoblots of the injured (+) and the sham-treated (–) mice were prepared and probed with the anti-phosphorylated tau mAb AT8. The immunoblot assays were performed as described in the legend to Figure 1

DISCUSSION

The mAbs AT8, RT97 and PHF1 immunoblot experiments revealed that tau hyperphosphorylation in apoE-deficient mice is epitope-specific. Further experiments utilizing additional anti-tau mAbs (e.g. AT270 and SMI32; to be published) suggest that tau epitopes which reside in the vicinity of that of mAb AT8 are also hyperphosphorylated (not shown), implying that tau of apoE-deficient mice contains a hyperphosphorylated 'hot spot' which resides just N-terminally to the microtubule binding domain of tau. This tau hyperphosphorylation may be due to distinct enzymatic changes which shift the balance between protein kinase and phosphatase activities in favor of the phosphorylated tau state. Alternatively the observed tau hyperphosphorylation may be due to changes in the accessibility of the 'hot spot' tau domain of the apoE-deficient mice to neuronal kinase and phosphatase activities.

The finding that the mAb AT8 epitope, which is hyperphosphorylated in apoE-deficient mice (Figure 1), is preferentially dephosphorylated in these mice following treatment with the muscarinic agonist AF150(S) (Figure 2), and that the levels of phosphorylation of the RT97 and PHF1 epitopes are unaffected by this treatment, suggests that epitopes which reside at or near the hyperphosphorylated tau 'hot spot' are particularly sensitive to experimental manipulation. Indeed, closed head injury also has a selective effect on the AT8 tau epitope. However, in this case the resulting effect is hyperpolarization, whose magnitude 24 h after injury is more pronounced in the apoE-deficient mice (Figure 3). The similarity of the tau epitopes which are affected by M_1 muscarinic activation and by closed head injury, and the vast difference between the pathophysiological effects of these treatments, suggest that what is altered in the apoE-deficient mice is the accessibility of some of the tau epitopes to phosphorylating and dephosphorylating enzymatic activities (e.g. AT8), and not the activities of these enzymes. It is not yet known, however, whether these structural alterations in tau of apoE-deficient mice are due to direct tau conformational changes or to alterations in other proteins which can bind to tau and thereby modulate its accessibility to kinase and phosphatase activities.

Two correlations were observed between the levels of tau phosphorylation and the performance of the apoE-deficient mice: namely, that (a) treatment of apoE-deficient mice with the M_1 muscarinic agonist AF150(S) reverses their cognitive and neurochemical deficits [17] and reduces the extent of their tau hyperphosphorylation (Figure 2); and (b) that closed head injury, to which the apoE-deficient mice are particularly susceptible [5], also results in preferential hyperphosphorylation of their neuronal tau. These correlations suggest that the extent of tau hyperphosphorylation in apoE-deficient mice is a measure of the extent of neuronal stress and dysfunction of these mice.

In summary, this present study shows that tau of apoE-deficient mice contains a distinct, hyperphosphorylated domain, whose levels of phosphorylation are particularly susceptible to distinct pharmacological and brain injury paradigms. This model provides a novel system for studying the mechanisms underlying the effects of apoE on tau phosphorylation *in vivo* and for evaluating the functional and neuropathological ramifications of tau hyperphosphorylation.

CONCLUSIONS

In summary, apolipoprotein E (apoE)-deficient mice have distinct memory deficits which are associated with specific neurochemical changes and with hyperphosphorylation of the tau epitope recognized by mAb AT8. In addition, these mice are particularly susceptible to closed head injury. In the present study we further characterized the extent of tau hyperphosphorylation in apoE-deficient mice and examined the effects thereon of experimental paradigms which either improve or hamper the performance of the mice. This revealed that tau of apoE-deficient mice contains a hyperphosphorylated 'hot spot' which resides near the microtubule binding domain of tau and that the levels of phosphorylation of epitopes which flank this domain are normal. Prolonged treatment of the mice with the muscarinic agonist AF150(S), which has been shown to reverse the cognitive and cholinergic deficits of these mice, results in preferential dephosphorylation of tau of the apoE-deficient mice. In the case of mAb AT8, this results in a marked reduction of the difference in tau phosphorylation between the apoE-deficient and control mice. In contrast, closed head injury resulted in hyperphosphorylation of the AT8 epitope, whose extent 24 h after injury was more pronounced in the apoE-deficient mice. Taken together, these findings suggest that apoE deficiency results in specific alterations in the accessibility of distinct tau domains to phosphorylating and dephosphorylating reactions. This model provides a novel system for studying the mechanisms underlying the effects of apoE on tau phosphorylation and for evaluating the functional and neuropathological ramifications of tau hyperphosphorylation.

ACKNOWLEDGEMENTS

We thank Dr P. Davies for kindly providing us with mAb PHF1. This work was supported in part by grants to DMM from the US–Israel Binational Science Foundation (Grant No. 95/16); from the Joint German–Israeli Research Program (Grant No. 1626); from the Eichenbaum Foundation; and from the Revah-Kabelli Fund. D.M.M. is the incumbent of the Myriam Lebach Chair in Molecular Neurodegeneration at Tel Aviv University.

REFERENCES

1. Poirier J. Apolipoprotein E in animal models of CNS injury and in Alzheimer's disease. Trends Neurosci 1995; 17: 525–30.
2. Roses AD. Apolipoprotein E is a genetic locus that affects the role of Alzheimer's disease expression: β-amyloid burden is a secondary consequence dependent on apoE genotype and duration of disease. J Neuropathol Exp Neurol 1994; 53: 429–37.
3. Gordon I, Grauer E, Genis I, Sehayek E, Michaelson DM. Memory deficits and cholinergic impairment in apolipoprotein E-deficient mice. Neurosci Lett 1995; 199: 1–4.
4. Chapman S, Michaelson DM. Specific neurochemical derangements of brain projecting neurons in apolipoprotein E-deficient mice. J Neurochem 1998; 70: 708–14.
5. Chen Y, Lomnitzki L, Michaelson DM, Shohami E. Motor and cognitive deficits in apolipoprotein E-deficient mice after closed head injury. Neuroscience 1997; 80: 1255–62.
6. Goedert M. Tau protein and the neurofibrillary pathology of Alzheimer's disease. Trends Neurosci 1993; 11: 460–65.
7. Mandelkow E-M, Mandelkow E. Tau as a marker for Alzheimer's disease. Trends Biochem Sci 1993; 18: 480–83.
8. Strittmatter WJ, Saunders AM, Goedert M, Weisgraber KH, Dong LM, Jacks R, Huang DY, Schmechel D, Pericak-Vance M, Roses AD. Isoform specific interaction of apolipoprotein E with the microtubule-associated protein tau: implications for Alzheimer's disease. Proc Natl Acad Sci USA 1994; 91: 243–9.
9. Roses AD. A model for susceptibility polymorphisms for complex diseases: apolipoprotein E and Alzheimer's disease. 1997; 1: 3–11.
10. Genis I, Gordon I, Sehayek E, Michaelson DM. Phosphorylation of tau in apolipoprotein E-deficient mice. Neurosci Lett 1995; 199: 5–8.
11. Kosik KS, Orecchio LD, Binder L, Trojanowski J, Lee VM-Y, Lee G. Epitopes that span the tau molecule are shared with paired helical filaments. Neuron 1988; 1: 817–25.
12. Goedert M, Spillantini MG, Jakes R, Rutherford D, Crowther RA. Multiple isoforms of human microtubule-associated protein tau: sequences and localization in neurofibrillary tangles of Alzheimer's disease. Neuron 1989; 3: 519–26.
13. Brion J-P, Couck A-M, Robertson J, Loviny TLF, Anderton BH. Neurofilament monoclonal antibodies RT97 and 8D8 recognize different modified epitopes in paired helical filament tau in Alzheimer's disease. J Neurochem 1993; 60: 1372–82.
14. Mawal-Dewan M, Henley J, Van de Voorde A, Trojanowski JQ, Lee VM-Y. The phosphorylation state of tau in the developing rat brain is regulated by phosphoprotein phosphatase. J Biol Chem 1994; 269: 30981–7.
15. Lichtenberg-Kraag B, Mandelkow E-M, Biernat J, Steiner B, Schröter C, Gutske N, Meyer HE, Mandelkow E. Phosphorylation-dependent epitopes of neurofilament antibodies on tau protein and relationship with Alzheimer tau. Proc Natl Acad Sci USA 1992; 89: 5384–488.
16. Mercken M, Vandermeeren M, Lubke U, Six J, Bioos J, Van de Voorda A, Martin J, Gheuen J. Monoclonal antibodies with selective specificity for Alzheimer tau are directed against phosphatase-sensitive epitope. Acta Neuropathol 1992; 84: 262–72.

17. Fisher A, Brandeis R, Chapman J, Pittel Z, Michaelson DM. M_1 muscarinic agonist treatment reverses cognitive and cholinergic impairments of apolipoprotein E-deficient mice. J Neurochem 70: 1991–7.

Address for correspondence:
Daniel M. Michaelson,
Department of Neurobiochemistry,
The George S. Wise Faculty of Life Sciences,
Tel Aviv University, Tel Aviv 69978, Israel
Tel: 972 3 6409624 or 6426102; fax: 972 3 6407643;
e-mail: dmichael@ccsg.tau.ac.il

85 CSF Tau Protein Levels Before and After Tacrine Therapy in Patients with Dementia of Alzheimer's Type

MAGDA TSOLAKI, PARASKEVI SAKKA,
OLGA CHATZIZISI, GEORGE KYRIAZIS,
JOHN PAPANASTASIOU AND ARISTIDES KAZIS

INTRODUCTION

Alzheimer's disease (AD), as is well known, is the leading cause of dementia in the elderly. Among all the progressive degenerative brain diseases leading to dementia, AD is the most common (about 75–80% of all cases). The diagnosis of AD in life remains difficult and a definite diagnosis of AD relies on histopathological confirmation at post mortem or by cerebral biopsy.

The brains of all patients with AD are characterized by abundant neurofibrillary tangles (NFT), neuropil threads, dystrophic neurites and senile plaques. NFT represent intracellular accumulations of paired helical filaments (PHF) which are also shared with neuropil threads and dystrophic neurites. The abundant presence of both senile plaques and tangles in the brains of AD patients is the only accepted criterion for the unequivocal diagnosis of AD.

Immunocytochemical and biochemical studies showed that the major component of PHF found in the NFT in the brains of patients with AD is the microtubule-associated protein tau in a highly phosphorylated state [1, 2]. Although this protein was found to be clearly elevated in AD brain tissue [3], its presence in cerebrospinal fluid has been initially difficult to establish. Furthermore, this protein was shown to be indistinguishable from highly phosphorylated forms of microtubule-associated tau [4]. Additional studies have shown that tau is elevated in AD brain homogenates relative to control tissues [5]. During recent years, two other studies, one from Sweden [6] and the other from Japan [7], have found significant differences in CSF tau protein between controls and AD patients.

Alzheimer's Disease and Related Disorders
Edited by K. Iqbal, D.F. Swaab, B. Winblad and H.M. Wisniewski
© 1999 John Wiley & Sons Ltd

Many studies have shown that CSF tau protein levels are increased in patients with dementia of Alzheimer's type. Unfortunately, the specificity of this biochemical test is low, so tau protein levels can not be used as a diagnostic marker for AD. A recent study showed that concentrations of CSF tau were stable at 1 year follow-up in both patients with AD and patients with vascular dementia [8]. Our initial thought was that perhaps CSF tau levels could be used as an objective marker to follow up patients after different treatments. So, the aim of this work was to study CSF tau protein levels before and after treatment with tacrine, the first approved drug for AD patients, and to correlate this possible change with cognitive deterioration. If so, then we would have another more objective way to follow up different therapeutic managements. As far as we know, this is the first study that uses CSF tau protein as an objective marker to follow up patients with AD under anticholinesterase treatment. We examined 20 CSF samples of patients (mean age = 65, 18 ± 6, 27) with AD according to the DSM-IV criteria before and after 6–12 months' treatment with tacrine and 10 CSF samples of AD patients before and after 6–12 months' therapy with nootropics. We recorded MMSE, CAMCOG and FRSSD before and after both treatments. The results showed that CSF tau protein levels were decreased after 6–12 months of treatment with tacrine in AD patients (p = 0.001) while they were not changed after nootropics (p = 0.64). No statistical difference was noticed in all the neuropsychological scales before and after tacrine therapy, while a significant deterioration was noticed in the second group.

MATERIALS AND METHODS

Twenty CSF samples of patients with AD before and after tacrine treatment and 10 CSF samples of patients with AD before and after therapy with other medication were examined by immunoassay hTAU-Ag [9]. Altogether, 241 CSF samples of patients with AD and 81 CSF samples of patients with other neurological disorders were examined during the last 3 years in two different laboratories. Fourteen samples of the same patients were examined in both laboratories to assess the reliability of the method. No statistical difference was noticed between the results (p = 0.26). The diagnosis of AD was according to DSM-IV and NINCDS–ADRDA criteria. MMSE, CAMCOG and FRSSD were used before and after treatment in both groups for the cognitive (MMSE, CAMCOG) and functional (FRSSD) assessment. Hematological, biochemical, serum B12 levels, serum folic acid levels, T3, T4, TSH, VDRL, CT scan or MRI and neurological examinations were performed on all patients.

Table 1 shows the characteristics of the two treatment groups. As can be seen, there are no significant differences between the two groups as far as age, MMSE, CAMCOG, FRSSD and tau protein levels are concerned.

Table 1. Characteristics of the two treatment groups before treatment

Group	Age	MMSE	CAMCOG	FRSSD	Tau
Tacrine	65.18 ± 6.27	14.68 ± 6.67	48.36 ± 23.7	14.38 ± 10.9	266.41
Other medication	65 ± 6.04	14 ± 5.41	39.05 ± 17.6	13.94 ± 7.49	199.58
	p = 0.9	p = 0.72	p = 0.16	p = 0.88	p = 0.16

STATISTICS

Wilcoxon matched pairs test was used for statistical analysis between the two groups.

RESULTS

Table 2 shows the mean and standard deviation of all parameters studied in this work, before and after treatment. There was a significant decrease (p = 0.001) in CSF tau protein levels in the tacrine group and no significant change (0.64) in CSF tau protein levels in the group with other medication. No statistical difference was noticed in any of the neuropsychological scales before and after tacrine therapy, while a significant deterioration was noticed in the second group.

Table 2. All parameters before and after treatment in both groups

Group		MMSE	CAMCOG	FRSSD	Tau
Tacrine	Before	14 ± 6.6	48 ± 23	14 ± 10	266.4 ± 105
	After	13.6 ± 5	42 ± 20	16.4 ± 8	177.8 ± 101
p Value		p = 0.8	p = 0.17	p = 0.4	p = 0.001
Other medication	Before	14 ± 5.4	39 ± 17	13.9 ± 7	199.5 ± 124
	After	10 ± 6.9	28 ± 23	18 ± 10	216 ± 106
p Value		p = 0.0014	p = 0.0048	p = 0.003	p = 0.64

DISCUSSION

It is well-known that CSF tau protein levels are increased in patients with AD. Our results of all samples which were examined also confirm these previous data. Until now there was no objective marker to follow up AD patients who take medication, apart from neuropsychological scales. The results from this study open a new chapter on this direction.

There is some evidence that CSF tau levels are significantly increased during a follow-up period [10] while other authors report that concentrations of CSF tau remain stable at 1 year follow-up [8]. The present study confirms the second finding. From the new data of this study, tacrine seems to stop further possible destruction of brain for a short period of life and inhibits both cognitive and functional deterioration. The question is, how tacrine can stop this cellular destruction. As is well known, the pharmacology of tacrine has been widely studied since it was first synthesized in 1945 by Albert and Gledhill. In a recent review, tacrine, except for the inhibition of cholinesterases *in vitro* and *in vivo*, seems to have interactions with muscarinic receptors, interactions with ion channels—Na^+, K^+ and Ca^{++}—and interactions with the release and uptake of neurotransmitters other than ACh, so we could say that tacrine prevents the destruction of brain cells, like GABA (inhibits the release of GABA), 5-hydroxytryptamine, noradrenaline, histamine, and dopamine evokes the release of these neurotransmitters [11], if we accept the recent observation that a significant K^+ outflow is observed during apoptosis [12] and the phosphorylation status of proteins is dependent on changes in intracellular Ca^{2+} [13]. On the other hand, tacrine is rapidly taken up into the brain and shows regional localization to cortex, hippocampus, thalamus and striatum. Regional uptake into the brain also does not correlate consistently with the distribution of AChE [14]. All these data support the hypothesis that tacrine having all these effects on the brain tissue can inhibit further cellular destruction, decrease the release of tau protein and perhaps retard the progression of the disease.

REFERENCES

1. Grundke-Iqbal I, Iqbal K, Quilan M, Tung Y-C, Ziada MS, Wiesniewski HM. Microtubule-associated protein tau: a component of Alzheimer paired helical filaments. J Biol Chem 1986; 261: 6084–9.
2. Wolozin B, Pruchnicki A, Dickson DW, Davies P. A neural antigen in the brains of Alzheimer patients. Science 1986; 232: 648–50.
3. Ghanbari HA, Miller BF, Haigler HJ et al. Biochemical assay of Alzheimer's disease-associated protein(s) in human brain tissue. JAMA 1990; 263: 2907–10.
4. Ksiezak-Reding H, Davies P, Yen S. Alz-50, a monoclonal antibody to AD antigens, crossreacts with tau proteins in bovine and normal human brain. J Biol Chem 1988; 263: 7943–6.
5. Khatoon S, Grundke-Iqbal I, Iqbal K. Brain levels of microtubule-associated protein tau are elevated in Alzheimer's disease: a radioimmuno-blot assay for nanograms of the protein. J Neurochem 1992; 59: 750–53.
6. Jensen M, Basun H, Lannfelt L. Increased cerebrospinal fluid tau in patients with Alzheimer's disease. Neurosci Lett 1995; 186: 189–91.
7. Hiroyuki A, Terajima M, Miura M, Higuchi S, Muramatsu T, Machida N, Seiki H, Takese S, Clark C, Lee VM-Y, Trojanowski JQ, Sasaki H. Tau in cerebrospinal fluid: a potential diagnostic marker in Alzheimer's disease. Ann Neurol 1995; 38: 649–52.

8. Andreasen N, Vanmechelen E, Van-de-voorde A, Davidsson P, Hesse C, Tarvonen S, Raiha I, Sourander L, Winblad B, Blennow K. Cerebrospinal fluid tau protein as a biochemical marker for Alzheimer's disease: a community-based follow-up study. J Neurol Neurosurg Psychiat 1998; 64: 298–305.
9. Tsolaki M, Chatzizisi O, Iakovidou V, Kyriazis G, Kazis A. Elevation of tau protein in patients with AD. South-East European Society for Neurology and Psychiatry, 11th Conference, Thessaloniki, Greece, 25–28 September 1996.
10. Arai H, Terajima M, Miura M, Higuchi S, Muramatsu T, Matsushita S, Machida N, Nakagawa T, Lee VM-Y, Trojanowski JQ, Sasaki H. Effect of genetic risk factors and disease progression on the cerebrospinal fluid tau levels in Alzheimer's disease. J Am Geriat Soc 1997; 45: 1228–31.
11. Freeman SE, Dawson RM. Tacrine: a pharmacological review. Progr Neurobiol 1991; 36: 257–77.
12. Dallaporta B, Hirsch T, Susin SA, Zamzami N, Larochette N, Brenner C, Marzo I, Kroemer G. Potassium leakage during the apoptotic degradation phase. J Immunol 1998; 160: 5605–15.
13. Roeper J, Lorra C, Pongs O. Frequency-dependent inactivation of mammalian A-type K^+ channel KV1.4 regulated by Ca^{2+}/calmodulin-dependent protein kinase. J Neurosci 1997; 17: 3379–91.
14. McNally W, Roth M, Young R, Bockbrader H, Chang T. Quantitative whole-body autoradiographic determination of tacrine tissue distribution in rats following intravenous or oral dose. Pharmaceut Res 1989; 6: 924–30.

Address for correspondence:
Magda Tsolaki,
Assistant Professor of Neurology,
Aristotle University of Thessaloniki,
Despere 3, Thessaloniki 54621, Greece
Fax: +3031 283973, 357603; e-mail: tsolakim@med.auth.gr

IX Non-pharmacological Treatments

86 Decreased Neuronal Activity and Therapeutic Strategies Directed towards Reactivation in Alzheimer's Disease

D.F. SWAAB, P.J. LUCASSEN, A. SALEHI,
E.J.A. SCHERDER, E.J.W. VAN SOMEREN AND
R.W.H. VERWER

Alzheimer's disease (AD) is a multifactorial disease in which APOE-ε4 and age are important risk factors. In addition, various mutations play a role. There is evidence in favor of the hypotheses that: (a) the neuropathological Alzheimer changes cannot all be explained by a cascade starting with amyloid (β/A4) deposits; but that (b) the neuropathological hallmarks of AD are basically independent phenomena; and that (c) cell death in AD is generally not a major occurring phenomenon, but is restricted to a few brain areas; and (d) reduced neuronal activity is most probably one of the major characteristics of AD and may underlie the clinical symptoms of dementia, which makes it attractive to direct therapeutic strategies towards restimulation of neuronal metabolism and repair mechanisms.

The amyloid cascade hypothesis constitutes a major, but controversial, working hypothesis in current AD research. The 'congophilic' components of neuritic plaques (NPs) are assumed to arise from the amorphic Congo red-negative amorphous plaques by aggregation of β/A4-protein fibrils. The neurotoxicity of β/A4 would induce NP formation, the occurrence of neuropil threads and dystrophic neurites, followed by neurofibrillary tangle (NFT) formation and, ultimately, cell death. Although there are certainly arguments in favor of the amyloid cascade hypothesis, there are also data from a large number of papers that do not fit this hypothesis (for reviews, see [1, 2]). The vast majority of AD cases (99.5%) is not linked to APP gene mutations or an extra copy of chromosome 21. The occurrence of familial AD cases linked to chromosomes other than chromosome 21, e.g. chromosome 14 or 1, as well as the cases linked to the APOE-ε4 locus on chromosome 19, are not directly

Alzheimer's Disease and Related Disorders
Edited by K. Iqbal, D.F. Swaab, B. Winblad and H.M. Wisniewski
© 1999 John Wiley & Sons Ltd

linked to the amyloid cascade hypothesis. Moreover, in transgenic mice with APP over-expression, amyloid did not appear to be acutely neurotoxic, or to induce NFTs or NPs.

The hippocampus and cerebral cortex of AD-demented boxers contain many amorphous plaques, NFTs and neuropil threads, but very few, if any, NPs. In addition, in several cases of familial and non-familial AD, NFTs have been found without amyloid deposition. The hypothalamic nucleus tuberalis lateralis (NTL) shows strong early cytoskeletal alterations in AD [3], while amyloid accumulation or silver-stained NPs are rare in the NTL [4]. These observations indicate that cytoskeletal changes may in principle occur independently of aggregated β/A4 fibril amyloid cores. In addition, cytoskeletal changes and amorphous plaques are not related in their localization. Furthermore, amorphous plaques are also found in neurodegenerative disorders other than AD, e.g. progressive supranuclear palsy, Parkinson's disease, Huntington's chorea and frontal lobe dementia. However, in these disorders they are not associated with the presence of NPs or neuropil threads as they are in AD. The most important argument against a transformation, however, is that plaque types that should represent intermediate forms between amyloid plaques and NPs have never been reported [2]. Moreover, 30% of the demented senile 'Alzheimer patients' with plaques in the neocortex appeared to lack tangles in this brain area [5]. These observations suggest that the occurrence of classical NPs and NFTs are phenomena that occur independently of each other.

The last step of the amyloid cascade hypothesis implied that neurons that show cytoskeletal changes are indicative of impending neuronal death and that the process of cell death would be induced by the neurotoxic NPs. Indeed, neurons are lost in a limited number of areas, such as the locus coeruleus [6], the areas CA1 and CA4 of the hippocampus [7] and the superior temporal sulcus, but it should be mentioned that no relationship was found with the number of NPs or NFTs [8]. The earlier reported loss in the large-sized cholinergic neurons in the nucleus basalis of Meynert (NBM) in AD could be explained by cell shrinkage, reduced activity, and loss of cholinergic cell markers, rather than by cell loss [9]. Regeur et al. [10] showed that global neocortical cell loss does not take place in the cortex of AD patients, providing strong evidence that neuronal shrinkage rather than cell death is a major phenomenon in this neurodegenerative disorder. In addition, the Alz-50 staining of the NTL of AD patients is so abundant that it can even be seen with the unaided eye, although the neuron number in AD is not different from that in control subjects [4]. We chose CA1 to study the question of whether or not NPs may induce local cell death. Our study [11] showed that, indeed, there is a slightly lower neuronal density around NPs. However, the contribution of the effect of the neighborhood of a plaque to the total cell death in the CA1 area was very limited, i.e. 2.6% out of the reported cell death of 70%. This study, therefore, again supports the notion that the occurrence of NPs and cell death are for the most part two independent phenomena.

DECREASED NEURONAL ACTIVITY IS A MAJOR HALLMARK OF AD

Various observations indicate that decreased neuronal activity is an essential characteristic of AD, either as a risk factor or as a direct pathogenetic factor, and that high or enhanced neuronal activity would protect against the degenerative changes of aging and of AD, an hypothesis paraphrased as 'use it or lose it' [12]. It has been reported that the AD brain contains a lower total amount of protein, a clear reduction in total cytoplasmic RNA and messenger RNA, reduced glucose metabolism (especially in temporal and parietal lobes, as shown by positron emission tomography, PET), a smaller cell size (such as the somatostatin neurons in the cortex), and a small size of the neuronal Golgi apparatus (GA), indicative of decreased metabolic activity in AD ([9, 13, 14]; for references, see [2]). The changes in regional cerebral glucose metabolism, as measured by PET in the temporoparietal, frontal and occipital cortex, were correlated with a change of the Mini-Mental State Examination score in probable AD patients, suggesting that clinical deterioration and metabolic impairment are closely related [15]. The activity of cytochrome oxidase (CO) was reduced in the hippocampus of AD patients [16].

As to the issue of hypometabolism being an early event, an important observation is that of Foster et al. [17], who demonstrated that a substantial decrease in cerebral glucose metabolism may precede cognitive impairment. This observation was supported by Small et al. [18] and Reiman et al. [19], who found that late middle-aged, cognitively normal subjects who were homozygous for the APOE-ε4 allele, and thus at risk for AD, already had reduced glucose metabolism in the precise region of the brain that is later affected in patients with probable AD.

RELATIONSHIP BETWEEN AD NEUROPATHOLOGY AND DECREASED METABOLISM

Using the size of the Golgi apparatus (GA) as a histological parameter of chronic activity changes in neurons, we studied the neuronal activity in areas with different types of neuropathological AD changes.

The supraoptic nucleus (SON) of the hypothalamus is generally spared in AD. As shown by Lucassen et al. [20], there was indeed a significant increase in activity of vasopressinergic neurons of the SON during aging, both in controls and AD patients, supporting the idea that activation of neurons is accompanied by an absence of AD pathologies [12].

The NBM is severely affected in AD. A significantly decreased size of the GA was also found in NBM neurons in AD, suggesting that protein synthetic activity of NBM neurons is strongly reduced in this brain area [9]. It is of great interest to our hypothesis that the metabolic reduction is APOE type-dependent. AD patients with one or two ε-4 alleles have a stronger decrease in neuronal metabolic rate in the NBM [11]. As shown by Salehi et al. [14], metabolic activity of tuberomamillary (TM) neurons, an area of the hypothalamus which is clearly affected by NFTs, is significantly reduced in AD, which again supports the existence of a relationship between the occurrence of AD pathology and decreased neuronal activity. The same holds for the CA1 area of the hippocampus, which is strongly affected by AD changes and where, as shown by Salehi et al. [13], neuronal activity was strongly decreased in AD patients.

The next step was to study the causality of the relationship between the presence of NPs and NFT in a brain area with decreased metabolic activity. For this purpose we compared metabolic activity of CA1 neurons that did contain NFTs with those that did not. There appeared to be no difference in the size of the GA between these two groups of neurons. The presence of NFT does not seem to decrease the general metabolic rate of a neuron [13]. If a neuritic plaque contains neurotoxic compounds inhibiting neuronal activity, one would expect that the closer a neuron is situated to the plaque, the lower its metabolic rate would be. However, there appeared to be no relationship between either the density of NPs or the distance of each NP to the metabolic activity of neighboring neurons [11]. These findings support the idea that neuronal metabolism and NPs are two basically independent phenomena.

NEURONAL ACTIVATION IN OLDER SUBJECTS

Other data in favor of the 'use it or lose it' hypothesis are provided by studies on the infundibular nucleus of the hypothalamus of elderly men and postmenopausal women. Strong activational changes were found in neurons expressing estrogen receptor mRNA, as judged from the pronounced neuronal hypertrophy and the occurrence of larger and double nucleoli. Also, marked increases in tachykinin gene expression were found in this nucleus in postmenopausal women [21]. These changes are probably related to the loss of negative steroid hormone feedback as a result of ovarian failure in postmenopausal women. Interestingly, recent information suggests that the postmenopausal activation of the infundibular (= arcuate) nucleus in women prevents the formation of AD changes in this area. The sex-specific AD changes in the median eminence and infundibular nucleus occurred in most men over the age of 60 years but were seldom found in women of the same age [22]. The activation of the infundibular nucleus in postmenopausal women was much more pronounced than in men of the same age [21]. This observation may, therefore, serve as an extremely good example of the 'use it or lose it' concept and illustrates, in addition, that it is quite possible to stimulate a neuronal population successfully in the second half of life.

REACTIVATION AS A MEANS OF RESTORING NEURONAL FUNCTION IN AD

The present review shows that there is a clear reduction in neuronal metabolic activity in various brain areas in AD patients. Consequently, one may assume that restoration of the activity of neurons, either by pharmacological or non-pharmacological stimuli, would lead to diminished cognitive impairment [12]. Recent data show that reactivation of neurons may, in principle, indeed be beneficial to AD patients. The application of moderately long-acting cholin-esterase inhibitors such as tacrine (tetrahydroaminoacridine, THA), has signifi-cant effects on cognitive functioning in AD patients and has even been claimed to slow down the progress of the disease. Furthermore, the increases in glucose metabolism following tacrine treatment are paralleled by improvements in neu-ropsychological performance and EEG [23]. These observations support the concept of AD as a hypometabolic disorder and indicate that enhanced func-tional brain activity can be obtained in AD after application of an appropriate stimulus.

Various older studies showed that reality orientation—a long-term program of formal didactic group therapy—improved cognitive functioning of demented elderly people [24–26]. Also exercise therapy improved cognition in institu-tionalized geriatric mental patients [27]. In two studies, elderly demented pa-tients, including AD patients, received an 'integrity-promoting care' program consisting of increased emotional and intellectual communication and physical activation [28, 29]. After applying this program for 2 months, short-term memory and visual perception had improved in the experimental group, while they had deteriorated in the control group [28]. Moreover, compared to the experimental group, concentration declined and absent-mindedness increased significantly in the control group. An important additional finding was that the experimental group showed an increase in their mean CSF level of the neuropeptide somatostatin, whereas the control group showed a decrease. In the other study, AD patients and patients with multi-infarct dementia (MID) received the 'integrity-promoting care' program for 3 months [29]. Short-term memory, dress-ing ability and physical activity improved, whereas confusion diminished. More-over, the reduced CSF level of somatostatin had been elevated in the experimental group. In a series of experiments, Scherder found positive effects of increased somatosensory input by means of various types of peripheral nerve stimulation [i.e. transcutaneous electrical nerve stimulation (TENS), tactile nerve stimulation and a combination of both types of stimuli] on memory, and on independent and affective functioning of patients in a relatively early stage of AD [30]. In one study, transcranial electrostimulation in elderly patients with multi-infarct dementia was also found to decrease wandering and nocturnal delirium and to enhance the patients' interaction with others [31]. The authors suggest that the transcranial electrical stimulus might partly be mediated through the somatosensory system.

The suprachiasmatic nucleus (SCN)—the biological clock of the brain—is of critical importance in the circadian modulation of behavior and physiology. In aging, and even more so in AD, a marked reduction in the number of vasopressin-expressing neurons was found. The combined anatomical, physiological and behavioral findings suggest that a dysfunctional clock may underlie the sleep–wake pattern fragmentation [2, 3, 32], and we therefore employed a number of strategies designed to stimulate the circadian timing system in order to promote preservation of neuronal functioning of the circadian timing system, and thereby to enhance the functionality of the clock. Increased input to the circadian timing system can, among other things, be effected by means of bright environmental light, TENS and increased levels of physical activity. Additional bright light indeed improved the coupling of rest–activity rhythms to stable environmental clues (so-called 'Zeitgebers') in patients with intact vision, but not in patients with severely compromised sight (partial blindness, cataract) [33]. These results agree with other studies that show improved circadian rhythms and decreased behavioral disorders in AD patients treated with bright light.

In conclusion, an increasing number of observations indicate that neuronal activation may have positive effects on degenerative changes in aging and AD. The observations that glucose administration or increasing glucose availability by hyperinsulinemia enhances memory in patients with probable AD [34, 35] not only support the view that AD is basically a hypometabolic disease, but also indicate that the focus on metabolic stimulation of neurons appears to be a fruitful strategy. The best way to prove that decreased metabolic activity indeed plays a major role in the development of dementia would, of course, be to show that reversing decreased neuronal metabolism would lead to considerable improvement of cognitive functions. The first series of data support this idea.

ACKNOWLEDGEMENTS

Brain material used was obtained from The Netherlands Brain Bank in The Netherlands Institute for Brain Research, Amsterdam (coordinator, Dr R. Ravid). We are grateful to Dr M.A. Hofman for his critical remarks, and to Ms W.T.P. Verweij for her excellent secretarial support. P.J.L. is supported by NWO Grant No. 904-34-132. P.J.L. and A.S. are supported by the Internationale Stichting Alzheimer Onderzoek (ISAO).

REFERENCES

1. Van de Nes JAP, Kamphorst W, Swaab DF. Arguments for and against the primary amyloid local induction hypothesis of the pathogenesis of Alzheimer's disease. Ann Psychiat 1994; 4: 95–111.
2. Swaab DF, Lucassen PJ, Salehi A, Scherder EJA, Van Someren EJW, Verwer RWH. Reduced neuronal activity and reactivation in Alzheimer's disease. In:

van Leeuwen FW, Salehi A, Giger RJ, Holtmaat AJGD, Verhaagen J (eds) Progress in Brain Research, vol 117. Amsterdam: Elsevier, 1998; 343–77.

3. Swaab DF, Grundke-Iqbal I, Iqbal K, Kremer HPH, Ravid R, Van de Nes JAP. Tau and ubiquitin in the human hypothalamus in aging and Alzheimer's disease. Brain Res 1992; 590: 239–49.

4. Kremer HPH. The hypothalamic lateral tuberal nucleus: normal anatomy and changes in neurological diseases. In: Swaab DF, Hofman MA, Mirmiran M, Ravid R, van Leeuwen FW (eds) The Human Hypothalamus in Health and Disease: Progress in Brain Research, vol 93. Amsterdam: Elsevier, 1992; 249–63.

5. Terry RD, Hansen LA, DeTeresa R, Davies P, Tobias H, Katzman R. Senile dementia of the Alzheimer type without neocortical neurofibrillary tangles. J Neuropath Exp Neurol 1987; 46: 262–8.

6. Hoogendijk WJG, Pool CW, Troost D, Van Zwieten EJ, Swaab DF. Image-analyzer-assisted morphometry of the locus coeruleus in Alzheimer's disease, Parkinson's disease and amyotrophic lateral sclerosis. Brain 1995; 118: 131–43.

7. West MJ, Coleman PD, Flood DG, Tronsoco JC. Differences in the pattern of hippocampal neuronal loss in normal ageing and Alzheimer's disease. Lancet 1994; 344: 769–72.

8. Gómez-Isla T, Hollister R, West H, Mui S, Growdon JH, Petersen RC, Parisi JE, Hyman BT. Neuronal loss correlates with but exceeds neurofibrillary tangles in Alzheimer's disease. Ann Neurol 1997; 41: 17–24.

9. Salehi A, Lucassen PJ, Pool CW, Gonatas NK, Ravid R, Swaab DF. Decreased neuronal activity in the nucleus basalis of Alzheimer's disease as suggested by the size of the Golgi apparatus. Neuroscience 1994; 59: 871–80.

10. Regeur L, Jensen GB, Pakkenberg H, Evans SM, Pakkenberg B. No global neocortical nerve cell loss in brains from senile dementia of Alzheimer's type. Neurobiol Aging 1994; 15: 347–52.

11. Salehi A, Pool CW, Mulder M, Ravid R, Gonatas NK, Swaab DF. Limited effect of neuritic plaques on neuronal density in the hippocampal CA1 area of Alzheimer patients. Alzheimer's Dis Assoc Disord 1998 (in press).

12. Swaab DF. Brain aging and Alzheimer's disease: 'wear and tear' versus 'use it or lose it'. Neurobiol Aging 1991; 12: 317–24.

13. Salehi A, Ravid R, Gonatas NK, Swaab DF. Decreased activity of hippocampal neurons in Alzheimer's disease is not related to the presence of neurofibrillary tangles. J Neuropathol Exp Neurol 1995a; 54: 704–9.

14. Salehi A, Heyn S, Gonatas NK, Swaab DF. Decreased protein synthetic activity of the hypothalamic tuberomammillary nucleus in Alzheimer's disease as suggested by a smaller Golgi apparatus. Neurosci Lett 1995b; 193: 29–32.

15. Mielke R, Herholz K, Grond M, Kessler J, Heiss WD. Clinical deterioration in probable Alzheimer's disease correlates with progressive metabolic impairment of association areas. Dementia 1994; 5: 36–41.

16. Simonian NA, Hyman BT. Functional alterations in Alzheimer's disease: diminution of cytochrome oxidase in the hippocampal formation. J Neuropathol Exp Neurol 1993; 52: 580–85.

17. Foster NL, Chase TN, Mansi L, Brooks R, Fedio P, Patronas NJ, Di Chiro G. Cortical abnormalities in Alzheimer's disease. Ann Neurol 1984; 16: 649–54.

18. Small GW, Mazziotta JC, Collins MT, Baxter LR, Phelps ME, Mandelkern MA, Kaplan A, La Rue A, Adamson CF, Chang L, Guze BH, Corder EH, Saunders AM, Haines JL, Pericak-Vance MA, Roses AD. Apolipoprotein E type 4 allele and cerebral glucose metabolism in relatives at risk for familial Alzheimer disease. JAMA 1995; 273: 942–7.

19. Reiman EM, Caselli RJ, Yun LS, Chen K, Bandy D, Minoshima S, Thibodeau SN, Osborne D. Preclinical evidence of Alzheimer's disease in persons homozygous for the ε4 allele for apolipoprotein E. N Engl J Med 1996; 334: 752–8.

20. Lucassen PJ, Salehi A, Pool CW, Gonatas NK, Swaab DF. Activation of vasopressin neurons in aging and Alzheimer's disease. J Neuroendocr 1994; 6: 673–9.
21. Rance NE. Hormonal influences on morphology and neuropeptide gene expression in the infundibular nucleus of post-menopausal women. In: Swaab DF, Hofman MA, Mirmiran M, Ravid R, van Leeuwen FW (eds) Progress in Brain Research. Amsterdam: Elsevier, 1992; 221–35.
22. Schultz C, Braak H, Braak E. A sex difference in neurodegeneration of the human hypothalamus. Neurosci Lett 1996; 212: 103–6.
23. Nordberg A. Long-term treatment with tacrine: effects on progression of Alzheimer's disease as determined by functional brain studies. In Iqbal K, Mortimer JA, Winblad B, Wisniewski HM (eds) Research Advances in Alzheimer's Disease and Related Disorders. Chichester: Wiley, 1995; 293–8.
24. Woods RT. Reality orientation and staff attention: a controlled study. Br J Psychiat 1979; 134: 502–7.
25. Hanley IG, McGuire RJ, Boyd WD. Reality orientation and dementia: a controlled trial of two approaches. Br J Psychiat 1981; 138; 10–14.
26. Zanetti O, Frisoni GB, De Leo D, Della Buono M, Bianchetti A, Trabucchi M. Reality orientation in Alzheimer disease: useful or not? A controlled study. Alzheimer's Dis Assoc Disord 1995; 132–8.
27. Powell RR. Psychological effects of exercise therapy upon institutionalized geriatric mental patients. J Teratol 1974; 29: 157–64.
28. Karlsson I, Widerlöv E, Melin EV, Nyth A, Brane GAM, Rybo E, Rehfeld JF, Bissette G, Nemeroff CB. Changes of CSF neuropeptides after environmental stimulation in dementia. Nord Psykiat Tidssk 1985; 39: 75–81.
29. Widerlöv E, Bråne G, Ekman R, Kihlgren M, Norberg A, Karlsson I. Elevated CSF somatostatin concentrations in demented patients parallel improved psychomotor functions induced by integrity-promoting care. Acta Psychiat Scand 1989; 79: 41–7.
30. Scherder E, Bouma A, Steen L, Swaab D. Peripheral nerve stimulating in Alzheimer's disease: a meta-analysis. Alzheimer's Res 1995; 1: 183–4.
31. Hozumi S, Hori H, Okawa M, Hishikawa Y, Sato K. Favorable effect of transcranial electrostimulation on behavior disorders in elderly patients with dementia: a double-blind study. Intern J Neurosci 1996; 88: 1–10.
32. Swaab DF, Fliers E, Partiman T. The suprachiasmatic nucleus of the human brain in relation to sex, age and dementia. Brain Res 1985; 342: 37–44.
33. Van Someren EJW, Kessler A, Mirmiran M, Swaab DF. Indirect bright light improves circadian rest–activity rhythm disturbances in demented patients. Biol Psychiat 1997; 41: 955–63.
34. Manning CA, Ragozzino ME, Gold PE. Glucose enhancement of memory in patients with probable senile dementia of the Alzheimer's type. Neurobiol Aging 1993; 14: 523–8.
35. Craft S, Newcomer J, Kanne S, Dagogo-Jack S, Cryer P, Sheline Y, Luby J, Dagogo-Jack A, Alderson A. Memory improvement following induced hyperinsulinemia in Alzheimer's disease. Neurobiol Aging 1996; 17: 123–30.

Address for correspondence:
D.F. Swaab,
Netherlands Institute for Brain Research,
Meibergdreef 33, 1105 AZ Amsterdam, The Netherlands
Tel: (31) 20 5665500; fax: (31) 20 6961006

87 Effects of Environmental Stimulation with Bright Light and Transcranial Electrostimulation on Sleep and Behavior Disorders in Elderly Patients with Dementia

M. OKAWA, K. MISHIMA AND S. HOZUMI

CIRCADIAN RHYTHM ALTERATIONS IN AGING

Elderly patients with dementia due to organic brain syndrome are likely to show sleep disturbances as well as numerous behavior disorders during waking hours, such as wandering, aggressiveness, agitation, violent behaviors and/or delirium. In our previous researches [1, 2], which investigated circadian rhythm disorders in the sleep–wake cycle and body temperature in elderly patients with dementia, we concluded that sleep and behavior disorders in these patients might be due to circadian rhythm disorders.

Many previous reports have also indicated that there exists a dysfunction of the circadian time-keeping system among these patients which might be related to their sleep and behavior disorders [3]. Recently, we conducted a systematic study of serum melatonin rhythm in senile dementia of Alzheimer's type (SDAT) patients with disturbed sleep–wake cycles [4, 5]. These patients showed significantly disturbed melatonin rhythm. Melatonin is often used as a stable marker in assessing the functional properties of the circadian time-keeping system. Melatonin secretion rhythm disorders in demented elderly may play an important role in irregular sleep–wake cycles. For the treatment of sleep and behavior disorders, we have reported two novel treatments based on chronobiological principles.

Alzheimer's Disease and Related Disorders
Edited by K. Iqbal, D.F. Swaab, B. Winblad and H.M. Wisniewski
© 1999 John Wiley & Sons Ltd

BRIGHT-LIGHT THERAPY

Bright light has recently been suggested as a therapy for sleep disorders in the aging [6, 7]. We have also applied bright-light therapy to sleep disturbances and behavior disorders in demented elderly and have observed favorable results [1, 8]. However, there is a problem in determining the efficacy of bright-light therapy. Since the voluntary compliance of demented patients is minimal, continuous attendance by the nursing staff is necessary to keep patients in front of the light source. Thus, a placebo effect may be introduced by the simultaneous increase in attention to the patient by the nursing staff. To exclude such a placebo effect in evaluating bright-light therapy for these elderly patients, we recently conducted a randomized cross-over study using both dim light and bright light.

We examined the therapeutic efficacy on behavioral and rest–activity rhythm disorders in 12 patients with multi-infarct dementia (MID) and in 10 patients with SDAT. They were exposed to 2 weeks of bright light (5000–8000 lux) and 2 weeks of dim light (300 lux) in the morning (09.00–11.00 h) in a randomized cross-over design. A representative case who favorably responded to bright-light exposure is shown in Figure 1. The bright-light exposure induced a significant reduction in both night-time activity and in ratio (percentages) of night-time activity to total activity, as compared with the pretreatment period as well as with the dim-light condition in the MID group. Behavior disorders in MID patients were significantly decreased with bright-light therapy (Figure 2). On the other hand, SDAT patients did not show any significant change in either night-time activity or behavior disorder score. These findings support the assumption that the therapeutic efficacies of morning bright-light exposure are prominent in MID patients, and are mainly due to its photic effect rather than the non-photic effect of greater social interaction.

The underlying mechanism of the therapeutic effect produced by bright light is unclear. It is possible that our subjects were short of time cues to entrain some of their circadian rhythms, including the sleep–wake cycle. Bright-light therapy may enhance photic entrainment of the circadian rhythm. In our previous studies, bright light sometimes also had a favorable effect on disturbed body temperature rhythm, characterized by increased amplitude and rhythmicity [5]. This was considered to be a sympathomimetic effect of bright light. It is possible that this kind of arousal-producing (vigilance-elevating) effect of bright light may also play a role in reducing the daytime sleepiness and delirium often observed in dementia.

TRANSCRANIAL ELECTROSTIMULATION

Recently, transcranial electrostimulation with a new device (HESS-10, Homer Ion Co. Tokyo), based on results in experimental animal studies [9],

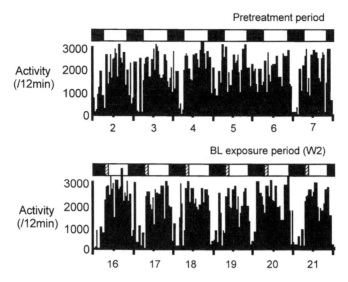

Figure 1. Raw data plots of rest–activity (R–A) rhythm for a representative 74 year-old female patient with multi-infarct dementia who responded favorably to bright-light (BL) exposure. R–A data were monitored in 1 min periods using an actigraph and are illustrated in a convenient style ($\times 10^3$ counts/12 min). Horizontal black and white bars indicate night-time (21.00–06.00 h) and daytime (06.00–21.00 h), respectively. Shaded columns in the day–night bars on the bottom panel indicate periods of bright-light exposure (09.00–11.00 h) during the second week of the treatment

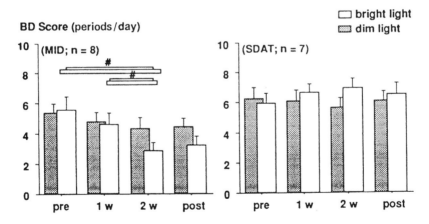

Figure 2. The results of bright light (8000 lux) and dim light (300 lux) exposure for behavior disorders in eight patients with MID and seven patients with SDAT. Behavior disorder was recorded every 30 min for the pretreatment period, during the 1st and 2nd weeks of light exposure and post-treatment. Behavior disorder score was defined as the average number of periods per day in which behavior disorders were observed. $^\#$ p < 0.01

has been introduced for preventing drowsiness while driving a car or working. Transcranial stimulation with this device has been shown to induce arousal from sleep in normal human subjects and cats [9]. We conducted a double-blind study of transcranial electrostimulation in 27 demented MID patients with sleep and behavior disorders [10].

Electrostimulation (6–8 V, increasing frequency 6–80 Hz) was delivered for 20 min from 10.00 h in the morning for 2 weeks. In the active therapy group, there were significant improvements in motivation, behavior disorders, sleep disorders and subjective complaints. Sleep disorders were improved by both active and placebo therapy, and there was no significant difference between the two groups. Electroencephalograms showed improvements characterized by the appearance or increased frequency of alpha waves and a decrease in or disappearance of theta waves. A representative case is shown in Figure 3.

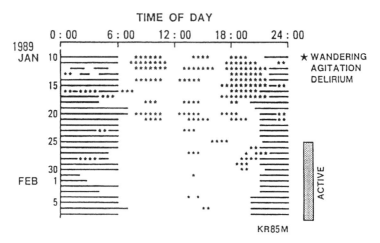

Figure 3. Clinical course of transcranial electrostimulation in an 85 year-old male with MID. Thick horizontal lines indicate sleep, asterisks episodes of behavior disorder. The patient displayed frequent episodes of behavior disorder during both day and night, and an irregular sleep–wake pattern before institution of active therapy. The number of behavior disorder episodes decreased markedly and the sleep–wake pattern became regular during active therapy

This study demonstrates the efficacy of transcranial electrostimulation for disorders of behavior, motivation and sleep in elderly demented patients. The effects of electrostimulation may be explained by elevated daytime vigilance levels, an explanation supported by the finding of improved background activity in electroencephalography.

The mechanism by which our transcranial electrostimulation improves vigilance levels is unknown. High-frequency electric current has been shown to directly stimulate the brain arousal system in experimental animals [9].

Recently, Scherder et al. [11] observed significant effects of transcutaneous electrical nerve stimulation on memory and affective behavior in probable Alzheimer's patients. In addition, the patients became more active and more alert, with increased social contact. Electrical stimulation is considered to be a new therapeutic strategy to improve the quality of life of demented patients.

Despite the lack of an explanation on the mechanism of chronobiological non-pharmacological treatments, the mere findings of circadian rhythm enhancement are of clinical importance. Time cues seemed to decrease in institutionalized elderly people. Moreover, since the suprachiasmatic nucleus in the elderly shows functional and structural degeneration, many of the time cues in daily life for elderly people should be more intensively enhanced than for young people. Both environmental stimulation and electrical stimulation seem to be effective in enhancing the amplitude of circadian rhythm, which results in increased activity during the daytime and better sleep at night. These chronobiological treatments appear to be promising as a way of improving the quality of life of the elderly.

REFERENCES

1. Okawa M, Mishima K, Hishikawa Y et al. Circadian rhythm disorders in sleep–waking body temperature in elderly patients with dementia and their treatment. Sleep 1991; 14: 478–85.
2. Mishima K, Okawa M, Satoh K et al. Different manifestations of daily rest–activity and body temperature rhythms in patients with senile dementia of Alzheimer's type and multi-infarct dementia. Neurobiol Aging 1997; 18: 105–9.
3. Witting W, Kwa IH, Eikelenboom P et al. Alterations in the circadian rest–activity rhythm in aging and Alzheimer's disease. Biol Psychiat 1990; 27: 563–72.
4. Mishima K, Hishikawa Y, Okawa M. Randomized, dim-light controlled, cross-over test of morning bright-light therapy for behavioral and rest–activity rhythm disorders in patients with vascular dementia and dementia of Alzheimer's type (in press).
5. Mishima K, Hishikawa Y. Chronotherapy for circadian rhythm disorders in elderly patients with dementia. In: Hayaishi O, Inoué S (eds) Sleep and Sleep Disorders: From Molecule to Behavior. Tokyo: Academic Press, 1996; 177–91.
6. Bunnell DE, Treiber SP, Phillips NH et al. Effects of evening bright light exposure on melatonin, body temperature and sleep. J Sleep Res 1992; 1: 17–23.
7. Satlin A, Volicer L, Ross V et al. Bright light treatment of behavioral and sleep disturbances in patients with Alzheimer's disease. Am J Psychiat 1992; 149: 1028–32.
8. Mishima K, Okawa M, Hishikawa Y et al. Morning bright light therapy for sleep and behavior disorders in elderly patients with dementia. Acta Psychiat Scand 1994; 89: 1–7.
9. Matsumoto H, Morita Y, Seno H. Transitional mechanism from sleep to arousal in cats. Neuroscience 1988; 14: 353–63.

10. Hozumi S, Hori H, Okawa M et al. Favorable effect of transcranial electrostimulation on behavior disorders in elderly patients with dementia: a double-blind study. Int J Neurosci 1996; 88: 1–10.

11. Scherder EJA, Bouma A, Steen AM. Effects of short-term transcutaneous electrical nerve stimulation on memory and affective behaviour in patients with probable Alzheimer's disease. Behav Brain Res 1995; 67: 211–19.

Address for correspondence:
  M. Okawa,
  National Institute of Mental Health, NCNP,
  Akita University School of Medicine,
  Akita, Japan

88 Effects of Transcutaneous Electrical Nerve Stimulation (TENS) on Mood and Cognition in Alzheimer's Disease

ERIK J.A. SCHERDER, ANKE BOUMA,
EUS J.W. VAN SOMEREN, DICK F. SWAAB

INTRODUCTION

Given the progressive character of Alzheimer's disease (AD), one might well ask what the best therapeutic strategy may be. It has been pointed out that in AD patients brain atrophy, the main hallmark in AD, is based upon shrinkage of cells rather than on cell death, and that shrunken cells may still be subject to plastic changes during ageing and AD by stimulation of neuronal systems [1–3]. This hypothesis, paraphrased as 'use it or lose it' [2], was the basis for electrical stimulation in AD.

In a recent human experimental study, transcranial electrostimulation in elderly patients with multi-infarct dementia was found to be effective in, among others, decreasing sleep and wake disturbances [4]. These authors suggest that transcranial electrostimulation is partly mediated by the somatosensory system. In another study, transcutaneous electrical nerve stimulation (TENS) improved neglecting hemianaesthesia in right brain-damaged patients [5]. The findings of these studies suggest that peripheral electrical stimuli, through the somatosensory system, could influence supra-spinal areas. Indeed, TENS could activate the hippocampus and the hypothalamus which play a role in memory and mood, respectively [6], and are affected in AD [7, 8] by direct and indirect pathways [9–11].

RESEARCH QUESTIONS

Based on the above-mentioned studies, it was investigated in our clinical studies whether TENS in the presence of the therapist, applied for 6 h or 30 min/day, and a 30 min/day treatment with TENS in the absence of the

Alzheimer's Disease and Related Disorders
Edited by K. Iqbal, D.F. Swaab, B. Winblad and H.M. Wisniewski
© 1999 John Wiley & Sons Ltd

therapist, could improve disturbances in memory, and independent and affective functioning in patients in an early stage of AD. Furthermore, it was examined whether TENS also had a beneficial influence on patients in a midstage of AD. Finally, it was investigated whether possible treatment effects could be maintained after a 6 week period without stimulation.

OVERVIEW OF METHODOLOGY

SUBJECTS

The patients in our clinical studies were either in a relatively early stage [12–14], i.e. stage 5 of the Global Deterioration Scale [15], or midstage [16], i.e. stage 6 of the GDS, of late-onset AD (onset at the age of 65 or after). The subjects, drawn from a sample of 500 persons who lived in a residential home for elderly people, met the NINCDS–ADRDA criteria for the clinical diagnosis of probable AD [17]. Patients with a history of depression or other psychiatric disorders, alcoholism, cerebral trauma, cerebrovascular disease, hydrocephalus, neoplasm, epilepsy, disturbances of consciousness, or focal brain abnormalities were excluded from participation in our studies. In each study, the subjects were randomly divided into an experimental and a control group. Both groups were matched with respect to level of cognitive functioning, age and sex (for details, see [12–14, 16]).

MATERIALS AND PROCEDURE

Neuropsychological Tests

The patients underwent a number of neuropsychological tests in order to evaluate the effects of treatment on various aspects of memory, including verbal and visual short-term and long-term memory, and semantic memory: Digit Span and Visual Memory Span from the Wechsler Memory Scale-Revised (WMS-R) [18]; Eight Words Test [19]; Face and Picture Recognition from the Rivermead Behavioural Memory Test (RBMT) [20]; and Word Fluency from the Groninger Intelligence Test [21] (for details on the tests, see [13]).

Observation Scales

One observation scale was a standard factor-analysed rating scale for elderly patients (Beoordelingsschaal voor Oudere Patiënten: BOP [22]), divided into six subscales, i.e. Need of Help, Aggressiveness, Physical Invalidity, Depressed Behaviour, Mental Invalidity, and Inactivity. As the BOP scale is particularly suitable to assess patients' independent functioning in activities of daily life, the Behaviour Inventory was administered to evaluate patients' affective behaviour. This Inventory includes 12 main traits, i.e. depression, elation, shyness, mood, anger, tiredness, activity, anxiety, conscience, indifference, cognition, and contact. In order to investigate whether treatment improved overall affective behaviour, a total score of changes was calculated by summing up the scores of all items employed in the Behaviour Inventory.

Stimulation

TENS was applied to patients of the experimental groups by an electrostimulator, type Premier 10s. The control groups received a placebo treatment with the same electrostimulator, i.e. no current was administered to the patients. The patients of the experimental group and control group were treated 5 days/week, during a 6 week period, followed by the same period without stimulation.

CLINICAL STUDIES

Table 1 presents the effects (p-values) on memory, independent and affective functioning of patients in an early and midstage of AD, by TENS, both in the presence and absence of the therapist.

LONG-TERM TENS

In a first pilot study, the effects of TENS, applied for 6 h/day (long-term TENS), were examined only on memory of eight patients (four in the experimental group and four in the control group) in a relatively early stage of AD [12]. The results reveal that TENS improves patients' ability to learn new verbal information (the subtests Immediate Recall and Recognition of the 15 Words Test) and to retrieve familiar, categorized information from their memory store (Verbal Fluency). Although the number of participating subjects was small, the results were promising enough to warrant further research.

SHORT-TERM TENS

In the second study, a 30 min/day treatment with TENS (short-term TENS) was applied to 16 AD patients (eight in the experimental group and eight in the control group) [13]. Compared to long-term TENS [12], short-term TENS particularly improved recognition memory (the subtest Recognition of the Eight Words Test, Face and Picture Recognition), for which much less complex memory function is required. In addition, stimulated patients participated more independently in daily life activities and tended to look for more social contacts (BOP subscales Need of Help, Physical Invalidity, and Inactivity). Also, patients' overall affective behaviour improved after treatment.

Table 1. Effects (p-values) on memory, independent and affective functioning of patients in an early and mid-stage of AD by TENS, in both the presence and absence of the therapist

	Early AD			Midstage AD
	Presence of the therapist		Absence of the therapist	Presence of the therapist
	Long-term TENS[1] p	Short-term TENS[2] p	Isolated TENS[3] p	TENS[4] p
Neuropsychological tests				
Digit span				
Visual memory		0.08	0.002	0.004
8/15 Words Test*				
Immediate recall	0.03			0.06
Delayed recall				
Recognition	0.05	0.05		
Face recognition		0.01	0.04	
Picture recognition		0.001	0.08	
Verbal fluency	0.04		0.03	
BOP subscales				
Need of help		0.01	0.04	
Aggressiveness				
Physical invalidity		0.02		
Depressed Behaviour				
Mental invalidity				
Inactivity		0.07		
Behaviour inventory				
Overall affective behaviour		0.03		

* The 15 Words Test was only applied in the long-term TENS study. [1] Reference [12]; [2] reference [13]; [3] reference [14]; [4] reference [16]

'ISOLATED' TENS

In the two studies mentioned above, the therapist was present during the treatment of both the experimental and control group. Hence, a positive effect of the combination of (sham) stimulation and interpersonal communication (between patient and therapist) could not be excluded. Therefore, the effects of TENS, in the absence of the therapist ('isolated' TENS), were examined in 18 AD patients (nine in the experimental group and nine in the control group) [14]. The improvements in cognition and independent functioning of AD patients who were treated paralleled those observed after short-term TENS [13]. However, only the combination of TENS with interpersonal communication appeared to result in an additional improvement in 'overall' affective behaviour.

TENS IN MID-STAGE AD

So far, the participating patients were in a relatively early stage of AD, i.e. stage 5 of the GDS [15]. In this study, it was investigated whether TENS would still exert beneficial effects in 16 patients (eight in the experimental group and eight in the control group) at a more advanced stage of AD, i.e. stage 6 of the GDS [16]. A significant treatment effect was observed only for non-verbal short-term memory (Visual Memory). TENS appeared to have no effect on patients' independent and affective functioning.

Analyses of the data obtained after 6 weeks without stimulation revealed that the majority of the treatment effects observed in the above-mentioned studies disappeared.

DISCUSSION

Comparison of the effects of short-term TENS with 'isolated' TENS suggests that the most efficient treatment strategy in AD seems to be TENS in combination with interpersonal communication. TENS may act on different neurotransmitter systems (cf. [13]), including the cholinergic system [23]. It is therefore interesting to note that although physostigmine, a cholinesterase inhibitor, improved recognition memory when applied separately [24], physostigmine combined with lecithine, a cholinergic precursor, enhanced patients' performance on more complex tasks, e.g. learning new verbal information [25]. In other words, a combination of various types of intervention may have a surplus value, i.e. TENS + interpersonal communication has an additional treatment effect on affective behaviour, physostigmine + lecithine enhances more complex cognitive processes. The effect of TENS seems to be stage-dependent, a finding that might be related to the observation that the restorative effect of sprouting declines during the course of the disease [26]. The finding that the majority of the observed treatment effects disappeared after a treatment-free period of 6 weeks might imply that TENS should be applied continuously. Finally, it should be emphasized that TENS does not claim to cure AD but its effects are in the same range as those of the current pharmacological therapies.

REFERENCES

1. Regeur L, Badsberg Jensen G, Pakkenberg H, Evans SM, Pakkenberg B. No global neocortical nerve cell loss in brains from patients with senile dementia of Alzheimer's type. Neurobiol Aging 1994; 15: 347–52.
2. Swaab DF. Brain aging and Alzheimer's disease, 'wear and tear' versus 'use it or lose it'. Neurobiol Aging 1991; 12: 317–24.
3. Swaab DF, Hofman MA, Lucassen PJ, Salehi A, Uylings HBM. Neuronal atrophy, not cell death, is the main hallmark of Alzheimer's disease. Neurobiol Aging 1994; 15: 369–71.

4. Hozumi S, Hori H, Okawa M, Hishikawa Y, Sato K. Favorable effect of transcranial electrostimulation on behavior disorders in elderly patients with dementia: a double-blind study. Int J Neuroscience 1996; 88: 1–10.

5. Vallar G, Rusconi ML, Bernardini B. Modulation of neglect hemianesthesia by transcutaneous electrical stimulation. J Int Neuropsychol Soc 1996; 2: 452–9.

6. Salzmann E. Importance of the hippocampus and parahippocampus with reference to normal and disordered memory function. Fortschr Neurol Psychiat 1992; 60: 163–76.

7. Scheltens PH, Leys D, Barkhof F, Huglo D, Weinstein HC, Vermersch P, Kuiper M, Steinling M, Wolters E, Valk J. Atrophy of medial temporal lobes on MRI in 'probable' Alzheimer's disease and normal ageing: diagnostic value and neuropsychological correlates. J Neurol Neurosurg Psychiat 1992; 55: 967–72.

8. Swaab DF. Neurobiology and neuropathology of the human hypothalamus. In: Bloom FE, Björklund A, Hökfelt T (eds) Handbook of Chemical Neuroanatomy, vol 13, The Primate Nervous System, part I. Amsterdam: Elsevier Science, 1997; 39–136.

9. Burstein R, Giesler GJ. Retrograde labeling of neurons in spinal cord that project directly to nucleus accumbens or the septal nuclei in the rat. Brain Res 1989; 497: 149–54.

10. Giesler GJ, Katter T, Dado RJ. Direct spinal pathways to the limbic system for nociceptive information. Trends Neurosci 1994; 17: 244–50.

11. Höhmann C, Antuono P, Coyle JT. Basal forebrain cholinergic neurons and Alzheimer's disease. In: Iversen LL, Iversen SD, Snijder SH (eds) Handbook of Psychopharmacology. New York: Plenum, 1988; 69–106.

12. Scherder EJA, Bouma A, Steen AM. Influence of transcutaneous electrical nerve stimulation on memory in patients with dementia of the Alzheimer type. J Clin Exp Neuropsychol 1992; 14: 951–60.

13. Scherder EJA, Bouma A, Steen AM. Effects of short-term transcutaneous electrical nerve stimulation on memory and affective behaviour in patients with probable Alzheimer's disease. Behav Brain Res 1995; 67: 211–19.

14. Scherder EJA, Bouma A, Steen AM. Effects of 'isolated' short-term transcutaneous electrical nerve stimulation on memory and affective behaviour of patients with probable Alzheimer's disease. Biol Psychiat 1998 (in press).

15. Reisberg B, Ferris SH, De Leon MJ, Crook T. The Global Deterioration Scale for assessment of primary dementia. Am J Psychiat 1982; 139: 1136–9.

16. Scherder EJA, Bouma A, Steen AM. Effects of transcutaneous electrical nerve stimulation on memory and behaviour in Alzheimer's disease may be stage-dependent. Biol Psychiat 1998 (in press).

17. McKhann G, Drachman D, Folstein M, Katzman R, Price D, Stadlan EM. Clinical diagnosis of Alzheimer's disease: reports of the NINCDS–ADRDA workgroup under the auspices of the Department of Health and Human Services task force on Alzheimer's disease. Neurology 1984; 34: 939–44.

18. Wechsler D. Wechsler Memory Scale—Revised. New York: The Psychological Corporation, 1987.

19. Lindeboom J, Jonker C. Amsterdamse Dementie-Screeningstest, Handleiding. Lisse: Swets & Zeitlinger, 1989.

20. Wilson B, Cockburn J, Baddeley A. The Rivermead Behavioural Memory Test. Titchfield: Thames Valley Test Company, 1987.

21. Snijders JTH, Verhage F. Groninger Intelligentie Test. Lisse: Swets & Zeitlinger, 1983.

22. Van der Kam P, Mol F, Wimmers MFHG. Beoordelingsschaal voor Oudere Patiënten. Deventer: Van Loghum Slaterus, 1971.

23. Dutar P, Lamour Y, Jobert A. Activation of identified septohippocampal neurons by noxious peripheral stimulation. Brain Res 1985; 328: 15–21.
24. Christie JE, Shering A, Ferguson J, Glen AJM. Physostigmine and arecoline: effects of intravenous infusions in Alzheimer presenile dementia. Br J Psychiat 1981; 138: 46–50.
25. Thal IJ, Fuld PA, Masur DM et al. Oral physostigmine and lecithin improve memory in Alzheimer's disease. Ann Neurol 1983; 13: 491–6.
26. Geddes JW, Cotman CW. Plasticity in Alzheimer's disease: too much or not enough? Neurobiol Aging 1991; 12: 330–33.

Address for correspondence:
Erik J.A. Scherder, PhD,
Department of Clinical Psychology, Vrije Universiteit,
De Boelelaan 1109, 1081 HV Amsterdam, The Netherlands
Tel: (31) 20 4448770; fax: (31) 20 448758;
e-mail: EJA.Scherder@psy.vu.nl

89 Stimulation of the Circadian Timing System in Healthy and Demented Elderly

EUS J.W. VAN SOMEREN, ERIK J.A. SCHERDER AND
DICK F. SWAAB

INTRODUCTION

Circadian rhythms, i.e. rhythms of approximately 24 h, are present in many physiological and behavioural phenomena. They are crucial in the adaptation to the day–night differences in the environment. In ageing, and even more so in Alzheimer's disease, the circadian rhythms in many behavioural and physiological variables are less prominent or even absent. A decrease in circadian modulation has, amongst others, been observed in hormone levels, temperature, electroencephalographic (EEG) activity, alertness and sleep [1]. Elderly people start napping during the day and often complain of disturbed sleep during the night. In Alzheimer's disease (AD), this fragmentation of the sleep–wake pattern is even more pronounced, and may even closely resemble the pattern that is found in animal studies after lesions of the hypothalamic suprachiasmatic nucleus (SCN), the biological clock of the brain. Several correlative studies suggest that the severity of circadian rhythm disturbances in AD patients is related to the severity of agitation and 'sundowning' [2–5]. Since sleep disturbances, sundowning and agitation are primary factors in caregiver stress and in the decision of the responsible relatives to have a family member institutionalized [5–9], the study of underlying mechanisms and treatment possibilities is of clinical and economical importance.

POSSIBLE MECHANISM UNDERLYING CIRCADIAN RHYTHM DISTURBANCES IN ALZHEIMER'S DISEASE

The SCN is of critical importance in the circadian modulation of behaviour and physiology. Although the isolated SCN *in vitro* is capable of retaining an

Alzheimer's Disease and Related Disorders
Edited by K. Iqbal, D.F. Swaab, B. Winblad and H.M. Wisniewski
© 1999 John Wiley & Sons Ltd

endogenous rhythm of about 24 h, in the intact animal it uses several sources of input to synchronize the internal clock to the external 24 h light–dark cycle. The strongest input originates in retinal ganglion cells, which project directly to the SCN through the retinohypothalamic tract and inform the SCN about the intensity of environmental light. Other probable sources of input, the relative significance and mechanisms of which are at present less clear, include the pineal hormone melatonin, physical activity, and possibly also temperature and somatosensory input [10, 11].

It is hypothesized that a reduced input from these sources to the SCN may play an important role in the deterioration of the SCN. The 'use it or lose it' hypothesis states that activation of nerve cells by internal or external stimuli prevents their degeneration and may even restore functions in ageing or AD [12]. As a metaphor, a comparison could be made to muscle atrophy resulting from disuse, which is associated with decreased protein synthesis, whereas exercise restores both atrophy and induces increased protein synthesis [13]. In ageing, and even more so in Alzheimer's disease, the markedly reduced presence of one of the major peptides, i.e. vasopressin, in SCN neurons [14] may be related to a reduced SCN activation. Our studies in aged rats have demonstrated improvement of both functional and anatomical signs of degeneration of the circadian timing system after pro-longed environmental stimulation. Witting et al. [15] demonstrated that the decreased amplitude in the circadian distribution of sleep and wakefulness, as is present in old rats, could be restored to the level of young rats by means of increasing the intensity of daytime environmental light. Lucassen et al. [16] demonstrated that such increased light input counteracted the age-related decrease in the number of vasopressin-expressing neurons in the rat SCN.

A reduced input to the circadian timing system appears to be present al-ready before the start of the clinical manifestation of Alzheimer's disease [17]. In a study of the history of patients and controls, AD patients had been suffering from cataracts three times more often and had been engaged in outdoor activities two times less often than healthy controls. Furthermore, AD patients had been engaged in various physical activities two to ten times less often than healthy controls. These findings indicate a reduced input to both light- and activity-sensitive parts of the circadian timing system, even before the clinical manifestation of dementia, and such an attenuated input is thought to contribute to degeneration.

In subjects in which the dementia has become manifest, less exposure to environmental light [18, 19], increased incidence of cataract and macula de-generation [20] and increased retinal ganglion cell degeneration and optic nerve atrophy [21, 22] have been reported in addition to the age-related attenuation of light transmission through the eye caused by a reduced pupil diameter and yellowing of the lens [23, 24]. All these factors limit the input to the SCN normally resulting from exposure to bright light. Other inputs to the circadian timing system are likewise attenuated. Elderly people engage less in vigorous physical activity [25], and feedback from the pineal hormone melatonin is also reduced [26–34].

TREATMENT POSSIBILITIES

Based on the 'use it or lose it' concept [12], we have tried a number of strategies presumed to *stimulate* the circadian timing system in order to promote the activity and preservation of neurons in the circadian timing system, and thereby enhance the functionality of the biological clock. Increased input to the circadian timing system can, amongst other means, be effected by means of bright environmental light, peripheral nerve stimulation and increased levels of physical activity (Figure 1).

In healthy and demented elderly people, we have used the rest–activity rhythm as a marker of the functionality of the circadian timing system, because this variable can easily be assessed using actigraphy. An actigraph is a small wrist-worn solid state recorder that continuously assesses the activity level, resulting in a time series from which the strength of the circadian rhythm can be calculated.

In a correlational study, we first investigated which constitutional and environmental factors were related to the severity of rhythm disturbances in Alzheimer patients. Regression analyses showed the most severe rest–activity rhythm disturbances in patients with a sedentary rather than physically active life style, and in patients exposed to low levels of environmental light [35].

Consequently, we investigated the effect of additional bright light on rest–activity rhythm disturbances in demented patients. Additional bright light improved the coupling of rest–activity rhythms to stable environmental clues (so-called 'Zeitgebers') in patients with relatively intact vision, but not in patients with severely compromised sight (partial blindness, cataract [36]). An example is given in Figure 2.

The effect of additional physical activity was investigated in healthy elderly subjects, since fitness training appeared unfeasible in most demented subjects. Fitness training improved the fragmentation of periods of rest and activity that has been found both during normal ageing and, more pronounced, after SCN lesions [37].

Whereas the effect of light and activity on the circadian timing system is well documented, the possible effect of somatosensory input to the SCN has only recently been suggested by our group [11]. The available data from rat and squirrel monkey studies suggest that the SCN is innervated by direct spino-hypothalamic projections conveying somatosensory information [38, 39]. We have therefore investigated whether additional somatosensory input (by means of transcutaneous electrical nerve stimulation, or TENS) would

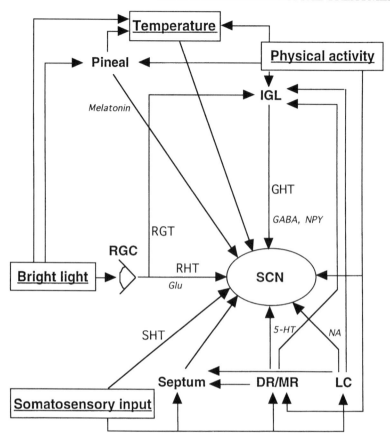

Figure 1. Schematic overview of the inputs to the suprachiasmatic nucleus, and their interactions, that may be relevant for the concept of SCN stimulation. For reasons of clarity, temperature input is only shown for the SCN, whereas thermosensitivity has in fact been demonstrated in the pineal, SCN, septum, raphe nuclei, locus coeruleus and somatosensory afferents. Inputs are underlined, structures are in bold font, tracts are in normal font and neurotransmitters and hormones in italics. 5-HT = 5-hydroxytryptamine (serotonin); DR = dorsal raphe nucleus; GABA = γ-aminobutyric acid; GHT = geniculohypothalamic tract; Glu = glutamate; IGL = intergeniculate leaflet; LC = locus coeruleus; MR = median raphe nucleus; NA = noradrenalin; NPY = neuropeptide Y; RGC = retinal ganglion cells; RGT = retinogeniculate tract; RHT = retinohypothalamic tract; SCN = suprachiasmatic nucleus; SHT = spinohypothalamic tract. Reproduced with permission from reference [10]

provide an alternative means for the activation of SCN neurons. In early-stage demented elderly patients, repeated TENS was indeed found to improve the coupling of rest–activity rhythms to 'Zeitgebers', whereas placebo treatment was ineffective [11]. A similar improvement was found after treating mid-stage demented elderly patients with TENS [40].

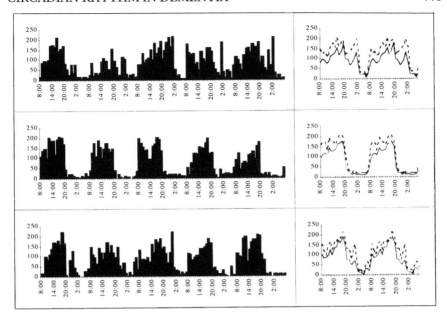

Figure 2. Raw activity data (left panels) of a patient with Alzheimer's disease assessed three times for five days: before (upper left panel), during (middle left panel) and after (lower left panel) light treatment. The right panels show double plots of the average 24 h activity level (solid line) and one standard deviation above this level (dashed line). Note the decreased variability and the smoother average during light treatment. Reproduced with permission from reference [36]

CONCLUSION

The anatomical and functional findings from the reported studies confirm the previous notion that the SCN is a structure in which plasticity is highly preserved throughout the life span [41] and even in dementia. In support of the 'use it or lose it' concept, a reduced input to the SCN appears to contribute to the severity of AD-related circadian rhythm disturbances. Increasing the input to the SCN by means of non-pharmacological strategies appears effective in the management of these disturbances. However, in the studies performed by us and others (e.g. [3, 42–44]) only a limited number of variables has been assessed, usually mainly for evaluating the functionality of the circadian timing system. As is the case for pharmacological treatment evaluation, future studies should include a more diverse assessment of the impact of the treatment on various aspects of the quality of life of the patient and caregiver. It is therefore advised to include a parsimonious observation and test battery in order to evaluate the effects of the treatments on cognitive, behavioural and affective disturbances.

In the selection of appropriate evaluation scales, note should be taken of the developmental course of observed sleep disturbances and actigraphically assessed rhythm disturbances. Circadian rhythm disturbances are most likely to present in the mid-stage of dementia. Reisberg et al. [45] found that the incidence of sleep disturbances shows an inverted U relation with the degree of dementia. Hopkins et al. [46] demonstrated a similar inverted U relation between the duration of the dementia and the incidence of 'sundowning' behaviour (peaking at approximately 9 years after the estimated onset of symptoms). Likewise, fragmentation of the circadian rest–activity rhythm was found to be most severe in mid-stage demented Alzheimer patients [35]. Thus, contrary to many of the presently used assessment instruments for cognitive, behavioural and affective disturbances, scales which do not show floor effects in the range of moderate to severely demented should be selected. A standardized assessment protocol is presently under development, and interested research groups can contact E.J.W. Van Someren at The Netherlands Institute for Brain Research. The use of this protocol by several research groups will facilitate the comparability of results and pooling of data.

In summary, circadian rhythm disturbances appear to be involved in nocturnal restlessness and 'sundowning' in patients suffering from Alzheimer's disease (AD). These behavioural problems are often difficult to treat with currently available pharmaceuticals and place a severe burden on the quality of life of patients and caregivers. Stimulation of the circadian timing system by means of bright light, physical activity and somatosensory input enhances its functionality and improves day–night rhythms.

REFERENCES

1. Van Someren EJW, Mirmiran M, Swaab DF. Non-pharmacological treatment of sleep and wake disturbances in aging and Alzheimer's disease: chronobiological perspectives. Behav Brain Res 1993; 57: 235–53.
2. Cohen-Mansfield J, Marx MS. The relationship between sleep disturbances and agitation in a nursing home. J Aging Health 1990; 2: 42–57.
3. Hozumi S, Okawa M, Mishima K, Hishikawa Y, Hori H, Takahashi K. Phototherapy for elderly patients with dementia and sleep–wake rhythm disorders—a comparison between morning and evening light exposure. Japan J Psychiat Neurol 1990; 44: 813–14.
4. Rebok GW, Rovner BW, Folstein MF. Sleep disturbance and Alzheimer's disease: relationship to behavioral problems. Aging 1991; 3: 193–6.
5. Lebert F, Pasquier F, Petit H. Sundowning syndrome in demented patients without neuroleptic therapy. Arch Gerontol Geriat 1996; 22: 49–54.
6. Sanford JR. Tolerance of debility in elderly dependents by supporters at home: its significance for hospital practice. Br Med J 1975; 3: 471–3.
7. Rabins PV, Mace NL, Lucas MJ. The impact of dementia on the family. JAMA 1982; 248: 333–5.
8. Pollak CP, Perlick D. Sleep problems and institutionalization of the elderly. J Geriat Psychiat Neurol 1991; 4: 204–10.

9. Gallagher-Thompson D, Brooks JOD, Bliwise D, Leader J, Yesavage JA. The relations among caregiver stress, 'sundowning' symptoms, and cognitive decline in Alzheimer's disease. J Am Geriat Soc 1992; 40: 807–10.

10. Van Someren EJW. Rest–Activity Rhythms in Aging, Alzheimer's Disease and Parkinson's Disease. Methodological Developments and Therapeutic Interventions. PhD Thesis, Medical Faculty of the University of Amsterdam, University of Amsterdam, Amsterdam.

11. Van Someren EJW, Scherder EJA, Swaab DF. Transcutaneous electrical nerve stimulation (TENS) improves circadian rhythm disturbances in Alzheimer's disease. Alzheimer's Dis Assoc Disord 1998; 12: 114–18.

12. Swaab DF. Brain aging and Alzheimer's disease, 'wear and tear' versus 'use it or lose it'. Neurobiol Aging 1991; 12: 317–24.

13. Tucker KR, Seider MJ, Booth FW. Protein synthesis rates in atrophied gastrocnemius muscles after limb immobilization. J Appl Physiol 1981; 51: 73–7.

14. Swaab DF, Fliers E, Partiman TS. The suprachiasmatic nucleus of the human brain in relation to sex, age and senile dementia. Brain Res 1985; 342: 37–44.

15. Witting W, Mirmiran M, Bos NP, Swaab DF. Effect of light intensity on diurnal sleep–wake distribution in young and old rats. Brain Res Bull 1993; 30: 157–62.

16. Lucassen PJ, Hofman MA, Swaab DF. Increased light intensity prevents the age-related loss of vasopressin-expressing neurons in the rat suprachiasmatic nucleus. Brain Res 1995; 693: 261–6.

17. Kondo K, Niino M, Shido K. A case-control study of Alzheimer's disease in Japan—significance of life-styles. Dementia 1994; 5: 314–26.

18. Campbell SS, Kripke DF, Gillin JC, Hrubovcak JC. Exposure to light in healthy elderly subjects and Alzheimer's patients. Physiol Behav 1988; 42: 141–4.

19. Sanchez R, Ge Y, Zee PC. A comparison of the strength of external Zeitgebers in young and older adults. Sleep Res 1993; 22: 416.

20. Ancoli-Israel S, Klauber MR, Gillin JC, Campbell SS, Hofstetter CR. Sleep in non-institutionalized Alzheimer's disease patients. Aging Clin Exp Res 1994; 6: 451–8.

21. Blanks JC, Schmidt SY, Torigoe Y, Porrello KV, Hinton DR, Blanks RHI. Retinal pathology in Alzheimer's disease. 2. Regional neuron loss and glial changes in GCL. Neurobiol Aging 1996; 17: 385–95.

22. Blanks JC, Torigoe Y, Hinton DR, Blanks RHI. Retinal pathology in Alzheimer's disease. 1. Ganglion cell loss in foveal/parafoveal retina. Neurobiol Aging 1996; 17: 377–84.

23. Hughes PC, Neer RM. Lighting for the elderly: a psychobiological approach to lighting. Human Factors 1981; 23: 65–85.

24. Teresi J, Lawton MP, Ory M, Holmes D. Measurement issues in chronic care populations: dementia special care. Alzheimer's Dis Assoc Disord 1994; 8 (suppl 1): S144–83.

25. Van Someren EJW, Lijzenga C, Mirmiran M, Swaab DF. Effect of physical activity on the circadian system in the elderly. In: Mallick BN, Singh R (eds) Environment and Physiology. New Delhi: Narosa, 1994; 153–63.

26. Kabuto M, Otsuka T, Saito K, Maruyama S. A preliminary report on the levels and rhythmicity of urinary melatonin in the patients with senile dementia of the Alzheimer type. Mental Health Res 1982; 29: 65–77.

27. Nair NPV, Hariharasubramanian N, Pilapil C, Thavundayil JX. Plasma melatonin rhythm in normal aging and Alzheimer's disease. J Neural Transm 1986; 21 (suppl): 494.

28. Sack RL, Lewy AJ, Erb DL, Vollmer WM, Singer CM. Human melatonin production decreases with age. J Pineal Res 1986; 3: 379–88.

29. Nair NP, Hariharasubramanian N, Pilapil C, Isaac I, Thavundayil JX. Plasma melatonin—an index of brain aging in humans? Biol Psychiat 1986; 21: 141–50.
30. Sharma M, Palacios-Bois J, Schwartz G, Iskandar H, Thakkur M, Quirion R, Nair NPV. Circadian rhythms of melatonin and cortisol in aging. Biol Psychiat 1989; 25: 305–19.
31. Skene DJ, Vivien-Roels B, Sparks DL, Hunsaker JC, Pevet P, Ravid D, Swaab DF. Daily variation in the concentration of melatonin and 5-methoxytryptophol in the human pineal gland: effect of age and Alzheimer's disease. Brain Res 1990; 528: 170–74.
32. Uchida K, Okamoto N, Ohara K, Morita Y. Daily rhythm of serum melatonin in patients with dementia of the degenerate type. Brain Res 1996; 717: 154–9.
33. Mishima K, Hishikawa Y. Chronotherapy for circadian rhythm disorders in elderly patients with dementia. In: Sleep and Sleep Disorders: From Molecule to Behavior. Takeda Science Foundation, 1997; 177–91.
34. Nair NPN, Schwartz G, Ng Ying Kin NMK, Thakur M, Thavundayil JX. Melatonin and cortisol circadian rhythms in Alzheimer's disease patients and normal elderly subjects. In: Touitou Y (ed) Biological Clocks: Mechanisms and Applications. Amsterdam: Elsevier, 1998; 357–60.
35. Van Someren EJW, Hagebeuk EEO, Lijzenga C, Scheltens P, De Rooij SEJA, Jonker C, Pot A-M, Mirmiran M, Swaab DF. Circadian rest–activity rhythm disturbances in Alzheimer's disease. Biol Psychiat 1996; 40: 259–70.
36. Van Someren EJW, Kessler A, Mirmiran M, Swaab DF. Indirect bright light improves circadian rest–activity rhythm disturbances in demented patients. Biol Psychiat 1997; 41: 955–63.
37. Van Someren EJW, Lijzenga C, Mirmiran M, Swaab DF. Long-term fitness training improves the circadian rest–activity rhythm in elderly males. J Biol Rhythms 1997; 12: 146–56.
38. Cliffer KD, Burstein R, Giesler GJ Jr. Distributions of spinothalamic, spino-hypothalamic, and spinotelencephalic fibers revealed by anterograde transport of PHA-L in rats. J Neurosci 1991; 11: 852–68.
39. Newman HM, Stevens RT, Apkarian AV. Direct spinal projections to limbic and striatal areas: anterograde transport studies from the upper cervical spinal cord and the cervical enlargement in squirrel monkey and rat. J Comp Neurol 1996; 365: 640–58.
40. Scherder EJA, Van Someren EJW, Swaab DF. Transcutaneous electrical nerve stimulation (TENS) improves the rest–activity rhythm in midstage Alzheimer's disease (submitted).
41. Rutishauser U, Landmesser L. Polysialic acid in the vertebrate nervous system: a promoter of plasticity in cell–cell interactions. Trends Neurosci 1996; 19: 422–7.
42. Okawa M, Mishima K, Shimizu T, Iijima S, Hishikawa Y, Hozumi S, Hori H. Sleep–wake rhythm disorders and their phototherapy in elderly patients with dementia. Japan J Psychiat Neurol 1989; 43: 293–5.
43. Satlin A, Volicer L, Ross V, Herz L, Campbell S. Bright light treatment of behavioral and sleep disturbances in patients with Alzheimer's disease. Am J Psychiat 1992; 149: 1028–32.
44. Lovell BB, Ancoli-Israel S, Gevirtz R. Effect of bright light treatment on agitated behavior in institutionalized elderly subjects. Psychiat Res 1995; 57: 7–12.
45. Reisberg B, Franssen E, Sclan SG, Kluger A, Ferris SH. Stage specific incidence of potentially remediable behavioral symptoms in aging and Alzheimer's disease: a study of 120 patients using the BEHAVE-AD. Bull Clin Neurosci 1989; 95–112.

46. Hopkins RW, Rindlisbacher P, Grant NT. An investigation of the sundowning syndrome and ambient light. Am J Alzheimer's Care Related Disord Res 1992; 7: 22–7.

Address for correspondence:
E.J.W. Van Someren,
Netherlands Institute for Brain Research,
Meibergdreef 33, 1105 AZ Amsterdam, The Netherlands
Tel: 31 20 566 5500; fax: 31 20 696 1006;
e-mail: E.van.Someren@nih.knaw.nl

90 Exercise Program in Patients with Alzheimer's Disease

C. MOUZAKIDIS, M. TSOLAKI, J. THEODORAKIS,
E. EFREMIDOU AND C. KAMPITSIS

INTRODUCTION

Alzheimer's disease (AD) is a progressive, degenerative disease of the brain which results in impaired memory, thinking and behaviour [3, 4, 14]. AD is distinguished from other forms of dementia by characteristic changes in the brain that are visible only upon microscopic examination. Reduced production of certain brain chemicals, especially acetylcholine, norepinephrine, serotonin and somatostatin, have also been observed. These chemicals are necessary for normal communication between nerve cells. AD is more likely to occur as a person gets older. The disease occurs in middle age as well. In Greece, according to an epidemiological study, 50 000 people aged 70 and over are affected by AD. At this time there is no treatment that can stop or reverse the mental deterioration of AD. New drugs are used and being studied to find out whether they can slow the progression of the disease or improve memory for even a small period of time.

Many studies concerning aged people have suggested that *physical exercise* is beneficial because it improves their functional abilities and cardiovascular capacity, increases their cognitive and psychological functions and increases the production of brain chemicals (norepinephrine, serotonin, etc.) [1, 5, 7, 10, 13, 16]. Although exercise has frequently been incorporated into the activity programs of many nursing homes, there are few indicators about what type of exercise program is most suitable or what groups of elderly residents benefit from these activities.

In a study of patients with dementia, Schwab et al. [9] described how participation in simple stretching and motion exercises elicited a variety of positive responses among patients. Some were taken off psychotropic drugs, some ceased noisy disruptive behaviour and some showed increased interaction with others. Another study [12] with AD patients focused on changes in the cognitive ability of patients residing in two long-term care facilities as they took part in a group exercise therapy program. Results indicated that an exercise program

Alzheimer's Disease and Related Disorders
Edited by K. Iqbal, D.F. Swaab, B. Winblad and H.M. Wisniewski
© 1999 John Wiley & Sons Ltd

seems to increase cognitive ability through increased cardiovascular benefits and emotional stimulation. A recent study [8] formulated a program suited for mildly and moderately impaired patients residing in an AD centre. The study confirmed that the exercise program was both feasible and desirable for patients with AD and that it reduced some of the adverse behaviours of the patients.

According to the literature [2, 5–8, 11, 12, 15–17], most studies on exercise programmes have been conducted with institutionalized patients. There are fewer studies which have been conducted with AD patients and none of them with outpatients.

The main purpose of the present study was to work out exercise programs for outpatients with AD, in order to find out which form of exercise best fits the needs of these patients according to their cognitive, functional and be-havioural level. Thus, this pilot research had four purposes:

1. To work out and form an individualized exercise program for AD outpatients.
2. To evaluate the effectiveness of this program.
3. To determine any changes occurring in the mobility and the fitness level of AD patients.
4. To determine the effectiveness of this programme on the behavioural, cogni-tive and functional state of the AD patient and the progression of the disease.

METHOD

SUBJECTS

Five AD patients (three men and two women), aged 50–71 (mean age = 60.6 years), participated in this pilot study.

PROCEDURES

All subjects were evaluated by the clinical diagnostic team of the Third De-partment of Neurology of the Aristotle University of Thessaloniki, in 'G. Papanikolaou' General Hospital, and were found to meet the DSM-IV and NINCDS–ADRDA criteria for clinically probable senile dementia of the AD type (MMSE = 4–20; mean score = 14.6). The scientific team consisted of a neurologist, a psychologist, a general practitioner and a fitness instructor.

MATERIAL

The exercise program was conducted in (a) the physiotherapy room of the hospital, which was modified for the purposes and needs of the exercise pro-gram, and (b) a municipal gymnasium in the centre of the city.

We used simple exercising equipment such as coloured easily controlled balls, sticks, hoops of different sizes, plastic bottles, soda cans, static bicycles and a mechanical treadmill.

A battery of psychomotor, flexibility, upper and lower limbs strength, endurance and agility tests were used at the beginning and end of the program, in order to evaluate the general ability of each patient.

DURATION

The program lasted 16 weeks (3 days/week, every other day). Every exercise session lasted 60 min.

EXERCISE PROGRAM

The exercise program consisted of a warm-up period (10 min), a main exercise period (40–45 min) and a cool-down period (5–10 min). Each patient was exercised alone. During the exercise session extra assistance was given to the patients by three physiotherapists who had been trained especially for these patients.

The *warm-up* period consisted of a series of safe range-of-motion exercises designed to gently stretch each major muscle group and increase flexibility in order to prepare the body for exercise and decrease the chance of injury. The protocol was a combination of standing and sitting exercises with one or two trials and five to eight repetitions per trial.

The *cool-down* period consisted of the same protocol, its main purpose being to allow the heart rate to return to normal and the body to relax.

In the main exercise period, exercise routines were chosen to improve flexibility, strength of upper and lower limbs, endurance, orientation, memory, dexterity and agility of the patients. The exercises can be modified to the needs and the abilities of each patient. Each exercise was repeated five times, increasing according to the attainment level of each patient.

RESULTS

1. There were improvements in the flexibility, the strength of upper and lower limbs, the coordination and the agility of the patients.
2. The varying levels of dementia did not make a notable difference in exercise performance. In one case (Patient 5) we had to modify the program because of his weak lower limbs.
3. The patients enjoyed exercising. They cooperated with the staff and had fun. They were anxious about the time and the day of the exercise program.

4. Conducting one-to-one exercises allowed the staff to give more attention to the patients.
5. The patients' self-efficacy and self-esteem were improved. Their attention to the program was improved.
6. We started to bring together in the exercise room two patients (Patient 2 and Patient 3), between the 12th and 16th weeks of the pilot program. We had the impression that they enjoyed the exercise more when they were together. They told us that they had more fun and that they would like to exercise together from now on.
7. We were informed by their caregivers that the patients showed a considerable decrease in disruptive behaviour and became more socialized. One caregiver told us that his wife started her household activities again.
8. We were also informed that there were improvements in the quality of sleep in these patients.

Table 1 shows the increase in MMSE in three of the five patients.

Table 1. MMSE before and after exercise program

Patients	Sex	Age	MMSE (before)	MMSE (after)
1	Female	50	20	22
2	Male	51	20	25
3	Male	71	19	20
4	Female	63	10	10
5	Male	69	04	04

CONCLUSIONS

- AD patients are able to participate in an exercise program.
- Improvements in their strength and their flexibility as well as in their cognitive and behavioural function are feasible.
- More research has to be done to evaluate the effectiveness of an exercise intervention on cognitive function, physical abilities and psychological effects in an AD patient.

This research was a pilot project with individualized exercise intervention in order to formulate and discover the most suitable exercise routines for AD patients. The results have shown us that an exercise intervention specially designed for patients with dementia is feasible. Our future concern is to compare a group intervention with an individualized one and in two different populations in Greece and the UK.

ACKNOWLEDGEMENTS

The project is supported by the European Commission, Grant No. SOC 97 201421 05F03.

REFERENCES

1. Blumenthal J, Emery C, Madden D, George L, Coleman E, Riddle MW, McKee DC, Reasoner J, Williams RS. Cardiovascular and behavioral effects of aerobic exercise training in healthy older men and women. J Gerontol 1989; 44: 147–57.
2. Bowlby C. Therapeutic Activities with Persons Disabled by Alzheimer's Disease and Related Disorders. Gaithersburg, MD: Aspen, 1993; 150–54.
3. Cohen-Mansfield J, Billing N. Agitated behaviors in the elderly: I. J Am Geriat Soc 1986; 34: 711–21.
4. Coons DH. Wandering. Am J Alzheimer's Care Rel Disord Res 1988; 3: 31–6.
5. Hopkins DR, Murrah B, Hoeger WW, Rhodes C. Effect of low-impact aerobic dance on the functional fitness of elderly women. Gerontologist 1990; 30: 189–92.
6. McGrowder-Lin R, Bhatt A. A wanderer's lounge program for nursing home residents with Alzheimer's disease. Gerontologist 1988; 28: 607–9.
7. Molloy D, Beerschoten D, Borrie M, Crilly R, Cape RD. Acute effects of exercise on neuropsychological function in elderly subjects. J Am Geriat Soc 1988; 36: 29–33.
8. Namazi KH, Gwinnup PB, Zadorozny CA. A low intensity exercise/movement program for patients with Alzheimer's disease: the TEMP-AD protocol. J Aging Phys Activity 1994; 2: 80–92.
9. Schwab M, Rader J, Doan J. Relieving the anxiety and fear in dementia. J Gerontol Nursing 1985; 11: 8–15.
10. Shephard RJ. The scientific basis of exercise prescribing for the very old. J Am Geriat Soc 1990; 83: 62–70.
11. Poser CM, Ronthal M. Exercise and Alzheimer's disease, Parkinson's disease and multiple sclerosis. Physician Sportsmed 1991; 19: 85–92.
12. Lindenmuth G, Moose B. Improving cognitive abilities of elderly Alzheimer's patients with intense exercise therapy. Am J Alzheimer's Care Rel Disord Res 1990; 5: 31–3.
13. Binder EF, Brown M, Craft S, Schechtman KB, Birge SJ. Effects of a group exercise program on risk factors for falls in frail older adults. J Aging Phys Activity 1994; 2: 25–37.
14. Goldsmith SM, Hoeffer B, Rader J. Problematic wandering behavior in the cognitively impaired elderly. A single-subject case study. J Psychosoc Nurs Ment Health Serv 1995; 33(2): 6–12.
15. Miziniak H. Persons with Alzheimer's: effects of nutrition and exercise. J Gerontol Nurs 1994; 20(10): 27–32.
16. Fiatarone MA, O'Neill EF, Ryan ND, Clements KM, Solares GR, Nelson ME et al. Exercise training and nutritional supplementation for physical frailty in very elderly people. N Engl J Med 1994; 330: 1769–75.

17. Emery CF, Gatz M. Psychological and cognitive effects of an exercise program for community residing older adults. Gerontologist 1990; 30(2): 184–8.

Address for correspondence:
    Chris A. Mouzakidis,
    Department of Physical Education & Sport Science,
    Democritus University of Thrace,
    40 Mikras Asias Str. 55 132, Kalamaria,
    Thessaloniki, Greece

X   Psychosocial

91 The Circle Model—Support for Relatives of People with Dementia*

WALLIS JANSSON, BRITT ALMBERG,
MARGARETA GRAFSTRÖM AND
BENGT WINBLAD

For most people with dementia, the home is the primary setting in which care is provided. There, the majority of disabled elderly receive the bulk of their personal care and support from family members [1, 2].

The effects of dementia are not limited to the sufferer. The involvement of relatives in the care of a person with dementia has consequences for their lives and well-being. The family caregivers of cognitively impaired elderly often experience high levels of physical, psychological and emotional strain due to their caregiving role (for review, see [3]). These experiences, which collectively are known as 'caregiver burden', were also reported from the Kungsholmen Project, which is an epidemiological population-based study carried out at the Stockholm Gerontology Research Center in Sweden. In this study, relatives of elders with and without dementia have been followed by interviews for several years [2, 4–7].

The results collected from interviews with the family caregivers participating in the Kungsholmen Project indicated that information about dementia and accessibility of support available from the community were needed. A frequent request which arose from the caregivers was the availability of respite from the care-providing routine. For these reasons, an intervention study, called the 'Circle Model', was carried out.

The purpose of the intervention study was to develop and test a model to meet the desires of the family caregivers, and also to assess the experiences of each group of Circle Model participants. Participating in the study were relatives of people with dementia, volunteers and parish deacons. Their experiences were assessed on the following objectives:

* The text of this chapter was originally published as part of an article in Int J Geriat Psychiat 1998; 13: 674–681. Reproduced by permission.

Alzheimer's Disease and Related Disorders
Edited by K. Iqbal, D.F. Swaab, B. Winblad and H.M. Wisniewski
© 1999 John Wiley & Sons Ltd

- The training and care relief services provided by the study.
- The participation and experiences of the volunteers.
- The parish deacons serving as trainers and group leaders.

Collaboration was initiated between the Stockholm Gerontology Research Center, the Church of Sweden Commission of Congregational Life, the Ersta diakonisällskap (Ersta association for deaconal work), the National Dementia Association in Sweden and the Swedish Christian Educational Association.

The study was conducted in several stages (Figure 1):

- *Stage 1.* Fifteen deacons within the Swedish Church from nine localities in Sweden were trained in an overview course in dementia (equivalent to 5 weeks of full-time studies) at the Stockholm University College of Health Sciences.
- *Stage 2.* The deacons recruited, from their respective congregations, primary family caregivers and volunteers willing to participate in the study. Collaboration with the social services provided contacts with the relatives. The volunteers were, in most cases, recruited from the voluntary network within the Swedish Church. Twenty-seven relatives and the same number of volunteers were recruited.
- *Stage 3.* The relatives and the volunteers were trained together in study circles consisting of 8–10 participants, with the deacons as leaders and in collaboration with the Swedish Christian Educational Association. The groups met weekly for 3 h on five occasions and focused on the following pertinent topics: (a) aspects of dementia; (b) guidelines for interaction and establishment of contact with persons suffering from dementia; (c) community resources and services available; and (d) ethical and confidentiality issues. At the completion of five training study circle sessions, suitable assignment of a volunteer to fit the family's needs was based on close and personal network established between the relative and the volunteer.
- *Stage 4.* The volunteers began providing respite care services. The volunteer's task was to provide companionship for the elderly person, not to perform the normal social service tasks. The relief care phase of this study was implemented for 4–5 h/week for 4 months. During this stage, the deacons provided support for the volunteers and the relatives. The study circle continued with monthly meetings.

Before the study circle and after the relief care phase, the research leaders conducted interviews with the participants of the study. The questionnaires used in the interviews contained open-ended questions. All the interviews were tape recorded, transcribed and analysed by coding and categorization (italicized in the following text).

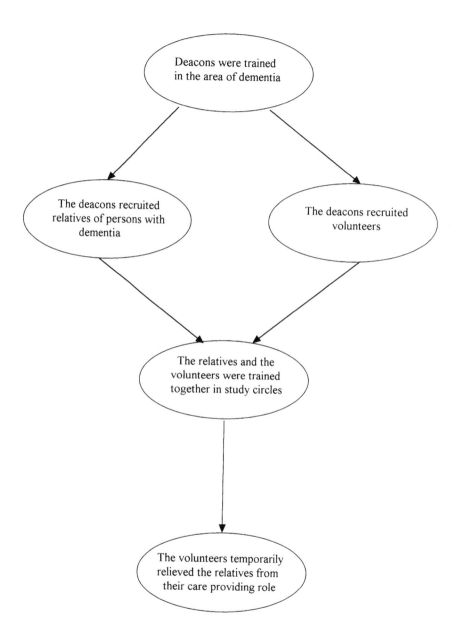

Figure 1. The Circle Model

HOW DID THE CIRCLE MODEL PARTICIPANTS EXPERIENCE THE TRAINING AND THE RELIEF CARE SERVICES?

THE RELATIVES

The relatives emphasized *experience exchanges* as being very important. Many of them had not previously had the opportunity to express and share their feelings with others. The study circle experiences were expressed in positive statements such as the following:

> All have been able to talk about their situations and, in particular, exchange experiences. One hears that others have in fact had similar and equally stressful problems.

The relatives reported acquiring increased *knowledge* about dementia and support available from the community. This category, together with exchanges of experiences, had led to better *coping strategies*:

> I have become more tolerant towards Karl since I started this course. I didn't know anything about this previously.

They expressed experiencing a spirit of *community* which emerged among the study circle group members:

> This group is the best there is. We have become very good friends.

The *feelings of security* and *relaxation* were also described by the relatives with regard to the temporary relief care service provided by the volunteers:

> I felt secure. It is great if one can have someone at home.

> I could relax completely when she was here. I felt that I could rely on Karin.

THE VOLUNTEERS

The volunteers were highly satisfied with their participation in the study. They appreciated the *theoretical* as well as the *practical* knowledge which they had received during the study circles. Much of the practical knowledge which the volunteers gained was the result of listening to the relatives' verbal accounts of personal experiences:

> This close contact with the relatives has been very profitable because, whatever the circumstances, one cannot get an understanding of their situation by reading a book. One must come closer to them in order to understand how extensive their problems really are and how tied up they in fact are.

Prior to this intervention study the volunteers had had little or no contact with a person suffering from dementia. Therefore some of them felt *concerned* and uncertain at the initial relief care session:

> It went well but I was nervous that it would not work out from a human point of view. One knows that some people do not fit in well together because of their different personalities.

The volunteers were able to apply theoretical knowledge to lessen the elders' memory deficits by listening to the recounting of past events and considering their special interests. They were good at finding common *meeting places*. One of the volunteers said, for instance:

> The dialogues between us go really well if we keep the topics of conversation within certain familiar subjects. For example, we talk about places they have lived, their hobbies and experiences in the past. We speak about Tranås (a small town in Sweden), Hyland (a television personality in Sweden) and furniture styles.

The volunteers did not receive any remuneration for their efforts; nevertheless, the volunteer work was reported as rewarding. They obtained *satisfaction* from their efforts in providing a period of relaxation for the relatives and by doing something valuable for another person. The volunteer work for them was not only a matter of giving, but also encompassed reciprocity [8, 9]. The experience was expressed as:

> It is a mutual give and take.

The intervention was time-limited but the group meetings have continued beyond the originally planned sessions, indicating that both the recipients and the volunteers perceived benefits from the activity.

THE DEACONS

The deacons' experiences of linking prospective participants to the project, of being leaders of the study circles and having a supportive role during the period of relief care can be summarized in one quotation:

> It has been good, it has been exciting, but it has also been hard work since one wants to do as good a job as possible. One feels the responsibility because it is human beings whom one takes care of.

CONCLUSION

It is necessary that family caregivers receive considerable support and assistance on an individualized basis to prevent them from being overburdened, and to prolong the time the person with dementia can remain at home. Indeed, effective interventions that will fit the preferences of the family caregivers are increasingly needed to reduce the stress of caregiving.

A variety of interventions for family caregivers is reported in the literature (for review, see [10]) but to our knowledge, the Circle Model is unique in that family caregivers and respite care volunteers are educated together. It provides the caregivers with necessary training and regular time off from the day-to-day care of a relative with dementia. An advantage with the model is the training preceding the care replacement period. This phase provides the necessary knowledge for dealing with the complexity and severe nature of dementia. It also provides an insight for those providing the respite care into what the family caregivers are experiencing. Another advantage of this model is that persons suffering from dementia can remain in their homes, in an environment which is familiar to them.

The Circle Model brings new dimensions to the home care services. The fully developed model provides an effective complementary service to those existing support social services.

REFERENCES

1. Johansson L. Caring for the next of kin. On informal care of the elderly in Sweden. Comprehensive summaries of Uppsala Dissertations from the Faculty of Medicine. Acta Universitatis Upsaliensis 1991.
2. Grafström M, Fratiglioni L, Sandman P-O, Winblad B. Health and social consequences for relatives of demented and nondemented elderly: a population-based study. J Clin Epidemiol 1992; 45: 861–70.
3. Dhooper SS. Caregivers of Alzheimer's disease patients: a review of the literature. J Gerontol Soc Work 1991; 18: 19–37.
4. Grafström M, Norberg A, Winblad B. Abuse is in the eye of the beholder. Reports by family members about abuse of demented persons in home care. A total population-based study. Scand J Soc Med 1993; 21: 247–55.
5. Grafström M, Winblad B. Family burden in the care of the demented and nondemented elderly—a longitudinal study. Alzheimer's Dis Assoc Disord 1995; 9: 78–86.
6. Almberg B, Grafström M, Winblad B. Caring for a demented elderly person—burden and burnout among caregiving relatives. J Adv Nurs 1997; 25: 109–16.
7. Jansson W, Grafström M, Winblad B. Daughters and sons as caregivers for their demented and non-demented elderly parents. A part of a population-based study carried out in Sweden. Scand J Soc Med 1997; 25: 289–95.
8. Dorfman LT, Rubenstein LM. Paid and unpaid activities and retirement satisfaction among rural seniors. Phys Occup Ther Geriat 1993; 12: 45–63.
9. Smith JD. Volunteering in Europe: opportunities and options for the next decade. Soc Med Tidskr 1994; 9: 386–91.
10. Bourgeois MS, Schulz R, Burgio L. Interventions for caregivers of patients with Alzheimer's disease: a review and analysis of content, process and outcomes. Int J Aging Hum Devel 1996; 43: 35–92.

Address for correspondence:
Wallis Jansson,
Stockholm Gerontology Research Center,
Box 6401, SE–113 82 Stockholm, Sweden
Tel: 46 8 690 58 06; fax: 46 8 33 52 75;
e-mail: Wallis.Jansson@ebox.tninet.se

92 Support Program for Demented Patients and Their Carers: The Role of Dementia Family Care Coordinator Is Crucial

ULLA ELONIEMI-SULKAVA, JUHANI SIVENIUS AND
RAIMO SULKAVA

INTRODUCTION

The major problems in home care of demented patients are carers' distress and patients' behavioural and functional problems [1–5], which often leads patients to institutional long-term care. Training programs and therapeutic group meetings have been used in supporting carers, with positive results [6–8]. Some recent studies show that it is also possible to conduct programs for demented patients which improve their functional capacity [9, 10].

The public service system is often complicated and carers have to contact different professionals for different needs and problems. Demented patients and their primary carers need a care coordinator who would take a comprehensive responsibility for services they need. This coordinator would make possible a 'one-stop shopping' principle in service organization [11].

The intervention provided by professionals has been efficiently used previously among elderly people living in the community [12–14]. The post of a Stroke Family Care Worker has been evaluated in supporting both a patient and a carer [15]. This type of intervention measure has not previously been studied among demented patients and their carers. We conducted a prospective randomized intervention study in 1993–1996 with the aim of evaluating the effect of support from a Dementia Family Care Coordinator (DFCC) in prolonging home care. In addition, patients and carers participated in yearly training courses.

Alzheimer's Disease and Related Disorders
Edited by K. Iqbal, D.F. Swaab, B. Winblad and H.M. Wisniewski
© 1999 John Wiley & Sons Ltd

METHODS

SUBJECTS

The study patients were drawn from the list of the patients of the National Pension Institution entitled to payment for home care because of dementing disease in the area of five communes in eastern Finland (total population 124 000). The payment for home care (USD 70–300/month, depending on the need for care) is tax-free and independent of income. It can be obtained on the basis of a medical certificate, stating that the patient needs help on a regular basis in order to be able to live at home. All patients with dementing disease and requiring regular care are eligible for the payment.

The patients were eligible for the study if they were 65 years or over, living at home with the primary support of an informal carer and were without any other severe disease (e.g. severe stroke, cancer) possibly leading to institutionalization in the near future. We excluded those who were prevented from participation in yearly courses with the carer.

A total of 141 demented patients were found to be eligible for the study. Of these, 26 refused and 15 were unable to participate in the yearly courses. No significant differences could be seen in clinical features between the study patients and drop-outs. The study patients (n = 100) were randomly allocated to the intervention group (n = 53) and the control group (n = 47). Before randomization all patients were diagnosed by a neurologist according to the DSM-IIIR criteria [16].

Before randomization the study patients and their carers gave written consent to participate in the study. The study was approved by the ethics committee of the National Pensions Institution and the Board of Health Authorities in the home cities of the study subjects.

INTERVENTION

The control patients received services from the municipal social and health care system or from the private sector as usual. The 2 year support program was provided for the intervention patients. The program consisted of two types of intervention. The main intervention was the comprehensive support provided by a DFCC, who had access to a physician. The DFCC gave continuous and systematic counselling, conducted follow-up calls and in-home visits as well as arranging social and health care services. She acted as a dementia expert and an advocate for the patients and the carers. However, she had no funds to buy services for the patients. Thus, only services which were in the financial range of the carers and patients were used.

The other type of intervention came through annual courses, in which both the patients and the carers participated (8–10 patients with their carer on each course). The first course was at the beginning of the study, lasting for 10 days. The following two courses were 1 and 2 years later, lasting for 5 days. The purpose of the courses was to support the functional capacity and adaptation of both patients and carers. They included medical check-ups, psychological assessments, lectures, therapeutic group meetings and different kinds of physical, mental and social stimulation. The rehabilitation team made the service plan for each family. The DFCC arranged the planned services with the patient's and his/her carer's permission and at their expense.

MAIN OUTCOME MEASURES

The end point of the study was either the death or the long-term institutional care of a patient. Main outcome measures were institutionalization and the period in home care from enrollment of patients in the study to moving to long-term institutional care.

STATISTICAL ANALYSES

Statistical analyses were performed using SPSS for Windows 6.1. The differences in continuous variables within and between the groups were compared by Student's t-test. The chi-squared test was used for dependences of variables.

RESULTS

There were no drop-outs in the study during the 2-year follow-up. The baseline characteristics of the patients and their carers are shown in Tables 1 and 2. No significant differences could be found in characteristics between the groups.

LONG-TERM INSTITUTIONAL CARE AND DEATH

There were no significant differences in the number of the patients having moved to long-term institutional care and that of deaths between the groups during the 2-year study. After the first year, four patients (8%) from the intervention group and nine patients (19%) from the control group moved to the long-term institutional care (p = 0.09). Six (11%) intervention patients and three control patients (6%) had died (p = 0.39) during home care. At the end of the second year, 17 intervention patients (32%) and 14 control patients (30%) had moved to long-term institutional care (p = 0.80). Nine (17%) intervention and eight (17%) control patients had died in home care.

Table 1. Base-line characteristics of study patients (n = 100) at the beginning of intervention. Percentages in brackets

	Intervention patients (n = 53)	Control patients (n = 47)
Mean age (years); range	78.8; 65–97	80.1; 67–91
Gender		
Female	26 (49)	27 (57)
Male	27 (51)	20 (43)
Diagnosis		
Alzheimer's disease	30 (57)	24 (51)
Vascular dementia	16 (30)	19 (40)
Other	7 (13)	4 (9)
MMSE score (mean ± SD)	14.4 ± 6.2	15.3 ± 5.5
Barthel Index score (mean ± SD)	85.3 ± 13.6	79.8 ± 21.0
MARDS score (mean ± SD)	9.6 ± 6.4	11.7 ± 6.8
Living arrangement		
Alone	6 (11)	3 (6)
With a carer	47 (89)	44 (94)

Table 2. Base-line characteristics of the carers in the intervention and control group. Percentages in brackets

	Intervention group (n = 53)	Control group (n = 47)
Mean age (years); range	64.8; 34–83	63.3; 40–86
Gender		
Female	40 (75)	29 (62)
Male	13 (25)	18 (38)
Relationship		
Spouse	32 (60)	24 (51)
Child	14 (27)	20 (43)
Other	7 (13)	3 (6)
Health		
Good	33 (62)	31 (66)
Moderate	15 (28)	11 (23)
Poor	5 (10)	5 (11)
GHQ score (mean ± SD)	4.3 ± 3.6	3.9 ± 3.1

PERIOD IN HOME CARE

The median time of home care in those who were institutionalized was 233 days longer in the intervention group (473 days) than in the control group (240 days) (p = 0.02).

JOB DESCRIPTION OF DEMENTIA FAMILY CARE COORDINATOR

The DFCC had a public health nurse background. At the beginning and during the study she was given a wide range of training regarding dementia care.

The first main task of the DFCC was to take comprehensive responsibility in supporting the patients and their primary carers during difficult situations in home care (Table 3). It was emphasized to the carers to contact the DFCC in the case of any problem arising. The DFCC was available 24 h/day via mobile phone. Typical contacts were due to patients' health problems, sleep disturbances or anxiety. The DFCC would respond by making a home visit aiming to evaluate the causes of the problem and support the carer to live through the problem. Patients' unsuitable medication, pain and low blood pressure and a carer's burden of unbroken duties were the most common causes of problems. Often the DFCC had to be persistent in trying to find solutions. The doctor could be contacted for consultation and medical care. During the process of problem solving the carer was strongly supported.

Table 3. Tasks of Dementia Family Care Coordinator (DFCC)

Follow-up calls
In-home visits
Arranging social and health care services with the goal of 'one-stop shopping'
Problem solving in crises threatening home care
Psychological support

The second main task was to coordinate patients' services. The patients and carers could contact the DFCC with all kinds of problems. The DFCC collaborated with the municipal social and health care system in order to get proper, good quality services for patients and their carers. Services from a physiotherapist were often crucial for a patient's functional capacity. During the service delivery (e.g. institutional respite care) she followed the quality of the service. The goal was a 'one-stop shop'. As an advocate the DFCC worked for families, respecting their needs and wishes rather than those of the social and health care system.

The DFCC has to be an expert in dementia care. She has to be a positive, flexible and persistent person. She has to be able to take responsibility and to work independently.

COMMENT AND CONCLUSIONS

Our prospective randomized intervention study showed that the period in home care can be prolonged through the support from a DFCC. Based on our results, it can be estimated that during the 2 years of intervention, the period of home care is 6 years longer per 100 patients than without intervention.

The patients were drawn from the list of patients of the National Pension Institution entitled to a payment for home care. All community-living demented patients requiring regular care are entitled to the payment. Recruitment from the list of a national organization covering all Finns makes it likely that the results can be fairly well generalized to concern all demented Finnish people aged 65 years and over, living at home with primary support of an informal carer.

To our knowledge, our study is the first prospective randomized study where the long-term intervention was directed both to the demented patients and their carers. This kind of intervention provided by home care professionals has been used earlier, e.g. among elderly people and stroke patients living in the community [12–15, 17].

The annual courses were conducted to provide knowledge, stimulation and rehabilitation for the patients and their carers. Service plans based on individual needs assessments of the patients and their carers were made. According to our experience, the courses should take place more frequently (2–3 times a year) and they could be shorter (3–5 days).

The intervention in our study could be conducted within the municipal social and health care system. In the study area, with a population of 124 400 (13% aged 65 years and over), there were 141 demented patients living with their carers who would have needed the type of intervention used in our study. Our experience shows that one DFCC is able to support at least 50 demented patients and their primary carers. We can estimate that one coordinator is needed for a population of 7000 aged 65 years and over. We would like to emphasize that successful work of the DFCC demands a wide range of knowledge and skill regarding dementia care. The coordinator needs continuous training and support and she should have access to a physician for consultation. Home care intervention used in our study is suitable for all demented patients, regardless of the aetiology and stage of dementia.

Home care is usually the best solution for demented patients, if they have somebody to take care of them. It is often preferred by carers even at more advanced stages of dementia. Home care provides the opportunity for financial savings. In 1993 we started the community-based, randomized study, 'Support of home care of demented patients'. The aim of the intervention study was to evaluate whether it was possible to prolong home care by providing systematic support to demented patients and their carers. The subjects of the study consisted of 100 demented patients living at home with the primary support of the informal carer. The patients were randomly allocated to the intervention group (n = 53) and the control group (n = 47). Main outcome measures were institutionalization and period in home care from enrollment of patients in the study to moving to long-term institutional care. The 2 year support program was provided for the intervention group. This program consisted of systematic support from a dementia family care coordinator (DFCC) and yearly courses for the patients and carers. The control patients received their standard services from the municipal social and health care system or from the private sector. After 2 years, 17 (32%) intervention and 14 (30%) control patients had ended up in long-term care. The number of deaths was the same. The median time of home care before institutionalization was 233 days longer in the intervention than in the control group (p = 0.02). Thus, we were able to prolong the period of home care of demented patients by providing proper supporting services to both the patients and their carers. Our results during the 2 years of support indicate that the period of home care is 6 years longer per 100 patients than without intervention.

REFERENCES

1. Gold DP, Reis MF, Markiewicz D, Andres D. When home caregiving ends: a longitudinal study of outcomes for caregivers of relatives with dementia. J Am Geriat Soc 1995; 43: 10–16.
2. Gibbons P, Cannon M, Wrigley M. A study of aggression among referrals to a community-based psychiatry of old age service. Int J Geriat Psychiat 1997; 12: 384–8.
3. Juva K, Mäkelä M, Sulkava R, Erkinjuntti T. One-year risk of institutionalization in demented outpatients with caretaking relatives. Int Psychogeriat 1997; 9: 175–82.
4. Scott WK, Edwards KB, Davis DR, Cornman CB, Macera CA. Risk of institutionalization among community long-term clients with dementia. Gerontologist 1997; 37: 46–51.
5. Vernooij-Dassen M, Felling A, Persoon J. Predictors of change and continuity in home care for dementia patients. Int J Geriat Psychiat 1997; 12: 671–7.
6. Brodaty H, Gresham M, Luscombe G. The Prince Henry Hospital dementia caregivers training program. Int J Geriat Psychiat 1997; 12: 183–92.
7. Graham C, Ballard C, Sham P. Carers' knowledge of dementia, their coping strategies and morbidity. Int J Geriat Psychiat 1997; 12: 931–6.
8. Mittelman MS, Ferris SH, Shulman E, Steinberg G, Levin B. A family intervention to delay nursing home placement of patients with Alzheimer's disease. J Am Med Assoc 1996; 276: 1725–31.
9. Eloniemi U, Tervala J, Sulkava R. Special care units (SCUs) are efficient in respite care of demented patients. Res Pract Alzheimer's Dis 1998; 1: 223–32.
10. Rosewarne R, Bruce A, McKenna M. Dementia programme effectiveness in long-term care. Int J Geriat Psychiat 1997; 12: 173–82.
11. Katofsky L, Levin E. Community-based formal support services. In: Gauthier S (ed) Clinical Diagnosis and Management of Alzheimer's Disease. London: Martin Dunitz, 1996; 305–17.

12. Rich MW, Beckham V, Wittenberg C, Leven CL, Freedland KE, Carney RM. The multidisciplinary intervention to prevent the readmission of elderly patients with congestive heart failure. N Engl J Med 1995; 333: 1190–95.
13. Rudd AG, Wolfe CDA, Tilling K, Beech R. Randomised controlled trial to evaluate early discharge scheme for patients with stroke. Br Med J 1997; 315: 1039–44.
14. Stuck AE, Aronow HU, Steiner A, Alessi CA, Bula CJ, Gold MN, Yuhas KE, Nisenbaum R, Rubenstein LZ, Beck JC. A trial of annual in-home comprehensive geriatric assessments for elderly people living in the community. N Eng J Med 1995; 333: 1184–9.
15. Dennis M, O'Rourke S, Slattery J, Staniforth T, Warlow C. Evaluation of stroke family care worker: results of a randomized controlled trial. Br Med J 1997; 314: 1071–6.
16. American Psychiatric Association. Diagnostic and Statistical Manual of Mental Disorders, 3rd edn, revised (DSM-IIIR). Washington, DC: American Psychiatric Association, 1987.
17. Bernabei R, Landi F, Gambassi G, Sgadari A, Zuccala G, Mor V, Rubenstein LZ, Carbonin PU. Randomised trial of impact of model of integrated care and case management for older people living in the community. Br Med J 1998; 316: 1348–51.

Address for correspondence:
Ulla Eloniemi-Sulkava
Department of Public Health and General Practice,
University of Kuopio,
PO Box 1627, 70211 Kuopio, Finland
Fax: +358 17 162 937; e-mail: ulla.eloniemi@uku.fi

93 Reducing Stress and Turnover in Professional Caregivers of Alzheimer's Disease Patients

MARY GUERRIERO AUSTROM AND
FREDERICK W. UNVERZAGT

Providing care to patients with Alzheimer's disease (AD) is burdensome and stressful. While it has been well documented that the majority of family caregivers seek institutional care for their loved one at some point in the disease, it is becoming increasingly apparent that professional caregivers also experience stress when providing care to AD patients [1, 2, 3]. Nursing in long-term care (LTC) facilities is physically and emotionally demanding. High levels of morbidity and mortality in the patient population increase the stressful and exhausting nature of the job. In addition, many LTC employees work for near minimum wages, have limited education and limited opportunity for career advancement or for collegial recognition [4, 5, 6]. Although nurses in LTC function with greater autonomy and address very complex patient care needs, they are usually viewed as being less skilled than nurses in acute care settings and not valued as important members of the health care team [3]. If one does not feel valued, it becomes difficult to provide quality, compassionate care to others [4]. The extremely high rates of staff turnover in the LTC industry further underscore the demanding and stressful nature of the job and are making it difficult for facilities to provide the quality, consistent care for AD patients that family caregivers are seeking [1, 2]. The purpose of this paper is to identify issues contributing to staff stress and turnover and to describe a comprehensive staff development and dementia training program which was used as an intervention strategy to increase staff morale and reduce turnover.

INTERVENTION

ASSESSMENT OF TRAINING NEEDS

While most LTC administrators and directors of nursing believe that their staff members are in need of more education about AD in order to do their

Alzheimer's Disease and Related Disorders
Edited by K. Iqbal, D.F. Swaab, B. Winblad and H.M. Wisniewski
© 1999 John Wiley & Sons Ltd

jobs, few administrators take the time to ask the staff what they believe they need to know about AD to do a better job. Fewer still ask their employees what they believe are key issues or concerns affecting their jobs. However, research on adult learners indicates that they will be more motivated to learn and will retain more information if they are involved in the decision making process about the material to be learned [1]. To address the range of needs, we developed a more comprehensive approach, one that not only provides training on the nature of AD but also addresses the working environment and management systems. Our approach includes an assessment, implementation of management development workshops and staff development sessions for the service providers. Finally, we evaluated the impact of this process on several outcome measures.

The assessment process consisted of individual interviews with members of the management team and two focus groups with staff members. The interview questions included: What do you like about working in the health care center? What gets in the way of being as effective as possible in your job? What will it take to keep you here? The assessment revealed a general perception of low morale, lack of leadership and poor communication among front-line staff and their supervisors. Factors that staff reported contributed to stress and turnover included:

- They did not feel trusted and genuinely respected.
- They did not feel their talents were valued, especially prior experience.
- Lack of recognition for a job well done.
- Lack of teamwork.
- Compensation; CNAs wanted pay increases.
- Not enough development opportunities.
- Heavy use of negative reinforcement.
- Not having any control or being involved in decisions directly affecting them.
- Being reprimanded when they did not know what was expected in the first place.
- Lack of role clarity.
- Lack of up-to-date job descriptions, policy manuals and procedures.
- Poorly defined and confusing roles and responsibilities.
- Few staff members who knew the jobs well enough to train others.
- Lack of timely feedback or performance appraisals which delayed compensation for good performance.

MANAGEMENT INTERVENTION

To the management's credit, they decided it was necessary to address the underlying issues prior to beginning the dementia specific training program. A management team retreat was held at which the issues raised in the assessment were addressed and a manageable plan for dealing with the root causes of the staff's complaints was developed and implemented. The management team intervention included sessions on clarifying the mission and vision of the health care center; team building skills, identifying and addressing barriers to effective leadership and communication and increasing goal-setting skills. In addition, the management team was charged with meeting bi-weekly and systematically monitoring the issues raised in the assessment phase. Prior to the introduction of the training program, the management team had never met as a team.

IMPLEMENTATION OF STAFF DEVELOPMENT AND AD TRAINING

Based upon the assessment phase, the training program was expanded to include information on teamwork, effective communication, attitudes and goal-setting, as well as extensive material on AD and patient management techniques. A key component to the training program was that management team members were expected to attend all sessions with their employees. In order for all staff members to attend the program, training sessions were repeated weekly so that half of the staff would attend one week and the other half the following week. Sessions were 2 hours in length and the entire training program took 4 months to complete. We found that short, frequent sessions of training result in higher retention of new information. Staff were able to use new patient management techniques and then report on their effects or ask for clarification at the next session [1, 2]. Specific topics covered in the training program have been described in detail elsewhere [1, 2].

EVALUATION

All departments within the facility participated in the training program, including Administration/Management (n = 14), Nursing (licensed nursing staff not in a management position, n = 10), Nursing Assistants (n = 15), and Support Services (n = 11). Demographic data and baseline measures of general physical health, life satisfaction (adapted from the Physical Health Section of the Older Americans Research and Service Center Instrument, OARS) [7, 8], job satisfaction (Job Descriptive Index, JDI) [9, 10], and depression (Beck Depression Inventory, BDI) [11] were collected prior to the training program and repeated 6 months later. The sample, measures and results are described in detail elsewhere [12].

RESULTS OF THE INTERVENTION

In the pre-test, the Nursing group reported significantly lower scores in life satisfaction, significantly higher levels of depressive symptoms and the lowest scores in job satisfaction as compared to the other three groups. Important qualitative data was gained through focus groups held with staff members during the assessment, implementation and evaluation phases of the program. In general, focus groups held with the staff at 6 months post-training indicated increased levels of job satisfaction and improved morale. Staff members reported finding the staff development program beneficial in a number of ways. The meeting time allowed them to air their concerns and grievances in a safe environment and gave them the opportunity to develop a sense of team with their co-workers. Learning new information about AD and appropriate patient management techniques was particularly helpful. Facility turnover rates decreased dramatically during and following the completion of the program (106% at baseline compared with 70% post-training). However, when the post-test data was collected at 6 months, of the 35 completed questionnaires, only nine were staff members from the original 50. Results from this small sub-sample indicated that those nine individuals scored higher on job and life satisfaction than at the pre-test. One individual was more depressed at follow-up but it is difficult to determine the reason for that increase.

DISCUSSION

ADVANTAGES OF THE PROGRAM

The needs assessment process was a valuable means of determining the underlying causes of staff stress, low morale and turnover in this LTC facility. The process afforded the management team the opportunity to meet as a team and focus their energies on a common goal, addressing the problems identified in the assessment. It is difficult for managers of the various departments in an LTC facility to address systemic concerns such as poor communication, low morale, turnover and communication if they never meet as a group to discuss possible solutions. Staff and management both agreed on the value of the meetings and focus groups held on a regular basis during the training intervention program. Staff members reported that they felt listened to and appreciated throughout the program. The training meetings, held on a bi-weekly basis, became in effect a support group for the staff where they were able to voice their concerns.

CHALLENGES

The challenge for this and other facilities remains sustaining the beneficial impact of training and intervention programs. Beyond the formal phase of this program, and once we were not meeting with groups on a regular basis, the management began to revert back to pre-training leadership styles. Successful LTC facilities will be those whose management teams are committed to developing their most valuable resource, their staff. Central to such a commitment is the realization that to affect any real changes in management or staff behavior will take time. The constant understaffing of LTC facilities, high rates of turnover, and challenging patient care issues result in high levels of stress as the staff and management always operate in crisis mode with little opportunity to plan ahead [4, 13, 14]. Due to the constant turmoil and turnover in staffing, management often looks for a 'quick fix' to staff stress and turnover issues. However, comprehensive staff development programs that include staff support and incentive programs to increase morale take time to implement and must be ongoing. In addition, adequate compensation and promotion packages must be put in place. Clearly articulated procedures, job descriptions and performance evaluations must be consistently presented and implemented. Perhaps most important is that staff members be treated with dignity and respect at all times.

ACKNOWLEDGEMENTS

This research was supported in part by NIA Grant No. P30AG10133-06.

REFERENCES

1. Austrom MG. Staff training and support: the key to a successful special care unity. In: Hoffman SB and Kaplan M (eds) Dementia Specific Care Programs: Strategies for Success. Baltimore, MD: Health Professions Press, 1996; 27–35.
2. Austrom MG, Hendrie HC. Preserving the dignity of the invisible person. Educating long term care staff about the care and treatment of Alzheimer disease patients. In: Morgan J (ed) Ethical Issues Dealing with the Aged and Dying. Toronto: Baywood Publishing, 1996; 79–91.
3. Hays AM, Dowling T. Perceptions of job satisfaction in a long term care facility: a comparison between a dedicated Alzheimer's unit and non-Alzheimer's units. Am J Alzheimer's Dis 1997; 12(1): 35–9.
4. Caudill M, Patrick M. Nursing assistant turnover in nursing homes and need satisfaction. J Gerontol Nursing 1989; 15: 24–30.
5. Helper S. Assessing training needs of nursing home personnel. J Gerontol Soc Work 1987; 11(112): 71–9.
6. Lyons JS, Hammer JS, Johnson N, Silberman M. Unit specific variation in occupational stress across a general hospital. Gen Hosp Psychiat 1987; 9: 435–8.
7. Szwabo PA, Stein AL. Professional caregiver stress in long term care. In: Szwabo PA, Grossberg GT (eds) Problem Behaviors in Long Term Care. Recognition, Diagnosis, and Treatment. New York: Springer, 1993.
8. Pfeiffer E. Multidimensional Functional Assessment: The OARS Methodology. Durham, NC: Center for the Study of Aging and Human Development.
9. Kane RL, Kane RA. Assessing the Elderly. Toronto: Rand Corporation, 1981.
10. Schultz DP, Schultz SE. Psychology and Work Today. New York: MacMillan, 1994.
11. Smith PC, Kendall L, Hulin CL. The Measurement of Satisfaction in Work and Retirement. Chicago: Rand McNally, 1969.

12. Beck AT, Ward CH, Mendelson M, Mock J, Erbaugh J. An inventory for measuring depression. Arch Gen Psychiat 1961; 4: 561–71.
13. Austrom MG, Class A, Unverzagt F. Life satisfaction, depression and job satisfaction in long term care staff. Paper presented at the 49th Annual Meetings of the Gerontological Society of America, Washington, DC, 1996.
14. Anderson MA, Haslam B. How satisfied are nursing home staff? Geriat Nursing 1991; March/April, 85–7.

Address for correspondence:
    Mary Guerriero Austrom,
    Department of Psychiatry and Indiana Alzheimer Disease Center,
    541 Clinical Drive, CL 590, Indiana University School of Medicine,
    Indianapolis, Indiana 46202-5111, USA

94 Effects of Caregiver Training and Behavioral Strategies on Alzheimer's Disease

LINDA TERI

For a majority of patients with Alzheimer's disease (AD), effective treatment is dependent upon care providers, who have the responsibility for initiating, establishing and maintaining an effective treatment regimen. Whether professional or non-professional, paid or unpaid, relative or not, these care providers are essential. Numerous psychosocial and educative programs have aimed at teaching caregivers effective ways to care better for patients with AD. While the majority of published reports are clinical descriptions, a number of controlled trials do exist and suggest that such approaches may be effective in ameliorating behavioral problems common among patients with AD (for more detailed reviews of these programs, see [1–3]). This paper will discuss some of the methodological challenges that are evident in the literature and then present data from a recently published controlled clinical trial that demonstrates these points and shows that caregivers can be trained to effectively reduce some of the troubling symptoms of AD.

METHODOLOGICAL CHALLENGES

Perhaps the biggest challenge facing studies designed to evaluate effectiveness and efficacy center around issues of definition: definitions of sample (patients and caregivers); definitions of treatments (active and controls); and definitions of outcomes.

SAMPLE DEFINITIONS

For the most part, studies have become increasingly more sophisticated about how patients are described. Often patients have been subjected to a comprehensive evaluation and standardized criteria (such as DSM-IV or

Alzheimer's Disease and Related Disorders
Edited by K. Iqbal, D.F. Swaab, B. Winblad and H.M. Wisniewski
© 1999 John Wiley & Sons Ltd

NINCDS–ADRDA [4, 5]). Unfortunately, the same rigor is not evident in definitions of caregivers or informants. Traditionally, caregiver education programs focus on family members. But 'family' is often broadly described to include those related by blood (e.g. adult children) or marriage (spouses, in-laws) or even unrelated (e.g. institutional or home aides). Often sample sizes preclude analysis of the impact of such differential caregivers, and all too often such differences are not addressed at all.

TREATMENT DEFINITIONS

A full continuum of training exists, from generally provided basic information, education and support to specialized and systematic behavioral and psychological techniques, with well-defined strategies available in training manuals with standardized instructions. While such diversity is needed in clinical settings, in research protocols it makes generalizations and replications difficult if not impossible to accomplish. The types of training included in active treatment and the details about control conditions are often lacking in published studies.

As may be expected, the intended primary outcomes of change for the various programs differ as well. Numerous programs have focused on caregivers themselves seeking to reduce caregiver burden, help them cope with the disease, improve their own well-being, and enhance their access to social support (e.g. [6–8]). Many of these have shown that caregivers enjoy participation in supportive and psycho-educational groups, but overall treatment effects have been modest and short-term. Other programs have focused on patient outcomes and have shown somewhat better success. For example, numerous reports have shown that caregivers were able to learn specific behavioral techniques and successfully reduce problematic behaviors (e.g. [8–10]). More recently, controlled trials have suggested the effectiveness of caregiver training programs in reducing behavioral problems and delaying institutionalization in patients with dementia [11–17].

OUTCOME DEFINITIONS

As is already evident from the preceding discussion, treatments vary tremendously as to which areas of patient or caregiver function they prioritize, treat and measure. While such heterogeneity is certainly understandable, given the diversity of needs of this patient population, it again makes comparison across studies difficult and raises questions as to whether strategies employed in one domain might be effective in another. Often, even when domains seem to be the same across studies (e.g. institutionalization), the manner in which they are assessed varies. Often subjective strategies are more common than objective data (e.g. asking caregivers what happened and relying on their retrospective reports vs. obtaining actual long-term admission data), and data on the psychometric properties of outcome measures all too often are not reported. Fortunately, more standardized measures are now available and more recent studies are taking advantage of these advances in measurement.

In summary, methodological issues of sample definition, treatment details and outcome measurement make generalizations of conclusions across studies difficult. However, recent sophisticated controlled trials suggest that caregiver-based education programs may be effective in reducing dementia problems and additional research on such programs is needed. One of these newer programs will now be described.

THE SEATTLE PROTOCOL

The Seattle Protocol for teaching caregivers behavioral strategies to reduce or eliminate problematic behaviors has been described elsewhere [18–21]. This protocol was first developed to target depression in patients with AD and was subjected to a controlled clinical trial [17]. It was also extended to include a video training program on an array of problematic behaviors [22] and adapted to focus on agitation in dementia [23]. The depression treatment study will be discussed here.

SAMPLE DEFINITION

Patients were each provided with a comprehensive medical and neuro-psychological evaluation to ensure they met NINCDS–ADRDA criteria for probable AD. In addition, since the focus of treatment was depression, patients were also provided with a comprehensive assessment of depression, using standardized caregiver-report and interviewer-report measures (additional information about these measures is available in [24]). Caregivers were restricted to spouses or adult children who lived with the patient and could therefore participate actively in treatment and provide detailed assessment information.

TREATMENT DEFINITION

A complete therapist manual and caregiver reader was developed to ensure standardization of protocol and facilitate future replication (this material is available by contacting the author—see address at the end of the chapter). In brief, treatment consisted of nine sessions, once a week for nine weeks. During this time, patients and caregivers were: (a) provided with education about AD and the rationale for behavioral intervention; (b) taught methods of behavior change; (c) given strategies for identifying and increasing patient pleasant activities; (d) instructed in methods to help understand and maximize the patient's remaining cognitive and functional abilities; (e) taught effective problem-solving techniques for the day-to-day difficulties of patient care, especially those related to depression behaviors; (f) given aid with caregiving responsibilities; and (g) provided with plans for maintaining and generalizing treatment gains, once treatment has ended. A series of papers describes this intervention in more detail [17–21].

OUTCOME DEFINITION

Patient depression was the primary outcome of interest. To assess the spectrum of depression adequately in a sample of AD patients, both caregiver-report and clinical interview data was obtained (for a more detailed discussion of the measurement strategies and issues in depression assessment of dementia patients, see [24, 25]). For the purposes of this paper, data are gathered on the primary outcome measure, the Hamilton Depression Rating Scale (HDRS) [26, 27], and a newly modified measure, the informant-based Beck Depression Inventory [24]. This latter measure represents an advance in depression assessment for patients with AD as it provides a reliable method for caregivers to assess patient depression. All assessments were conducted at baseline, post-treatment and, for the active conditions, at 6 months follow-up.

DESIGN AND RESULTS

Patients–caregiver dyads were randomly assigned to one of four treatment conditions: two active behavioral treatments, a typical care condition and a wait list control. Each active behavioral treatment condition followed the protocol outlined earlier. One treatment, 'Behavior Therapy—Pleasant Events', focused on improving patient depression by increasing pleasant events and using behavioral problem-solving strategies to alter contingencies which relate to depression and associated problems. The other, 'Behavior Therapy—Problem Solving', was more flexible, allowing caregivers more input into the content and flow of treatment. It did not focus on pleasant events, although this was included as appropriate.

Typical Care and Wait List were of equal duration to the behavioral treatments (9 weeks). In Typical Care, advice and support provided by services available in the community were provided. In Wait List, no contact was provided until after the 9 weeks.

Table 1 provides the demographic characteristics of the patients and caregivers involved in the study. As can be seen, patients and caregivers represent a well-educated sample, predominantly white, consistent with the clinical population from which they were drawn. Patients had an average duration of dementia of 3 years, with 1.5 years of depression. Also consistent with the clinical literature and the population from which they were drawn, caregivers were predominantly women (69%).

Table 1. Demographic characteristics

	Total (n = 72)
Patient	
Age	76.4 ± 8.2
Education	14.1 ± 2.9
Gender	
Female	34 (47%)
Male	38 (53%)
Dementia duration (months)	35.6 ± 24.2
Depression diagnosis	
Major	54 (75%)
Minor	18 (25%)
Depression duration (months)	19.4 ± 17.4
Living situation	
Private home	61 (86%)
Retirement home	4 (6%)
Adult group home	6 (8%)
Caregiver	
Age	66.9 ± 11.0
Education	14.2 ± 2.7
Gender	
Female	50 (69%)
Male	22 (31%)
Relationship	
Spouse	56 (79%)
Adult child	10 (14%)
Close friend	5 (7%)

Table 2 shows the change from pre-test to post-test for subjects in each of the active and control conditions on the primary outcome measure, the HDRS. Subjects in both behavior therapy conditions improved significantly, pre-test to post-test ($p < 0.01$), and improved significantly more than subjects in either the Typical Care or Wait List conditions. Investigating the degree of clinically significant improvement, 60% of subjects in behavior therapy improved pre- to post-therapy, compared to only 20% on Typical Care or Wait List (see Table 3). At 6 months follow-up, subjects in behavior therapy maintained their gains.

In summary, results indicated significant levels of improvement in patient depression after treatment, as measured by two measures of depression, the HDRS and the informant-based Beck Depression Inventory. Patients in the behavior therapy conditions improved significantly more than did those in Typical Care or Wait List conditions.

Table 2. Changes in patient depression

Treatment condition	Depression measures	
	Hamilton Depression Rating Scale	Informant-based Beck Depression Inventory
'Behavior Therapy—Pleasant Events' (n = 23)	−5.3 ± 4.0	−1.3 ± 6.3
'Behavior Therapy—Problem Solving' (n = 19)	−3.8 ± 2.3	−4.5 ± 4.5
Typical Care (n = 10)	−0.3 ± 4.7	1.9 ± 5.8
Wait List (n = 20)	0.3 ± 3.5**	0.5 ± 4.6*

*$p < 0.01$. **$p < 0.0001$.

Table 3. Clinically significant improvement pre- to post-treatment by treatment condition[a]

	'Behavior Therapy— Pleasant Events'	'Behaviour Therapy— Problem Solving'	Typical Care	Wait List
Improved	12 (52%)	13 (68%)	2 (20%)	4 (20%)
No change	11 (48%)	6 (32%)	6 (60%)	15 (75%)
Worse	0	0	2 (20%)	1 (5%)

[a]χ^2 (6, n = 72) = 18.48; $p < 0.005$.

CONCLUSIONS AND FUTURE DIRECTIONS

Numerous questions remain to be investigated in caregiver-based treatment programs. Future studies need to continue to subject clinical experience to controlled clinical trials. Effectiveness and efficacy need to be investigated. Differential efficacy needs to be addressed. How do caregiver-based treatments compare to pharmacotherapy for the problems that beset caregivers and patients? How can treatments be maximized to enhance therapeutic efficacy? How might definitions of samples, treatments, and outcomes be broadened or limited to facilitate study and enhance effectiveness?

These are just some of the many questions that can be asked of future studies. The past 5 years has seen a veritable explosion of new techniques for the care and treatment of patients with AD. It can only be hoped that the next 5 years will provide some answers to the very real questions raised by this devastating disease.

ACKNOWLEDGEMENTS

This study was supported in part by Grant No. 10845 from the National Institute of Aging.

REFERENCES

1. Zarit SH, Teri L. Interventions and services for family caregivers. Ann Rev Gerontol Geriat 1991; 11: 241–65.
2. Bourgeois MS, Schulz R, Burgio L. Interventions for caregivers of patients with Alzheimer's disease: a review and analysis of content, process, and outcomes. Int J Aging Hum Dev 1996; 43: 35–92.
3. Teri L, McCurry S. Psychosocial therapies. In: Coffey C, Cummings J (eds) Textbook of Geriatric Neuropsychiatry. Washington, DC: American Psychiatric Press, 1994; 662–82.
4. American Psychiatric Association. Diagnostic and Statistical Manual of Mental Disorders. Washington, DC: American Psychiatric Association, 1994.
5. McKhann G, Drachman D, Folstein M, Katzman R, Price D, Stadlem E. Clinical diagnosis of Alzheimer's disease: Report of the NINCDS–ADRDA Work Group under the auspices of Department of Health and Human Services Task Force on Alzheimer's disease. Neurology 1984; 34: 939–44.
6. Toseland RW, Smith GC. Effectiveness of individual counseling by professional and peer helpers for family caregivers of the elderly. Psychol Aging 1990; 5: 256–63.
7. Zarit SH, Anthony CR, Boutselis M. Interventions with caregivers of dementia patients: comparison of two approaches. Psychol Aging 1987; 2: 225–32.
8. Haley WE, Brown SL, Levine EG. Experimental evaluation of the effectiveness of group intervention for dementia caregivers. Gerontologist 1987; 27: 376–82.
9. Pinkston EM, Linsk N. Behavioral family intervention with the impaired elderly. Gerontologist 1984; 24: 576.
10. Aronson MK, Levin G, Lipkowitz R. A community based family/patient group program for Alzheimer's disease. Gerontologist 1984; 24: 339–42.
11. Schmidt GL, Bonjean MJ, Widem AC, Schefft BK, Steele DJ. Brief psychotherapy for caregivers of demented relatives: comparison of two therapeutic strategies. Clin Gerontologist 1988; 7: 109–25.
12. Robinson K, Yates K. Effects of two caregiver-training programs on burden and attitude toward help. Arch Psychiat Nurs 1994; 8: 312–19.
13. Mohide EA, Pringle DM, Streiner DL, Gilbert JR, Muir G, Tew M. A randomized trial of family caregiver support in the home management of dementia. J Am Geriat Soc 1990; 38: 446–54.
14. Mittelman M, Ferris S, Steinberg G et al. An intervention that delays institutionalization of Alzheimer's disease patients: treatment of spouse-caregivers. Gerontologist 1993; 33: 730–40.
15. Mittelman MS, Ferris SH, Schulman E et al. A comprehensive support program: effect on depression in spouse-caregivers of AD patients. Gerontologist 1995; 35: 792–802.
16. Mittelman MS, Ferris SH, Shulman E, Steinberg G, Levin B. A family intervention to delay nursing home placement of patients with Alzheimer's disease. J Am Med Assoc 1996; 276: 1725–31.
17. Teri L, Logsdon RG, Uomoto J, McCurry S. Behavioral treatment of depression in dementia patients: a controlled clinical trial. J Gerontol B: Psychol Sci 1997; 52B: P159–66.

18. Teri L, Uomoto J. Reducing excess disability in dementia patients: training care-givers to manage patient depression. Clin Gerontologist 1991; 10: 49–63.
19. Teri L. Behavioral treatment of depression in patients with dementia. Alzheimer's Dis Assoc Disord 1994; 8: 66–74.
20. Teri L. Depression in Alzheimer's disease. In: Hersen M, van Hasselt VB (eds) Psychological Treatment of Older Adults: An Introductory Text. New York: Plenum, 1996; 209–22.
21. Teri L. The relation between research on depression and a treatment program: one model. In: Rubinstein RL, Lawton MP (eds) Depression in Long Term and Residential Care: Advances in Research and Treatment. New York: Springer, 1997; 129–53.
22. Teri L. Managing and understanding behavior problems in Alzheimer's disease and related disorders. Seattle: University of Washington, 1990.
23. Teri L. Managing problems in dementia patients: depression and agitation. In: Khachaturian ZS, Radebaugh TS (eds) Alzheimer's Disease: Cause(s), Diagnosis, Treatment, and Care. Boca Raton, FL: CRC Press, 1996; 297–304.
24. Logsdon RG, Teri L. Depression in Alzheimer's disease patients: caregivers as surrogate reporters. J Am Geriat Soc 1995; 43: 150–55.
25. Teri L, Wagner A. Alzheimer's disease and depression. J Consult Clin Psychol 1992; 3: 379–91.
26. Hamilton M. A rating scale for depression. J Neurol Neurosurg Psychiat 1960; 23: 56–62.
27. Hamilton M. Development of a rating scale for primary depressive illness. Br J Soc Clin Psychol 1967; 6: 278–96.

Address for correspondence:
Linda Teri PhD,
Department of Psychosocial and Community Health,
Box 357263, University of Washington,
Seattle, WA 98195-7263, USA
Tel: (206) 543 0715; fax: (206) 685 9551;
e-mail: Lteri@u.washington.edu

Copies of the treatment manuals are available by contacting the author at this address.

95 Development of a Short Measurement of Individual Quality of Life (SEIQoL Short Form)

DENISE MEIER, VALÉRIE VODOZ AND RENÉ SPIEGEL

INTRODUCTION

Assessment of quality of life (QoL) is becoming increasingly important in medicine, nursing and behavioural and social science, particularly as an outcome variable in assessing the impact of disease and treatment. There is as yet no common definition of what constitutes QoL, neither is there a universally accepted gold standard measure. Despite the lack of consensus in QoL research, there is consensus about two fundamental aspects of the concept: subjectivity and its multidimensionality.

Most QoL questionnaires are based on a nomothetic approach and impose an external value system by using standard formats, questions and weights of preselected components of QoL derived from group data. The relevance of these standardized questionnaires to the individual has not been widely addressed. Specific goals or behaviours important to an individual's QoL are unlikely to be represented adequately by broad questions about physical mobility or general health. Apparently similar behaviours do not have the same significance for all individuals desiring to experience them, neither do events or functions necessarily retain the same salience for a given individual with the passage of time or over the course of an illness. The advantage of individualized measurements is the adequate assessment of the singularity of a person's QoL. A number of attempts have been made to incorporate the perspective of the individual into QoL assessment. One of them is the Schedule for the Evaluation of Individual Quality of Life (SEIQoL Long Form) [1, 2, 3].

The SEIQoL Long Form has been used in a variety of study populations, including healthy elderly, early dementia patients and their caregivers [4].

Alzheimer's Disease and Related Disorders
Edited by K. Iqbal, D.F. Swaab, B. Winblad and H.M. Wisniewski
© 1999 John Wiley & Sons Ltd

Results have shown that the SEIQoL Long Form is a reliable and valid instrument and sensitive to change, e.g. after total hip replacement or to measure the treatment effect of cognitive competence training [3, 5].

The interview procedure associated with the SEIQoL Long Form, specifically the judgement analysis (JA) section, is highly complex and not easy to understand, requires considerable time to complete (an average of 20–30 min) and asks for special computer software. Thus, the SEIQoL Long Form may be primarily suitable for research settings or clinical situations where the instrument is being used as part of the process of having the individual consider a range of options or outcomes in evaluating QoL. For other settings, its use is too time-consuming. A briefer instrument with a direct weighting procedure for QoL domains [6] may be more suitable for routine clinical use than JA. It imposes fewer demands on individuals, is easy to evaluate and can also be administered to patients with reduced cognitive functions. The aim of the present study was to validate a briefer (German) version of the SEIQoL (SEIQoL Short Form), namely a direct weighting procedure replacing the judgement analysis.

METHODS

STUDY POPULATION

Participants were 64 healthy elderly living in the community or in resident homes (see Table 1). Their cognitive status was assessed by the Mini-Mental State Examination (MMSE) [7], emotional status by the Geriatric Depression Scale (GDS) [8] (0 = no depression, 15 = depression). Inclusion criteria were a MMSE of 27–30 points and a GDS of 0–10 points. Dementia patients were excluded. All participants were interviewed with SEIQoL Long and Short Forms.

Table 1. Demographic variables

	Community	Resident home	Total
n	32	32	64
Gender	16 Male 16 Female	12 Male 20 Female	28 Male 36 Female
Age	75.9, SD 5.4	84.9, SD 6.6	80.4, SD 7.5
MMSE score (0–30)	28.6, SD 1.0	28.0, SD 0.9	28.3, SD 1.0
GDS score (0–15)	1.8, SD 1.3	2.2, SD 1.5	2.0, SD 1.5

SEIQoL LONG AND SHORT FORMS

The SEIQoL Long and Short Forms are designed to measure three elements of QoL: (a) those aspects of life a person considers crucial to his/her QoL; (b) current functioning/satisfaction with each aspect; and (c) the relative importance of each aspect. The SEIQoL Long Form includes an implicit weighting procedure by judgement analysis, the Short Form an explicit weighting procedure. The latter consists of a pie-chart, where the relative size of each of five coloured segments (representing the five domains nominated as important to QoL) may be adjusted and readjusted by the subject, until the proportion of the pie-chart given to each QoL domain represents the relative weight attached by the individual to that domain.

The SEIQoL is intended primarily as an individual measure. For group comparisons, a global index is calculated with both forms that may be used in within- or between-subject study designs. This index is a continuous measure ranging from 0 (worst QoL) to 100 (best QoL), calculated by multiplying the levels by the weights and then summing these products across the five cues.

RESULTS

GLOBAL QoL INDEX

Global QoL indexes determined by the two approaches were calculated and shown to be very similar (r = 0.95, p < 0.0001) (Table 2). There was no difference between QoL scores of people living in the community and in resident homes.

Table 2. Global QoL indexes by SEIQoL Long and Short Forms

	QoL (SEIQoL Long Form)	QoL (SEIQoL Short Form)
Community	77.9, SD 9.8	77.5, SD 9.4
Resident home	77.6, SD 9.8	77.9, SD 9.1
Total	77.7, SD 9.8	77.7, SD 9.2

IMPORTANT QoL ASPECTS

A variety of 32 different life aspects were nominated. The most frequent aspects were health (75%), social contacts (56.3%), family (54.7%), finances (40.6%) and housing conditions (31.3%). Participants living in the community nominated family more often (68.8% and 40.6%, χ^2 = 4.1, p < 0.05) and social contacts less often (68.8 and 40.6%, χ^2 = 5.1, p < 0.05) than people living in resident homes. Interestingly, 22% of participants living in resident homes but none of the persons living in the community nominated 'cognitive abilities' (χ^2 = 7.9, p < 0.01).

CONCORDANCE OF IMPLICIT (SEIQoL LONG FORM) AND
EXPLICIT (SEIQoL SHORT FORM) WEIGHTING PROCEDURE

The concordance of the weights given in the SEIQoL Long and Short Forms
(Table 3) was calculated by several different methods:

- Rank pair differences: 80% of rank pairs (community and resident home)
  differed by 0 or 1 rank. This means that only one-fifth of weights differed
  by more than 1 rank.
- Mean difference value of weights as established by the SEIQoL Long and
  Short Forms was 7.2, SD 2.8 (0 = maximum concordance, 40 = maximum discordance); 95% of mean difference values were between 1.6 and
  12.8 points.
- Cohen's Kappa was 0.44 (–1 = maximum discordance, +1 = maximum
  concordance).
- Kendall's Tau was 0.49 (–1 = perfect negative rank correlation, +1 =
  perfect positive rank correlation).

Table 3. Concordance of implicit (SEIQoL Long Form) and explicit (SEIQoL Short
Form) weighting procedure

	Community	Resident home	Total
Mean difference values (0–40)	6.7, SD 2.8	7.6, SD 2.9	7.2, SD 2.8
Cohen's Kappa (–1–+1)	0.45, SD 0.39	0.43, SD 0.35	0.44, SD 0.37
Kendall's Tau (–1–+1)	0.49, SD 0.44	0.49, SD 0.42	0.49, SD 0.43

DISCUSSION

The assessment of individual QoL by SEIQoL Long and Short Forms was
successfully administered to cognitively healthy elderly living in the community
or in resident homes. The wide variety of aspects considered important by
different individuals in the evaluation of their QoL demonstrates the necessity of
elicitation, rating and weighting of individually chosen QoL aspects.

Results showed almost identical global QoL scores with the SEIQoL Long
and Short Forms. The difference between the SEIQoL Long and Short Forms
lies in the weighting procedure: the Long Form comprises an implicit (judgement analysis), the Short Form an explicit procedure (pie-chart). With several
different statistical methods a high concordance of the Long and Short SEI-
QoL Forms was demonstrated; 80% of rank pairs differed by only 0 or 1 rank.
This means that only one-fifth of weights differed by more than 1 rank. Mean
difference value of weights as established by SEIQoL Long and Short Forms
was 7.2, SD 2.8 (0 = maximum concordance, 40 = maximum discordance).
Kendall's Tau was 0.49, Cohen's Kappa 0.44.

The advantage of the Long procedure is the possibility of controlling internal validity and reliability of judgements; its limitation lies in the complex and time-consuming method of administration. The advantage of the SEIQoL Short Form is its practicability: it could be very useful in clinical practice. The instrument is less time-consuming, colourful, handy, easy to understand and especially appropriate for elderly people, even for those with beginning to present moderate dementing disease.

ACKNOWLEDGEMENTS

This study is an excerpt from an unpublished Master's Thesis (Lizentiatsarbeit), University of Basel (Switzerland), 1997.

REFERENCES

1. McGee HM, O'Boyle CA, Hickey A, O'Malley K, Joyce CRB. Assessing the quality of life of the individual: the SEIQoL with a healthy and a gastroenterology unit population. Psychol Med 1991; 21: 749–59.
2. O'Boyle CA, McGee HM, Hickey A, O'Malley K, Joyce CRB. Reliability and validity of judgement analysis as a method for assessing quality of life. Br J Pharmacol 1989; 27: 155pp.
3. O'Boyle CA, McGee HM, Hickey A, O'Malley K, Joyce CRB. Individual quality of life undergoing hip replacement. Lancet 1992; 339: 1088–91.
4. Meier D. Lebensqualität im Alter. Eine Studie zur Erfassung der individuellen Lebensqualität von gesunden Aelteren, von Patienten im Anfangsstadium einer Demenz und ihren Angehörigen. Europäischer Verlag der Wissenschaften. Bern: Peter Lang AG, 1995.
5. Meier D, Ermini-Fünfschilling D, Monsch AU, Stähelin HB. Kognitives Kompetenztraining mit Patienten im Anfangsstadium einer Demenz. Z Gerontopsychol Psychiat 1996; 3: 207–17.
6. Browne JP, O'Boyle CA, McGee HM, McDonald NJ, Joyce CRB. Development of a direct weighting procedure for quality of life domains. Qual Life Res 1997; 6: 301–9.
7. Folstein MF, Folstein SE, McHugh PR, 'Mini Mental State'—a practical method for grading the cognitive state of patients for the clinician. J Psych Res 1975; 12: 189–98.
8. Sheikh JA, Yesavage JA. Geriatric Depression Scale (GDS): recent findings and development of a shorter version. In Brink TL (ed) Clinical Gerontology: A Guide to Assessment and Intervention. New York: Haworth, 1986; 165–73.

Address for correspondence:
Denise Meier,
Memory Clinic, Geriatric University Clinic,
Hebelstrasse 10, 4031 Basel, Switzerland

Author Index

Subject Index

Note: Page numbers in *italics* refer to figures; those in **bold** to tables

Indexes compiled by Maria Rayson, Indexing Specialists, Hove, UK